Amygdala: The Study of Dexterity of the Brain

Edited by **Noah Martin**

hayle medical

New York

Published by Hayle Medical,
30 West, 37th Street, Suite 612,
New York, NY 10018, USA
www.haylemedical.com

Amygdala: The Study of Dexterity of the Brain
Edited by Noah Martin

International Standard Book Number: 978-1-63241-039-9 (Hardback)

Printed in China.

Contents

Preface

This book was inspired by the evolution of our times; to answer the curiosity of inquisitive minds. Many developments have occurred across the globe in the recent past which has transformed the progress in the field.

This book illustrates up-to-date information regarding amygdala and studies the dexterity of the brain. Among the various constituents of the limbic system, the amygdala is an intriguing structure that is involved in the procedures of liking and disliking and in the manners our emotions drive our actions and affect the strength of our memories. Integrated with novel conceptual breakthroughs, the most recent information acquired by veteran experts in amygdala function from all over the world has been reviewed in this book. This information should help the readers to comprehend how the amygdalae contribute to these procedures as well as to a variety of neuropsychiatric and neurological pathologies. Due to the accelerating rate of research development, the information in this book accurately corresponds to various important questions addressed by veterans employing extremely specific techniques. Analysis from distinct research areas which are necessary for consideration in discussing the role of amygdala in memory and emotion has been compiled in this book. The aim of this book is to acquaint and inform beginners and experts with latest information in the field of brain structures involved in mechanisms underlying emotional learning and memory and also help to stimulate discussion on the functional role of amygdala and connected brain structures in these mechanisms.

This book was developed from a mere concept to drafts to chapters and finally compiled together as a complete text to benefit the readers across all nations. To ensure the quality of the content we instilled two significant steps in our procedure. The first was to appoint an editorial team that would verify the data and statistics provided in the book and also select the most appropriate and valuable contributions from the plentiful contributions we received from authors worldwide. The next step was to appoint an expert of the topic as the Editor-in-Chief, who would head the project and finally make the necessary amendments and modifications to make the text reader-friendly. I was then commissioned to examine all the material to present the topics in the most comprehensible and productive format.

I would like to take this opportunity to thank all the contributing authors who were supportive enough to contribute their time and knowledge to this project. I also wish to convey my regards to my family who have been extremely supportive during the entire project.

Editor

Chapter 1

Amygdala and Emotional Learning in Vertebrates – A Comparative Perspective

Juan Pedro Vargas, Juan Carlos López and Manuel Portavella

Additional information is available at the end of the chapter

1. Introduction

The mammalian amygdala is a telencephalic structure of complex embryonic origin, composed of several nuclei that proceed from both the telencephalic pallial wall and the striated sheet, settling a border or transition zone between the telencephalic pallium and subpallium. In primates, the amygdala is located in the anterior temporal lobe, and in other mammals occupies a topologically equivalent position. Klüver & Bucy (1939) described a syndrome after bilateral ablation of the temporal lobes of rhesus monkeys which, among other symptoms, caused a dramatic decrease in the emotional reaction of fear, an effect attributed primarily to the ablation of the amygdaline system rather than other structures. This effect sparked interest in studying the possible involvement of the amygdala in emotional responses, such as learning and emotional memory that has been developed since the second half of the 20th century. In fact, bilateral lesions to the amygdala (or its equivalent anatomical structure) in other vertebrate groups (reptiles, birds, and non-primate mammals) cause serious interference with the normal development of emotional responses characteristic of the species such as aggressive, sexual, or parental behavior (Kling & Brothers, 1992). Studies about emotional and avoidance (active or passive) conditioning show that the complete or partial injury to amygdala causes serious disorders in these learned responses (LeDoux, 1995). Moreover, the amygdala is involved in memory and attention processes (Kapp et al., 1992), in the emotional evaluation of stimuli (Davis, 1992; Gallagher & Chiba, 1996; Gallagher & Holland, 1992; Halgren, 1992; LeDoux, 1992, 1995) and in emotional aspects of dreams (Calvo et al., 1987). In the past, its intricate structure and the paradoxical experimental results that sometimes were obtained in both humans and animals (Phelps & Anderson, 1997) have been especially confusing when trying to clearly identify its functions. Although, a common factor found in these data is its emotional aspect. It has now become clear that it is also involved in humans' social learning of fear and in anxiety disorders (Olsson & Phelps, 2007). In fact, it appears that stimuli that are not consciously perceived activate the amygdala; this provides a fast and automatic processing of the stimuli for social cognition (Adolphs, 2009), especially with regard to facial expression (Adolphs et al., 1994).

As stated above, the amygdala is not a uniform structure, not only in terms of the structural differences but also by the intrinsic and extrinsic pattern of afferents and efferents of its different nuclei, including the divisions of the subnuclei (Amaral et al., 1992; Pitkänen et al., 1997), which also appears to be involved in different functions for different circuits. Lesion and stimulation studies may lead to varying results depending on the affected circuit, but always shows implicit emotional factors (Davis, 1992; Gallagher & Chiba, 1996; Gallagher & Holland, 1992; Killcross et al., 1997; LeDoux, 1992). In the human case, the amygdala could be considered an essential part of the brain involved in surveillance tasks of potentially ambiguous or unpredictable stimuli (Whalen, 1999).

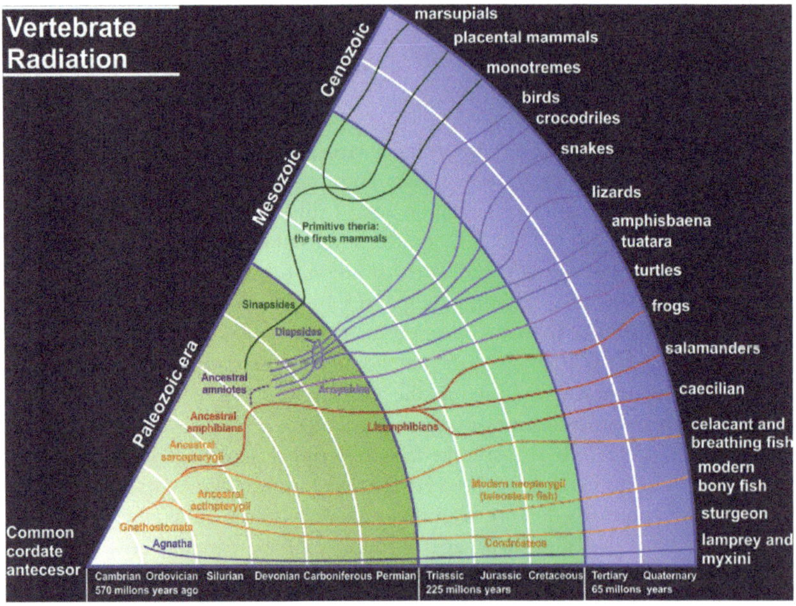

Figure 1. Phylogeny of vertebrates represented in a cladogram. Although the first fossil records are from the Ordovician period, the existence of vertebrates in the Cambrian is very likely. Fishlike vertebrates gave rise to the agnatha (jawless fish) and gnathostomes (jawed fish). The current vertebrates descended from one of these two groups. Gnathostomes were diversified into different classes, such as reptilians, birds, and mammals. Current bony fishes present brain structures with a cytoarchitecture and function very close to the amygdala in mammals. This data indicates that most likely a common ancestor to vertebrates had a brain with a structure functionally similar to the amygdala, and because of its adaptive value, it was conserved throughout the phylogeny.

It is considered that the amygdala is not an exclusive structure of mammals, since genoarchitectonic, neurochemical, embryological, anatomical, and behavioral studies in a comparative perspective (Aggleton, 1992; Bruce & Neary, 1995; Macphail, 1996; Medina et al., 2011; Moreno & González, 2006; 2007; Parent, 1986; Sriedter, 1997; Wulliman & Rink, 2002) have proposed several homologies for this structure in other vertebrate groups (fish, amphibians, reptiles, and birds). Although there has been no complete agreement on the homology of all parts of this structure (pallial and subpallial portion) among all vertebrate groups over time (Braford, 1995; Bruce & Neary, 1995; Northcutt, 1995; Sriedter, 1997), the existence of a basic scheme of the amygdala in fish, reptiles, birds, and mammals, irrespective of the diverse differentiation of this structure along the evolution of the different groups of tetrapods has been established by examining the comparative genoarchitecture (Medina et al., 2011; Moreno & González, 2006; 2007). In this sense, it is possible that the amygdala or analogous structure was present in an ancestor of current vertebrates. Its function was necessary for the adaptative processes, and it was conserved along the vertebrate radiation (figure 1).

2. The amygdala. Homologies among vertebrates

As noted previously, the amygdala of mammals and other tetrapods is divided into two main parts, one pallial or cortical, and another subpallial or striated. In addition, it is divided into different nuclei, and these divisions also seem to be found in groups other than mammals, such as reptiles and birds (Bruce & Neary, 1995; DeOlmos et al, 1985; Lohman & Smeets, 1990; McDonald, 1992; Medina et al., 2011; Moreno & González, 2007; Northcutt, 2008; Striedter, 1997; Wulliman & Rink, 2002; Zeier & Karten, 1971). In the case of chondrichthyan fish the so-called Nucleus A is recognized as a possible homologue of the tetrapod pallial amygdala, both for its position and its pattern of connectivity (Northcutt, 1995; 2008; Smeets, 1990). In actinopterygians, the telencephalon undergoes an eversion process that raises a serious difficulty in establishing homologies with the amygdala (Braford, 1995; Gage, 1983; Scalia & Ebbesson, 1971). However, the cytoarchitecture, the neurohistochemistry, studies of embryonic development, the pattern of connectivity and topological studies (Braford, 1995; Chanconie & Clairambault, 1975; Morgan, 1974a, 1974b; Murakami et al., 1983; Northcutt, 1981; 1995; Northcutt & Braford, 1980) suggest that the region Dmv of the teleost telencephalon is a good candidate to be considered the homologue of the pallial amygdala (Northcutt, 1995; Northcutt & Braford, 1980), although other authors suggest that Dmv could be homologous to the basal ganglia or the hippocampus of mammals (Murakami et al., 1983; Parent et al., 1978). Moreover, the pattern of connectivity, with strong sensory thalamic inputs and reciprocal connections with the hypothalamus, gives a distinctly limbic character to Dmv (Braford, 1995; Echteler & Saidel, 1981; Ito et al., 1986; Murakami et al, 1983; Striedter, 1991). Another circumstance that would support the homology of Dmv with the pallial amygdala is its topological situation. The Dmv telencephalon is located between the ventral subpallial area (possible striated region) and the dorsoposterior area (main olfactory receptor area), a similar position to the pallial amygdala of other vertebrates, between the olfactory cortex and the subpallial amygdala (Braford, 1995; Bruce & Neary, 1995; Neary, 1990; Neary & Bruce, 1993; Northcutt & Kicliter, 1980). Other authors (Kyle & Peter, 1982; Kyle et al., 1982) have pointed to the region VspVv (ventral area supracomisural ventral-ventral area) as homologous to the corticomedial amygdala, based on the fact that it receives olfactory afferents (Oka, 1980), the concentration of steroid hormone receptors (Kim et al., 1978; see Medina et al., 2011 for a review of steroid hormone-regulated as a component of the amygdala), and the results of electrolytic lesions (Kyle et al., 1982). This data is also supported by functional data as damage to this structure affects the male reproductive behavior and other signs of social interest such as parental care or aggressive behavior, the same pattern of deficits that is found with lesions of the corticomedial amygdala in mammals (Isaacson, 1976; Kling & Brothers, 1992). In fact, it has been proposed that the most medial region of the ventral area of the telencephalon in teleosts fish correspond to the subpallial amygdala (Northcutt, 1995; 2008; Northcutt & Braford, 1980).

3. Functions of the amygdala in emotional learning and memory in mammals

3.1. Amygdala and fear conditioning

The conditioning of the fear response in short delay procedures is affected by the lesion of specific areas of the amygdala, mainly the central, basal, and lateral nucleus (Davis, 1992; LeDoux, 1992; 1995). This conditioned fear response is established very easily and this characteristic seems to be preserved through evolution in all vertebrate groups (LeDoux 1992; Portavella et al, 2004a), and consists of three components: behavioral (eg usually appears a "freezing" response), autonomic (eg bradycardia response) and hormonal (eg increased levels of ACTH) (Davis, 1992). In the human case, the involvement of the amygdala in fear conditioning has been shown by both consciously and unconsciously processed stimuli (Morris et al., 1989). Thus, the lesion of the amygdala produces a serious effect on the ability to recognize expressions of fear (Adolphs et al., 1994; 2005), and thus interferes seriously in the early detection of emotional stimuli. Recent studies using functional imaging techniques have analyzed the role of different parts of the human limbic system in the processing of emotional discrimination of faces and natural scenes (Fusar-Poli et al., 2009; Sabatini et al., 2011)

To better understand the role of the amygdala in fear conditioning, it is necessary to know how the main efferents and afferents of the amygdalar structures are organized and their intrinsic connections (Amaral et al., 1992; Pitkänen et al., 1995; Pitkänen et al., 1997; Savander et al., 1995). In fact, the study of the function and the connectivity go hand in hand, since not all lesions nor interventions have the same effects in different amygdaloid nuclei; although some pallial nuclei (lateral, basal and accessory basal nuclei) and subpallial (central nucleus) appear to be more decisive in this type of conditioning (see LeDoux, 2000 for a review). In mammals, the lateral nucleus receives direct thalamic afferents from different sensory modalities (eg intralaminar nuclei, supregeniculate nucleus and medial division of the medial geniculate nucleus), so it receives somesthetic, visual, and auditory thalamic afferents (Campeau & Davis, 1995; Gallagher & Chiba, 1996; Rogan & LeDoux,

1995). The lesion of this nucleus produces a severe deficit in the expression of conditioned fear response, and also an inability to learn it (see Rosen, 2004). Also specific neurotoxic lesions in the basolateral complex (lateral and basal nuclei) prevent the animal from acquiring a conditioned fear response (Campeau & Davis, 1995; Rabinak & Maren, 2008). Inputs from cortical regions to the lateral nucleus send processed information of the same stimuli (sensory, association, and polymodal cortex), through a thalamo-cortico-amygdala via (for a review see Sah et al., 2003). The importance of the thalamus-amygdala via is proven by the fact that ablation or disconnection of sensory cortical region does not prevent fear conditioning to a single sound stimulus (DiChara et al., 1970; LeDoux et al., 1986). However, when the set of stimuli is more complex (such as in a program of differential conditioning where there are two different sounds as stimuli or a reinforced conditioned stimulus (CS +) and a non-reinforced one (CS-), and the animal during the training and reversal has to learn which one is paired with the EI (electric footshock), the lesion to this circuit disrupts the performance on this type of differential learning tasks (Jarrell et al., 1987). It has also been shown that the context can become a fundamental cue for learning. This contextual conditioning has been established when for example, the fear response occurs without the presence of the CS or the US (unconditioned stimulus), by merely placing an animal in the box in which it has been receiving these two paired stimuli. In this case, the presence of certain structures such as the hippocampus and related structures is essential, because the lesion of this structure is sufficient to block the fear response to the context (Nadel, 2008; Phillips & LeDoux, 1992; Selden et al., 1991; Wiltgen et al., 2006). Lesions of retrosplenial cortex (Keene & Bucci, 2008) and of the entorhinal cortex (Ji & Maren, 2008) also disrupt contextual fear conditioning. The entorhinal cortex is implicated in processing background contextual information given that NMDA lesions impair the processing of contextual background fear conditioning but not the fear conditioned to an auditory stimulus (Majchrzak et al., 2006). The hippocampus maintains connections to the lateral and basal nucleus via subiculum and with the basal nuclei (Ottersen, 1982). In this sense, the mere disconnection of this afferent or lesion to the hippocampus is enough to prevent and suppress emotional conditioning context (Maren & Fanselow, 1995; Phillips & LeDoux, 1992). All available data point to the lateral nucleus as a nucleus of sensory input to the amygdala (Rogan & LeDoux, 1995), which according to LeDoux (1995) could act as an interface and a major site for integration of information from the different inputs of sensory information during the conditioning of the fear response. The afferents of the lateral nucleus are directed to other amygdalar structures including the pallial basal and basal accessory nuclei too (Pitkänen & Amaral, 1991).

The basal nucleus (basal and basal accessory) receives input from the hippocampus and cortical association areas such as inferotemporal cortex and other structures (Amaral et al., 1992), and sends efferents to the sensory association cortex and the central nucleus (Aggleton, 1985; Amaral et al., 1992; Price & Amaral, 1981). Electrolytic or NMDA-induced lesion of the basolateral complex of the amygdala blocked fear conditioning to both visual and auditory CSs (Campeau & Davis, 1995). The use of substances that produce temporal inactivation such as muscimol (a GABA type A agonist) has introduced some controversy, since some studies show that injecting this substance in the basal and lateral nuclei produced different results depending on the time of injection. If the drug is injected before conditioning it results in acquisition deficits, although the same manipulation made immediately after conditioning has no effect (Helmstetter & Bellgowan, 1994). Nevertheless, with a similar design Muller et al. (1997) showed that injecting muscimol to functionally inactivate the basal or the lateral nucleus produced little conditioned fear to contextual or auditory conditioned stimuli. Herry et al. (2008) and Amano et al. (2010) have also shown that inactivation of the basal nuclei with muscimol does not block the expression of the conditioned fear. Fanselow & Kim (1994) did the same with the local infusion of d-APV (a NMDA receptor antagonist), obtaining similar results. Cousens & Otto (1998) analyzed the relation between the fear response to olfactory and contextual stimuli. The results showed that excitotoxic lesions (infusion of high concentration of NMDA) disrupted the conditioned response to odor and context. All the data supports the involvement of the amygdala in the acquisition of a conditioned fear response, such as in its expression, once conditioning is established.

The central nucleus, in contrast, has essentially extra-amygdala efferents, and maintains important connectivity with brainstem nuclei and areas, such as the periaqueductal gray matter, and lateral hypothalamus (Davis, 1992), which in turn control the response patterns that involve the emotional response of fear. In fact, the neurotoxic lesion of this structure impairs the learning of a conditioned fear response (Campeau & Davis, 1995).

3.2. Plasticity in the amygdala and fear conditioning

In rats, the plastic processes that take place in amygdala structures during learning of fear conditioning have been studied on the presence of postsynaptic long-term potentiation (Clugnet et al., 1990; Sah et al., 2008). Some of these studies found that these processes were not mediated by NMDA receptors (Chapman & Bellavance, 1992), as occurs in the hippocampus (Bliss & Collingridge, 1993; Hicks, 1995; Lynch et al., 1991; Madison et al., 1991; Malenka & Nicholl, 1993; McEntee & Crook, 1993; Morris et al, 1989; Witkin, 1995). Nevertheless, later studies found the existence of long-term potentiation processes mediated by NMDA receptors located in the lateral amygdala (Gean et al., 1993). Furthermore, these receptors located in the lateral amygdala are implicated in the processing of the conditioned stimulus in fear conditioning (Farb & LeDoux, 1997; Li et al., 1996). The use of antagonists of these receptors causes serious interference in the conditioning of the fear response to simple stimuli as the context, but not retention or expression of a learned response (Fanselow & Kim, 1994; Gerwirtz & Davis, 1997; Maren et al., 1996). "In vivo" and "in vitro" studies show how fear conditioning induces a process of long-term potentiation (LTP) mediated by NMDA receptors (Rogan et al., 1997; McKernan & Shinnick-Gallagher, 1997). It has also been shown that NMDA receptor blockade interferes with the process of extinction of a conditioned fear response (Falls et al., 1992). These results and their relationship to learning processes are parallel to those found in the hippocampus, and indicate that a long-term depression (LTD) also mediated by NMDA receptors, which has been linked to the extinction of responses acquired in other structures like the hippocampus, takes place in the amygdala too (Dudek & Bear, 1992). In fact, it has been proposed (LeDoux, 1995), that the convergence of sensory information of the conditioned and the unconditioned stimuli in the amygdala would follow Hebbian patterns (Hebb, 1949) and it would affect other areas involved in the process of emotional conditioning. In the last 20 years, a great amount of evidence (Johansen et al., 2011) showed that two kinds of molecular mechanisms are responsible for fear conditioning in the amygdala, specifically in the lateral amygdala: hebbian plasticity and neuromodulatory processes. In this sense, studies of fear conditioning to auditory stimuli suggest the existence of response potentiation in the lateral nucleus after learning. In addition, these plastic changes have also been observed in the auditory cortex. This change would be mediated by the circuit thalamus - lateral nucleus – basal nucleus - central nucleus - nucleus basalis of Meynert, since this latest nucleus sends a strong cholinergic innervation to the cerebral cortex (Price & Amaral, 1981; Russchen et al., 1985). It is very probable that this circuit has a key role in producing fast brain activity rhythms of low voltage (Bukasi et al., 1988). These results has been verified in studies that analyzed the involvement of the central nucleus of the amygdala in brain activation (Kapp et al, 1984; 1990; 1992) showing that activation of the amygdala and the prosencephalic basal nucleus produced cerebral asynchrony mediated by this cholinergic innervation. Therefore, the neuromodulatory processes in the glutamate amygdalar circuits (Ferry & McGaugh, 2008; Johansen et al., 2011) are mediated by monoamine transmitters (adrenaline, norepinephrine, and dopamine). The consolidation of this learning is dependent on plastic changes of amygdala synapses. The synthesis of a broad amount of proteins underlies consolidation of fear conditioning, such as receptor glutamate subunits, calmodulin, protein-kinases, and signaling pathway (see Helmstetter et al., 2008).

Experimental results show that the specific lesion of a thalamic region (that sends its efferents to the amygdala as the medial division of medial geniculate nucleus) can prevent the animal to be conditioned to a stimulus of that sensory modality (auditory), but not to another of different modality, such as visual (Campeau & Davis, 1995). On the other hand, different results show that the thalamo-amygdala and the thalamo-cortico-amygdala pathways are equipotential with the facilitation of classical conditioning to a simple stimulus (Johansen et al., 2011). These data indicate that there may be multiple and multi-modal representation of the CS-US associations in the amygdalar structure and the intrinsic circuits for fear conditioning (Gallagher & Chiba, 1996; LeDoux, 1995).

The neural system proposed by several authors for fear conditioning (Davis, 1992; LeDoux, 1995; Pitkänen et al, 1997) gives a central role to the amygdala as a receiving center of different information about stimuli, such as features of the stimuli (thalamus-lateral nucleus), perceptual phenomena (sensory association areas-lateral nucleus), spatial location and/or contextual and explicit memory (hippocampus-parvocellular division of the basal and lateral nucleus), polymodal representations (polymodal association cortex-lateral nucleus), and proprioceptive information (hypothalamus-medial nucleus). In this way, the response elicited by the circuit through the central nucleus would be induced by multiple representations of the existing stimulus in various structures, including the amygdala (Johansen et al., 2011).

3.3. Amygdala and avoidance conditioning

The studies on the involvement of the amygdala in avoidance learning performed between the decades of the 50's and the 70's were somewhat confusing (Brady et al., 1954; Campenot, 1969; Caruthers, 1969; Fonberg, 1973; Grossman, 1972; Grossman et al., 1974;, Isaacson, 1976; Kaada, 1972; Kling et al., 1960; McGaugh & Gold, 1976; Pellegrino, 1968; Ursin, 1965). After a critical reading of these works many of the lesions performed in the different studies affect more than one area, the procedures were not exactly comparable to one another, and it was unclear what the animals were really learning and in what context. However, while some results appear contradictory, it seems that it can be establish the differential involvement of some of the amygdaloid nuclei in the different types of avoidance behavior: passive, discriminative active -lever press- or one-way and two-way active discrimination (Ambrogli et al., 1991; Fonberg, 1973; Grossman et al., 1974; Handwerker et al., 1974; Horvath, 1963; Killcross et al., 1997; Liang & McGaugh, 1983; McIntery & Stein, 1973; Roozendaal et al., 1997; Sanchez-Riolobos 1986; van-der-Zee et al., 1997; Werka et al., 1978; Wiersma et al., 1998). The contradictory results mentioned above could be due to the fact that the amygdala has been considered a functional structure instead of a set of functional subsystems. The most important issues to consider when interpreting the different results on different types of avoidance behaviors are the result of overtraining, and hence the degree of consolidation of learning, individual differences (high-level avoidance animals and low-level avoidance animals within the same strain of animals), and of course, the verification of experimental procedures.

In addition, the similarity of lesions between different species, and defining which structures are affected are important data to analyze, since it has been shown that all these factors can dramatically influence the effects on acquisition or retention of this learned avoidance responses on apparently similar procedures as is exposed below.

3.4. Amygdala and olfactory conditioning

Fear conditioning studies have been directed primarily to analyzing the relationship between visual/auditory cues and the US, with little attention to olfactory cues. Studies with these types of cues are relatively recent although olfactory cues are of great evolutionary importance for laboratory animals such as rats. As with visual and auditory cues, studies that have used odors as CS associated with a foot-shock have recorded a strong emotional response, showing even greater resistance to extinction processes (Richardson et al. 2002). Electrophysiological studies also showed that the synaptic modifications in the BLA are dependent on the contingency between CS and US (Rosenkranz & Grace, 2002). Furthermore, this plasticity is also dependent of NMDA receptors during the acquisition process and is dependent of AMPA during recovery (Walker et al. 2005).

In addition to the BLA, other areas like the mPFC, perirhinal cortex and hippocampus specifically influence the expression of activity of the amygdala during fear conditioning odor. While the perirhinal cortex is essential for the initial processing of odor stimulus (Herzog & Otto, 1998), CA1 and CA3 of the hippocampus have been linked to the encoding and retrieval of context information (Hunsaker & Kesner, 2008). The subiculum is the principal structure linking the hippocampus with the entorhinal cortex and many other cortical and subcortical areas. Specifically, the v-Sub may act as an interface between the hippocampus as a contextual information processor and cortical and subcortical processing systems related to motivation such as the ventral striatum and amygdala (Floresco et al., 2001; Quintero et al, 2011; Traverso et al, 2010). Parsons & Otto (2008) showed that the inactivation of dorsal hippocampus using an olfactory contextual conditioning, caused acquisition and retrieval deficits. In addition, neurons from mPFC are essential to acquire the association between CS and UC. These neurons show strong activity to foot-shock odor association. This activity is dopamine dependent, given that selective blockade of dopamine receptors reduces emotional response to the CS (Laviolette et al. 2005).

3.5. Effects of lesions to the amygdala

Kaada (1972) postulated that there were two different regions in the amygdala for the control of active avoidance behavior in rats, the defense amygdalar region, and the basolateral complex. Partial or total lesion to the defense amygdalar region (in rats and cats including the ventral part of the internal capsule and the ventral amigdalofugal pathway and pallial and subpallian structures), suppressed defense responses including the escape response (Blanchard & Blanchard, 1972; Kemble et al., 1984; 1990; Ursin et al., 1981). So, in their view it would have to block active avoidance responses in a classical active avoidance response paradigm. In contrast, lesion to the basolateral complex, which had inhibitory influences, impairs passive avoidance behavior but it does not affect the performance in an active avoidance paradigm behavior. Several experimental results support this view: in cats, both the electrolytically lesion of the anterior portion of the lateral nucleus and the interruption of the amigdalofugal ventral pathway produced a severe deficit in active avoidance conditioning, but not in passive avoidance (Ursin, 1965). Also, electrolytic lesion to the central nucleus and to the adjacent and dorsal regions to the basolateral complex in cats affected the retention of a two-way active avoidance response, but it did not affect one way active avoidance nor passive avoidance (Horvath, 1963). Similar data were obtained in rats (Pellegrino 1968). In this study, a lesion to the basolateral complex produced a severe disability for the maintenance of a passive avoidance response. Also, in mice, a large electrolytic lesion produces a severe deficit in both active and passive avoidance responses (Takashina et al., 1995). According to Werka et al. (1978) a lesion to the lateral cortex and central and lateral nuclei described deficits in the retention of one-way active avoidance. Killcross et al. (1997) demonstrated a process that allowed them to separate two responses related to fear conditioning (a conditioned suppression response to an aversive stimulus and an active avoidance response to the harmful stimulus) that lesions to the central nucleus affect the maintenance of the conditioned suppression response, but not the acquisition of the active avoidance response. In contrast, lesions to the basolateral nucleus produced the opposite effect. This latest result would establish a parallel processing of two types of fear dependent response, indicating that in the amygdala there are different mechanisms and different areas for processing the stimuli and the fear response. This idea would lead to a more critical discussion about the nature of avoidance responses, but what concerns us is that the amygdala is establishing an important relationship with this type of learning. Other studies present conflicting results, for instance Brady et al. (1954), showed that a large electrolytic lesion to the amygdala impairs cats to acquire an active avoidance response, but if the lesion was done after the learning, it did not affect the maintenance of the response. Similar results were obtained with passive avoidance procedure after bilateral electrolytic lesions (Liang et al., 1982). Also, in rats the lesion to the central nucleus produced a deficit in the acquisition but not in the retention of the response (Davis, 2000; Grossman et al., 1974; McIntery & Stein, 1973). In addition, different molecular processes seem underlying to acquisition and retention in central amygdala. While the inhibitory consolidation processes are under control of NMDA and cannabinoid CB1 receptors (Ghiasvand et al., 2011), serotonergic system is involved in the modulation of retention in the passive-avoidance task (Schneider et al., 2003). Another set of results have raised deeper questions about the involvement of various amygdaloid nuclei, where the amygdaloid cortex lesion severely affected the acquisition of one and two-way active avoidance response. In contrast, lesions of the cortical, medial, central, intercalated, lateral, and basolateral nucleus did not affect active avoidance, although lesions to the central, intercalated, and basolateral nucleus impair passive avoidance learning (Grossman et al., 1974). A recent electrophysiological study shows that the expression of conditioned freezing depends on increased activity levels of the medial region of the central amygdala but it does not depend on the activity of the lateral region (Duvarci et al., 2011). These differences in results could be due to various reasons (e.g. lesion differences, collaterally affected areas, use of different strains, etc). Another cause is the effect of overtraining, since according to Fonberg et al. (1962) it prevents the effects of the lesion on the amygdala. At the same line, Thatcher & Kimble, (1966) showed no effect on the retention of a learned avoidance response after overtraining. In contrast, a recovery deficit is observed in absence of overtraining (Goldstein, 1974; Thatcher & Kimble, 1966). It is possible to observe a very similar case in inhibitory avoidance. Reversibly inactivation or lesion to the amygdala affects retention if it is done soon after the training, but has no effect if it is performed much later (Liang et al., 1982; McGaugh et al., 2000; Parent & McGaugh, 1994; Wilensky et al., 2000; 2006).

However, although the amygdala is believed to be essential for the acquisition of Pavlovian fear conditioning, studies using excitotoxic lesions have recently called this view into question. Thus, different nuclei of the amygdala could contribute to the modulation of memory consolidation of an avoidance response (active or passive) in a different way:

a. Pallial amygdala. Lesions to the basolateral nucleus (lateral, basal, and accessory basal) produce severe deficits in the acquisition of both active and passive avoidance, although the effects on retention are lower in the passive than in the active (Ambrogli et al., 1991). The same lesions have no effect on the conditioned response nor in a passive avoidance response with contextual cues (Selden et al., 1991). A previous study comparing the effects of electrolytic lesions to those produced by ibotenic acid showed that only the electrolytic lesions by radiofrequency impairs for an active avoidance response (Jellestad & Cabrera, 1986). Nevertheless, this study did not define what amygdalar structures were indeed damaged. Moreover, it postulates the idea of the involvement of a pathway through the nucleus instead of the cell groups present in those structures.

b. Subpallial amygdala. Lesions to the central nucleus produce deficits in both an active avoidance response (Riolobos & Garcia, 1987) and a two-way active avoidance (Sánchez-Riolobos, 1986).

All these data together support the differential involvement of pallial and subpallial nuclei in active avoidance learning (McGaugh et al., 2000; Wilensky et al., 2000; 2006).

3.6. Effects of electrical stimulation

Early studies showed that electrical stimulation of the amygdala induced amnesia for different learning processes (Grossman, 1972; Isaacson 1976; Kaada, 1972) included avoidance learning. The specific stimulation of the central nucleus, immediately after training in an avoidance task, produced a large deficit in the retention of that task and a blockade of fear conditioning (Gold et al., 1975; McDonough & Kesner, 1971). The same results were observed in the retention of passive avoidance tasks (Gold et al, 1973a; Kesner, 1982), and in a one-way active avoidance after unilateral stimulation in the basomedial nucleus (McGaugh & Gold 1974). Gold et al. (1973) showed that 1 hour after training, stimulation produced a deficit in the avoidance response, but 6 hours later produced no effect in the same avoidance test. This data suggests that there is a plastic phenomenon related to learning, which would be disrupted by the stimulation shortly after training, but not once its effects are consolidated. Other studies also described amnesic effects in both one-way avoidance and discriminated avoidance (press a lever) after post-training stimulation (Hanwerker et al., 1974; McGaugh & Gold, 1976). Nevertheless, other studies have found memory facilitating effects after stimulation in passive avoidance tests with a weak shock (Gold & Van Buskirk, 1975). In other studies, a low intensity shock showed similar results in tasks such as conditioned emotional response. Lidsky et al. (1970), Gold & McGaugh (1975), and McGaugh & Gold (1976) proposed that the different motivational state caused by a severe or a mild shock condition would produce the differential effect of electrical stimulation. Subsequent studies have exposed as the amnesic effects of electrical stimulation can be modulated by hormone levels, which would support this hypothesis. The removal of the adrenal gland (decline on systemic levels of catecholamines) showed that electrical stimulation does not induce amnesia but showed an improvement in the retention of an inhibitory avoidance response in both active and passive condition (Bennett et al., 1985). Also, in a similar study, Liang et al. (1985) injected norepinephrine immediately after training and just before intraamygdaline electrical stimulation. Animals without adrenal medulla showed the same deficits as the control animals, which could determine a modulation of systemic norepinephrine on memory through or in connection with the amygdala.

In fact, we know the involvement between the amygdala (mainly central nucleus) and the CHR (corticotrophin releasing hormone) - ACTH (adrenocorticotropic hormone) - corticosteroids cascade and norepinephrine release, and its correlation with the response of fear, anxiety and stress (Davis 1992). Several studies have linked the conditioning of stressful situations, amygdalar lesions and intraamygdaline inoculation of systemic ACTH or CHR. Bush et al. (1973) showed that an electrolytic lesion of the amygdala produced extensive damage to a passive avoidance response, and this effect was reversed by systemic injection of ACTH. Krivanek (1971) showed that injection of norepinephrine, pentylenetetrazole (GABAergic antagonist) and ACTH produced a facilitation of avoidance behavior. Moreover, in an experiment with adrenalectomized rats, intra amygdalin electrical stimulation produced an amnesic effect in active and passive avoidance in control animals, while animals without adrenals improved their performance and retention in these tasks (Bennett et al., 1985). Another series of studies have combined individual differences in avoidance tasks and hormone action in the amygdala. Wiersma et al. (1998) determined that the animals of the RHA strain (high rate of avoidance) and the RLA (low avoidance rate) had different behavioural, physiological, and neurobiological responses under stress-free conditions after CRH microinfusion into the central nucleus of the amygdala. RHA increased heart-rate activity and decreased resting only in a stressful situation (inescapable shock) while a slight behavioral activation was observed in RLA. These results show a correlation between the ability to learn avoidance tasks, intra-individual differences, and hormonal regulation in the amygdala in an emotional context.

3.7. Social and neuroimage studies of primates and humans

In the studies of mammals (see above) it appears that the amygdala is involved in normal (LeDoux, 2012; Parkes & Westbrook, 2011; Phelps & LeDoux, 2005) and pathological (Magdaleno-Madrigal et al., 2010, Roozendaal et al., 2009) emotional processing. In primates including humans it integrates more complex functions of social and cognitive nature: such as anxiety disorders (Holzchneider & Mulert, 2011; Kim et al., 2011), decision making (Seymour & Dolan, 2008) or fear, and social learning (Olsson & Phelps, 2007). In species with a highly complex social environment, like in the human case, the amygdala has a crucial role. Neuroimaging studies has been shown that the amygdala functions as a relevance detector that allows humans to perceive incongruence in the emotional expressions, or fear (Phelps & LeDoux, 2005), although others argue that the amygdala activation is more indirect in these cases (van der Gaag et al., 2007). In humans, the amygdala shares common functions with other species, and also acquires more subtle properties in the management of emotional content information that can be shared at least in part with other social primates (Pessoa & Adolphs, 2010), in which circuit model "low road" and "high road" of emotional processing becomes more complicated in terms of increased complexity of sensory processing and perception in humans and primates, taking in this case a greater involvement of the cortex. However, there is a general conservation of function, with an implementation of new features that accompany human neural development itself (Adolphs, 2009; LeDoux, 2012; Olsson & Phelps, 2007; Pessoa & Adolphs, 2010). Likewise, in the pathological aspect of emotion, fMR studies have shown correlated changes in volume of the amygdala and secretion of cortisol in psychiatric disorders such as unipolar depression (Schuhmacher et al. 2012) and other behavioral disorders as described in other chapters of the present book.

4. Function of the amygdala homologous in non mammals vertebrates

Lesions or stimulation of the amygdala in reptiles and birds (or structures considered homologous to the amygdala) produce changes in social behavior or learning processes (Martínez-García et al, 2007). These changes are similar and show a comparable function to the amygdalar system of mammals. In the case of crocodilian reptiles (*Caiman sclerops*), lesions of the amygdala results in decreased frequencies of aggressive patterns (Keating et al., 1970). Likewise, lesions to the areas considered homologous to the amygdala in a iguanide in a social environment (*Sceloporus occidentalis*) caused a syndrome similar to that of mammals as it produced deficits in attention and response (loss of initiative), in patterns of dominance and submission, and a decrease in the response to fear stimulus (Tarr, 1977). Reproductive and aggressive behaviors, as well as associated seasonal variations, have been the main object of study in snakes (*Thamnophis sirtalis parietalis*). These studies show that the sphericus, considered homologous to the amygdala in these reptiles (Bruce & Neary, 1995; Sriedter, 1997), presents sexual dimorphism which is more evident of the males (Crews et al., 1993). Moreover, when the nucleus sphericus is lesioned before the start of the stage of hibernation, there is a facilitation of courtship patterns in the male after the hibernation that correlates with increased blood levels of androgens, indicating a potential facilitating effect of the lesion (Krohner & Crews, 1987).

Zeier & Karten (1971) have argued that the posteromedial portion of the archistriatum, now called arcopallium (The Avian Brain Nomenclature Consortium, 2005), is the homologous to pallial amygdala (basolateral amygdala) in birds. The experimental results support the homology proposal (Dafters, 1975; Goodson & Bass, 2001; Lowndes & Davies, 1994).

In the case of the turtle dove (*Streptopelia risoria*), it is known that electrical stimulation of archipallium produces emotional responses of fear, offense, and defense (The Avian Brain Nomenclature Consortium, 2005; Vowles & Beasley, 1974). In addition, lesions to this structure abolish the conditioned emotional response (as the cardiac acceleration that occurs paired with a shock) in *Columba livia* (Cohen, 1975, Dafter, 1976). When an active avoidance is used, the arquipallial lesion produces the same deficit for the acquisition of a avoidance response that the lesion of the mammalian amygdala (Dafter, 1975). In the case of active avoidance, the arquipallial lesion produces the same deficit in the acquisition of the avoidance response that lesion of the mammalian amygdala (Dafter, 1975). Phillips & Youngren (1968) showed that unilateral excitotoxic lesions of this structure in chicks that are 5 days old showed a decrease in distress vocalizations (the chirp). Anatides have a similar effect, since in the mallard (*Anas platyrhynchos*) lesions to archipallium produce a generalized effect as defined by author of "domestication" or put in another way, lack of fear of emotional reactivity (Phillips, 1964; The Avian Brain Nomenclature Consortium, 2005). The same effect occurs in *Columba livia* after lesions of the posterior portion of archipallium. In contrast, lesions to the anterior portion facilitate the emotional reaction of fear (Zeier, 1971). In a study in chickens (*Gallus gallus*), Maser et al. (1973) showed that lesions to the anterolateral portion produced an increase in reactive immobility typical of fear responses.

In psittacidae (*Agapornis roseicolis*), lesions of the medial part induces a decrease of fear, and it facilitates the approach toward dangerous stimuli of the animal (Phillips, 1968). These results seem to clearly differentiate two portions of the birds' medial archipallium, with opposite functions from the point of view of control of emotional responses. This is corroborated by the results of a study of a fringillidae, the zebra finch (*Taenopigya guttata*). In this study the activity of brain areas was measured by the uptake of 2-deoxyglucose-C14, after subjecting male animals to various stressful circumstances (Bischof & Herrmann, 1986). One group was housed alone in a cage. Animals with experience in courtship were assigned to a second group. A third group of subjects did not have experience in courtship and a fourth group was subjected to a situation in which the experimenter pretended to try to catch them in their cages. The analysis showed a high rate of uptake in the caudal portion of archistriapallium in the group without experience in courtship and the one of capture inside the cage: the two most stressful situations. Also lesions to the taenia nucleus of the amygdala (homologous to part of the medial amygdala of mammals) seriously affect the socio-sexual behavior of male Zebra finches (Ikebuchi et al., 2009).

In the case of teleosts fish, the results from the experiments of telencephalic lesions and stimulation that produce alterations in reproductive and aggressive behaviors (de Bruin, 1980; Kyle & Peter, 1982; Kyle et al., 1982) present a picture of behavioral changes that can be easily compared to changes mediated by the amygdala function. For instance, the agonistic behavior of male Betta fish has been widely studied. The sight of another male typically stimulates a series of agonistic behavioral displays toward the intruder often followed by physical aggression. The context used in these studies is known as agonistic context. The partial ablation of the dorsomedial telencephalon (Dm) in *Betta splendens* produces a loss of reactivity (facilitation of habituation) in an agonistic context (Marino-Neto & Sabbatini, 1983). However, lesion experiments often extend the damage to the basal portion of Dmv. If we admit the existence of telencephalic structures with limbic function equivalent to those of tetrapods, we would also have to admit that lesions in different limbic areas produce similar effects in fish and tetrapods.

The results of ablation studies in teleost fish show that the Dmv region, proposed as homologous to the pallial amygdala of land vertebrates, has a key role in Pavlovian conditioning. These studies showed a clear lesion effect in both the acquisition and maintenance of a two-way active avoidance behavior (Portavella et al., 2004a, 2004b; Portavella & Vargas, 2005). Thus, lesions to the Dmv region produce a deficit equivalent to those described in the case of complete ablation of the telencephalon in earlier studies in Pavlovian conditioning (Aronson, 1948; de Bruin, 1977; 1980; Fiedler, 1967; 1968; Hale, 1956; Kamrin & Aronson, 1954; Karamyan et al., 1967; Kassel & Davis, 1977; Kassel et al., 1976; Noble, 1939; Noble & Bourne, 1941; Overmier & Gross, 1974;; Segaar, 1961; 1965; Segaar & Nieuwenhuys, 1963; Ribbink, 1972). Also, the deficit showed in both the acquisition and retention in avoidance behavior cannot be attributed to the lack of activity or initiative of the animal after lesion, because the level of escape is very high. In addition, the absence of effects on spatial memory or motor response (Portavella & Vargas, 2005) rules out a possible functional homology with the hippocampus and basal ganglia of tetrapods (Braford, 1995; Braford et al., 1992; 1993; Echteler & Saidel, 1981; Murakami et al., 1983; Nieuwenhuys & Verrijdt, 1983; Northcutt, 1995; Northcutt & Braford, 1980; Parent, 1986; Parent et al., 1978). Thus, we concluded that the lesion produced a deficit in the associative process between the discriminative stimulus and the shock (Portavella et al, 2002; 2004a, 2004b; Portavella & Vargas, 2005; Vargas et al., 2009). Other results in fear context conditioning have showed that lesions of the dorsomedial telencephalic portion in *Betta splendens* produced a facilitation of habituation to the context (Marino-Neto & Sabbatini, 1983) and variations in levels of aggression (de Bruin, 1980). Taken as a whole, these data indicate that the Dm telencephalon area shares a great similarity with pallial amygdaloid nuclei and homologous structures in reptiles (Crews et al., 1993; Keating et al., 1970; Krohner & Crews, 1987; Tarr, 1977), birds (Cohen, 1975; Dafter, 1975; 1976; Ikebuchi et al., 2009; Martínez-García, et al., 2002; Phillips 1968; Phillips & Youngren, 1968; Vowles & Beasley, 1974; Zeier, 1971), and mammals (Ambrogli et al, 1991; Fonberg, 1973; Grossman et al., 1974; Hanwerker et al., 1974; Horvath, 1963; Killcross et al., 1997; Liang & McGaugh, 1983; McIntery & Stein, 1973; Pellegrino, 1968; Roozendaal et al., 1993; Sanchez-Riolobos, 1986; Takashina et al., 1995; van-der-Zee et al., 1997; Werka et al., 1978; Wiersma et al., 1998). These amygdala lesions affect not only the avoidance conditioning, but also the fear conditioning in mammals and birds (Cohen, 1975; Dafter, 1976).

One of two main approaches on the theories of avoidance in fish (Flood et al., 1976; Zhuikov et al., 1994) is a model adapted from the theory of the two processes of Mowrer (1947). This model recognizes the existence of a two processes. One of them is the conditioning process of a motivational state (fear). That is crucial to the Pavlovian conditioning. The other one is the association between the CS and the shuttling response (Zhuikov et al, 1994). Given these results, it could be postulated that the lesion in the dorsomedial region deprives the fish of such capacity, and it would be one of the causes of the main deficit for the maintenance of avoidance behavior (Portavella et al, 2002; 2004a, 2004b; Portavella & Vargas, 2005; Vargas et al., 2009).

5. Conclusion

Learning theories for the function of the amygdalar system are not an organized body of various alternatives, but show a set of nuclei that receive any type of sensory or perceptual relevant information inducing changes in the neuroendocrine system, and the emergence of emotional patterns mediated by this structure (autonomic, humoral, and behavioral). This set of nuclei would in turn form a central part of the emotional learning processes (Aggleton, 1992; Davis, 1992; Gallagher & Chiba, 1996; Gallagher & Holland, 1992; Halgren, 1992; Killcross et al., 1997; LeDoux, 1992; 1995; Olsson & Phelps, 2007; Phelps & Anderson, 1997). Likewise, though being intrinsically a very complex structure (Amaral et al., 1992; Pitkänen et al., 1997), it is clear that lesions of a large part of the nucleus of the pallial amygdala (basolateral amygdala) and also the subpallial part seriously affect all type of emotional learning. In fish, the ablation of Dmv telencephalon induced a clear deficit in a conditioned avoidance behavior, similar to that produced after a complete ablation of the telencephalon (Portavella et al., 2004a, 2004b; Portavella & Vargas, 2005; Vargas et al., 2009). These data coupled with the effects of Dm lesions on aggressive behavior, breeding, habituation in situations of aggression in a resident/intruder paradigm (de Bruin, 1980; Marino-Neto & Sabbatini, 1983), as well as data from electrical stimulation of Dm in *Carassius* that show facilitation and inhibition of aggressive and reproductive patterns or startle response and escape (Savage, 1971), support the homology of the fish telencephalic Dmv with the pallial amygdala of mammals. This idea have been proposed on the basis of neuroanatomical and neurohistochemical evidence of similarities between the two structures developing an evolution-based model of brain organization (Braford, 1995; Echteler & Saidel, 1981; Hornby et al., 1987; Ito et al., 1986; Medina & Reiner, 1995; Murakami et al., 1983; Northcutt, 1995; 2008; Piñuela & Nortcutt, 1994; Reiner & Northcutt, 1992; Striedter, 1991; Wulliman & Rink, 2002) and that of reptiles (Crews et al., 1993; Keating et al., 1970; Krohner & Crews, 1987; Tarr, 1977), birds (Cohen, 1975; Dafter, 1975; 1976; Ikebuchi et al., 2009; Phillips 1968; Phillips & Youngren, 1968; Vowles & Beasley, 1974; Zeier, 1971), and mammals (Ambrogli et al., 1991; Fonberg, 1973; Grossman et al., 1974; Hanwerker et al., 1974; Horvath, 1963; Killcross et al., 1997; Liang & McGaugh, 1983; McIntery & Stein, 1973; Pellegrino, 1968; Roozendaal et al., 1993; Sanchez-Riolobos, 1986; Takashina et al., 1995; van-der-Zee et al., 1997; Werka et al., 1978; Wiersma et al., 1998).

This exhibition along with the data of the previous sections would support the fact that structures homologous to the amygdala of the different groups of vertebrates, including humans, share similar functions, at least in terms of information processing of emotional content, which is essential for the survival of the species (LeDoux, 2012). This idea is based on results from genoarchitectonical studies showing the consistancy of genetical markers along vertebrates' brains evolution. In the case of amygdala of tetrapods (Medina et al., 2011) is composed of four different regions: ventral pallial amygdala (i.e. basal amygdala of mammals, dorsal ventricular ridge in reptiles and birds), striatal amygdala (i.e. the central nucleus in different groups), pallidal amygdala (medial amygdala of amniotes) and hypothalamical part present in different vertebrates groups (i.e. bed nucleus and extended amygdala). A part of specific gene expression of these four divisions is present in mammals, birds, reptiles, and amphibians. In the case of teleost fish, behavioral approaching (Portavella et al., 2004a, 2004b; Portavella & Vargas, 2005) showed similar learning deficits after brain lesions on homologues areas to mammalian amygdala, and genetical studies showed constancy in the expression of pallial and subpallial genes, and the presence of, at least, a medial amygdala (Gonzalez & Northcutt, 2009) and the hypothalamical components (Eaton et al., 2008). The behavioral studies commented in previous sections of this chapter show how essential functions for species survival such as fear conditioning, escape and avoidance behavior, aggressive, and sexual behaviors are dramatically impaired after mammalian amygdala lesions, or homologues structures in the case of birds, reptiles, amphibians, or teleost fish (see sections II and III of this chapter). These behavioral data and genetical studies, together with evidence of homologies seem to support the existence of a basic bauplan in the vertebrates' line, including man, which has been broadly conserved during evolution of the vertebrate nervous system, including structures such as the amygdala.

Author details

Juan Pedro Vargas, Juan Carlos López and Manuel Portavella
Laboratory of Behavioral Neuroscience, Department of Experimental Psychology, University of Seville, Spain

Acknowledgement

This study was supported by PSI2009-12761 and RyC2006/1284 (Spanish Government) grants. We thank Paola Revilla for technical assistance and Brittany Adams for her helpful comments on the manuscript.

6. References

Adolphs, R. (2009). The social brain: neural basis of social knowledge. *Annual Reviews of Psuychology, 60*, 693-716.

Adolphs, R., Gossein, F., Buchanan, T. W., Tranel, D., Schyns, P. & Damasio, A. R. (2005) A mechanism for impaired fear recognition after amygdala damage. *Nature, 433*, 68-72

Adolphs, R., Tranel, D., Damasio, H. & Damasio, A. (1994) Impaired recognition of emotion in facial expressions following bilateral damage to human amygdala. *Nature, 372*, 669-672

Aggleton, J. P. (1985). A description of intraamygdaloid connections in the old world monkeys, *Experimental Brain Research, 57*, 390-399.

Aggleton, J. P. (1992). *The amygdala: neurobiological aspects of emotion, memory, and mental dysfunction*. Wiley-Liss, New York.

Amano, T., Duvarci, S. & Paré, D. (2010). The basal nuclei of the amygdala are involved in conditioned fear extinction but not expression. *Society for Neuroscience Abstract, 36*, 808, 24

Amaral, D. G., Price, J. L., Pitkänen, A. & Carmichael, S. T. (1992) Anatomical organization of tje primate amygdaloid complex. In: J. P. Aggleton (Ed.). *The Amygdala: Neurobiological Aspects of Emotion, Memory, and Mental Dysfunction*. Wiley-Liss, New York.

Ambrogi-Lorenzini, C., Bucherelli, C., Giachetti, A., Mugnai, L. & Tassoni, G. (1991). Effects of nucleus basolateralis amygdalae neurotoxic lesions on aversive conditioning in the rat. *Physiology and Behavior, 49*, 765-770.

Aronson, L. R. (1948). Problems in the behavior and physiology of a species of African mouthbreeding fish. *Transactions of the New York Academy of Sciences, 11*, 33-42.

Bennett, C., Liang, K. C. & McGaugh, J. L. (1985). Depletion of adrenal catecholamines alters the amnestic effect of amygdala stimulation. *Behavioral Brain Research, 15*, 83-91.

Bischof, H. J. & Herrmann, K. (1986). Arousal enhances ^{14C}2-deoxyglucose uptake in four forebrain areas of the zebra finch. *Behavioral Brain Research, 21*, 215-221.

Blanchard, D. C. & Blanchard, R. J. (1972). Innate and conditioned reactions to threat in rats with amygdaloid lesions. *Journal of Comparative and Physiological Psychology, 81*, 281-290.

Bliss, T. V. P. & Collingridge, G. L. (1993). A synaptic model of memory: long-term potentiation in the hippocampus. *Nature, 361,* 31-39.

Brady, J. V., Schreiner, L., Geller, J. & Kling, A. (1954). Subcortical mechanisms in emotional behavior: The effect of rhinencephalic injury upon acquisition of a conditioned avoidance response in cats. *Journal of Comparative and Physiological Psychology, 47,* 179-196.

Braford, M. R. (1995). Comparative aspects of forebrain organization in ray-finned fishes: touchstones or not? *Brain Behavior and Evolution, 46,* 259-274.

Braford, M. R., Jensen, A. A. & Russell, R. W. (1992). Some connections of the torus longitudinalis in the osteoglossomorph teleost, *Xenomystus nigri. Society for Neuroscience Abstracs, 18,* 326.

Braford, M. R., Prince, E. & McCormick, C. A. (1993). A presumed acoustic pathway from the ear to the telencephalon in an osteoglossomorph teleost. *Society for Neuroscience Abstracs, 19,* 160.

Bruce, L. L. & Neary, T. J. (1995). The limbic system of tetrapods: A comparative analysis of cortical and amygdalar populations. *Brain, Behavior and Evolution, 46,* 224-234.

Bukasi, G. Bickford, R. G., Ponomareff, G., Thal, L. J. Mandel, R. & Gage, F. H. (1988). Nucleus basalis and thalamic control of neocortical activity in freely moving rat. *Journal of Neuroscience, 8,* 4007-4026.

Bush, D. F., Lovely, R. H. & Pagano, R. R. (1973). Injection of ACTH induces recovery from shuttle-box avoidance deficits in rats with amygdala lesions. *Journal of Comparative and Physiological Psychology, 83,* 168-172.

Calvo, J. M., Badillo, S., Morales-Ramírez, M. & Palacios-Salas, P. (1987). The role of the temporal lobe amygdala in ponto-geniculo-occipital activity and sleep organization in cats. *Brain Research, 403,* 22-30.

Campeau, S. & Davis, M. (1995). Involvement of the central nucleus and basolateral complex of the amygdala in fear conditioning measured with fear-potentiates startle in rats trained concurrently with auditory and visual conditioned stimuli. *Journal of Neurociences, 15,* 2301-2311.

Campenot, R. B. (1969) Effect of amygdaloid lesions upon active avoidance acquisition and anticipatory responding in rats. *Journal of Comparative and Physiological Psychology, 69,* 492-497.

Caruthers, R. P. (1969). Deficits in shock-avoidance performance after amygdala-hippocampus separation. *Journal of Comparative and Physiological Psychology, 67,* 547-554.

Chanconie, M. & Clairrambault P. (1975). Développment du télencephale de *Salmo irideus Gib. Journal of Comparative Neurology, 208,* 107-126.

Chapman, P. F. & Bellavance, L. L. (1992). NMDA receptors-independent LTP in the amygdala. *Synapse, 8,* 145-149.

Clugnet, M. C., LeDoux, J. E. & Morrison S. F. (1990). Unit responses evoked in the amygdala and striatum by electrical stimulation of the medial geniculate body. *Journal of Neuroscience, 10,* 1055-1061

Cohen, D. H. (1975). Involvement of the avian amygdala homologue (archistriatum posterior and mediale) in defensively conditioned heat rate change. *Journal of Comparative Neurology, 160,* 13-36.

Cousens, G. & Otto, T. (1998). Both pre- and posttraining excitotoxic lesions of the basolateral amygdala abolish the expression of olfactory and contextual fear conditioning. *Behavioral Neuroscience, 112,* 1092–1103

Crews, D., Robker, R. & Mendoca, M. (1993). Seasonal fluctuations in brain nuclei in the red-side garter snake and their hormonal control. *Journal of Neuroscience, 13,* 5356-5364.

Dafters, R. (1975). Active avoidance behavior following archistriatal lesions in pigeons. *Journal of Comparative and Physiological Psychology, 89,* 1169-1179.

Dafters, R. (1976). Effect of medial archistriatal lesions on the conditioned emotional response and on auditory discrimination performance of the pigeon. *Physiology and Behavior, 17,* 659-665.

Davis, M. (1992). The role of the amygdala in conditioned fear. In: J. P. Aggleton (Ed.). *The amygdala: neurobiological aspects of emotion, memory, and mental dysfunction.* Wiley-Liss, New York. Pp. 55-305.

Davis, M. (2000). The role of the amygdala in conditioned and unconditioned fear and anxiety. In: J. P. Aggleton (Ed.). *The Amygdala.* Oxford University Press, Oxford, UK. Pp. 213–288.

de Bruin, J. P. C. (1977). *Telencephalic functions in the behavior of the Siamese fighting fish,Betta splendens* Regan (Pisces, Anabantidae). PhD Dissertation. University of Amsterdam.

de Bruin, J. P. C. (1980). Telencephalon and behavior in teleost fish. A neuroethological approach. In S. O. E. Ebbesson (Ed.). *Comparative neurology of the telencephalon.* Plenum, New York. Pp. 175-201.

DeOlmos, J., Alheid, G. F. & Beltramino, C. A. (1985). Amygdala. In: G. Paxinos (Ed.). *The rat nervous system. Vol. 1.* Academic Press, New York. Pp. 223-334.

DiCara, L., Braun, J. J. & Pappas, B. (1970). Classical conditioning and instrumental learning of cardiac and gastrointestinal responses following removal the neocortex in the rat. *Journal of Comparative and Physiological Psychology, 73,* 208-216.

Dudek, S. M. & Bear, M. F. (1992). Homosynaptic long-term depression in area CA1 of hippocampus and effects of N-methyl-D-aspartate receptor blockade. *Proceedings of National Academy of Sciences, 89,* 4363-4367.

Duvarci, S., Popa, D. & Paré, D. (2011). Central amygdala activity during fear conditioning. *Journal of Neurosciences, 31,* 289-294.

Eaton, J. L., Holmqvist, B. & Glasgow, E. (2008): Ontogeny of vasotocin-expressing cells in zebrafish: selective requirement for the transcriptional regulators orthopedia and singleminded 1 in the preoptic area. *Developmental Dynamics, 237,* 995–1005.

Echteler, S. M. & Saidel, W. M. (1981). Forebrain projections in the goldfish support telencephalic homologies with land vertebrates. *Science, 212,* 683-685.

Falls, W. A., Miserendino, M. J. D. & Davis, M. (1992). Extinction of fear-potentiated startle: blockade by infusion of an NMDA antagonist into the amygdala. *Journal of Neuroscience, 12,* 854-863.

Fanselow, M. S. & Kim, J. J. (1994). Acquisition of contextual Pavlovian fear conditioning is blocked by application of an NMDA receptor antagonist D,L-2-amino-5-phosphono-valeric acid to the basolateral amygdala. *Behavioral Neuroscience, 108,* 210-212.

Farb, C. R. & LeDoux, J. E. (1997). NMDA and AMPA receptors in the lateral nucleus of the amygdala are postsynaptic to auditory thalamic afferents. *Synapse, 27,* 106-121.

Ferry B. & McGaugh J. L. (2008). Involvement of basolateral amygdala alpha2-adrenoceptors in modulating consolidation of inhibitory avoidance memory. *Learning and Memory, 3,* 238-43.

Fiedler, K. L. (1967). Ethologische und neuroanatomische Auswirkungen von Vorderhirnexstirpationen bei Meer brassen (*Diplodus*) and Lippfischen (*Crenilabrus,* Perciformes, Teleostei). *Journal für Hirnforschung, 9,* 481-563.

Fiedler, K. L. (1968). Verhaltenswirksame Strukturen im Fischgehirn. *Zoologischer Anzeiger, 31,* 602-616.

Flood, N. B., Overmier, J. B. & Savage, G. E. (1976). The teleost telencephalon and learning: An interpretative review of data and hypotheses. *Physiology & Behavior, 16,* 783-798.

Floresco, S. B., Todd, C. L. & Grace, A. A. (2001). Glutamatergic afferents from the hippocampus to the nucleus accumbens regulate activity of ventral tegmental area dopamine neurons. *Journal of Neuroscience, 21,* 4915-22

Fonberg, E. (1973). The normalizing effect of lateral amygdalar lesions upon dorsomedial amygdalr syndrome in dogs. *Acta Biologiae Experimentalis, 33,* 449-466.

Fonberg, E., Brutkowski, S. & Mempel (1962). Defensive conditioned reflexes and neurotic motor reactions following amygdalectomy in dogs. *Acta Biologiae Experimentalis, 22,* 51-57.

Fusar-Poli, P., Placentino, A., Carletti, F., Allen, P., Landi, P., Abbamonte, M., Barale, F., Perez, J., McGuire, P. & Politi, P. L. (2009). Laterality effect on emotional facesprocessing: ALE meta-analysis of evidence. *Neuroscience Letters, 452,* 262–267.

Gage, S. P. (1893). The brain of *Diemyctylus viridescens* from larval to adult life and comparison with the brain of Amia and Petromyzon. In: *Wilder Quarter Century Book.* Ithaca, New York.

Gallagher, M. & Chiba, A. (1996). The amygdala and emotion. *Current Opinion in Neurobiology, 6,* 221-227.

Gallagher, M. & Holland, P. C. (1992). Understanding the function of the central nucleus: Is simple conditioning enough?. In: J. P. Aggleton. (Ed.). *The Amygdala: Neurobiological Aspects of Emotion, Memory, and Mental Dysfunction.* Wiley-Liss, New York, pp 307-321.

Gean, P. W., Chang, F. C., Huang, C. C., Lin, J. H. & Way, L. J. (1993). Long-term enhancement of EPSP and NMDA receptor-mediated synaptic transmission in the amygdala. *Brain Research Bulletin, 31,*7-11.

Gewirtz, J. C. & Davis, M. (1997). Second-order fear conditioning prevented by blocking NMDA receptors in amygdala. *Nature, 388,* 471-473.

Ghiasvand, M., Rezayof, A, Zarrindast, MR., & Ahmadi, S. (2011). Activation of cannabinoid CB1 receptors in the central amygdala impairs inhibitory avoidance memory consolidation via NMDA receptors. *Neurobiology of Learning and Memory, 96,* 333-338.

Gold, P. E., Hanskins, L., Edwards, R., Chester, J. & McGaugh, J. L. (1975). Memory interference and facilitation with posttrial amygdala stimulation: Effect on memory varies with footshock level. *Brain Research, 86,* 509-513.

Gold, P. E., Macri, J. & McGaugh, J. L. (1973a). Retrograde amnesia gradients: Effects of direct cortical stimulation. *Science, 179,* 1343-1345.

Gold, P. E., Macri, J. & McGaugh, J. L. (1973b). Retrograde amnesia produced by subseizure amygdala stimulation. *Behavioral Biology, 9,* 671-680.

Gold, P. E. & McGaugh, J. L. (1975). A single-trace, two-process view of memory storage processes. In: D. Deutsch & A. J. Deutsch (Eds.). *Short Term Memory.* Academic Press, New York.

Gold, P. E. & Van Buskirk, R. B. (1975). Facilitation of time-dependent memory processes with posttrial epinephrine injections. *Behavioral Biology, 13,* 145-153.

Goldstein, M. L. (1974). The effect of amygdalectomy on long-term retention of an undertrained classically conditioned fear response. *Bulletin of Psychonomic Society, 4,* 548-550.

González, A. & Northcutt, R. G. (2009). An immunohistochemical approach to lungfish telencephalic organization. *Brain Behavior and Evolution, 74,* 43–55.

Goodson, J. L. & Bass, A. H. (2001). Social behavior functions and related anatomical characteristics of vasotocin/vasopressin systems in vertebrates. *Brain Research Reviews, 35,* 246-265

Grossman, S. P. (1972). The role of the amygdala in escape-avoidance situations. In: B. E. Eleftheriou (Ed.). *The Neurobiology of the Amygdala. Advances in Behavioral Biology, Volume* 2. Plenum Press, New York, pp. 537-551.

Grossman, S. P., Grossman, L. & Walsh, L. (1974). Functional organization of the rat amygdala with respect to avoidance behavior. *Journal of Comparative and Physiological Psychology,* 88, 829-850.

Hale, E. B. (1956). Effects of forebrain lesions on the aggressive behavior of green sunfish. *Lepomis cyanellus. Psysiological Zoology, 29,* 107-127.

Halgren, E. (1992). Emotional neurophysiology of the amigdala within the contex of human cognition. In: J. P. Aggleton (Ed.). *The Amygdala: Neurobiological Aspects of Emotion, Memory, and Mental Dysfunction.* Wiley-Liss, New York, pp. 191-228.

Handwerker, M., Gold, P. E. & MacGaugh, J. L. (1974). Effects of posttrial electrical stimulation of the amygdala on retention of an active avoidance response. *Brain Research, 75,* 324-327.

Hebb D. O. (1949). *The Organization of Behavior,* Wiley: New York.

Helmstetter, F. J. & Bellgowan, P. S. (1994). Effects of the muscimol applied to de basolateral amygdala in acquisition and expression of contextual fear conditioning in rats. *Behavioral Neuroscience, 108,* 1005-1009.

Helmstetter, F. J., Parsons, R. G. & Gafford, G. M. (2008). *Neurobiology of Learning of Memory, 89,* 324-337.

Herry, C., Ciocchi, S., Senn, V., Demmou, L., Müller, C. & Lüthi, A. (2008) Switching on and off fear by distinct neuronal circuits. *Nature, 454,* 600–606.

Herzog C. & Otto T. (1998). Contributions of anterior perirhinal cortex to olfactory and contextual fear conditioning. *Neuroreport, 9,* 1855–59.

Hicks, T. P. (1995). The role of glutamate receptor and its receptors in synaptic transmission. In: T. W. Stone (Ed.). *CNS Neurotransmitters and Neuromodulators: Glutamate.* CRS Press, Boca Raton, Florida, pp. 201-218.

Holzschneider, K. & Mulert, C. (2011) Neuroimaging in anxiety disorders. *Dialogues in Clinical Neuroscience, 13,* 453-461.

Hornby, P., Piekut, D. T. & Demski, L. S. (1987). Localization of immunoreactive tyrosine hydroxylase in the goldfish brain. *Journal of Comparative Neurology,* 261, 1-14.

Horvath, F. E. (1963). Effects of basolateral amygdalectomy on three types of avoidance behavior in cats. *Journal of Comparative and Physiologycal Psychology,* 56, 380-389.

Hunsaker MR & Kesner RP. (2008). Dissociations across the dorsal-ventral axis of CA3 and CA1 for encoding and retrieval of contextual and auditory-cued fear. *Neurobiology of Learning & Memory, 89,* 61-69.

Ikebuchi, M., Hasegawa, T. & Bischof, H. J. (2009). Amygdala and socio-sexual behavior in male zebra finches. *Brain, behavior and Evolution, 74,* 250-257.

Isaacson, R. I. (1976). Experimental brain lesions and memory. In: M. R. Rosenzweigand E. L. Bennet (Eds.). *Neural mechanisms of learning and memory.* The MIT Press, Cambridge, Massachusetts.

Ito, H., Murakami, T., Fukuoka, T. & Kishida, R. (1986), Thalamic fiber connections in a teleost (*Sebastiscus marmoratus*): Visual somatosensory, octavolateral, and cerebellar relay region to the telencephalon. *Journal of Comparative Neurology, 250,* 215–227.

Jarrel, T. W., Gentile, C. G. Romanski, L. M., McCabe, P. M. & Schneiderman, N. (1987). Involvement of cortical and thalamic auditory regions in retention of differential bradycardia conditioning to acoustic conditioned stimuli in rabits. *Brain Research, 412,* 285-294.

Jellestad, F. K. & Cabrera, I. C. (1986). Exploration and avoidance learning after ibotenic acid and radio-frequency lesions in the rat amygdala. *Behavioral and Neural Biology, 46,* 195-215.

Ji, J. & Maren, S. (2008). Lesions of the entorhinal cortex or fornix disrupt the context-dependence of fear extinction in rats. *Behavioral Brain Research, 194,* 201-6.

Johansen, J. P., Cain, C. K., Ostroff, L. E. & LeDoux,J. E. (2011). Molecular mechanism of fear learning and memory. *Cell, 28,* 509-524.

Kaada, B. R. (1972). Stimulation and regional ablation of the amygdaloid complex with reference to functional representations. In: B. E. Eleftheriou (Ed.). *The Neurobiology of the Amygdala. Advances in Behavioral Biology, Volume 2.* Plenum Press, New York, pp. 205-281.

Kamrin, R. P. & Aronson, L. R. (1954). The effects of forebrain lesions on mating behavior in the male platyfish, *Xiphophorus maculatus. Zoologica, 39,* 133-140.

Kapp, B. S., Pascoe, J. P. & Bixler, M. A. (1984). The amygdala: a neuroanatomical system approach to its contributions to aversive conditioning. In: N. Butlersand & L. R. Squire (Eds.). *Neuropsychology of Memory.* Guilford Press, New York, pp. 473-488.

Kapp, B. S., Whalen, P. J, Supple, W. F. & Pascoe, J. P. (1992). Amygdaloid contributions to conditioned arousal and sensory information processing. In: J. P. Aggleton (Ed.). *The amygdala: neurobiological aspects of emotion, memory, and mental dysfunction.* Wiley-Liss, New York, pp. 229-254.

Kapp, B. S.,Wilson, A. Pascoe, J. P. Supple, W. F. & Whalen, P. J. (1990). A neuroanatomical systems analysis of conditioned bradycardia in the rabits. In: M. Gabrieland & J. Moore (Eds.). *Learning and computational neuroscience: foundations of adaptative networks.* MIT Press, Cambridge, Massachussett, pp. 53-90.

Karamyan, A. I., Malukova, I. V. & Sergeev, B. F. (1967). Participation of the telencephalon of bony fish in the accomplishment of complex conditioned-reflex and general behavior reactions. In *Behavior and Reception in Fish.* Academy of Science, USSR, Moscow (translated by Bureau of Sport Fisheries and Wildlife, EEUU).

Kassel, J. & Davis, R. E. (1977). Recovery of function following simultaneous and serial telencephalon ablation. *Behavioral Biology, 21,* 489-499.

Kassel, J., Davis, R. E. & Schwagmeyer, P. (1976). Telencephalic lesions and behavior in the teleost *Macropodus opercularis*: further analysis of reproductive and operant behavior in the male. *Behavioral Biology, 18,* 179-188.

Keating, G. E., Kormann, S. & Horel, A. (1970). The behavioral effects of stimulating and ablating the reptilian amygdala. *Physiology and Behavior, 5,* 55-59.

Keene, C. S. & Bucci, D. J. (2008). Neurotoxic lesions of retrosplenial cortex disrupt signaled and unsignaled contextual fear conditioning. *Behavioral Neurosciences, 122,* 1070-7.

Kemble, E. D., Blanchard, D. C. & Blanchard, R. J. (1990). Effects of regional amygdaloid lesions of flight and defensive behaviors of wild black rats (*Rattus rattus*). *Physiology and Behavior, 48,* 1-5.

Kemble, E. D., Blanchard, D. C., Blanchard, R. J. & Takush, R. (1984). Taming in wild rats following medial amygdaloid lesions. *Physiology and Behavior, 32,* 131-134.

Kesner, R. P. (1982). Brain stimulation: Effects on memory. *Behavioral Brain Biology, 36,* 315-367.

Killcross, S., Robbins, T. W. & Everitt, B. J. (1997). Different types of fear-conditioned behaviour mediated by separate nuclei within amygdala. *Nature, 388,* 377-380.

Kim, M. J., Loucks, R. A., Palmer, A. L., Brown, A. C., Solomon, K. M., Marchante, A. N. & Whalen, P. J. (2011). The structural and finctional connectivity of the amygdala: From normal emotion to pathological anxiety. *Behavioural Brain Research, 223,* 403-410.

Kim, Y. S., Stumpf, W. E. & Sar, M. (1978). Topography of estrogen target cells in the forebrain of goldfish, *Carassius auratus. Journal of Comparative Neurology, 197,* 611-620.

Kling, A. J., Orbach, J., Schwartz, N. & Towne, J. (1960). Injury to the limbic system and associated structures in cats. *Archives of General Psychiatry, 3,* 391-340.

Kling, A. S. & Brothers, L. A. (1992). The Amygdala and Social Behavior. In: J. P. Aggleton (Ed.). *The amygdala: neurobiological aspects of emotion, memory, and mental dysfunction.* Wiley-Liss, New York, pp, 353-377.

Klüver, H. & Bucy, P. C. (1939). Preliminary analysis of the temporal lobes in monkeys. *Archives of Neurology and Psychiatry, 42,* 979-1000.

Krivanek, J. (1971). Facilitation of avoidance learning by pentylenetetrazol as a function of task difficulty, deprivation and shock level. *Psychopharmacologia, 20,* 213-229.

Krohmer, R. W. & Crews, D. (1987). Facilitation of courtship behavior in the male red-sided garter snake (*Thamnophis sirtalis parietalis*) following lesions of the septum or nucleus sphericus. *Physiology and Behavior, 40,* 759-765.

Kyle, A. L. & Peter, R. E. (1982). Effects of brain lesions on spawning behaviour in the male goldfish. *Physiology and Behavior, 28,* 1103-1109.

Kyle, A. L., Stacey, N. E. & Peter, R. E. (1982) Ventral telencephalic lesions: Effects on bisexual behavior, activity, and olfation in the male goldfish. *Behavioral and Neural Biology, 36,* 229-241.

Laviolette S. R., Lipski W. J. & Grace A. A. (2005). A subpopulation of neurons in the medial prefrontal cortex encodes emotional learning with burst and frequency codes through a dopamine D4 receptor-dependent basolateral amygdala input. *Journal of Neuroscience, 25,* 6066–75.

LeDoux, J. E. (1992). Brain mechanisms of emotion and emotional learning. *Current Opinion in Neurobiology, 2,* 191-198.

LeDoux, J. E. (1995). Emotions: Clues from the Brain. *Annual Review of Psychology, 46,* 209-235.

LeDoux, J. E. (2000). Emotion circuits in the brain. *Annual Review of Neuroscience, 23,* 155–184.

LeDoux, J. E. (2012) Rethinking the Emotional Brain. *Neuron, 73,* 653-676.

LeDoux, J. E., Sakaguchi, A., Iwata, J. & Reis, D. J. (1986). Interruption of projections from medial genicualte nuclesu mediate emotional responses conditioned by acoustic stimuli. *Journal of Neuroscience, 4,* 683-698.

Li, X. F., Stutzmann, G. E. & LeDoux, J. E. (1996). Convergent but temporally separated inputs to lateral amygdala neurons from the auditory thalamus and auditory cortex use different postsynaptic receptors: *in vivo* intracellular and extracellular recordings in fear conditioning pathways. *Learning and Memory, 3,* 229-242.

Liang, K. C., Bennett, C. & McGaugh, J. L. (1985). Peripheral epinephrine modualtes the effects of posttraining amygdala stimulation on memory. *Behavioral Brain Research, 15,* 93-100.

Liang, K. C. & McGaugh, J. L. (1983). Lesion of the stria terminalis attenuate the amnestic effect of amygdaloid stimulation on avoidance responses. *Brain Research, 274,* 309-318.

Liang, K. C., McGaugh, J. L., Martínez, J. L., Jensen, R. A., Vázquez, B. J. & Messing, R. B. (1982). Posttraining amygdaloid lesions impair retention of an inhibitory avoidance response. *Behavioral Brain Research, 4,* 237-249.

Lidsky, T. I., Levine, M. S., Kreinick, C. J. & Schwartz-Baum, J. (1970). Retrograde effects of amygdaloid stimulation on conditioned suppression (CER) in rats. *Journal of Comparative and Physiological Psychology, 73,* 135-149.

Lohman, A. H. M. & Smeets, W. J. A. J. (1990). The dorsal ventricular ridge and cortex of reptiles in historical and phylogenetic perspective. In B. L. Finlay, G. Innocenti & H. Scheich (Eds.). *The neocortex: ontogeny and phylogeny.* Plenum Press, New York, pp. 59-74.

Lowndes M. & Davies D. C. (1994). The effects of archistriatal lesions on one-trial passive-avoidance learning in the chick. *European Journal of Neuroscience, 6,* 525-530.

Lynch, G., Larson, J., Staubli, U. & Granger, R. (1991). Variants of synaptic potentiation and different types of memory operations in hippocampus and related structures. In: L. Squire, N. M. Weinberger, G. Lynchand & J. L. McGaugh (Eds.). *Memory: organization and locus of change.* Oxford University Press, New York, pp. 330-363.

Macphail, E. M. (1996). Cognitive function in mammals: the evolutionary perspective. *Cognitive Brain Research, 3,* 279-290.

Madison, D. V., Malenka, R. C. & Nicoll, R. A. (1991). Mechanisms underlying long-term potentiation of synaptic transmission. *Annual Review of Neuroscience, 14,* 379-397.

Magdaleno-Madrigal, V. M., Martinez-Vargas, D., Valdés-Cruz, A., Almazán-Alvarado, S. & Fernández-Mas, R. (2010). Preemptive effect of nucleus of the solitary tract stimulation on amygdaloid kindling in freely moving cats. *Epilepsia, 51,* 438-444.

Majchrzak, M., Ferry, B., Marchand, A. R., Herbeaux, K., Seillier, A. & Barbelivien A. (2006). Entorhinal cortex lesions disrupt fear conditioning to background context but spare fear conditioning to a tone in the rat. *Hippocampus 16,* 114–124.

Malenka, R. C. & Nicoll, R. A. (1993). NMDA-receptor-dependent synaptic plasticity: multiple forms and mechanisms. *Trends in Neurociences, 16,* 521-527.

Maren, S., Aharonov, G. & Fanselow, M. S. (1996). Retrograde abolition of conditional fear after excitotoxic lesions in the basolateral amygdala of rats: Absence of a temporal gradiente. *Behavioral Neuroscience, 110,* 718-726.

Maren, S. & Fanselow, M. S. (1995). Synaptic plasticity in the basolateral amygdala induced by hippocampal formation stimulation *in vivo. Journal of Neuroscience, 15,* 7548-7564.

Marino-Neto, J. & Sabbatini, R. M. (1983). Discrete telencephalic lesions accelerate the habituation rate of behavioral arousal responses in Siamese fighting fish (*Betta splendens*). *Brazilian Journal of Medical and Biological Research, 16,* 271-278.

Martínez-García, F., Novejarque, A. & Lanuza, E. (2007). Evolution of the amygdala in vertebrates. In: J. H. Kaas (Ed.) *Evolution of Nervous Systems, Vol. 2: The Evolution of Nervous Systems in Non-Mammalian Vertebrates.* Academic Press, Oxford, pp. 255-334.

Maser, J. D., Klara, J. W. & Gallup, G. G. (1973). Archistriatal lesions enhance tonic immobility in the chicken (*Gallus gallus*). *Physiology and Behavior, 11,* 729-733

McDonald, A. J. (1992). Cell types and intrinsic connections of the amygdala. In: Aggleton, J. P. (Ed). *The amygdala: Neurobiological aspects of emotion, memory and mental disfunctions.* Wiley-Liss, New York, pp. 67-96.

McDonough, J. H. & Kesner, R. P. (1971). Ammesia produced by brief electrical stimulation of the amygdala or dorsal hippocampus in cats. *Journal of Comparative and Physiological Psychology, 77,* 171-178.

McEntee, W. J. & Crook, T. H. (1993). Glutamate: its role in learning, memory and aging brain, *Psychopharmacology,* 111, 391-401.

McGaugh, J. L., Ferry, B., Vazdarjanova, A., & Roozendaal, B. (2000). Amygdala: Role in modulation of memory storage. In J. P. Aggleton (Ed.), *The amygdala.* Oxford University Press, London, England, pp. 391–423.

McGaugh, J. L. & Gold, P. E. (1974). The effects of drugs and electrical stimulation of the brain on memory storage processes. In: R. D. Myers & R. R. Drucker-Colin (Eds.). *Neurohumoral coding of brain function*. Plenum Press, New York, pp. 189-206.

McGaugh, J. L. & Gold, P. E. (1976). Modulation of memory by electrical stimulation of the brain. In: M. R. Rosenzweigand & E. L. Bennett (Eds.). *Neural mechanisms of learning and memory*. The MIT Press, Cambridge, Massachusetts.

McIntyre, M. & Stein, D. G. (1973). Differential effects of one- versus two-stage amygdaloid lesions on activity, exploration, and avoidance behavior in the albino rat. *Behavioral Biology*, 9, 451-465.

McKernan, M. G. & Shinnick-Gallagher, P. (1997). Fear conditioning induces a lasting potentiation of synaptic currents *in vitro*. *Nature, 390,* 607-611.

Medina, L., Bupesh, M. & Abellán, A. (2011). Contribution of genoarchitecture to understanding forebrain evolution and development, with particular emphasis on the amygdala. *Brain, Behavior and Evolution*, 3, 216-236.

Medina, L. & Reiner, A. (1995). Neurotransmitter organization and connectivity of the basal ganglia in vertebrates: implications for the evolution of basal ganglia. *Brain, Behavior and Evolution, 46,* 235-258.

Moreno, N. & González, A. (2006). The common organization of the amygdaloid complex in tetrapods: new concepts base don developmental, hodological ans neurochemical data in anuran amphibians. *Progress in neurobiology, 78,* 61-90.

Moreno, N. & González, A. (2007). Evolution of the amygdaloid complex in vertebrates, with special reference to the anamnio-amniotic transition. *Journal of Anatomy, 211,* 151-163.

Morgan, G. C. (1974a). The early development of the telencephalon of the marine catfish, *Galeichtys felis. Journal fur Hirnforsch, 15,* 427-447.

Morgan, G. C. (1974b). The late embryology and maturation of the telencephalon of the catfish, *Galeichtys felis. Journal fur Hirnforsch, 15,* 449-468.

Morris, R. G. M., Davis, S. & Butcher, S. P. (1989). The role of NMDA receptors in learning and memory. In: C. J. Watkinsand G. L. Collingridge (Eds.). *The NMDA receptor*. Oxford University Press, Oxford, IRL Pressand.

Mowrer, O. H. (1947). On the dual nature of learning: A reinterpretation of "conditionning"and "problem-solving". *Harvard Educational Review, 17,* 102-150.

Muller, J., Corodimas, K. P., Fridel, Z. & LeDoux, J. E. (1997). Functional inactivation of the lateral and basal nuclei of the amygdala by muscimol infusion prevents fear conditioning to a explicit conditioned stimulus and to contextual stimuli. *Behavioral Neuroscience, 111,* 683-691.

Murakami, T., Morita, Y. & Ito, H. (1983). Extrinsic and intrinsic fiber connections of the telencephalon in a teleost, *Sebasticus marmoratus. Journal of Comparative Neurology, 216,* 115-131.

Nadel, L. (2008). The Hippocampus and Context Revisited. In S. J. Y. Mizumori (Ed.). *Hippocampal place fields: relevance to learning and memory*. Oxford University Press, New York.

Neary, T. J. (1990). The pallium of anuran amphibians. En Jones, E. G. & Peters, A. (Eds). *Cerebral Cortex, Vol. 8A, Comparative Structure and Evolution of Cerebral Cortex,* Part I. Plenum Press, New York.

Neary, T. J. & Bruce, L. (1993). Comparisons of forebrain groups among tetrapods. *Society for Neuroscience Abstracs, 19,* 997.

Nieuwenhuys, R. & Verrijdt, P. W. Y. (1983). Structure and connections of the telencephalon of the teleostfish *Xenomystis nigri*. II. The area dorsalis. *Acta Morphologica Neerlandaise Scand., 21*:330

Noble, G. K. (1939). Neural basis of social behavior in vertebrates. *Collecting Net, 14,* 121-124.

Noble, G. K. & Borne, R. (1941). The effect of forebrain lesions on the sexual and fighting behavior of *Betta splendens* and other fishes. *Anatomical Record* (Suppl.), *79,* 49.

Northcutt, R. G. (1981). Localization of neurons afferent to the telencephalon in a primitive bony fish, *Polypterus palma. Neuroscience Letters, 22,* 219-222.

Northcutt RG (1995) The forebrain of gnathostomes: in search of a morphotype. *Brain Behavior and Evolution,* 46, 275-318.

Northcutt RG (2008), Forebrain evolution in bony fishes. *Brain Research Bulletin, 75,* 191-205.

Northcutt, R. G. & Braford, M. R. (1980). New observations on the organization and evolution of the telencephalon in actinopterygian fishes. In S. O. E. Ebbesson (Ed.) *Comparative neurology of the telencephalon.* Plenum Press, New York, pp: 41-98.

Northcutt, R. G. & Kicliter, E. (1980). Organization of the amphibian telencephalon. In: S. O. E. Ebbesson (Ed.). *Comparative Neurology of the Telencephalon.* Plenum Press, New York.

Oka, Y. (1980). The origin of the centrifugal fibers to the olfactory bulb in the goldfish, *Carassius auratus*: An experiment study using the fluorescent dye primuline as a retrograde tracer. *Brain Research, 185,* 215-225.

Olsson, A. & Phelps, E. A. (2007). Social Learning of fear. *Nature Neuroscience, 10,* 1095-1102

Ottersen, O. P. (1982). Connections of the amygdala of the rat. IV: corticoamygdaloid and intra- amygdaloid connections as studied with axonal transport of horseradish peroxidase. *Journal of Comparative Neurology, 205,* 30-48.

Overmier, J. B. & Gross, D. (1974). Effects of telencephalic ablation upon nest-building and avoidance behaviors in East African mouth breeding fish, *Tilapia mossambica. Behavioral Biology, 12,* 211-222.

Parent, A. (1986). *Comparative neurobiology of the basal ganglia.* Wiley. New York.

Parent, A. L., Dubé, M. R., Braford, M. R. & Northcutt, R. G. (1978). The organization of monoamine-containing neurons in the brain of the sunfish (*Lepomis gibbosus*) as revealed by fluorescence microscopy. *Journal of Comparative Neurology, 182,* 495-516.

Parent, M. B., & McGaugh, J. L. (1994). Posttraining infusion of lidocaine into the amygdala basolateral complex impairs retention of inhibitory avoidance training. *Brain Research, 661,* 97–103.

Parkes, S. L. & Westbrook, F. (2011). Role of the basolateral amygdala and NMDA receptors in higher-order conditioned fear. *Review of Neurocience, 22,* 317-333.

Parsons T. C. & Otto T. (2008). Temporary inactivation of dorsal hippocampus attenuates explicitly nonspatial, unimodal, contextual fear conditioning. *Neurobiology of Learning & Memory, 90,* 261–68.

Pellegrino, L. (1968). Amygdaloid lesions and behavioral inhibition in the rat. *Journal of Comparative and Physiological Psychology*, 65, 483-491.

Pessoa, L. & Adolphs, R. (2010). Emotion processing and the amygdala: from a 'low road' to a 'many roads' of evaluating biological significance. *Nature Reviews Neuroscience, 11,* 773-782.

Phelps, E. A. & Anderson, A. K. (1997). Emotional memory: What does the amygdala do? *Current Biology, 7,* R311-R314.

Phelps, E. A. & LeDoux, J. E. (2005) Contributions of the amygdala to emotion processing : From animal models to human behavior. *Neuron, 48,* 175-187.

Phillips, R. E. (1964). "Wildness" in the mallard duck: effects of brain lesions and stimulation on "escape behavior" and reproduction. *Journal of Comparative Neurology, 122,* 139-155.

Phillips, R. E. (1968). Approach-withdrawal behavior of peach-faced lovebirds, *Agapornis roseicolis,* and its modification by brain lesions. *Behaviour, 31,* 163-184.

Phillips, R. G. & LeDoux, J. E. (1992). Differential contribution of amygdala and hippocampus to cued and contextual fear conditioning. *Behavioral Neuroscience, 106,* 274-85.

Phillips, R. E. & Youngren, O. M. (1968). Unilateral kainic acid lesions reveal dominance of right archistriatum in avian fear behavior. *Brain Research, 377,* 216-220.

Piñuela, C. & Northcutt, R. G. (1994). Immunohistochemical organization of the forebrain in the white sturgeon. Society for Neuroscience Abstracs, 20, 997.

Pitkänen A, & Amaral DG. (1991). Demonstration of projections from the lateral nucleus to the basal nucleus of the amygdala: a PHA-L study in the monkey. *Experimental Brain Research, 83,* 465-70.

Pitkänen, A., Savander, V. & LeDoux, J. E. (1997) Organization of intra-amygdaloid circuitries in the rat: an emerging framework for understanding functions of the amygdala. *Trends in Neurosciences, 20I,* 517-523.

Pitkänen, A., Stefanacci, L., Farb, C. R., Go, G-G., LeDoux, J. E. & Amaral, D. G. (1995). Intrinsic connections of the rat amygdaloid complex: Projections originating in the basal nucleus. *Journal of Comparative Neurology, 356,* 288-310.

Portavella, M. Torres, B. & Salas, C (2004a) Avoidance response in goldfish: emotional and temporal involvement of medial and lateral telencephalic pallium. *The Journal of Neuroscience 24,* 2335-2342

Portavella, M., Torres, B., Salas, C. & Papini, M. R (2004b). Lesions of the medial pallium, but not of the lateral pallium, disrupt spaced-trial avoidance learning in goldfish (*Carassius Auratus*). *Neuroscience Letters, 362,* 75-78.

Portavella, M. & Vargas, JP. (2005). Emotional and spatial learning in goldfish is dependent on different telencephalic pallial systems. *European Journal of Neuroscience, 21,* 2800-2806.

Portavella, M., Vargas, JP., Torres, B. & Salas, C. (2002) The effects of telencephalic pallial lesions on spatial, temporal, and emotional learning in goldfish. *Brain Research Bulletin, 57,* 397-399.

Price, J. L. & Amaral, D. G. (1981). An autoradiographic study of the projections of the central nucleus of the monkey amygdala. *Journal of Neuroscience, 1,* 1242-1259.

Quintero E, Díaz E, Vargas JP, de la Casa LG & Lopez JC. (2011). Ventral subiculum involvement in latent inhibition context specificity. *Physiology and Behavior, 102,* 414-420.

Rabinak, C. A. & Maren, S. (2008). Associative structure of fear memory after basolateral amygdala lesions in rats. *Behavioral Neuroscience, 122,* 1284-94.

Reiner, A. & Northcutt, R. G. (1992). An immunohistochemical study of the telencephalon of the Senegal bichir (*Polypterus senegalus*). *Journal of Comparative Neurology, 319,* 359-386.

Ribbink, A. J. (1972). The behaviour and brain function of the cichild fish *Hemihaplochromis philander*. *Zoologica. Africanis, 7,* 21-41.

Richardson, R., Tronson, N., Bailey, G. K. & Parnas, A. S. (2002). Extinction of conditioned odor potentiation of startle. *Neurobiology of Learning & Memory, 78,* 426–440.

Riolobos, A. S. & Garcia, A. I. M. (1987). Open field activity and passive avoidance responses in rats after lesions of the central amygdaloid nucleus by electrocoagulation or ibotenic acid. *Physiology and Behavior, 39,* 715-720.

Rogan, M. T. & LeDoux, J. E. (1995). LTP is accompanied by commensurate enhancement of auditory-evoked responses in fear conditioning circuit. *Neuron, 15,* 127-136.

Rogan, M. T., Stäubli, U. V. & LeDoux, J. E. (1997). Fear conditioning induces associative long-term potentiation in the amygdala. *Nature,* 390, 604-607.

Roozendaal, B., Koolhaas, J. M. & Bohus, B. (1993). The central amygdala is involved in conditioning but not in retention of active and passive shock avoidance in male rats. *Behavioral and Neural Biology, 59,* 143-149.

Roozendaal, B., McEween, B. S. & Chattarji, S. (2009). Stress, memory and the amygdala. *Nature reviews, 10,* 423-430.

Roozendaal, B., van der Zee, E. A., Hensbroek, R. A., Maat, H. Luiten, P. G., Koolhaas, J. M. & Bohus, B. (1997). Muscarinic acetylcholine receptor immunoreactivity in the amygdala I. Fear-induced plasticity. *Neuroscience, 76,* 75-83.

Rosen, J. B. (2004). The neurobiology of conditiones and unconditioned fear: a neurobehavioral system analysis of the amygdala. *Behavioral and Cognitive Neuroscience Reviews, 3,* 23-41.

Rosenkranz J. A. & Grace A. A. (2002). Dopamine-mediated modulation of odour-evoked amygdala potentials during pavlovian conditioning. *Nature, 417,* 282–87.

Russchen, F. T., Amaral, D. G. & Price, J. L. (1985). The afferent connections of the substantia innominata in the monkey, *Macaca fascicularis*. *Journal of Comparative Neurology, 242,* 1-27.

Sabatinelli, D., Fortune, E. L., Li, Q., Siddiqui, A. P., Krafft, C., Oliver, W., Beck, S., & Khublai, J. (2011). Emotional perception: Meta-analyses of face and natural scene processing. *NeuroImage, 54,* 2524-2533.

Sah, P., Faber, E. S. L, Lopez de Armentia, M. & Power, J. (2003). The Amygdaloid Complex: Anatomy and Physiology. *Physiological Reviews, 83,* 803-834.

Sah, P., Westbrook, R. F. & Lüthi, A. (2008). Fear conditioning and long-term potentiation in the amygdala. *Annals of New York Academy of Sciences, 1129,* 88-95.

Sánchez-Riolobos, A. (1986). Differential effect of chemical lesion and electrocoagualtion of the central amygdaloid nucleus on active avoidance responses. *Physiology and Behavior, 36,* 441-444.

Savage, G. E. (1971). Behavioural effects of electrical stimulation of the telencephalon of the goldfish, *Carassius auratus. Animal Behaviour, 19,* 661-668.

Savander, V., Go, C. G., LeDoux, J. E. & Pitkänen, A. (1995). Intrinsic connections of the rat amygdaloid complex: projections originating in the accessory basal nucleus. *Journal of Comparative Neurology, 374,* 291-313.

Scalia, F. & Ebbesson, S. O. E. (1971). The central projections of the olfactory bulb in a teleost, (*Gymnothorax funebris*). *Brain, Behavior & Evolution, 4,* 376-399.

Schneider,AM., Wilkins,E., Firestone,A., Everbach, EC., Naylor, JC. & Simson, PE. (2003). Enhanced retention in the passive-avoidance task by 5-HT1A receptor blockade is not associated with increased activity of the central nucleus of the amygdala. *Learning & Memory, 10,* 394-400.

Schuhmacher, A., Mössner, R., Jessen, F., Scheef, L., Block, W., Belloche, A. C., Lennerts, L., Welper, H., Höfels, S., Pfeiffer, U., Wagner, M., Maier, W., Schwab, S. & Zobel, A. (2012). Association of amygdala volumes with cortisol secretion in unipolar depressed patients. *Psychiatry research, 31,* 96-103.

Segaar, J. (1961). Telencephalon and behavior in *Gasterosteus aculeatus. Behaviour, 18,* 256-287.

Segaar, J. (1965). Behavioural aspects of degeneration and regeneration in fish brain: A comparison with higher vertebrates. *Progress in Brain Research, 14,*143-231.

Segaar, J. & Nieywenhuys, R. (1963). New etho-physiological experiments with male *Gasterosteus aculeatus,* with anatomical comment. *Animal Behaviour, 11,* 331-344.

Selden, N. RW., Everitt, B. J., Jarrad, L. E. & Robbins, T. W. (1991). Complementary roles for the amygdala and hippocampus in aversive conditioning to explicit and contextual cues. *Neuroscience, 42,* 335-350.

Seymour, B., Dolan, R. (2008). Emotion, decision making, and the amygdala. *Neuron, 58,* 662-671.

Smeets, W. J. (1990). In E. G. Jones & A. Peters (Eds.). *Comparative Structure and Evolution of Cerebral Cortex*. Plenum Press.

Striedter, G. F. (1991). Auditory, electrosensory and mechanosensory lateral line pathways through the forebrain of channel catfishes. *Journal of Comparative Neurology, 312,* 311-331.

Striedter, G. F. (1997). The telencephalon of tetrapods in evolution. *Brain Behavior and Evolution, 49,* 179-213.

Takashina, K., Saito, H. & Nishiyama, N. (1995). Preferential of avoidance performances in amygdala-lesioned mice. *Japanish Journal of Pharmacology, 67,* 107-115.

Tarr, R. S. (1977). Role of the amygdala in the intraspecies aggressive behavior of the iguana lizard, *Sceloporus occidentalis. Physiology and Behavior, 18,* 1153-1158.

Thatcher, R. W. & Kimble, D. P. (1966). Effect of amygdaloid lesions on retention of an avoidance response in overtrained and nonovertrained rats. *Psychonomic Science, 6,* 9-10.

The Avian Brain Nomenclature Consortium (2005). *Nature Review Neuroscience, 6(2),* 151-159

Traverso, L. M., Quintero, E., Vargas, J. P., De la Casa, L. G. & López, J. C. (2010). Taste memory trace disruption by AP5 administration in basolateral amygdala. *Neuroreport, 21,* 99-103.

Ursin, H. (1965). Effect of amygdaloid lesions on avoidance behavior and vision discrimination in cats. *Experimental Neurology, 11,* 298-317.

Ursin, H., Jellestad, F. & Cabrera, I. G. (1981). The amygdala, exploration and fear. In: Y. Ben-Ari (Ed.). *The Amigdaloid Complex.* Elsevier, Amsterdam, pp. 317-329.

van der Gaag, C., Minderaa, R. B. & Keysers, C. (2007) The BOLD signal in the amygdala does not differentiate between dynamic facial expressions. *Social Cognitive and Affective Neuroscience, 2,* 93-103.

van der Zee, E. A., Roozendaal, B., Bohus, B., Koolhaas, J. M. & Luiten, P. G. (1997). Muscarinic acetylcholine receptor immunoreactivity in the amygdala I. Cellular distribution correlated with fear-induced behavior. *Neuroscience, 76,* 63-73.

Vargas, J. P., Lopez, J. C. Portavella, M. (2009). What are the functions of fish brain pallium? *Brain Research Bulletin, 79,* 436-440

Vowles, D. M. & Beasley, L. D. (1974). The neural substrate of emotional behavior in birds. In: I. J. Goodmanand & M. W. Schein (Eds.). *Birds: Brain and Behavior.* Academic Press, New York.

Walker D. L., Paschall G. Y. & Davis M. (2005). Glutamate receptor antagonist infusions into the basolateral and medial amygdala reveal differential contributions to olfactory vs context fear conditioning and expression. *Learning & Memory, 12,* 120–29.

Werka, T., Skar, J. & Ursin, H. (1978). Exploration and avoidance in rats with lesions in amygdala and piriform cortex. *Journal of Comparative and Physiological Psychology, 92,* 672-681.

Whalen, P. J. (1999) Fear, vigilance, and ambiguity: initial neuroimaging studies of the human amygdala. *Current Directions in Psychological Science, 7,* 177-187.

Wiersma, A., Konsman, J. P., Knollema, S., Bohus, B. & Koolhaas, J. M. (1998). Differential effects of CHR infusion into the cetral nucleus of the amygdala in the Roman high-avoidance and low-avoidance rats. *Psychoneuroendocrinology, 23,* 261-274.

Wilensky, A. E., Schafe, G. E., Kristensen, M. P., & LeDoux, J. E. (2006). Rethinking the fear circuit: the central nucleus of the amygdala is required for the acquisition, consolidation, and expression of Pavlovian fear conditioning. *Journal of Neuroscience, 26,* 12387–12396.

Wilensky, A. E., Schafe, G. E., & LeDoux, J. E. (2000). The amygdala modulates memory consolidation of fear-motivated inhibitory avoidance learning but not classical fear conditioning. *Journal of Neuroscience, 20,* 7059–7066.

Wiltgen, B. J., Sanders, M. J., Anagnostaras, S. G., Sage, J. R. & Fanselow M. S. (2006). Context fear learning in the absence of the hippocampus. *Journal of Neuroscience, 26,* 5484-91.

Witkins, J. M. (1995). Role of NMDA receptors in behavior and behavioral effects of drugs. In: T. W. Stone (Ed.). *CNS Neurotransmitters and Neuromodulators: Glutamate.* CRS Press, Boca Raton, Florida, pp, 323-350.

Wulliman, M. F & Rink, E. (2002). The teleostean forebrain: A comparative and developmental view based on early proliferation, *Pax6* activity and catecholaminergic organization. *Brain Research Bulletin, 57,* 363-370.

Zeier, H. (1971). Archistriatal lesions and response inhibition in the pigeon. *Brain Research, 31,* 327-339.

Zeier, H. & Karten, H. J. (1971). The archistriatum of the pigeon: Organization of afferent and efferent connections. *Brain Research, 31*, 313-326.

Zhuikov, AY, Couvillon, PA & Bitterman, ME. (1994). Quantitative two-process analysis of avoidance conditioning in goldfish. *Journal of Experimental Psychology: Animal Behaviour Processes, 20*, 32-43.

Chapter 2

Neuroimaging of the Amygdala: Quantitative Mechanistic Approach

Miguel Ángel Bertoni

Additional information is available at the end of the chapter

1. Introduction

Radiology has evolved fantastically since the discovery of X-rays on 8th November 1989, when William Roentgen amazed the world with a new source of energy, the X rays, capable of penetrating opaque matter making it transparent to non-invasive observation.

Radiology Imaging has counted with constantly improving technology that boosted this great evolution, not only because of science but also due to the influence of strong economic components operating in health and biology sciences, probably considering the massiveness of potential applicability and its vast and always growing field of action.

Neuroimaging technology has been part of these changes increasing its potential more dramatically in the last decades; everything indicates these continuous improvements will not decrease. Little did we know two decades ago that we would be able to assess in the same exam, in a totally non-invasive manner, morphology, biochemistry and function of the Central Nervous System with the degree of accuracy, detail and image quality we can in fact obtain nowadays. Constantly evolving technology will help us to do it even better, faster, and with a much more exquisite level of detail, allowing us to reach our challenge of generalization and reproducibility of findings that patients deserve, science pursues and we expect.

Since the very beginning radiology imaging has mostly been a qualitative visual based discipline capable of studying opaque matter, internal structures, otherwise not observable in a non-invasive manner. It has helped scientists, clinicians and technicians to know more about the human body in general and the central nervous system in particular, interfering less with the studied object, by means of a diversity of devices, producing images of remarkable quality.

Radiology has demonstrated to be an excellent qualitative tool to assess the central nervous system's normal features. However and since not long ago, it has started a firm transformation from being a mere qualitative observation technique to become a precise quantitative discipline, at present able to study volume changes throughout time, with an excellent level of precision, capable of registering physiology-induced image variations, which lead to become a mechanistic specialty.

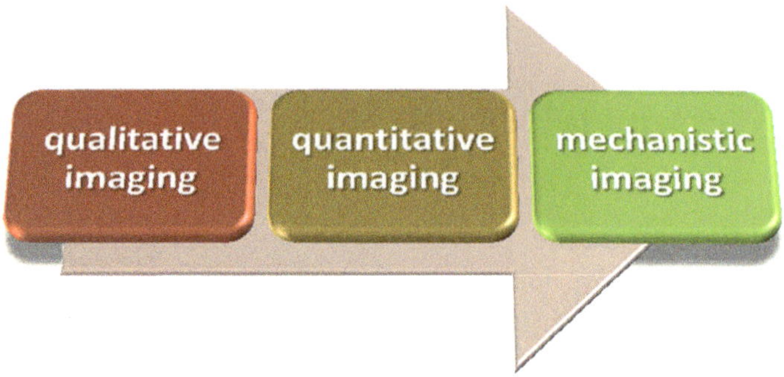

Figure 1. Paradigm shift in Brain Imaging

Imaging improvements have been dramatic in the last few years during which a paradigm shift has taken place, evolving from not only obtaining good images of the central nervous system but also accurately identifying precise boundaries of brain tissue, quantifying its volume, assessing neural connections, feeding vessels, hemodynamics, perfusion parameters, molecular and biochemical properties, and CNS functions, becoming mechanistic radiology [Fig 1] (Buckler, et al. 2011).

The changes leading to mechanistic imaging are also referred to as functional or molecular imaging. The new paradigm of quantification is reshaping the qualitative picture taking model of imaging in use until not long ago, by adopting concrete measurement-making processes not only in research but also in usual clinical practice.

In recent years, reputed authors in the field of radiology formally commenced a robust discipline of quantification in diagnostic imaging, formerly used to assess quality more or less vaguely –or with less reproducibility and precision- now named Quantitative Radiology, in all possible radiology imaging modalities, although more emphatically in computed tomography (qCT) and magnetic resonance imaging (qMRI). The latter, quantitative Magnetic Resonance Imaging (qMRI), is the modality of choice to image the amygdala. The amygdala, or *corpus amygdaloideum* in Latin, from Greek "almond", is a large nuclear complex situated in the dorsomedial portion of the temporal lobe adjacent to and richly connected with the hippocampus. Both form an essential part of the Limbic System (Nieuwenhuys et al 1988). The functions of the amygdala appear related to emotions and modulation of stimuli interpretation, also intervening in mood modulation. The limbic system regulates a number of essential behaviors controlling appropriate responses to stimuli with social, emotional or motivational relevance (Sokolowski and Corbin 2012). qMRI techniques permit to demonstrate cross sections and volumes, boundaries, signal intensity characteristics, topography, in vivo biochemical properties of neural tissue, connections, biochemistry and functionality of this important grey structure in the limbic system (Nieuwenhuys, Voogd and van Huijzen 1988) [Fig 2].

Magnetic resonance is the procedure of choice to image the amygdala and the remainder of the limbic system (Hirai, et al. 2000). Computed Tomography (CT) can be used to study the limbic system although to a lesser extent; besides, its grey-white matter dissociation is not has high as in MRI while it delivers ionizing radiation, to be avoided if possible, due to its biological effects. Extra consideration should be given to the administration of iodinated contrast material to enhance grey matter on CT since it has deleterious effects over the kidneys (Klatzberg and Barrett 2007).

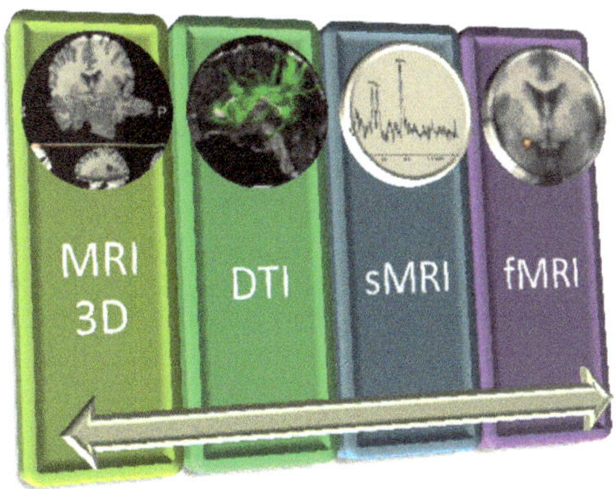

Figure 2. Usual possibilities of interrogating the subject with MR in neuroimaging the amygdala

Neuro imaging techniques to demonstrate the amygdala morphologically are therefore mainly and almost exclusively based on magnetic resonance imaging (MRI), capable of rendering a detailed neurostructural analysis, and also to assess neural connectivity, in vivo biochemical properties and functionality at a synchronous moment without moving the studied subject from the same imaging modality unit in which the exam is being performed. MRI also provides the essential capability of an excellent spatial (Jacobs, Ibrahim and Ouwerkerk 2007) and temporal resolution (Li, et al. 2002), remarkably important for mechanistic imaging. Other procedures based on nuclear medicine principles are single proton emission computed tomography or SPECT, positron emission tomography or PET (Karow, et al. 2010), the combination of PET with computed tomography, PET-CT, and magnetic resonance imaging or PET-MRI. The last ones are obtained in units capable of carrying out both modalities simultaneously, fusing images with a high degree of accuracy, reliability and reproducibility (Judenhofer, et al. 2007). However, temporal resolution remains as an essential element to be considered, being the capability to register stimuli in rapid succession, which is not doable with nuclear medicine technologies (Ranger, et al. 2007). The latter registers metabolic activity from a known amount of radiotracer administered to the subject before the exam. The nervous tissue is avid of glucose, its main feeding metabolite. If it is marked with a radiotracer, neural tissue becomes visible in direct proportion to its metabolic activity. Although signal fades with time, its rate is not as fast as needed in an adequate stimulus-response model. Given the temporal resolution drawback of nuclear medicine studies, functional exams are performed in a magnetoencephalography (MEG) or functional MRI (fMRI) unit.

Magnetoencepahlography (MEG) has an exquisite temporal resolution and a very good signal localization into space although needs to be fused to MRI obtained structural study to increase spatial resolution to the required level. Therefore an MRI must be obtained immediately before or after MEG, with appropriate skin markings to be untouched throughout both procedures. These skin markers will be essential to successfully fuse structural images from MRI to signal from MEG permitting a unified visual impression (Qingmao, et al. 2008).

MRI of the amygdala can be satisfactorily done at a variety of magnetic field strengths obtaining very good quality images from units with a magnetic field strength from 0.5, 1 to 1.5 Tesla (Maubon, et al. 1999). Although an important number of clinicians and researchers continue working at 1.5 Tesla (Korvenoja, et al. 2006), there is an increasing tendency to study subjects under 3 Tesla units (Spampinatto, et al. 2011), 7 Tesla and 9.3 Tesla in clinical settings. Preliminary results seem to suggest that ultra high field strength MR units will be able not only to improve signal to noise even more dramatically but also to obtain MR spectra from other elements as sodium, an apparent excellent marker of conditions as Alzheimer's type cognitive impairment years before the clinical onset, abnormality already proven to be detectable in brain tumors (Ouwerkerk, et al. 2003).

The amount of available signal in conventional magnetic resonance imaging (MRI) is inextricably tied to the static magnetic field strength (B_0) of the imaging system. Until recently, most clinical MRI scanners operated at field strengths at or below 1.5 Tesla, however, due in part to improvements in magnet design and shielding which ease siting requirements, 3 Tesla clinical scanners are now widely available and there is a push for even higher field whole body scanners (7- 11 Tesla) throughout the industry.

Single proton computed tomography (SPECT) and Positron emission tomography (PET) are nuclear medicine studies capable of rendering excellent functional images. However, the spatial and temporal resolution of both methods are not the best to assess the amygdala although in selected cases, as in mesial temporal sclerosis and other refractory seizure disorders, PET fused with CT may be of help. PET-MRI units are ready to enter the clinical field having passed several processes of assessment by selected centers and clinical researchers however not yet available to the vast majority of researchers, neuroscientists or clinical specialists.

2. MRI acquisition protocol

MRI acquisition protocol must be suitable to the purposes of the undertaken research. It varies whether it intends to be mainly structural, functional, combined or including aspects such as tissue biochemistry and connectivity.

Series	Description	Purpose
1	Ax T2	Neurostructural, pathology
2	Ax SPGR T1	Neurostructural
3	Ax GE	Susceptibility effect
4	Ax FLAIR	Water linked to macromolecules
5	Ax DWI >16 directions	Tractography
6	sMRI	Biochemistry
7	fMRI	Steady state and post stimuli

Table 1. General purpose MRI protocol. It may take 45-60 min depending on the MR unit, magnetic field strength, gradients, coils, software, sequences, operator and used paradigms for functional series (MRI: magnetic resonance imaging; Ax T1 3D: axial series T1 weighted 3 Dimensional; Ax T2. GE and FLAIR: axial series T2 weigthed, Gradient Echo T2 weighted, Fluid Attenuation Inversion Recovery; DWI>16 dir: Diffusion Weighted Images acquiring in sixteen directions or more; sMRI: spectroscopy MRI; fMRI: functional MRI)

The acquisition protocol concerning the amygdala and rest of the limbic system may be intended for pure anatomical evaluations including the assessment of intra and intercellular diffusion of water molecules, tissue biochemistry or tissue functionality. A standard protocol covering all aspects [Table 1] usually takes between 45 and 60 minutes, depending on factors such as magnetic field strength, gradients, receiver coils, software, pulse sequences, operator and used paradigms to assess functionality. Considering an initial adequate positioning and if the subject is beforehand explained as satisfactorily as possible about the study, the importance of being still throughout and clearly what he/she is expected to do during the delivery of stimuli in fMRI sequence, an acquisition study following the protocol mentioned in Table 1 would take approximately 75 minutes in a 1.5T and 60 minutes in a 3T unit.

It is crucial to discuss important aspects of the acquisition since results may vary significantly if they are neither strictly observed nor kept in mind at all times leading to potential error.

There are several important image parameters to assess quality being the most relevant magnetic field strength and Signal to Noise ratio, Contrast to Noise ratio, Modulation Transfer Factor, slice thickness and acquisition matrix.

The magnetic field strength is very important, influencing all of the others. Signal to noise ratio reflects signal intensity capable of forming image. It is considered a crucial parameter regarding image quality, although not the only one (Jacobs, Ibrahim and Ouwerkerk 2007). Contrast to noise ratio, type of coils, patient immobility, adequate positioning to minimize motion artifacts and pre saturation pulses to decrease artifacts from blood flowing from the heart with high kinetic energy are also relevant factors contributing to image quality (Brown and Semelka 1999). Other crucial factor to be kept in mind is the intrinsic noise of the system in use, quantitatively expressed by the Modulation Transfer Function or MTF (Ranger, et al. 2007). It is a ratio between existing and registered information, which by definition ranges between 0.99 and 0.01 being 1 the ideal and 0.01 the worst.

All of these factors affect the correct MRI assessment of amygdala's structure, connectivity, biochemistry and function. Neuroimaging of the limbic system as a whole or its components has usually a well-defined purpose, which helps to define the suitable study protocol.

Volume acquisitions are typically gradient echo sequences (GE) T1, Proton Density or T2 weighted images, prescribed in just one anatomical plane of axial, sagittal or coronal contiguous slices forming a volume composed by identical isovolumetric voxels usually ranging from 0.5 to 1 mm^3. If appropriate settings and algorithms are selected, high quality T1, Proton Density or T2 weighted images are obtained in 3 to 7 minutes, time that varies according to the MR unit, make, model and radiographer in charge, among other factors. The subject positioning and cooperation throughout the acquisition provide an additional quality factor. During the acquisition a *k*-space filling takes place, consistent in the initial data collection of each series to be used for reconstructing of the images. Its center represents image contrast while its periphery represents image anatomy. The *k*-space is an MRI concept naming where data forming the MR images are collected, in which morphology and contrast do not necessarily coincide in the same or adjacent point. As a practical consequence, if the subject moves near the end of the series, contrast may not be that affected as form. The subject must be still throughout the acquisition; the less motion affects scanned volume, the higher its imaging properties will be. These concepts are to be kept in mind by the research team especially to validate results testing consistency. Isovoxel based morphometry (IVBM), the technique used for manual, semi automated or fully automated segmentation, is based on signal intensity differences from voxels forming the volume. Therefore image quality factors influencing signal need to be thoroughly checked, mainly although not exclusively Modulation transfer factor (MTF), signal to noise ratio (SNR) and contrast to noise ratio (CNR).

The most common and useful series concerning neurostructural analysis are Gradient Echo T1 weighted series (with a narrow flip angle typically less than 20º). As other gradient echo sequences, they show high signal intensity (bright) within rapid flow vessels as carotid siphons, elements of the Circle of Willis and –usually- the initial segments of both mid cerebral arteries (MCAs). Grey-white matter differentiation is usually of remarkable high quality, suitable for post processing (Bertoni 1998; Bertoni 2010).

3. Assessing connectivity: MR tractography

Diffusion tensor images (DTI) obtained from diffusion-weighted images in at least 16 directions are usually a minimum requirement for a satisfactory tractography (N. Ratnarajah, A. Simmons, et al. 2012) capable of rendering 3D images of intra cerebral tracts with the quality of an atlas, a very useful initial approach to assess the whole neurostructure following techniques already described [Fig 4] (Catani 2008). For the limbic system, particularly the amygdala, the circuit of Papez is an important element to work on (Chan 1997, Kwon 2010), for which high resolution source diffusion weighted images (DWI) series are required as the source to post process, preferably in at least 64 directions (Ratnarajah 2011).

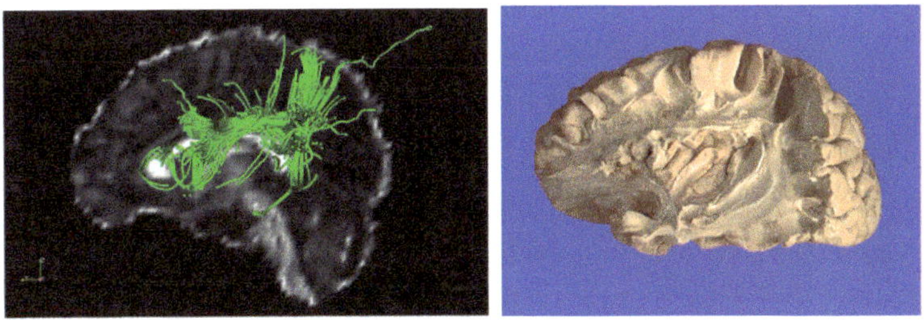

Figure 3. Demonstration of the arcuate fasciculus with DTI following Cattani's atlas technique for virtual dissection and Hojjatoleslami-Nagulan dual tensor technique to depict the tracts

Techniques vary according to the software in use and source images. Double tensor methods tend to provide useful tractography when compared with in vitro dissections (N. Ratnarajah, A. Simmons, et al., Residual bootstrapping on classified tensor morphologies 2011). Again, careful comparison of source images is crucial. It must be remembered that good source images should have enough number of directions and enough resolution, besides all the other essential factors mentioned before concerning image quality. These sets of will be several and composed by hundreds of images whose format source is DICOM, standing for Digital Imaging and Communications in Medicine, the accepted convention protocol to store and interact with medical images, containing not only the image but all the relevant subject and institutional identity, acquisition parameters and other relevant information concerning the procedure. Conversion from DICOM must be carried out carefully, especially when renaming the source images. Some software programs require standardization before running a tractography depiction. Newer MR units offer separate workstations including tractography-rendering software. However, some researchers prefer to carry them out under the same software program for all steps a mechanistic approach implies, to be able to fuse different post processing sets of images in a more flexible manner. Better results are usually obtained with dual tensor algorithms of reconstruction to carry out in vivo dissections like those already performed as in vivo dissections to form atlases of brain tractography (Catani and Thiebau de Schotten 2008).

4. Assessing biochemistry: MR spectroscopy (sMR)

Magnetic Resonance Spectroscopy, MRS or sMR, provides a measure of neural tissue chemistry. Resonance takes place by setting precession frequencies with hydrogen (^{1}H proton), sodium (^{23}Na) or phosphorus (^{31}P) for *in vivo* studies in human medicine. Hydrogen spectroscopy is the widest in use, easiest to perform with a much higher signal-to-noise ratio than the other two elements.

Metabolite	Indicates	ppm
Lipids	Brain catabolism	0.8 – 1.3
Lactate	Anaerobic glycolysis	1.3
NAA	Neuronal marker	2.0
Glutamine/GABA	Neurotransmitters	2.2 – 2.4
Creatine	Energy metabolism	3.0
Choline	Cell membrane	3.2
***myo*-Inositol**	Glial-cell marker	3.5
glucose	Intermediate metabolism	3.4 / 3.8

Table 2. Elements usually detected on spectroscopy MR of the brain, what they indicate and their concentration in parts per million

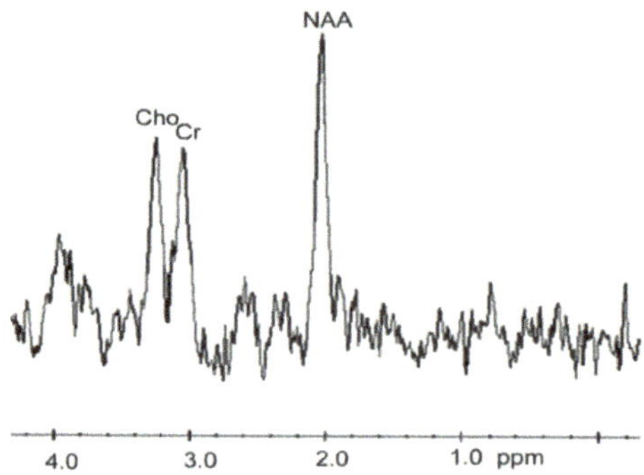

Figure 4. MR normal brain spectrum (Andre, et al. 2006)

In vivo spectroscopy can be performed in the range of 10 to 15 minutes being part as a usual MR protocol to study the brain. It can be used to determine and to monitor biochemical changes in normal brain and pathological conditions whether they are congenital, inflammatory, degenerative, neoplastic or even miscellaneous. MR spectra do not label diagnoses but must be interpreted within the appropriate clinical context, in the light of other neurostructural and functional findings.

sMRI implies measuring spectra in multiple voxels throughout the brain (multivoxel automated technique) or performing in selected areas always measuring the contralateral mirror area, as a manual technique. In the case of the amygdala, as for other components of the limbic system and considering their anatomy, the latter seems to be more convenient and reliable sMRI (Agarwal, et al. 2010), of increasing use in psychiatry.

Usually found peaks mark metabolites as lipids, lactate, N-acetyl aspartate, glutamine-gamma amino butyric acid, creatine, choline and *myo*-inositol. They tend to correlate or indicate brain destruction or catabolism, anaerobic glycolysis, neuronal tissue marker, neurotransmission, energy metabolism, cell membrane marker and glial cell marker, respectively (Smith, Smirniotopoulos and Rushing 2008).

The medial temporal lobe structures tends to show high levels of choline, presumably reflecting different cellular compositions between allocortex and neocortex (Arslanoglu, et al. 2004)

5. Assessing functionality: fMRI, MEG, SPECT, PET

Main neuroimaging MR techniques to assess in vivo functionality of neural structures are Magnetoencephalography or MEG, and functional MRI (fMRI), the latter within the acquisition protocol already described intended to study both, morphology and function [Fig 5].

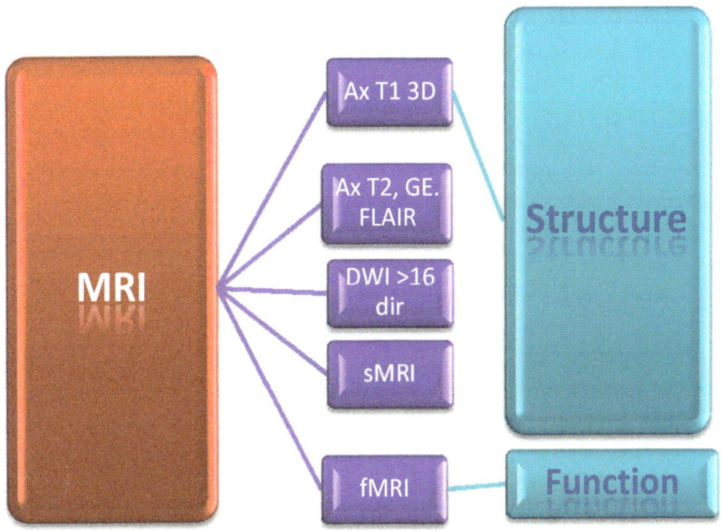

Figure 5. Standard acquisition protocol. MRI: magnetic resonance imaging; Ax T1 3D: axial series T1 weighted 3 Dimensional; Ax T2. GE and FLAIR: axial series T2 weigthed, Gradient Echo T2 weighted, Fluid Attenuation Inversion Recovery; DWI>16 dir: Diffusion Weighted Images acquiring in sixteen directions or more; sMRI: spectroscopy MRI; fMRI: functional MRI)

5.1. Magneto encephalography (MEG)

Magnetoencephalography or MEG measures electrical activity of the brain with similar principle to MRI , the Faraday's Law of induction (Bitar, et al. 2006), although registering and recording data as an electroencephalogram, frequently used to study epilepsy (Moore, et al. 2002) especially those cases refractory to treatment in which hippocampal sclerosis is suspected in view of a potential surgical approach to improve quality of life otherwise seriously compromised (Capizzano, et al. 2001).

It must be carried out in a separate and devoted MR unit, basically formed by a smaller but powerful magnet placed as a helmet in a Faraday's cage in which the subject is exposed to visual or auditory stimuli. Brain activity is registered and recorded with 120 channels according to Faraday's principle stating that every electrical current generates a magnetic field and vice versa. Stimuli are applied repeatedly throughout time with predetermined intervals.

Immediately before or after MEG the brain of the subject is studied with MRI to assess neurostructures. On both exams the subject wears the same set of external markings in pre-determined areas, usually nasion, occiput, temporal areas and vertex, which permit adequate post processing for image fusion, locating with precision where signal originates. Therefore, the exquisite spatial resolution of MRI and the reliable electrical signal from neural structures are depicted showing both, structure and function, usually color coded in a background of grey scale neuroimages, 2D or 3D.

5.2. Functional MRI (fMRI)

fMRI is carried out with an additional pulse sequence based in magnetic susceptibility effect that measures the rate of consumption of deoxy-hemoglobin (Chavand, et al. 2009) in a given amount of tissue. Magnetic susceptibility effect is obtained on $T2^*$ series, gradient echo pulse sequences with no rephasing pulse (Bitar, et al. 2006), what makes it particularly useful to detect elements distorting the magnetic field such as iron particles, being also sensible to other elements as calcium; it marks hydrogen distribution alteration in the vicinity of atoms from elements such as those mentioned before. Since changes can be detected rapidly varying throughout time, this is particularly useful for functional studies. Iron in the molecule of hemoglobin makes it prone to be detected. Its changes from deoxy-hemoglobin to oxy-hemoglobin indicate oxygen consumption by the brain tissue, a direct marker of activity. Nuclear medicine studies based in administering glucose marked with radiotracers, although exquisitely sensitive to mark metabolism, do not offer an identical temporal resolution to detect rapidly changing effects in the studied tissue, which makes it not suitable for functional studies (Jäger, et al. 2002).

Image fusion with neurostructural series does not require additional markings and the subject completes all required steps of the exam, morphology, biochemical, connectivity and functionality assessment, at the same time and in the same unit (Korvenoja, et al. 2006) without changing position, what enhances its advantages. Fusion can be thoroughly carried out without as many precautions required in other techniques. If a break is required in between series localizers must be obtained again and -preferably- an additional set of 3D for a precise image fusion.

There is an increasing tendency to study subjects with fMRI also in the steady state, not applying external stimuli, not only as a baseline series but also as a non-stimuli mediated investigation in normal and abnormal clinical scenarios. Steady state is a condition of equilibrium in between longitudinal and transverse magnetization when the subject is placed in the isocentre of a strong magnetic field (longitudinal magnetization), while receiving an external radiofrequency (transverse magnetization). Although applicable to other MRI concepts and sequences, for fMRI represents a relaxed, basal state hence suitable to be registered as a baseline and to compare with post stimuli registrations.

6. Stimuli

Paradigms can be predesigned in clinical settings by vendors of fMRI packages and workstations (Smiths, et al. 2006). Usually visual and auditory stimuli are applied in bursts with no stimuli gaps in between while the sequence is running. The patient has to respond generally by pressing buttons or by doing the required action. Pre exam discussion and subject cooperation play an essential role in these series. They do not significantly vary in either implementation or in interpretation if compared with other functional techniques (Faro and Mohamed 2006).

7. Post processing

Post processing encompasses all the processes taking place once data collection has been successfully carried out, usually on independent consoles or computers. It means transforming the available data to obtain further information. When applied to neuroimaging, post-processing purposes comprehend 3 dimensional image rendering, segmentation, evaluation of the cortex, evaluation of neural tracts and fusing images.

Segmentation, the process discussed in the following paragraphs, intends to thoroughly assess morphology of Central Nervous System in the endocranium, to measure volumes of grey matter (GM), white matter (WM) and Cerebro-spinal Fluid (CSF) with accuracy, precision and convenience in the totality or in the segments forming the CNS; and to assess the brain cortex. These objectives may vary among protocols, clinicians and researchers, depending on the clinical setting or type of research; their importance could be similar sometimes; or some could predominate over the others.

Neurostructural analyses are based in post processing of images carried out in independent consoles, usually by members of the research team. Workstations may be basically vendor provided or set by the clinical-research team. The former are usually designed by the vendor and less flexible, although straightforward and stable, i.e.: not prone to system crushes. The latter needs careful considerations regarding hardware, software and an adequate learning curve to maximize results. However, they have the remarkable advantage of flexibility. Hardware requirements are important for intended calculations of complex matrixes need to be considered. Most of the selected software programs explicitly mention minimum needs. PC, Linux and Mac computers are successfully used to run these calculations offering stable conditions to work through, satisfactory image rendering, good masking, segmentation and fusion options.

Quantitative magnetic resonance imaging of the brain to measure intracranial structures has become an essential clinical tool to evaluate and accurately assess both normal and abnormal individuals and a myriad of neuropsychiatric conditions in common practice permitting measurements with standardized techniques and procedures (Tofts 2004)

Volume loss of the brain versus age, involution changes and gender versus age, perinatal and childhood neurological anomalies, neurostructural analyses in patients with dementia (Krüger, Bertoni and Curran 2011), mainly those with Alzheimer's disease, frontotemporal dementia and Pick's disease, schizophrenia, subjects with refractory seizures and suspected mesial temporal sclerosis and those undergoing functional examinations of the brain to fuse images, tend to constitute the some of the groups of individuals more commonly examined with this technique.

Source images will almost invariably be in DICOM format (Digital Imaging and Communications in Medicine), which is computer language universally adopted and accepted in radiology imaging departments, standard for handling, storing, printing and transmitting information in medical imaging. The importance of DICOM lies not only in its universal applicability but also on the implied processes. DICOM archives are not only original processed signal or attenuation from the studied object as it was acquired but also much more information which is not part of the image but labels it adequately.

Once the study has been done, the images are transferred onto the DICOM archive and post-processing consoles can open them as part of the DICOM protocol. At this point, if an independent system is being used rather than a vendor provided one, images are to be downloaded to a separate archive. Studies have to remain completely anonymous, coded and transformed to formats suitable for post processing. It is essential to leave images with no traces of identifiable information but only a heading code to distinguish cases. Masking the identity of the subject data in DICOM images requires at least a reasonable degree of knowledge and expertise to be carried out effectively and to a bioethical acceptable extent. It must be remembered that DICOM archives are not just images but more complex collections of information, which may translate in images hence, extra care should be paid to these processes.

For segmentation, in general, the useful set of source images is provided by a high-resolution fast three-dimensional gradient echo T1 or T2-weighted pulse sequence (Jaume 2009). These series tend to produce a range of 160 to 180 slices which can be post processed on DICOM or other data formats, according to the software in use, to perform segmentation and sub segmentation of structures allowing appropriate volume measurements that can be carried out in manual, semi-automated or automated manner. Images should be formed by voxels of 1 or 0.5 mm with no gaps in between slices, which provide a satisfactory data collection for further three-dimensional image. A second likewise essential element to consider is to achieve the best possible signal intensity grey-white matter differences leading to a correct segmentation (Abidi 2012)

There is a range of post-processing software with several excellent programs, academically available at no cost, developed by reputed research centers, universities and institutes, including FLS, Surfer, Brain Suite 2, MIPAV (McAuliffe 2012) and Slicer, among others. Most of them are explicitly downloadable not for clinical but for research purposes. Their relevance, usefulness and reliability may vary. It is crucial that the team members become familiar with them perhaps using one as the main post processing tool and a second one to validate. Platforms they operate on are PC, Linux and Mac.

7.1. Source images

Several centers and authors prefer to change DICOM to other formats assigning them a coded number to identify and to differentiate between studies without breaching confidentiality of both, subject and institution, a legal and ethical bond which must be always carefully observed. This conversion usually facilitates building up and maintaining an appropriate database. Usual image formats could be ANALYZE™, hdr, img, nii, NIfTI and several others as [seriesname].mmr in the case of files created with Slicer.

Most databases can usually swap and convert from one format to another although extra care should be paid not only to avoid loosing information in the transformation but also to check anonymity details and potential left-right flipping which is not infrequent and may well go undetected for a while as it happens with organs following mirror corresponding parts on both sides with only a subtle *petalia* principle to help differentiate dominant side (Chang Chui and Damasio 1980) not usually picked up by the untrained observer. At this point, it is useful to consider an internal validation process, where the research team performs segmentations in several known control subjects under the formats to be used, comparing consistency and results. Calculations could be carried out in validated cases such as the ones available on LONI. Once consistency is proven and taken for granted, the method should be continued without significant changes until new validations take place.

7.2. Alignment, homogenization and skull erosion

Homogeneity and orientation have to be checked initially. The former can be corrected in some software programs as MIPAV. For alignment purposes, the axis from the anterior to the posterior grey commissure is essentially anteroposterior. The one extending throughout the inter-hemispheric cisterns determines the sagittal orientation plane. When possible, the plane extending from one petro-mastoid ridge to the other marks the third plane to align volume properly. If marked asymmetries of the brain and skull are present, automated segmentation techniques will not be reliable and should be carried out manually of in a semi-automated manner with constant visual check throughout the whole procedure.

Then, skull erosion has to be carried out [Fig 8] deleting structures from the skin to the inner aspect of the *duramater*. Some software programs require these steps explicitly giving some choices when it comes up to erode the skull. Some others carry out the process just naming it in the background although in all of them results tend to be equivalent. An important factor to be kept in mind here is a thorough visual inspection of the resulting surface; not infrequently islets –on occasions more than islets- of high signal intensity soft the process of erosion run by the program cannot adequately delete tissues and, if small volume changes are determined, results may be altered significantly leading to error. Visual analyses, expectably by someone trained in neuroanatomy, are essential to take for granted that segmented and measured volumes do correspond to the anatomical structures they are meant to correspond.

7.3. Standardization of images

The obtained volume must be aligned properly in all three axes of space, which could be done automatically or manually. The latter requires marking structures as anterior and posterior commissures and inter-hemispheric cisterns. Marking the most anterior, most posterior, superior, inferior and each one of both laterals as Talairach coordinates, essential to confine the atlas voxels to the intended area, carries out further standardization. Images must be taken from source to AC-PC (anterior commissure to posterior commissure) alignment and then to Talairach space to apply the voxels. Once done, images are taken back to AC-PC alignment and then back to normal to calculate volumes of each structure. This process is explained in detail by MIPAV (Medical Image Processing, Analysis and Visualization) (McAuliffe 2012)

7.4. Masking

Further steps vary significantly depending on the type of program. MIPAV gives choices to segment with automated masking providing both images and figures with the results. Others run similar calculations with no visual representation in which case, visual control of each step is required [Fig 6].

Masking is reducing tissue signal intensity differences to three or four main ones following mathematical algorithms, which narrows ranges between different magnitudes as having a rather quantic scale rather than continuum-like one. Grey-white matter and CSF segmentation can be however carried out without masking, by selecting the range of signals the measured tissue presents statistically an expression of mean signal plus minus 1 standard deviation. Cases with normal volunteers tend not to represent particular difficulties. However, some cases with atrophy and/or conspicuous changes in signal intensity due to pathology require manual calculations and careful slice-by-slice evaluation of these processes in order not to miss register results. Masking on CNS images follows mathematical algorithms on images to obtain two, or three signal intensity differences corresponding to grey, white matter and cerebrospinal fluid, which try to mimic gross specimen stains in pathology to help with visual discrimination of tissues in CNS. If the studied subject has no obvious signal intensity alterations in grey matter forming hippocampus or amygdala, this could help. Usually, masking could lead to consider some of the temporal cortices adjacent to the amygdala in the resulting final image, to be carefully checked case by case. Validation between manual and automated measurements is a useful step to carry out to gain certainty especially before considering studying extensive cohorts.

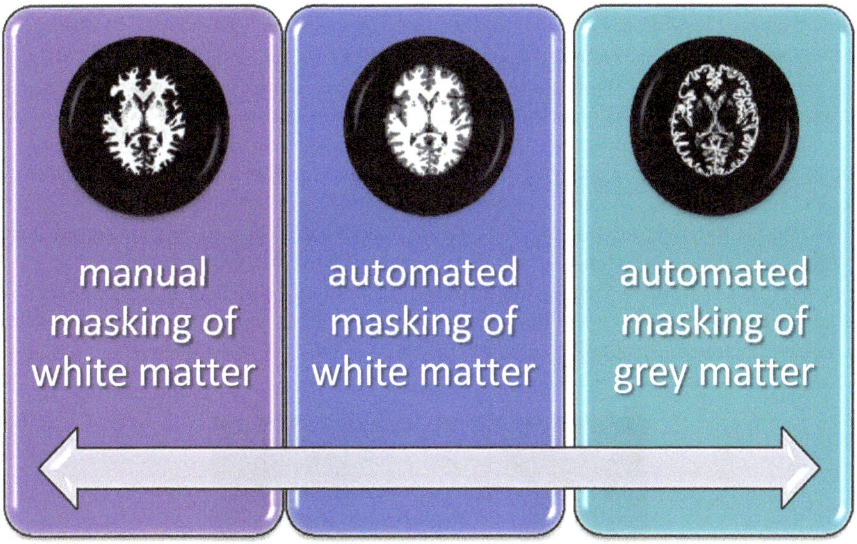

Figure 6. Masking for initial gross segmentation in grey matter, white matter and CSF

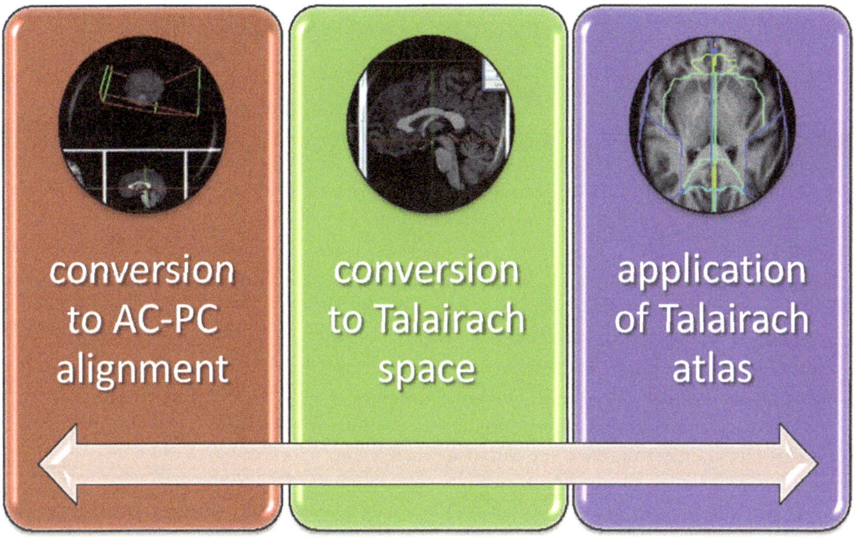

Figure 7. Alignment to anterior commissure-posterior commissure plane and further transformation into Talairach space before applying the atlas

3.2.5. Sub segmentation can carry on following an atlas, which usually is a validated one such as ICBM [Fig 9], Talairach, Talairach-Tournoux, Montreal, or even institution designed, the latter for as long as a rigorous validation process has taken place. Atlases will provide predetermined boundaries applied with precision from the central planes starting in sagittal, axial and coronal landmarks. Boundaries permit to measure volumes determined by signal intensity within the selected VOI (volume of interest), for automated processes [Fig 7]. Semi automated processes are based on moving the cursor throughout the slice to obtain graphs of isosignal intensity like isobars on a map. The observer accepts what he thinks is reasonable. Manual segmentation implies marking contours slice-by-slice measuring, as the other methods, signal intensity voxels within an accepted range. The latter is very useful in cases of frank signal intensity anomalies such as mesial temporal sclerosis affecting hippocampus and amygdala in which following Jack method (Jack, et al. 1992) is very helpful to determine a cutoff plane to divide parahippocampal gyrus from the hippocampal-amygdala complex. However, sub segmentation using Talairach atlas at an appropriate level carries it out automatically.

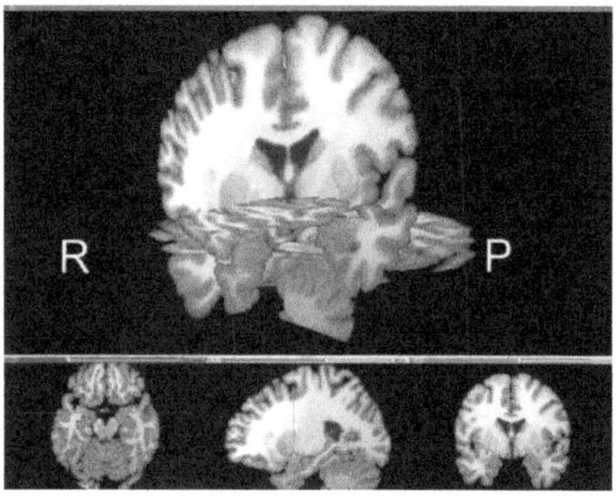

Figure 8. Segmentation with Slicer: skull erosion has already taken place

The study of the temporal lobe has been typically carried out in clinical settings for the study of refractory epilepsy, in most institutions, or all epilepsy cases in some others although tertiary centers do perform it as part of many other protocols with routine 3D acquisitions. High resolution T2 weighted images in coronal plane perpendicular to the Sylvian fissure are reliable to study signal intensity changes of the amygdalae and hippocampi, an essential assessment before attempting to carry out automated segmentation of the limbic system. It must be kept in mind that automated segmentation procedures are based on signal intensity differences. If the latter are not statistically significant any masking or not masking segmentation process may well be not reliable in which case it is better to carry out manual segmentation.

7.5. Manual segmentation

Carried out slice by slice by tracing contours of the amygdala, is the safest procedure when the researcher is trained enough in anatomy and imaging. (Bertoni 2010).

Any plane can be selected to depict the amygdala which, given its rounded-ovoid shape, permits a good delineation of boundaries in almost all possible planes, axial, coronal, saggital or oblique, to be used on manual segmentation method. However, segmentation must be carried out following the same plane throughout the manual procedure making sure that progressively increasing number of contiguous slices, contours are traced from the start to the end on each side. If further certainty is needed, the same researcher can calculate again following a different plane to check if results do match. Some structures are easier seen for segmentation purposes on one or two of all possible planes, which is influenced not only by researcher decisions but also his training and experience manipulating anatomical images. The hippocampal –amygdala complex volume calculations are usually carried out on oblique coronal images in most of the non-3D acquisitions to minimize boundaries determination errors on 2D slices, although at the same time, it implies that more slices are required to cover the whole of the anatomical area to be fully depicted. However, slices in the axial oblique reformatted plane from 3D source images tend to me much more useful in these regards being able to depict the entire hippocampal structure in fewer images (Bertoni 1998). Inter-observer and intra-observer variability are useful parameters to assess consistency of measurements as an initial evaluation of robustness of the method selected by the team.

7.6. Semi automated segmentation

Almost all the available post processing software programs permit to detect lines by highlighting sequences of points of identical signal intensity when the cursor is dragged on each image. Once the appropriate contour has been selected a click is usually enough to freeze it. Again, as it must be carried out in non-automated segmentation procedures, following the same plane throughout the calculation is essential.

7.7. Automated segmentation

Automated segmentation is based on the application of atlases on sets of images sequentially arranged, usually named "stack images" which the operator can scroll at will. Before applying any atlas, the operator must make sure all the required conditions are met to assure an adequate, precise, reproducible and thorough process in order to validate the results with certainty.

The basic principle to apply an atlas is to run a process of signal intensity measurement for which the source images must be of the highest possible quality, 3 dimensional, isovolumetric of not more than $1mm^3$, properly aligned and oriented, among other important conditions mentioned before.

In applying the atlas, the observer measures a volume of densities within a range (not masked) or a precise mathematical value (masked). Independently of choosing to calculate volumes from masked or unmaked pictures, images should be checked one by one before running the calculation, preferably by more than one observer to grant consistency before running any other subsequent validation method.

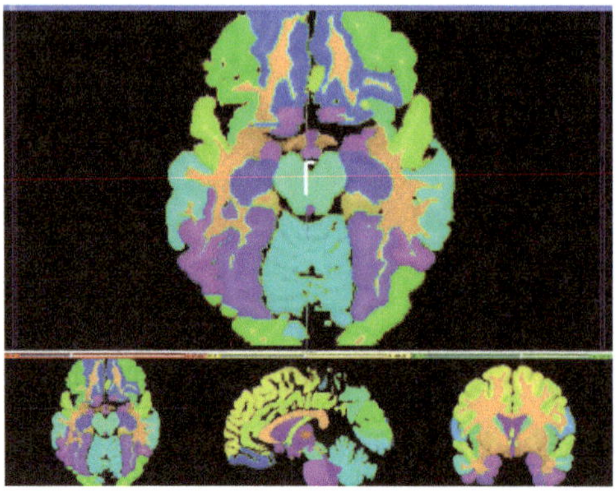

Figure 9. Segmentation and subsegmentation applying ICBM atlas on Slicer

A strong validation process usually results in publishing an academically available atlas. They vary according to the institution, research or clinical team, and author. Useful ones are Talairach, Talairach-Bazin, ICBM and Montreal, among others. There are normal and disease-specific ones. Their applicability may vary with the software program in use; the researcher should consider becoming very familiar with at least one, validating a reasonable number of cases by calculating structures with manual, semi-automated and automated procedures to gain certainty, skills and accuracy before trying to segment cohorts of larger numbers.

Some of them are intended to volumes and some are intended to neural tracts. All academically available segmentation software programs permit to carry out calculations based in atlases developed by the researcher which must fulfill the adequate internal and external validation requirements to be confidently used Although in the past only real dissections from post mortem specimens were doable and acceptable, technology available today permits to carry out in vivo dissections from source radiological images, which have also become the accepted source to demonstrate the whole of the neural structures including connectivity, mapping and functionality (The Human Connectome Projec) (LONI, UCLA 2012). Their essential principle is to apply volume of interest limits, slice by slice throughout the 3D series, to then measure signal intensity differences inside the selected volume. A proper alignment usually according to anterior-posterior grey commissures, inter-hemispheric cisterns and skull base-petrous planes are of crucial importance.

It is important to consider assessing selected images not only mathematically but also visually; signal intensity differences may lead to potential error if contours are not checked slice by slice throughout the entire selected volume. It is essential to consider that software programs can run mathematical calculations with precision; however, the appropriate determination of boundaries to avoid including unwished pieces of tissue which would lead to incorrect results, remains as a fundamental responsibility of the operator (Chen 2006).

The Talairach atlas (Nowinski, et al. 2005) offers a robust and validated process of segmenting and subsegmenting CNS structures, bilaterally or unilaterally. Once initial steps have been carried out including homogeneity check and skull erosion, an appropriate alignment according to anterior commissure (AC) to posterior commissure (PC) plane completed with selection of two points in the interhemispheric space to ensure a plane, after which Talairach coodinates are set to mark the most prominent points anteriorly, posteriorly, superiorly, inferiorly and on both sides. Images are taken from the source set to AC-PC plane and from it to Talairach space, mathematically created, normalized, to permit placement of different volumes of interest (VOIs) as each atlas level permits. As the VOIs are placed, the researcher must ensure no segment is left outside the area of interest, going through the whole set of images to check image boundaries. Then images with applied VOIs must be taken back to AC-PC and from it to the source set of pictures with all selected VOIs appropriately copied. Volume calculations for each VOI are then matter of selecting the appropriate signal intensity for grey or white matter in each volume. If the region selected, for instance, includes the amygdala, by selecting a signal intensity corresponding to grey matter, all those 1 mm^3 voxels having grey matter signal will be included in the result leaving aside all those with white matter signal. Signal intensity ranges for unmasked images (ie: 0-100 for cerebrospinal fluid, 150-250 for grey matter and 400-600 for white matter), or values for masked ones (1 for CSF, 2 for grey and 3 for white matter), need to be entered manually to determine each result in each voxel. This is what provides volume values for neural structures, voxel by voxel. If selected voxels include the whole of the boundaries of the brain, then segmentation values will show the totality of CSF, grey and white matter for the whole of the brain. If each hemisphere is selected and the voxel boundaries have been correctly set, each hemisphere , then results will be for each one of them. The same applies when subsegmentation takes place to determine volume for each lobe, region, subcortical structure and even Broadman areas, which can be calculated if level 5 segmentation is selected when using the Talairach atlas.

Unlike other imaging procedures based on attenuation of energy measured in standardized units with calibrated devices such as X Rays, computed tomography or ultrasound, MRI signal originates in resonance of hydrogen atoms placed in an external magnetic field and therefore intensity values for each pixel or voxel can vary from MR unit to MR unit, from one subject to the other or even within the same subject if his temperature of hydration change (Ramani, Hensen and Helpern 2006).

If multiple regions (several VOIs) are selected to calculate volumes from all of them simultaneously, the researcher should keep in mind the computing resources in use and the computer memory allocated to the calculation. More modern software program versions tend to be much more stable than earlier ones; likewise, more powerful computers and improved platforms result in a smother and successful calculation. In any case, some extra care should be paid to these details since this is sometimes the trickiest step in automated calculations. Validations against valid calculations or databases are similar demanding computer calculations.

ICBM atlas is other powerful resource to be considered by the research team. It runs smoothly on Slicer where fusion with uploaded volumes, subject-by-subject, result in an extremely useful step to facilitate correct VOIs placements. Calculations are then straightforward processes.

Independently from the chosen software program and for as long as the researchers are familiar and skilled operating it, if computing resources are adequate and internal-external validation processes take place, results will tend to be reliable, reproducible and consistent.

A careful analysis of all these factors will be of help to assess inconsistencies in results reported in the literature perhaps due to differences in cohorts numbers, field strength of the MR units, type of equipment, acquisition and calculation techniques.

Factors which may favorably influence robustness and confidence in segmentation results are the increasing availability of super high field MR units, larger cohorts of studied individuals and better software programs.

Several neuroscientists, authors and clinical researchers have carried out segmentation and functional studies of the amygdala with a diversity of purposes producing a very useful framework to consider. The study of the amygdala is of increasing interest to try to understand its role in cognition, impulses modulation, its participation in mood regulation and many other important aspects in the neurosciences field.

Neuroimaging the amygdala in the clinical domain has been more extensively dedicated to study its role in epilepsy, especially in refractory epilepsy causing dramatic alterations in lifestyle, therapeutic approach and outcome. Refractory epilepsy of medial temporal origin usually implies a thorough assessment of the amygdala-hippocampus complex because if a surgical therapeutic approach is accepted, resection of both structures take place aiming to improve quality of life.

Other important source of interest in the amygdala in the clinical domain originates in psychiatry. Cognitive impairment, memory problems and dementia constitute an increasing public health problem given today's extended life expectancy with its deep impact in individual, familiar and social life.

Clinical research concerning segmentation of the amygdala was initially based only on manual segmentation processes. They are very useful and accurate especially if there are signal intensity anomalies in the limbic system. They are also useful and accurate to study the hippocampus due to its intricate anatomy, and the amygdala given its proximity to the hippocampal head. The location of these two structures, not only adjacent to one another but also to the rest of the temporal cortex of the uncus and parahippocampal gyrus tend to be difficult to solve when volume calculations exclusively rely on automated segmentation processes. These calculations need to be corroborated manually to confirm consistency of results.

Volume changes have been found on a myriad of normal and abnormal conditions including mood disorders, schizophrenia, attention deficit disorder, depression, attention deficit disorder, anxiety and obsessive-compulsive as the main although not the exclusive entities linked to neurostrutural changes, biochemical and functional alterations (Goodwin 2000).

Familiarity with the anatomy, connections, neural biochemistry, functionality, MRI, image archiving and manipulation, software use, atlases application, image fusion to study morphology, biochemistry, connectivity and function are essential aspects to increase certainty, accuracy and testing results when studied cohort increase in number and quality.

A useful way of starting a robust process of segmentation is by carefully building and checking the database for image quality, noise and type of archives. DICOM format will always tend to be the most useful and universal, although perhaps not the most convenient for further post processing.

When the set of stack images has been selected, it should be copied from the archive to an ad-hoc folder in the computer in order to be used for calculations. Images must be checked one by one, usually in the range of 140 to 200. Axial plane is the most convenient to apply atlases on MIPAV such as Talairach, due to the original work carried out on Fleischig-type axial brain slices. ICBM as other atlases however, can be used in all three directions on the same screen simultaneously as it happens using Slicer.

Image noise, its homogeneity, positioning corrections and slice selection to include only slices from the base of the skull to the convexity are preliminary steps to be followed to grant a good quality control. Image preparation must be carried out independently to the software in use. The voxel dimensions and eventual resizing must be considered. In Mac environment, Osirix™ offers capability of resizing and rendering in a selected plane if source images have been obtained in a different plane or with a different voxel dimension. MIPAV offers that capability and can be conveniently implemented on PC.

Skull and soft tissue erosion usually represent the following step. Extra care should be paid to check results image by image in all three planes. Sometimes islets of fatty tissue are not satisfactorily removed due to their high signal intensity and positioning (as base of the skull , occiput or convexity) altering results, especially if little volume changes need to be detected. These cases do require manual removal because further erosion will probably delete noble tissue, necessary for a correct calculation.

3D sets of images cansubsequently be manipulated to study the surface of the brain identifying gyri and sulci with remarkable detail. Further reorientation is necessary for an adequate segmentation aligning the whole volume in the anterior commissure to posterior commissure plane to then mark Talairach coordinates, formed by the most superior, inferior, anterior, posterior and lateral planes.

It is safer to combine a sufficient number of studies doing two segmentation methods, for instance manual and automated, to look for consistency of results before validating them with external and more extensive databases.

Independently of these steps, a careful direct observation and measurement of signal intensities throughout the limbic system should be carried out before applying atlases in automated calculations to make sure measurements and boundaries delineation are consistent since they rely on signal intensity differences between adjacent areas.

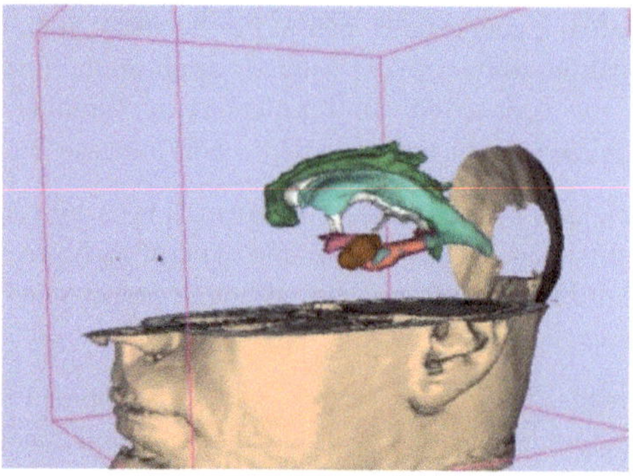

Figure 10. Subsegmentation of the amygdala with Slicer and ICBM atlas. The amygdala in shown in purple; hippocampus pink; pericallosal gyrus in green; corpus callosum in white; ipsilateral ventricle in light-blue

Manual measurements appear to be the safest method in present conditions to confirm that what we delineate and measure correspond to what the research team has intended to. Axial-oblique slices parallel to the largest head-tail hippocampal axis are a reliable method to manually delineate the amygdale, tracing its contours and studying its signal intensity (Bertoni, Sclavi and Sauer, Volumetry of hippocampus and amygdala with magnetic resonance imaging 1998). It is also a useful check up for consistency of results, randomly or systematically, in automated methods of segmentation (Bertoni and Sclavi, Isovoxel based morphometry of hippocampi and amygdalae: a comparison of manual and automated volume measurements 2010).

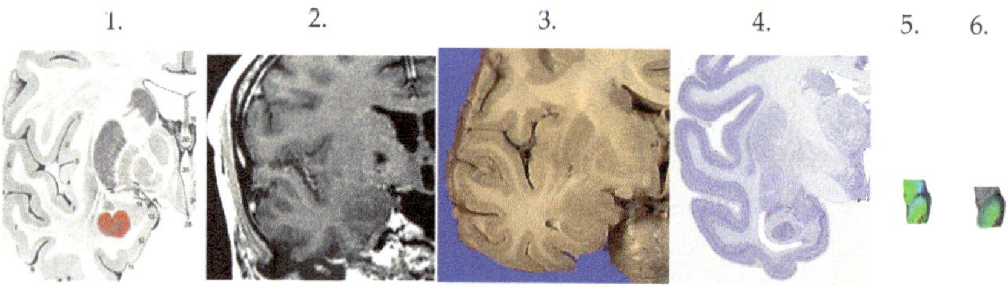

Figure 11. Right amygdala; coronal slices correlating atlas section, MRI, gross specimen, stained gross specimen, 3D reformat with part of the hippocampus and just the amygdala, with contours smoothed by the software

(1) Modified from Nieuwenhuys (Nieuwenhuys, Voogd and van Huijzen 1988); (2) coronal reformat MRI from source axial images; (3) gross specimen; (4) stained gross specimen, brainmaps.org, US; (5) Modified from Timoner (Timoner, et al. 2002)

Thorough assessment of signal intensities in the region of interest becomes essential in subjects with underlying neurostructural abnormalities. It should be remembered that in some cases of medial temporal sclerosis, for instance, as other neuropsychiatric conditions, a frankly abnormal range of signal measurements are obtained in areas of intricate anatomy.

Manual measurements provide an adequate method of reassurance in these difficult cases to avoid miss registration of volumes.

Mean normal volumes of the amygdala vary according to different authors, probably due to studied cohorts and technique differences. They vary in a range between 0.5 (Bertoni 1998) and 1.63cc (Bickart 2011). These volume variations may be due to differences in calculation procedures, techniques and MR units. Some of the technical details mentioned before concerning image quality parameters as noise, resolution, voxel dimensions, procedure of determining boundaries and validation are not thoroughly mentioned in all of the available research that provide volume measurements. Some series, however, include more extensive cohorts and therefore seem to give firmer bases to consider results. In any case, to study more extensive cohorts with strict quantitative mechanistic protocols and thorough validation processes are still due.

Disorder	Structural MR	DTI	fMR	sMR
Schizophrenia	1.Decreased frontotemporal and cerebral volumes, increased ventricular volume 2.Cortex thinning	Decreased prefrontal bundles, uncinate fas and corpus callosum	Decreased prefrontal, cerebellym and striate activity	1.Decreased NAA in prefrontal and cingulate 2.Increased Glu in prefrontal areas and hippocampus in risk subjects
Bipolar disorder	Increased T2 hyperintensity in white matter	Decreased prefrontal and corpus callosum bundles	Decreased prefrontal and cingulate activity	Decreased NAA in prefrontal
Major depressive disorder	Decreased prefrontal cortex, anterior cingulate, medial temporal and basal ganglia volumes	Decreased prefrontal bundles	Decreased cingulate, prefrontal and amygdala activity	Decreased NAA in prefrontal and hippocampus
Anxiety disorders	Decreased hippocampus	Decreased cortico striato cortical circuit	Decreased prefrontal and hippocampal activity	Decreased NAA in striatum
Attention deficit disorder	Decreased anterior cingulate, cortex thinning	Decreased frontostriatal bundles	Decreased prefrontal activity	Increased Glu in prefrontal and striatum

Figure 12. Reported findings in major psychiatric conditions (Agarwal, et al. 2010)

The increasing knowledge in the field of psychiatry has promoted more adequate, thorough and precise neuroimaging assessment of subjects with different conditions. Moreover, continuous updates on information permit to conceive systematic neurostructural stuydies to assess normal and abnormal subjects. These include detailed neurostructural analyses, whole brain and limbic system segmentation including the amygdala, extensive tractography for connectivity purposes, in vivo spectroscopy and functional studies in both, the steady state and post stimuli.

Multiple morbid and abnormal conditions are linked to amygdala volume and functional changes, including bipolar, depressive and anxiety disorders, schizophrenia and several others, among some of the most cited entities in which this limbic nucleus shows volume alterations, biochemical anomalies, altered neural connectivity and abnormal functionality in the steady state or after specific stimuli (Agarwal, et al. 2010).

8. Conclusion

Segmentation and volume determinations of the amygdala are image post processing techniques of increasing importance to assess healthy individuals and subjects with morbid conditions in neurosciences. A large number of studies have reported volume variations of the amygdala in usual physiological adjustment, neurobiology of mood, premorbid and pathological conditions reporting changes in a myriad of conditions. The latter include post traumatic stress, anxiety, depression and obsessive compulsive disorders, among others, probably the amygdala role in the modulation of emotions and sensory pathways. Although some studies have found sexual dysmorphism and different regression volume values of the amygdala depending of age (Bertoni 1998), others seem to suggest just the opposite (Hirai, et al. 2000).

Decreased volumes of the amygdale have been usually linked to almost all those cases with underlying pathological entities, from alcoholism (Thomas et al, 2011) and other addictions to schizophrenia (Wang, et al. 2008, Goodwin 2000).

Whether it be manual, semi-automated or fully-automated, segmentation results should be carried out not only thorough and carefully but also internally and externally validated. The former using at least two methods (manual and semi-automated or fully automated) and two different software programs until to grant consistency. External validation comparing results against more extensive databases is a further step to grant consistency, safer and more reliable results concerning neuroimaging the amygdala to assess its volume, boundaries, connectivity, metabolism and functionality.

Wider availability of high and very high magnetic field MR units, more powerful computing systems, systematic and more friendly quantitative mechanistic determinations and standardized paradigms of stimuli will probably facilitate and encourage further research in the near future to improve our present knowledge of the amygdala increasing the understanding of its complex modulatory functions influencing human behaviour

Author details

Miguel Ángel Bertoni
East Kent Hospitals University NHS Foundation Trust, University of Kent, UK

9. References

[1] Abidi, Ali. Advanced Segmentation of Brain MRI Images: An advanced Technique to Analysis Brain Structure. LAP Lambert Academic Publishing, 2012.

[2] Agarwal, Nivedita, John Port, Massimo Bazzocchi, and Perry Renshaw. "Update on the use of MR for assessment and diagnosis of psychiatric diseases." Radiology (The Radiological Society of North America) 255, no. 1 (April 2010): 23-41.

[3] Andre, E, et al. "MR spectroscopy in sinus mucocele: M-acetyl mimics of brina N-acetylaspartate." American Journal of Neuroradiology 27 (November 2006): 2210-2213.

[4] Arslanoglu, A, D Bonekamp, P B Barker, and A Horska. "Quantitative proton MR spectroscopic imaging of the mesial temporal lobe." J Magn Reson Imaging 20, no. 5 (2004): 772-8.

[5] Bertoni, Miguel Angel, and Nora Elsa Sclavi. "Isovoxel based morphometry of hippocampi and amygdalae: a comparison of manual and automated volume measurements." The Neuroradiology Journal (Centauro) 23, no. 6 (2010): 637-643.

[6] Bertoni, Miguel Angel, Nora Elsa Sclavi, and Harold Peter Sauer. "Volumetry of hippocampus and amygdala with magnetic resonance imaging." International Journal of Neuroradiology (Lippincott, Williams & Wilkins) 4 (1998): 291-295.

[7] Bickart, Kevin, Wright, Christopher, Dautoff, Rebecca, Dickerson, Bradford, and Barrett, LIsa. "Amygdala volume and social network size in humans." Nat Neurosci (Nature Publishing Group, a division of Macmillan Publishers) 14, no. 2 (February 2011): 163-164.

[8] Bitar, Richard, et al. "MR pulse sequences: what every radiologist wants to know but is afraid to ask." RadioGraphics (The Radiological Society of North America) 26 (March 2006): 513-537.

[9] Brown, Mark, and Richard Semelka. "MR imaging abbreviations, definitions, and description: a review." Radiology (The Radiological Society of North America) 213, no. 647-662 (1999).

[10] Buckler, Andrew, Linda Bresolin, N Dunnick, and Daniel Sullivan. "Quantitative imaging test approval and biomarquer qualification: interrelated but distinct activities." Radiology (The Radiological Society of North America) 259 (February 2011): 875-884.

[11] Capizzano, Aristides, et al. "Temporal lobe epilepsy: qualitative reading of 1H MR spectroscopic images for presurgical evaluation." Radiology (The Radiological Society of North America) 218 (January 2001): 144-151.

[12] Catani, Marco, and Michel Thiebau de Schotten. "A diffusion tensor imaging tractography atlas for virtual in vivo dissections." Cortex (Elsevier Masson), 2008: 1105-1132.

[13] Chan, Stephen, Joel Erickson, and Sidney Yoon. "Limbic system abnormalities associated with mesial temporal sclerosisL a model of chronic cerebral changes due to seizures." Radiographics (The Radiological Society of North America) 17 (1997): 1095-1110.

[14] Chang Chui, H, and R Damasio. "Human cerebral asymmetries evaluated by computed tomography." Jounal of Neurology, Neurosurgery and Psychiatry 43 (1980): 873-878.

[15] Chavand, Govin, Paul Babin, Bejoy Thomas, Manohar Shroff, and Kark Haacke. "Principles, techniques and applications of T2* based MR imaging and its special applications." Radiographics (The Radiological Society of North America) 29 (2009): 1433-1449.

[16] Chen, Lin. "Topology correction for brain atlas segmentation." In Bilverarbeitung für die Medizin, by Gudrun Wagenknecht, edited by Jan Ehrdart, 131-135. Springer-Verlag, 2006.

[17] Faro, Scott, and Feroze Mohamed. Functional MRI: Basic Principles and Clinical Applications. Springer, 2006.

[18] Goodwin, Guy. Neurobiological aetiology of mood disorders. Vol. 1, in New Oxford Textbook of Psychiatry, by Michael Gelder, Juan López-Ibor and Nancy Andreasen, edited by Michael Gelder, Juan López-Ibor and Nancy Andreasen, 711-724. Oxford: Oxford University Press, 2000.

[19] Hirai, Toshinori, Yukunori Korigi, Kazuhiro Yoshizumi, Yoshinori Shigematsu, Takeshi SUgahara, and Mutsumasa Takahashi. "Limbic lobe of the human brain: evaluation with turbo fluid-attenuated inversion-recovery MR imaging." Radiology (The Radiological Society of North America) 215 (May 2000): 470-475.

[20] Jäger, Lorenz, et al. "Focal epileptiform activity in the brain: detection with spike-related functional MR imaging-preliminary results." Radiology (The Radiological Society of North America) 223 (April 2002): 860-869.

[21] Jack, Clifford, Colleen Twomey, Alan Zinsmeister, Frank Sharbrough, Ronald Petersen, and Gregory Cascino. "Anterior temporal lobe and hippocampal formations: normative volumetric measurements from MR images in young adults." Radiology (The Radiological Society of North America) 172 (1989): 549-554.

[22] Jack, CR, F W Sharbrough, G D Cascino, K A Hirschorn, P C O'Brien, and W R Marsh. "Magnetic resonance image-based hippocampal volumetry: correlation with outcome after temporal lobectomy." Ann Neurol 31, no. 2 (February 1992): 138-46.

[23] Jacobs, Michael, Tamer Ibrahim, and Ronald Ouwerkerk. "MR imaging: brief overview and emerging applications." Radiographics (The Radiological Society of North America) 27 (2007): 1213-1229.

[24] Jaume, Sylvain. Topology Simplification Algorithm for Segmentation of Medical Scans: Application to the Segmentation of Brain MRI. LAP Lambert Academic Publishing, 2009.

[25] Judenhofer, Martin, et al. "PET/MR images acquired with a compact MR-compatible PET detector in a 7-T magnet." Radiology (The Radiological Society of North America) 244 (2007): 807-814.

[26] Karow, David, et al. "Relative capability of MR imaging and FGD PET to depict changes associated with prodromal and early Alzheimer disease." Radiology (The Radiological Society of North America) 256 (2010): 932-942.

[27] Klatzberg, Richard, and Brendan Barrett. "Risk of iodinated contrast material-induced nephropathy with intravenous administration." Radiology (The Radiological Society of North America) 243 (2007): 622-628.

[28] Korvenoja, Antti, Erika Kirveskari, Hannu Aronen, Sari Avikainen, Antii Branden, and Juha Huttunen. "Sensotimotor cortex localization: a comparison of magnetoencephalography, functional MR iaging and intraoperative cortical mapping." Radiology (The Radiological Society of North America) 241, no. 1 (October 2006): 213-222.

[29] Krüger, Sonja, Miguel Angel Bertoni, and Stephen Curran. "Early detection of dementia." In Practical Management of Dementia, by Stephen Curran and John Wattis, edited by Stephen Curran and John Wattis, 266. London: Radcliffe Publishing, 2011.

[30] Kwon, Hyeok Gyu, Hi Heon Hong, and Sung Ho Jang. "Mamillothalamic tract in human brain: diffusion tensor tractography study." Neurosciences Letters (Elsevier) 481, no. 1 (August 2010): 51-53.

[31] Laboratory of Neuroimaging, University of California at Los Angeles. The Human Connectome Project. 2012. http://www.loni.ucla.edu (accessed April 1, 2012).

[32] Li, Shi-Juang, Zhu Li, Waohong Gu, Mei-Jie Zhang, Malgorzata Franczak, and Piero Antuono. "Alzheimer disease: evaluation of a functional MR imaging index as a marker." Radiology (The Radiological Society of North America) 225 (2002): 253-259.

[33] Maubon, Antoine, Jean-Michel Ferru, Vincent Berger, Marie Colette Soulage, Mark DeGraeef, and Pierre Aubas. "Effect of field strenght on MR images: comparison of the same subject at 0.5, 1.0 and 1.5T." Radiographics (The Radiological Society of North America) 19 (1999): 1057-1067.

[34] McAuliffe, Matthew. MIPAV. United States of America Patent 12A/2029. 2012.

[35] Moore, Kevin, Michael Funke, Tawnya Constantino, Gregory Katzman, and Jeffrey Lewine. "Magnetoencephalographically directed review of high-spatial-resolution surface-coil MR images improves lesion detection in patients with extratemporal epilepsy." Radiology (The Radiological Society of North Amertica) 225 (2002): 880-887.

[36] Nieuwenhuys, Rudolf, Jan Voogd, and Chrstian van Huijzen. The Human Central Nervous System. Springer-Verlag, 1988.

[37] Nowinski, Wieslaw, et al. "Three-dimensional atlas of the brain anatomy and vasculature." infoRAD (The Radiological Society of North America) 25 (2005): 263-271.

[38] Ouwerkerk, Ronald, Karen Bleich, Joseph Gillen, Martin Pomper, and Paul Bottomley. "Tissue sodium concentration in human brain tumors as measured with 23Na MR imaging." Radiology (The Radiological Society of North America) 227 (May 2003): 529-537.

[39] Qingmao, Hu., Guoyu Qian, Michael Teistler, and Su Huang. "Automatic and adaptive brain morphometry on MR images." Radiographics (The Radiological Society of North America) 28 (March 2008): 345-356.

[40] Ramani, Anita, Jens Hensen, and Joseph Helpern. "Quantitative MR imaging in Alzheimer disease." Radiology (The Radiological Society of North America) 241 (October 2006): 26-44.

[41] Ranger, Nicole, Ehsan Samei, James Dobbins, and Carl Ravin. "Assessment of detective quantum efficiency: intercomparison of a recently introduced international standard with prior methods." Radiology (The Radiological Society of North America) 243, no. 3 (June 2007): 785-795.

[42] Ratnarajah, Nagulan, Andrew Simmons, Miguel Bertoni, and Ali Hojjatoleslami. "Multitensor random-walk probabilistic algorithms: analysis and tracking of complex fibre configurations." Magnetic Resonance Imaging (Elsevier), 2012.

[43] Ratnarajah, Nagulan, Andy Simmons, Miguel Angel Bertoni, and Ali Hojattoleslami. "Residual bootstrapping on classified tensor morphologies." Medical Image Understanding and Analysis. London: MIUIA, 2011. 87-91.

[44] Ratnarajah, Nagulan, Andy Simmons, Miguel Angel Bertoni, Mohamed Sakel, and Ali Hojattoleslami. "Two-tensor model-based bootstrapping on classified tensor morphologies: estimation of uncertainty in fibre orientation and probabilistic tractography." MICCAI 2011. Toronto: MICCAI-Workshop on Computational Diffusion MRI, 2011. 1-12.

[45] Smith, Alice, James Smirniotopoulos, and Elizabeth Rushing. "Central Nervous System infections associated with human immunodeficiency virus infection: radiologic-pathologic correlation." Radiographics (The Radiological Society of North America) 28 (November 2008): 2033-2058.

[46] Smiths, Marion, Evy Visch-Brink, Caroline Schraa-Tam, Peter Koudstaal, and Aad van der Lugt. "Functional MR imaging of language processing: an overview of easy-to-implement paradigms for patient care and clinical research." RadioGraphics (The Radiological Society of North America) 26 (October 2006): S145-S158.

[47] Sokolowski, K, and J Corbin. "Wired for behaviours: from development to function of innate limbic system circuitry." Front Mol Neurosci 5 (April 2012): 55.

[48] Spampinatto, Maria, Zoran Rumboldt, Robert Hosker, and Jacobo Mintzer. "Apolipoprotein E and gray matter volume loss in patients with mild cognitive impairment and Alzheimer Disease." Radiology (The Radiological Society of North America) 258, no. 3 (March 2011): 843-852.

[49] Thomas, Adam, Panos Koumellis, and Robert Dineen. "The fornix in health and disease: an imaging review." Radiographics (The Radiological Society of North America) 31 (July 2011): 1107-1121.

[50] Timoner, Samson, P Golland, R Kikinis, and M Shenton. "Performance issues in shape classification." MICCAI '02. LNCS, 2002. 355-362.

[51] Tofts, Paul. "Measurement and MR." In Quantitative MRI of the Brain, by P Tofts, edited by Paul Tofts, 3-16. Wiley, 2004.

[52] Wang, Lei, et al. "Progressive deformation of deep brain nuclei and hippocampal-amygdala formation in schizophrenia." Biological Psychiatry (Elsevier) 15, no. 64 (April 2008): 1060-1068.

Chapter 3

Cellular Mechanisms in the Amygdala Involved in Memory of Fear Conditioning

Ryong-Moon Shin

Additional information is available at the end of the chapter

1. Introduction

Natural disaster can occur in all countries of the world. Now Japan suffers triple disasters: massive earthquake, vast tsunami and the world`s worst nuclear crisis. The victims with fear in their minds deeply might fall into fear-related disorders in future.

Fear is a conserved emotion in response to danger and triggers some defensive mechanisms for adapting to threatening events for survival. Moreover, fear can lead to a number of anxiety disorders when aberrantly expressed. Defining the cellular and synaptic mechanisms underlying fear memory will enhance our understanding of biological mechanism to enemies, as well as our ability to develop treatments for individual afflicted with anxiety disorders, including posttraumatic stress disorder (PTSD).

The discovery of long-term potentiation (LTP), a phenomenon in which repetitive stimulation of afferent fibers results in a prolonged enhancement of synaptic strength provided the cellular mechanism to explain learning and memory formation. While LTP has been described at many synapses in different brain regions, it has been studied most intensively at glutamatergic synapses in the mammalian hippocampus. However, linking changes in synapse transmission of the hippocampus to specific behavioral changes has proved to be difficult largely because of the complex behaviors which the hippocampus is involved in.

We have to apply a simpler system to investigate such changes. Auditory fear conditioning induces LTP-like enhancement of synaptic transmission in cortical input to the principal neurons of the amygdala that both mimic and occlude LTP in acute slice induced with electrical stimulation, thus providing a simple linkage between changes of synaptic strength and behavior in auditory fear conditioning (Tsvetkov et al., 2002). The conservation of the anatomy and physiology of the amygdala between species allows studies in different animals to get potential implications for fear memory and associated disorders in human.

In the rat, one of the most important researches is the finding that auditory fear conditioning is linked to the persistent strength at glutamatergic synapse in both thalamic and cortical inputs to the principal cell of the amygdala (Rogan et al., 1997; McKernan & Shinnick-Gallagher, 1997).

It has been widely accepted that LTP in the amygdala is the basic factor in fear conditioning and better understanding mechanism for LTP will leads the mechanism for fear conditioning (Sah et al., 2008).

The aim of this chapter is to improve our understanding of cellular mechanism, in particular, synaptic mechanism underlying fear memory and permit rational development of better therapeutic treatments for PTSD and other anxiety disorders. We will focus on the lateral nucleus of amygdala (LA) because molecular and synaptic changes in this area have been shown to make essential contributions to the fear memory formation, storage, and expression of the learned fear (LeDoux, 1998).

To get a better understanding synaptic mechanism underlying the learned fear, we firstly will review auditory fear conditioning in detail and the basic anatomy and properties of synaptic transmission of the LA. Secondly we will summarize the molecular mechanisms that contribute to synaptic plasticity in the auditory fear conditioning.

Although neutral and aversive information enters via both thalamic and cortical inputs to the LA, the individual role of both inputs are still debated. Moreover there are a lot of studies about pre- and postsynaptic modifications in the induction and expression of LTP during auditory fear conditioning (Shin et al., 2010; Rumpel et al., 2005).

However, the specific roles of both modifications remain elusive.

Finally we review recent studies and discuss the two questions above.

2. The involvement of the amygdala in the learned fear

The most detailed behavioral studies from bilateral lesion of the primate temporal lobe suggest that the temporal lobe including amygadala is involved in processing emotion (Klüver & Bucy, 1937). In this study, monkeys with bilateral temporal lobe lesions tried to eat inedible objects, to copulate with same-sex partners or even with other species, and lost their fear of snakes. The key feature of this phenomenon, called psychic blindness by Klüver and Bucy (1937), was seemed to lose their emotional implications despite their fine visual perception. In experiment using functional magnetic resonance imaging, human amygdalae was preferentially activated by emotional stimuli such as fearful faces (Breiter et al. 1996). These reports suggested that the amygdala plays an important role on processing emotion in response to aversive stimulus.

In rodent experiment, anatomical tracing and lesion studies indicated the importance of the LA for encoding fear memory. In particular, bilateral infusion of N-methyl-D-aspartate (NMDA) receptor antagonist, D-2-amino-5-phosphonovaleric acid (D-AP5) into the rat LA decreased the amount of the learned fear (Miserendino et al., 1990). This result suggests two possibilities: the first is that we can confirm that the amygdala is the very important region which fear memory could be stored. The second is that NMDA receptor-dependent plasticity change can occur in the amygdala during fear memory formation. In 1996, two teams indicated that auditory fear conditioning is associated with persistent synaptic enhancement in auditory inputs to the LA: Rogan et al (1997) have shown the enhancement of evoked field potential in the LA of the conditioned rat in using *in vivo* recording; McKernan and Shinnick-Gallagher (1997) have reported that the probability of synaptic transmitter release in thalamic input to the principal neurons was increased in the acute slice prepared from the conditioned rat. Moreover, fear conditioning induced LTP-like enhancement of synaptic transmission in auditory input to the LA the occlude NMDA receptor-dependent LTP in acute slice induced by electrical stimulation (Tsvetkov et al., 2002). In addition, gastrin-releasin peptide suppressed NMDA receptor-dependent LTP induction by the enhanced excitability of local inhibitory interneuron, result in the decreased fear memory (Shumyatsky et al., 2002). These reports demonstrat that neural activity by NMDA receptor activation in the LA is involved in the encoding of fear memory.

Recently, Cho et al (2012) have been shown that the kainite receptor-dependent LTP was occluded in the slice of the conditioned rat and infusion of kainite receptor blockade into the LA attenuated auditory fear conditioning, indicating that the kainite receptor in the LA is essential to auditory fear conditioning by investigating LTP induction and behavioural experiments.

Overall neural activity induced by glutamatergic receptor activation in the LA can promote the encoding of fear memory, therefore, we review the relationship between excitability of the LA and fear memory in the following subchapters.

3. The animal model of fear memory: Auditory fear condtioning

Behavior related to fear could be relatively described in human; we can easily notice the fear from human face expression, however, it is very difficult to achieve when it concerns experimental animal. To assess the quantity of learned fear, a simpler behavioral method is required. Auditory fear conditioning provides an animal model that is commonly used to study associative learning, such as fear conditioning.

In the rat, fear conditioning learning consists to the presentation of an initially biologically insignificant conditioned neutral stimulus (CS; for example an auditory sound) that is paired with the presentation of an unconditioned aversive stimulus (US; for example an electric footshock). During conditioning, neutral stimulus to experimental animal is paired with an aversive stimulus. Following a single or a few such pairing, the neutral stimulus elicits a defensive response as if he is threatened by an aversive stimulus. Lesions of the amygdala disrupt both the acquisition and expression of fear conditioning. As subsequent presentation of the CS without the US elicits, in the conditioned animal, defensive behavioral responses (freezing responses), autonomic nervous system responses (change in blood pressure and heart rate) and neuroendocrine responses (release of hormones from the pituitary and adrenal glands). This simple form of learning is exceptionally robust and rapidly acquired, as it can be achieved as quickly as after a couple of trials (LeDoux, 1998; Whilensky et al., 2000; Repa et al., 2001). Some of these defensive responses are genetically determined: animals are innate species-specific responses to threats and express defensive responses automatically despite appropriate stimuli. In fear conditioning, therefore, when the CS is used as an initially biological insignificant stimulus, such as sound, light or touch, experimental animals can show learned "fear" that had never occurred in response to the neutral CS.

In the laboratory, the experimental cage for fear conditioning, equipped with stainless-steel shocking grids and a sound making apparatus, is placed in a sound-attenuating enclosure. On the training day the animal is placed in the chamber for a couple of minutes (habituation: Figure 1A) before the onset of the CS, auditory cue that is co-terminated with the US, footshock (fear conditioning: Figure 1B), and returns to its home cages after several CS-US pairings (paired group: Figure 1D). For unpaired control group (Figure 1E), animal receives tones and footshocks in an unpaired manner (tones and footshock are separated by random intervals of some minutes). During the test 24-72 hours after training, animals are placed in a novel cage in which the tone that had been presented during training is given after habituation period. Freezing scores are calculated as the fraction (percentage) of the total CS duration in which the animal remained immobile (Frozen) (Figure 1C).

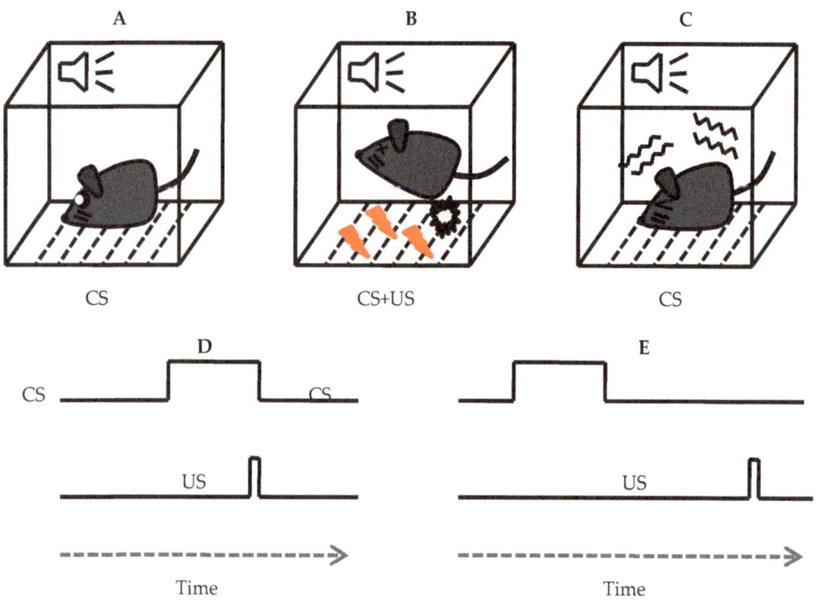

Figure 1. Auditory fear conditioning in rats.

The CS, only a single sensory modality or cue such as audible sound, light, smell or touch, can be unimodal. It is well established that unimodal (cued) fear conditioning is dependent on the amygdala but not the hippocampus by the results of behavioral studies utilizing pharmacological inactivation of the amygdala (Marea et al., 2001; Fanselow & LeDoux, 1999).

However, animals also exhibits fear response in the absence of CS when returned to the chamber in which the tone and footshock were paired or unpaired. This is called multimodal (contextual) fear conditioning and requires both the hippocampus and the amygdala (Dityatev & Bolshakov, 2005).

In a typical auditory fear conditioning procedure, rats are habituated to the chamber with the US (auditory sound) (A). During fear conditioning (B), the electric footshock (US) is paired with an auditory sound several times. The sound is presented alone in the test session to estimate the effects of conditioning (C). To assess the amount of learned fear, most researcher measure the time of "freezing" behavior elicited by the auditory sound alone. During fear conditioning, an auditory sound is co-terminated with a footshock (D: paired group). An unpaired group in which the auditory sound and electric footshock in a nonoverlapping manner (E).

4. The neural circuit of auditory fear memory

Recent studies indicate that some cortices are involved in fear memory formation during auditory fear conditioning; the disinhibition of pyramidal neurons of the auditory cortex is required for auditory fear conditioning (Letzkus et al., 2011); auditory fear memory is stored in the secondary auditory cortex in cue-specific manner (Sacco & Sacchetti, 2010).

The preceding section gives us a general scheme and better understanding for the neural circuit between the amygdala complex and other brain regions and /or within the amygdala complex in the acquisition of fear memory. Here, this section will summarize the neuronal network about the flow of CS (auditory sound) and US (electric footshock).

Anatomical tracing studies combined with single unit recording in experimental animals suggest that the LA is a site of convergence of somatosensory input carrying the information relative to the footshock US and afferent inputs carrying the CS information (whatever the sensory modality) (Pitkanen et al., 1997). Therefore, it has been suggested that the LA is the site, where the association of learned information about CS and US apparently occurs during fear conditioning (Fanselow & LeDoux, 1999).

During auditory fear conditioning, the sensory information that mediates the CS (an audible cue), reaches the LA by the two pathways, both of which are essential to the learned fear (Romanski & LeDoux, 1992). One input, consisting of the direct thalamo-amygdala projections, originates in the medial division of the thalamic medial geniclulate nucleus (MGm) and in the posterior intralaminar nucleus (PIN) of the thalamus (Dityatev & Bolshakov, 2005; Figure 2). The second input, the indirect cortico-amygdala projections, extends from the ventral division of the thalamic medial geniclulate nucleus (MGv) to the auditory cortex (TE) and includes further projections that relay the auditory information from the cortex to the LA (Maren, 2001). The LA is neither highly laminar structure nor homogenous: the LA is composed of at least three subnuclei: the dorsolateral (LAd), ventrolateral (LAvl), and medial division (LAm) (Pitkanen et al., 1997). Because auditory-evoked responses recorded in the different parts of the amygdala were the shortest in the LAd, it has been suggested that this part of the amygdala constitutes the entrance site to the fear conditioning (Bordi & LeDoux, 1992). After the information is processed in the LA, the final signals are sent to periaqueductal gary and brain stem via the central nucleu of the amygdala (CE), resulting in freezing, autonomic responses and release of stress hormones as the index of fear expression.

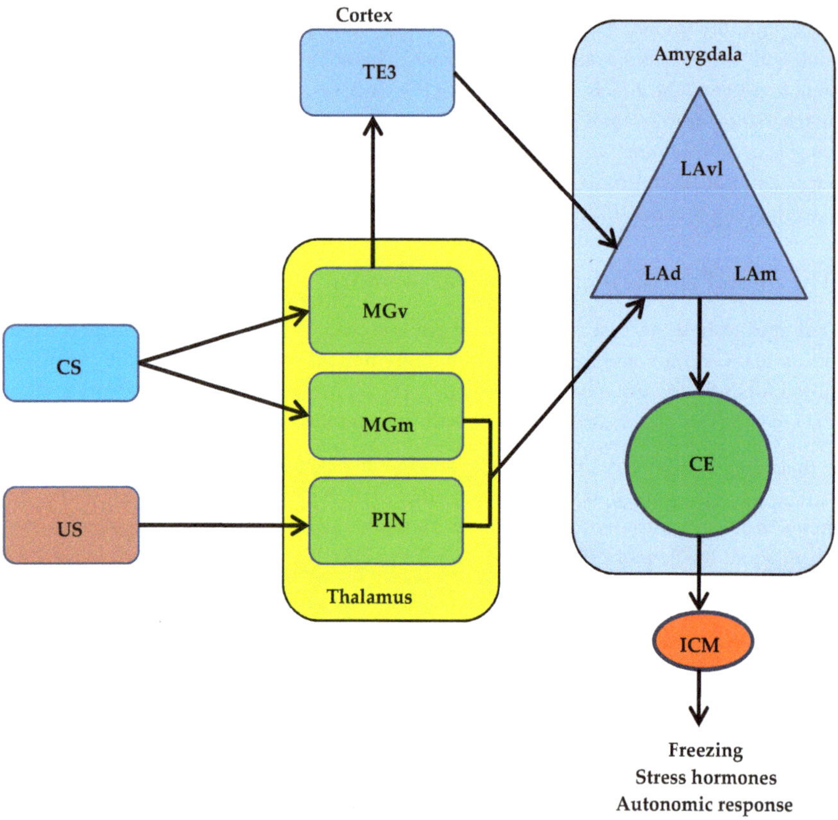

Figure 2. Auditory fear conditioning circuit

The CS (auditory sound) enters the LA directly via MGm and indirectly via MGm and TE.

The US (electric footshock) enters the LA via PIN. Convergence of CS and US enter in the LA, especially in the LAd, leading to synaptic plasticity. These signal processed in the LA projects to CE. The LA connects with CE directly and indirectly by way of other nucleus, such as ICM. Finally CE promotes some defensive responses, freezing, increased blood pressure and heart rate as the expression of conditioned fear by trigger of hypothalamic and brainstem areas. Abbreviation: LAd, LAvl,LAm: the dorsolateral, ventrolateral and medial division of the LA. MGv, MGm: the ventral and medial division of the thalamic medial geniclulate nucleus. PIN: the posterior intralaminar nucleus of the thalamus.ICM: intercalated cell masses. TE: the auditory cortex, CE: the central nucleus of the amygdala

5. The electrophysiological properties of the LA

We are just beginning to explore the properties of basic synaptic physiology in the LA for synaptic mechanism underling fear conditioning because the LA is the site where the CS and the US information convey and encoding fear memory is formed (LeDoux et al., 1990). LeDoux et al (1990) has reported that bilateral lesion of the LA impaired fear conditioning.

It is necessary to characterize the properties of neuron typing, excitatory and inhibitory synapse and neural network involving distinct types of neurons. I will describe the rules governing and modulation of synaptic plasticity in the next subchapter 6.

The whole-cell patch-clamp technique has widely been used to explore the synaptic character in the amygdala because the LA is not highly laminar, making field potential observations difficult.

5.1. Diversity of cell types dependent on electrophysiological classification

On the basis of neuronal morphology and chemical analysis, the LA contains two main cell types: (1) pyramidal-like shape projection neurons (principal neurons), which use glutamate as neurotransmitter, form the majority of the constituent neurons, and (2) non-pyramidal neurons, observed in far fewer numbers, function primarily as local inhibitory circuit by releasing γ-aminobutyric acid (GABA) (Shin et al., 2006; Faber et al., 2001).

In slice preparation, the cells are readily identifiable as principal neurons with the pyramidal shape of their soma and the ability to show spike frequency accommodation in response to prolonged current injections by using patch-clamp method (Figure 3A; Shin et al., 2006; Tsvetkov et al., 2002; Mahanty & Sah. 1998). In contrast, intenurons are identified as non-accommodation pattern, which show spiking at regular intervals for the duration of the depolarization and increasing spike frequency with increasing depolarization (Figure 3B; Shin et al., 2006; Mahanty & Sah. 1998).

The dendrites of interneruons of the LA lack spines and pyramidal neurons exhibit dendritic arbors without spatial polarization (Faber et al., 2001). By fine investigation of *in vitro* two-photon microscopy, the size of dendritic spines contacted by thalamic, with the ability large Ca^{2+} transients during action potential backpropagation, was larger than that by cortical input to the principal cell of the LA. This thalamic spine could induce Hebbian plasticity by activation of R-type voltage-dependent Ca^{2+} channel in input–specific manner (Humeau et al., 2005).

Recent report has demonstrated that fear conditioning increases the rate of spin elimination of layer-V pyramidal neurons of the mouse frontal association cortex connected to the LA using *in vivo* transcranial two-photon microscopy, indicating that fear conditioning can promote modification of fear conditioning-related neural circuit. (Lai et al, 2012).

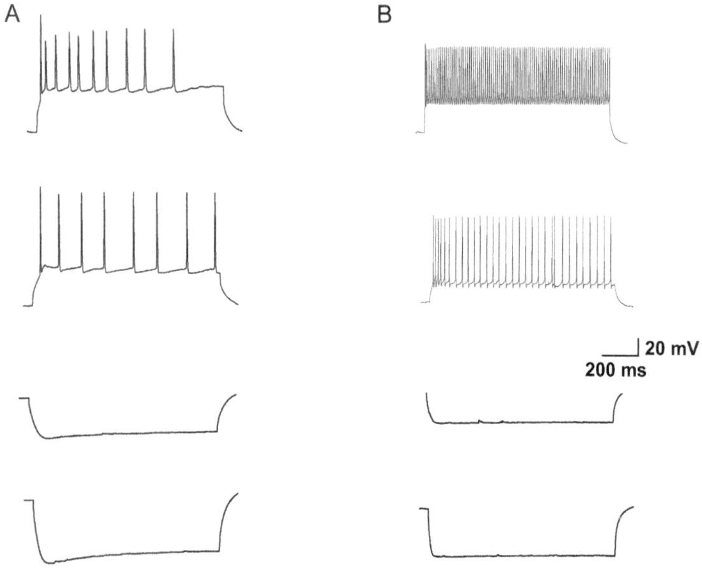

Figure 3. Membrane physiological characters of two representative cells of the LA. Typical firing patterns of the two neurons recorded under current-clamp mode in response to increasing current injection steps. The accommodation neuron (A) showed fewer action potentials per depolarization. By contrast, the nonaccommodation neuron (B) showed spiking at regular intervals for the duration of the depolarization and their spiking frequency was increased with the effect of depolarization.

5.2. Diversity in synaptic transmission: electrophysiological properties of LA neurons

5.2.1. Excitatory transmission

The early *in vitro* whole studies about excitatory and inhibitory synaptic transmission in the amygdala had done (Rainnie et al., 1991a, b). The afferent projections from thalamic nucleus or auditory cortex to the LA form excitatory synapses on both principal neurons and inhibitory interneurons (Rainnie et al., 1991a, b). The studies by using intracellular recording from rat acute slice indicated that postsynaptic potentials elicited stimulation of the LA is composed of excitatory postsynaptic potentials (EPSPs) followed by either a fast inhibitory postsynaptic potential (f-IPSP) only, or by a fast- and subsequent slow-IPSP (s-IPSP). The EPSPs at the resting membrane potential consisted of dual fast and slow, components. The f-EPSPs increased in amplitude with membrane hyperpolarization and was insensitive to the NMDA receptor antagonist, D-AP5, but was blocked non-NMDA receptor antagonist, 6-cyano-7-nitro-quinoxaline-2, 3-dione (CNQX). In contrast, the slow-EPSPs decreased with membrane hyperpolarization, were blocked APV but were insensitive to the CNQX receptor antagonist, indicating that slow-EPSPs are mediated by NMDA receptor activation (Rainnie et al., 1991a).

The stimulation of the cortical (auditory cortex) and thalamic (thalamus) afferent inputs that convey auditory information related to the CS during auditory fear conditioning induces synaptic response in principal neuron in the LA. In the presence of $GABA_A$ receptor antagonist, picrotoxin (PTX), such stimulation evokes a monosynaptic EPSP or excitatory postsynaptic currents (EPSC) with a short and constant latency in recorded cell in current- or voltage clamp mode at resting membrane potential (almost -70 mV) in brain slice (Shin et al., 2010, 2006; Kodirov et al., 2006; Shumyatsky et al., 2005, 2002; Tsvetkov et al., 2004, 2002; Weisskopf & LeDoux, 1999b). EPSC recorded by stimulation at either thalamic or cortical input was abolished by α- amino-3-hydroxy-5-methyl-4-isoxazole propionic acid (AMPA) receptor antagonist, CNQX, thus suggesting that EPSCs recorded in thalamic or cortical inputs are mediated by AMPA receptor (Tsvetkov et al., 2002; Weisskopf & LeDoux, 1999b).

Moreover, fine electrophysiological studies indicated that the glutamatergic input from both cortical and thalamic to principal cell of the LA do not differ in either their basal probability or quantal amplitude (Shin et al., 2006). Plus, both inputs do not overlap (Tsvetkov et al., 2004), indicating that both cortical and thalamic input to the LA are independent from each other. It has been reported that the vesicular Zn^{2+} released from cortical, but not thalamic afferents, to the principal cell of the LA can induce NMDA receptor-dependent LTP (Kodirov et al., 2006).

Some studies have been demonstrated that NMDA receptor-mediated components were identified in both thalamic and cortical afferent inputs to the principal neurons in the LA (Shin et al., 2006; Shumyatsky et al., 2005; Tsvetkov et al., 2004, 2002; Weisskopf & LeDoux, 1999b), and the NMDA receptors in both inputs play the important role on the induction of LTP (Shin et al., 2006; Tsvetkov et al., 2004, 2002).

NMDA receptor are also functionally expressed at both cortico- and thalamo- LA synapses becomes evident at membrane depolarization. NMDA receptors in the LA are represented by a complex of NR1, NR2A and NR2B subunits. Pharmacological studies using the selective NR2A antagonist ifenprodil and the NR2A antagonist NVP-AAM077 have indicated that subunit composition of synaptic NMDA receptors in cortical input is not different from that in thalamic pathway (Shin et al., 2006). However, there are distinct subsets mediated by NMDA receptor in thalamic input versus cortical input to the LA on the basis of voltage and Mg^{2+} sensitivity (Weisskopf & LeDoux, 1999b).

In contrast to pyramidal neuron, glutamatergic inputs to interneurons of the LA may not contain NMDA receptor (Mahanty & Sah. 1998). Synaptic response mediated by AMPA receptors in interneurons show inward rectification and sensitivity to external polyamines, indicating that GluR2 subunit-lacking AMPA receptor is permeable to Ca^{2+}.

5.2.2. *Inhibitory transmission*

As described above, Rainnie et al (1991a) showed that the EPSPs recorded in the LA are, followed by both fast- and slow-IPSPs. Both IPSPs were reduced the presence of APV, and were abolished by CNQX, indicating that both IPSPs were mediated by multi-synapse pathways. The CNQX-resistant fast-IPSPs were abolished by bicuculline methiodide, $GABA_A$ receptor antagonist, suggesting direct inhibition by local GABAegic circuit. The slow-IPSP, which reversal potential is deeper (-95 mV), was depressed by 2-hydroxy-saclofen, $GABA_B$ receptor antagonist (Rainnie et al., 1991b).

The afferent projections from thalamic nucleus or auditory cortex to the LA form excitatory synapses on both principal neurons and inhibitory interneurons (Rainnie et al., 1991a, b). The inhibitory interneurons send inhibitory inputs to principal neurons and other interneurons and their feedback and feed-forward GABAergic inputs to principal neurons determine how the information conveying to principal neurons are processed (Wang et al., 2001).

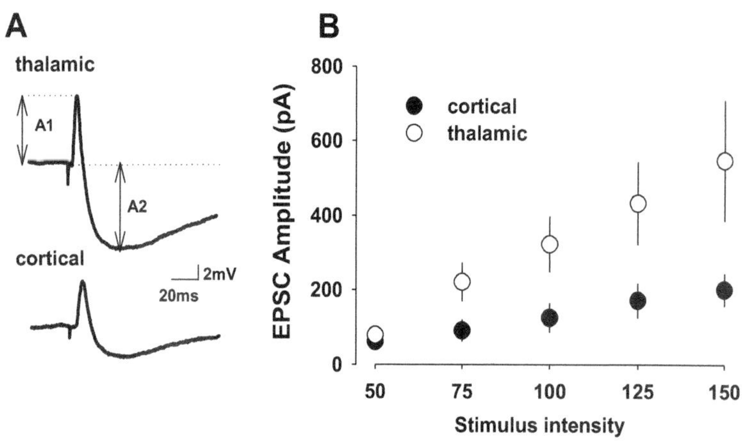

Figure 4. Feedfoward GABA receptor-mediated inhibition of principal neuron is stronger in thalamic input. (A) Examples of the EPSP/IPSP sequences recorded at a membrane potential of -55 mV in convergent cortical and thalamic pathways. (B) Input-output curves for the AMPA receptor-mediated EPSC recorded in interneurons at holding potential of -70 mV in the presence of $GABA_A$ receptor antagonist, PTX at convergent cortical and thalamic pathways. Reproduced with permission from Shin et al (Shin et al., 2006).

In Figure 4A, the EPSP/IPSP sequences elicited by both inputs to the same neuron display both monosynaptic glutamatergic EPSP (A1) and disynaptic GABAergic IPSP (A2). The ratios of each EPSP and IPSP amplitude (A2/A1) were enhanced in thalamic input when compared with cortical input. Strengthening of AMPA receptor-mediated inputs to interneurons leads to increased inhibition in principal cells in the LA (Mahanty & Sah, 1998). This suggests the possibility that input-specific differences in excitatory inputs to interneuron result in different inhibitory drives in individual pathway. In Figure 4B, the glutamatergic synaptic efficacies at convergent inputs (both thalamic and cortical input) to same interneuron were compared by analyzing two input-output curves of EPSCs. A leftward shift in the input-output curves obtained in thalamic input, as compared with those in cortical pathway was observed (Figure 4B). These results indicate the stronger inhibitory drive in thalamic pathway, as compared to cortical input.

6. Synaptic mechanism for fear memory

The hypothesis that NMDA-dependent LTP is involved in the cellular mechanism underlying fear conditioning arose initially from the finding that blockade of NMDA receptor within the LA decreased the amount of learned fear (Miserendino et al., 1990). Behavioral study combined with electrophysiological investigation showed that learned fear produced a persistent enhanced synaptic strength by both cortico- and thlamo-amygdala pathways (Tsvetkov et al., 2002; McKernan & Shinnick-Gallagher, 1997; Rogan et al., 1997). These synaptic modifications, observed along behavioural responses of learned fear, are mechanically similar to LTP induced artificially by electrical stimulation in acute slices of the LA. The NMDA receptor-dependent LTP induced by a pairing protocol (low-frequency presynaptic stimulation with postsynaptic depolarization) in the cortico-amygdala pathway was occluded in the acute slice of the conditioned rat (Tsvetkov et al., 2002). This result indicated that the NMDA receptors in the cortico-amygdala synapse are critical for fear conditioning. LTP induced by pairing protocol in the both the cortico- and thalmo-amygdala synapses required NMDA receptor activation (Shin et al., 2006). Other studies found that the LTP induced by a pairing protocol depended on both postsynaptic NMDA receptor and L-type voltage–dependent calcium channels (Tsvetkov et al., 2002; Weisskopf & LeDoux, 1999b; Huang & Kandel, 1998).

The NMDA receptor-mediated response in both cortical and thalamic input to principal cells is dependent on the NR1, NR2A and NR2B subunits. Despite the fact that NMDA receptor response in both inputs were largely mediated by NR2A-containing receptors (almost 75%), the blockade of NR2B subunit abolished pairing induced LTP in the LA (Shin et al., 2006). In addition, injection of NR2B subunit antagonist into the LA reduced the acquisition of fear conditioning without affecting expression of fear memories or basal synaptic transmission (Rodrigues et al., 2001). However, the activation of NMDA receptors in the LA following high frequency thalamic input stimulation is not necessary for the induction LTP (Weisskopf & LeDoux, 1999a).

By contrast, it has been shown that Ca^{2+} influx into interneurons resulting from the activation of AMPA receptor lacking GluR2 subunit may be implicated in the plasticity induction in the thalamic input (external capsule) to the amygdala interneuron (Mahanty & Sah, 1998).

In vivo electrophysiological recording of principal cells in the LA display unusually low firing pattern even during emotional arousal (Pare & Collins, 2000), providing that local GABAergic interneuron circuit`s tight inhibitory control on the excitability of principal neurons in the LA. Therefore, it is thought that LTP in the LA is significantly diminished when pairing protocol is delivered in the absence of $GABA_A$ receptor antagonist. However, by using a pairing protocol in the absence of PTX, ($GABA_A$ receptor antagonist), a cortical input stimulation was able to induce LTP in the principal cell of the LA, probably because the inhibitory circuits activated by the cortical inputs are weaker, as compared with thalamic input (Shin et al, 2006; Figure 5; see 5.2.2 Inhibitory transmission). Other electrophysiological studies have shown that norepinephrine and dopamine gate the LTP induction in the thalamo-amygdala synapse by suppressing excitability of feedforward GABAergic circuit in thalamic input to the LA (Tully et al., 2007; Bissiere et al., 2003). Moreover, Hu et al (2007) have reported that emotion can enhance memory via norepinephrine regulation AMPA receptor trafficking into glutamatergic synapse. In addition, the highly expressed gastrin-releasin peptide in the LA suppressed both the fear conditioning responses and the magnitude of LTP recorded in cortical input. This effect being probably due to an enhancement of the excitability of feedforward GABAergic circuit related to the cortical input (Shin et al., 2006; Shumyatsky et al., 2002).

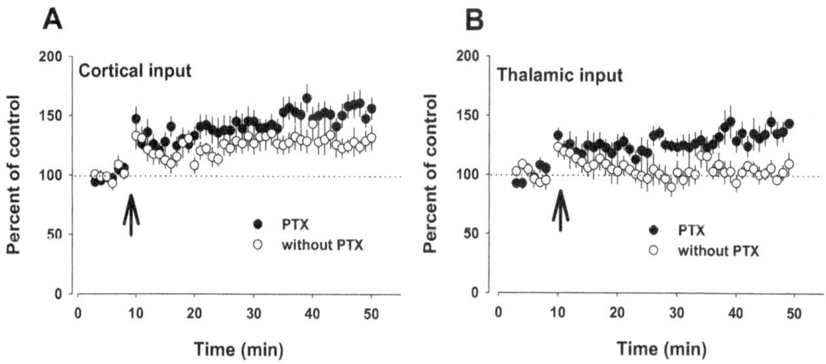

Figure 5. Pairing protocol induced LTP at the cortico-amygdala and thalamo-amygdal synapses. The graphs represent electrophysiological recordings of the LTP observed in cortical (A) and thalamic (B) inputs in the presence of PTX and without PTX. Reproduced with permission from Shin et al (Shin et al., 2006).

Most researchers have focused on postsynaptic modifications that occur in the principal cell of the LA during fear conditioning. However, some evidences also provided that presynaptic molecular alterations are important for encoding fear (Cho et al., 2012; Shin et al., 2010; Humeau et al., 2003; Tsvetkov et al., 2002; Pan et al, 2008; McKernan & Shinnick-Gallagher, 1997). Although the persistent increased synaptic strength in both thalamic and cortical inputs to the LA contributed to fear conditioning, the specific roles of both inputs are still debated. *In vivo* study revealed that the increased potential of the LA by stimulation of the auditory thalamus was observed, indicating that projections from the auditory thalamus to the LA are critical for auditory fear conditioning (Clugnet & LeDoux, 1990). According to this, it has been shown that the thalamic, but not cortical input to the LA, is essential for fear conditioning by using genetic methods (Humeau et al., 2007; Rumpel et al., 2005). In addition, rapid plasticity change occurred in the auditory thalamus rather than the auditory cortex during fear conditioning (Quirk et al., 1997). In contrast, some lesion studies have shown that either pathway alone is sufficient for auditory fear conditioning; the lesion of one of them being ineffective to disrupt learning of conditioned auditory fear (Romanski & LeDoux, 1992). Also, post-training lesion of cortical, but not thalamic input to the LA, abolished the learned fear, indicating that cortical input may be a dominant role in fear conditioning in intact brain (Campeau & Davis, 1997). Finally, combination of *in vivo* and *in vitro* studies has revealed that synaptic plasticity in cortical input was essential for fear conditioning (Cho et al., 2012; Tsvetkov et al., 2002). It has been reported that presynaptic GABA$_B$ receptor in the LA prevented the generalization of the learned fear via the regulation of LTP in cortical, but not thalamic input to the LA, by using genetic deletion technique (Shaban et al., 2006). Further, presynaptic GABA$_B$ receptor was also reported to suppress LTP in cortical input to the principal cell of the LA via the control of glutamate release in acute slice experiment (Pan et al., 2009).

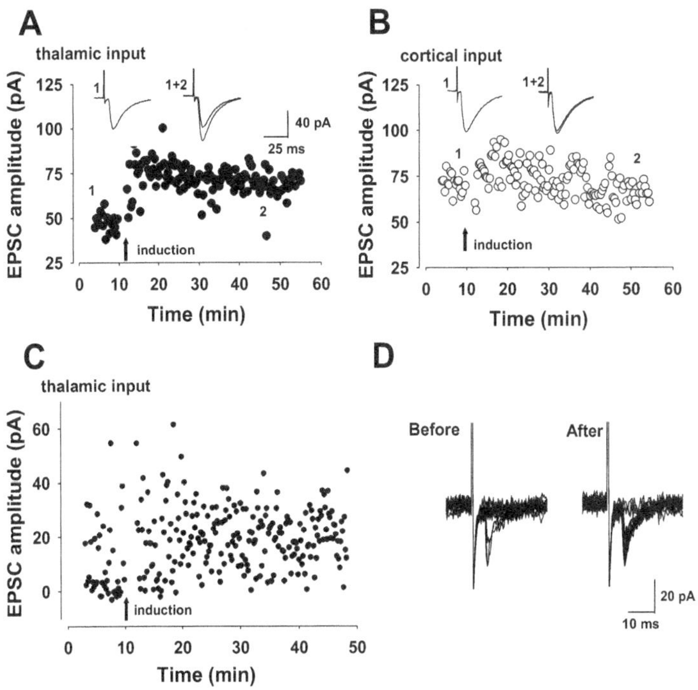

Figure 6. Properties of presynaptic form of LTP in thalamic input to the LA. LTP in thalamic input to the LA was induced by the presynaptic stimulation without postsynaptic depolarization (A). The same protocol did not induce LTP in cortical input (B). The course of LTP in thalamic input experiment by using unitary EPSAC recording (C). (D) Superimposed individual EPSCs before and after LTP experiment (C). Reproduced with permission from Shin et al (Shin et al., 2006).

Recently it has been found that LTP in thalamic, but not cortical input to the pyramidal neuron of the LA, expressed presynaptically, was resulted from low-frequency presynaptic stimulation in the absence of postsynaptic depolarization (Shin et al., 2010; Figure 6). In Figure 6C, D, same protocol above produced the increased probability of neurotransmitter release of glutamate in thalamic input to the LA in unitary recording, indicating that an expression of this LTP, observed in thalamic input alone, was presynaptic. Overall these studies revealed the possibility that each of the thalamic and cortical inputs may have distinct function in fear conditioning but their specific roles remain to be demonstrated.

7. Conclusion

Basic synaptic mechanisms in the amygdala that support auditory fear processes are now commonly known. However, in the light of recent findings some important questions remain to be answered. First: between the thalamic and cortical inputs, which is the afferent that control auditory fear conditioning? Second: Is it the pre- or postsynaptic modification of the induction and expression of LTP that is important during fear conditioning? I hope that young people or student will throw themselves into the research of fear conditioning.

Author details

Ryong-Moon Shin
National Institute of Radiological Sciences, Japan

8. References

Bissiere, S. Humeau, Y. & Lüthi, A. (2003). Dopamine gates LTP induction in lateral amygdala by suppressing feedforward inhibition. *Nature Neuroscience* 6, 587-592.

Bordi, F. & LeDoux, J.E. (1992). Sensory tuning beyond the sensory system: an initial analysis of auditory response properties of neurons in the lateral amygdaloid nucleus and overlying areas of the striatum. *Journal of Neuroscience* 12, 2493-2503.

Breiter, H.C. Etcoff, N.L. Whalen, P.J. Kennedy, W.A. Rauch, S.L. Buckner, R.L. Strauss, M.M. Hyman, S.E. Bruce, R. & Rosen, B.R. (1996). Response and Habituation of the Human amygdala during visual processing of facial expression. *Neuron* 17, 875-887.

Campeau, S. & Davis, M. (1995). Involvement of subcortical and cortical afferents to the lateral nucleus of the amygdala in fear conditioning measured with fear- potentiated startle in rats trained concurrently with auditory and visual conditioned stimuli. *Journal of Neuroscience* 15, 2312-2327.

Cho, J.H., Bayazitov, I.T., Meloni, E.G. Myers, K.M. Carlezon, W.A. Zakharenko, S.S. & Bolshakov, V.Y. (2012). Coactivation of thalamic and cortical pathways induces input timing-dependent plasticity in amygdala. *Nature Neuroscience* 15, 113-122.

Clugnet, M.C. & LeDoux , J.E. (1990). Synaptic plasticity in fear conditioning circuits: induction of LTP in the lateral nucleus of the amygdala by stimulation of the medial geniculate body. *Journal of Neuroscience* 10, 2818-2824.

Dityatev, A.E. & Bolshakov, V.Y. (2005). Amygadala, long-term potentiation, and fear conditioning. *Neuroscientist* 11, 75-88.

Faber, E.S. Callister, R.J. & Sah, P. (2001). Morphological and electrophysiological properties of principal neurons in the rat lateral amygdala in vitro. *Journal of Neurophysiology* 85, 714-723.

Fanselow, M.S. & LeDoux, J.E. (1999). Why we think plasticity underlying Pavlovian fear conditioning occurs in the basolateral amygdala. *Neuron* 23, 229-232.

Huang, Y.Y. & Kandel, E.R. (1998). Postsynaptic induction and PKA-dependent expression of LTP in the lateral amygdala. *Neuron* 21, 169-178.

Hu, H. Real, E. Takamiya, K. Kang, M. G. LeDoux, J. E. Hugani, R.L. & Malinow, R. (2007). Emotion Enhances Learning via Norepinephrine Regulation of AMPA-Receptor Trafficking. *Cell* 131, 160-173.

Humeau,Y. Reisel, D. Johnson , A. W. Borchardt, T. Jensen, V. Gebhardt, C. Bosch, V. Gass, P. Bannerman, D. M. Good, M. A. Hvalby, Ø. Sprengel, R. & Lüthi, A. (2007). A pathway- specific function for different AMPA receptor subunits in amygdala long-term potentiation and fear conditioning. *Journal of Neuroscience* 27, 10947-10956.

Humeau,Y. Herry, C. Kemp, N. Shaban, H. Fourcaudot, E. Bissiere, S. & Lüthi, A. (2005). Dendrite spine heterogeneity determines afferent-specific Hebbian plasticity in the amygdala. *Neuron* 45, 119-131.

Humeau,Y. Shaban, H. Bissiere, S. & Lüthi, A. (2003). Presynaptic induction of heterosynaptic associative plasticity in the mammalian brain. *Nature* 426, 841-845.

Klüver, H. & Bucy, P.C. (1937). Psychic blindness` and other symptoms following bilateral temporal lobectomy in rhesus monkeys. *American Journal of Physiology* 119, 352-353.

Kodirov, S.A. Takizawa, K. Joseph, J. Kandel, E.R. Shumyatsky, G.P. & Bolshakov, V.Y. (2006). Synaptically released zinc gates long-term potentiation in fear conditioning pathways. *PNAS* 103, 15218-15223.

LeDoux, J.E. Cicchetti, P. Xagoraris, A. & Romanski, L. M. (1990). The lateral amygdaloid nucleus: sensory interface of the amygdala in fear conditioning. *Journal of Neuroscience* 10, 1062-1069.

LeDoux, J.E. (1998). Fear and the brain: where have we been, and where are we going? *Biologcail Psychiatry,* 44, 1229-1238.

Lai, C.S. Franke, T.F. & Gan, W.B. (2012). Opposite effects of fear conditioning and extinction on dendritic spine remodelling. *Nature* 483, 87-91.

Letzkus, J.J. Wolff, S. B.E. Meyer, E. M. M. Tovote, P. Courtin. J. Herry, C, & Lüthi, A. (2011). A disinhibitory microcircuit for associative fear learning in the auditory cortex. *Nature* 480, 331-335.

Mahanty, N.K. & Sah, P. (1998). Calcium-permeable AMPA receptors mediate long-term potentiation in interneurons in the amygdala. *Nature* 394, 683-687.

Maren. S. (2001). Is There Savings for Pavlovian Fear Conditioning after Neurotoxic Basolateral Amygdala Lesions in Rats? Neurobiology of Learning and Memory 76, 268-283.

McKernan, M.G. & Shinnick-Gallagher, P. (1997). Fear conditioning induces a lasting potentiation of synaptic currents in vitro. *Nature* 390, 607-611.

Miserendino, M. J. Sanaes, C.B. Melia, K. R. & Davis, M. (1990). Blocking of acquisition but not expression of conditioned fear-potentiated startle by NMDA antagonists in the amygdale. *Nature 345*, 716-718.

Pan, B. X, Dong, Y. Ito, W. Yanagawa, Y. Shigemoto, R. & Morozov A. (2009). Selective gating of glutamatergic inputs to excitatory neurons of amygdala by presynaptic GABAb receptor. *Neuron* 61, 917-929.

Pan, B. X, Vautier, F. Ito, W. Yanagawa, Y. Bolshakov, V.Y. & Morozov A. (2008). Enhanced cortico-amygdala efficary and suppressed fear in absence of Rap 1. *Journal of Neuroscience* 28, 2089-2098.

Pare, D. & Collins, D. R. (2000). Neuronal Correlates of Fear in the Lateral Amygdala: Multiple Extracellular Recordings in Conscious Cats. *Journal of Neuroscience* 20, 2701-2710.

Pitkanen, A. Savander, V. & LeDoux, J.E. (1997). Organization of intraanygdaloid circuitries in the rat: an emerging framework for understanding function of the amygdala. *Trends in Neurosciences* 20, 517-523.

Quirk, G.J. Armony, J.L. & LeDoux, J.E. (1997). Fear Conditioning Enhances Different Temporal Components of Tone-Evoked Spike Trains in Auditory Cortex and Lateral Amygdala. *Neuron* 19, 613-624.

Rainnie, D.G. Asprodini, E.K. & Shinnick-Gallagher P. (1991a). Excitatory transmission in the basolateral amygdala. *Journal of Neurophysiology* 66, 986-998.

Rainnie, D.G. Asprodini, E.K. & Shinnick-Gallagher P. (1991b). Inhibitory transmission in the basolateral amygdala. *Journal of Neurophysiology* 66, 999-1009.

Repe, J.C. Muller, J. Apergi, S.J. Desrochers, T.M. Zhou, Y. & LeDoux, J.E. (2001). Two different lateral amygdala cell populations contribute to the initation and storage of memory. *Nature Neuroscience* 4, 724-731.

Rumpel, S. LeDoux, J. E. Zador, A. & Malinow, R. (2005). Postsynaptic receptor trafficking underlying a form of associative learning. *Science* 308, 83-88.

Rogan, M.T. Stäubli, U.V. & LeDoux, J.E. (1997). Fear conditioning induces associative long-term potentiation in the amygdale. *Nature 390*, 604-607.

Rodrigues, S.M. Schafe, G.E. & LeDoux, J.E. (2001). Intra-amygdala blockade of the NR2B subunit of the NMDA receptor disrupts the acquisition but not the expression of fear conditioning. *Journal of Neuroscience* 21, 6889-6896.

Romanski, L.E. & LeDoux, J.E. (1992). Equipotentiality of thalamo-amygdala and thalamo - cortico-amygdala circuits in auditory fear conditioning. *Journal of Neuroscience* 12, 4501-4509.

Sah, P. Westbrook, R.F. & Lüthi, A. (2008). Fear conditioning and long-term potentiation in the amygdale: what really is the connection? *Annals of the New York academy of science* 1129, 88-95.

Sacco, T. & Sachhtti, B. Role of secondary sensory cortices in emotional memory storage and retrieval in rats. *Science* 329, 649-655.

Shaban, H. Humeau, Y. Cyril, H.C. Cassasus, G. Shigemoto, R. Ciocchi1, S. Barbieri, S. Putten, H. Kaupmann, K. Bettler, B. & Lüthi1, A. (2006). Generalization of amygdala LTP and conditioned fear in the absence of presynaptic inhibition. *Nature Neuroscience* 9, 1028-1035.

Shin, R.M. Tsvetkov E. & Bolshakov V.Y. (2006). Spatiotemporal asymmetry of associative synaptic plasticity in fear conditioning pathways. *Neuron* 52, 883-896.

Shin, R.M. Tully, K. Li, Y. Cho, J. H. Higuchi, M. Suhara, T. & Bolshakov, Y. Y. (2010). Hierarchical order of coexisting pre- and postsynaptic forms of long-term potentiation at synapses in amygdale. *PNAS* 107, 19073-19078.

Shumyatsky, G.P Malleret, G. Shin, R.M. Takizawa, S. Tully, K. Tsvetkov, E. Zakharenko, S.S. Joseph, J. Vronskaya, S. Yin, D. Schubart, U.K. Kandel, E.R. & Bolshakov, V.Y. (2005). stathmin, a gene enriched in the amygdale, controls both learned fear and innate fear. *Cell* 123, 697-709.

Shumyatsky, G.P. Tsvetkov, E. Malleret, G. Vronskaya, S. Hatton, M. Hampton, L. Battey, J.F. Dulac, C. Kandel, E.R. & Bolshakov, V.Y. (2002). Identification of signaling network in lateral nucleus of amygdala important for inhibiting memory specifically related to learned gear. *Cell* 111, 905-918.

Tsvetkov, E. Shin, R.M. & Bolshakov, V.Y. (2004). Glutamate uptake determines pathway specificity of long-term potentiation in the neural circuitry of fear conditioning. *Neuron* 41, 139-151.

Tsvetkov, E. Carlezon, W.A. Benes, F.M. Kandel, E.R. & Bolshakov, V.Y. (2002). Fear conditioning occludes LTP-induced presynaptic enhancement of synaptic transmission in the cortical pathway to the lateral amygdale. *Neuron* 34, 289-300.

Tully, K. Li, Y. Tsvetkov, E. & Bolshakov, V.Y. (2007). Norepinephrine enables the induction of associative long-term potentiation at thalamo-amygdala synapses. *PNAS* 104, 14146-14150.

Wang, C. Wilson, W.A. & Moore, S.D. (2001). Role of NMDA, non-NMDA, and GABA receptors in signal propagation in the amygdala formation. *Journal of Neurophysiology* 86, 1422-1429.

Weisskopf, M.G. Bauer, E.P. & LeDoux, J.E. (1999a). L-type voltage-gated calcium channels mediate NMDA-independent associative long-term potentiation at thalamic input synapses to the amygdala. *Journal of Neuroscience* 19, 10512-10519.

Weisskopf, M.G. & LeDoux, J.E. (1999b). Distinct populations of NMDA receptors at subcortical and cortical inputs to principal cells of the lateral amygdala. *Journal of Neurophysiology* 81, 930-934.

Whilensky, A. E. Schafe, G. E. LeDoux, J. E. (2000). The amygdala modulates memory consolidation of fear-motivated inhibitory avoidance learning but not classical fear conditioning. *Journal of Neuroscience* 20, 7059-7066.

Chapter 4

The Role of the Amygdala in Anxiety Disorders

Gina L. Forster, Andrew M. Novick, Jamie L. Scholl and Michael J. Watt

Additional information is available at the end of the chapter

1. Introduction

1.1. Defining anxiety and fear

Anxiety is a term often used to encompass feelings of apprehension, dread, unease or similarly unpleasant emotions. Trait anxiety defines the affect of an organism over time and across situations, whereas state anxiety is the response or adaptation to a given situation [1]. Anxiety can be differentiated from fear, both biologically and behaviorally [see 1 for an extensive review]. Converging theories and evidence from clinical psychology and comparative neuroscience suggest that fear can be considered a negatively-valenced emotion that is brief, focused on the present, occurs in situations of specific threat, and aids in avoidance or escape [1,2]. Anxiety, on the other hand, is a negatively-valenced emotion that is characterized by sustained hyperarousal in response to uncertainty, is thus future-focused, and aids in defensive approach or risk assessment [1,2]. Both anxiety and fear are emotions experienced by all individuals and can serve to be adaptive in shaping decisions and behaviors related to survival of an organism [1,3]. However, when excessive, or pathological, or triggered inappropriately, fear and anxiety form the basis of a variety of anxiety disorders [3,4,5; Table 1]. As illustrated by Table 1, some anxiety disorders such as generalized anxiety disorder (GAD) or obsessive-compulsive disorder (OCD) are characterized by excessive anxiety as defined above [1]. However, other anxiety disorders are characterized, at least in part, by excessive and inappropriate fear, such as posttraumatic stress disorder (PTSD), specific phobias and social anxiety disorder [1,3; Table 1]. Thus, it is important to understand the neurobiology of both anxiety and fear to obtain a comprehensive picture of the physiological basis of anxiety disorders.

1.2. Anxiety disorders

One in three people will develop one of the anxiety disorders outlined by Table 1 within their life-time, with the life-time prevalence at least two times more likely for women [5,6].

Furthermore, individuals may present with one or more comorbid anxiety disorders, and anxiety disorders are highly likely to be comorbid with other psychiatric illnesses, such as major depressive disorder, psychosis, mania, and substance abuse disorder [4-6]. Several non-psychiatric disorders are also associated with anxiety disorders, and these include hyperthyroidism, Cushing's disease and mitral value prolapse [4,5]. Thus, anxiety disorders are one of the most prevalent psychiatric disorders, posing great personal, economic, and societal burdens [4-6].

Generalized Anxiety Disorder (GAD)
Excessive worry occurring more days than not over at least a 6 month period, accompanied by restlessness, fatigue, sleep disturbances, muscle tension or irritability.
Posttraumatic Stress Disorder (PTSD)
Characterized by a history of trauma and symptoms related to avoidance, re-experiencing, and physiological hyperarousal in the face of triggering cue.
Obsessive-Compulsive Disorder (OCD)
Compulsions (repeated actions) produced to reduce anxiety associated with obsessions (unwanted, intrusive thoughts).
Panic Disorder
Characterized by panic attacks; a period of intense fear or discomfort accompanied by a variety of physiological symptoms (e.g. sweating, trembling, chest pains, tachycardia).
Agoraphobia
Fear and avoidance of situations from which escape would be difficult in the event of having panic-like symptoms.
Specific Phobia
Excessive or unreasonable fear in anticipation or in response to a specific object or situation.
Social Anxiety Disorder (Social Phobia)
Excessive/unreasonable fear and avoidance of social situations (including performances) in which the person is exposed to unfamiliar people or possible scrutiny by others.

Table 1. Major Classes of Anxiety Disorders [4,5,7]

1.3. Goals of the current review

The neurobiological bases of anxiety and fear appear to be very similar across species [1], thus complementary findings from both animal models (most often rodents) and human studies can contribute to theories of the neurobiological basis of anxiety disorders. State fear within animal models is most often studied by measures of freezing and fear-potentiated startle, both acquired via classical conditioning of rodents [1,8]. State anxiety, on the other hand, is most often studied using apparatus such as an open field, elevated plus maze, or light-dark box, which all take advantage of the rodent's preference for familiar, dark, and/or enclosed areas [1,9]. Notably, these paradigms do not rely on the processes underlying classical conditioning, although McNaughton and Corr [2] caution against defining fear verses anxiety as conditioned versus unconditioned responses. While trait fear is not well-defined by animal studies [1], trait anxiety is often examined in animal models by the use of selective breeding, resulting in high- and low-anxiety strains and lines of rodents [for example, see 1, 10]. However, one can argue that experimental manipulations (such as early-life stress or amphetamine withdrawal) that drive a group of animals towards greater fear- and anxiety-like phenotypes also examine the underlying basis of trait fear or anxiety [e.g. 11, 12]. As noted by Sylver et al [1] clinical studies most often examine trait anxiety, whereas experiments involving animal models most often focus on state anxiety and fear, and then relate these findings to concepts associated with trait anxiety. Regardless, both human and animal studies suggest an important role for the amygdala, and subregions within, in mediating fear and anxiety, and in the manifestation of anxiety disorders (Sections 2 and 3). Therefore, the goals of this review are to first evaluate and integrate classical and recent findings from human studies and relevant animal models that reveal the specific role the amygdala plays in fear and anxiety, and then to elucidate how anxiolytic drugs may affect the amygdala function to ameliorate heightened fear and/or anxiety. This is important, given that traditional drug and cognitive behavioral therapy (CBT) are effective in reducing symptoms of the various anxiety disorders for many individuals, but often do not provide long-term relief, and relapse is a common post-treatment outcome [as reviewed by 3]. Therefore, the final goal of the current review is to identify future potential therapeutic targets for the treatment of anxiety disorders.

2. Human imaging studies: Amygdala hyperfunction and anxiety disorders

2.1. Amygdala reactivity and anxiogenic or fearful stimuli

Human imaging studies that explore the neurobiological bases of anxiety or fear processing typically use functional magnetic resonance imaging (fMRI) or positron emission tomography (PET) as measures of neural activity or cerebral blood flow. Imaging experiments that are designed to study neural reactivity to fearful stimuli utilize either conditioned fear paradigms similar to those used in animal models, or involve the presentation of unconditioned stimuli such as fearful faces [1]. It has become clear that masked stimuli can elicit conditioned and unconditioned fear responses from human subjects, suggesting unconscious, implicit processing of these cues [as reviewed by 1]. Similarly, increased activity of the amygdala is observed in response to both conditioned and unconditioned fearful stimuli, independent of whether the subject is aware of the stimulus [1,13-16].

Comparable studies that have examined neural correlates of anxiety in healthy controls are limited. One of the reasons for this is that many studies use fearful stimuli, such as the fearful faces or conditioned fear paradigms [1], blurring the distinction between fear and anxiety. Therefore, conclusions regarding neural bases of anxiety are better drawn from studies that include trait anxiety as a variable while utilizing fearful stimuli, or those fewer studies in which an anxiogenic situation is created within the experimental design. Like for studies of fear processing, the majority of these studies show a relationship between trait anxiety and greater amygdala reactivity [as reviewed by 17]. For example, a study of healthy subjects found that reactivity of the amygdala was positively correlated with anticipatory anxiety, and when the anticipated event was imminent, amygdala activation positively correlated with the degree of trait anxiety [18]. Furthermore, college students who scored in the upper 15th percentile for trait anxiety show greater amygdala reactivity to emotional faces as compared to students who scored in the normative range, suggesting that anxiety-prone individuals have greater amygdala reactivity [19]. A similar hyperactivity of the amygdala in high trait anxiety participants is noted when a masked emotional faces or unattended faces paradigm are used [20,21], suggesting the individual does not need to be aware of the stimulus to exhibit heightened amygdala activity. Interestingly, Etkin et al., [21] differentiate between different subregions of the amygdala (see Section 3.1 for more details on amygdala subregions), with the basolateral amygdala activated during masked presentations of emotional faces while the dorsal/central amygdala was activated during unmasked presentations. Thus, there may be subregion specificity within the amygdala when processing unconscious versus conscious emotionally-valenced stimuli.

When gender has been examined as a factor in populations of healthy subjects, higher trait anxiety is associated with greater amygdala responses to unattended fearful faces in female but not male participants [22]. A further factor potentially mediating the relationship between trait anxiety and amygdala reactivity appears to be perceived social support. To illustrate, Hyde et al. [17] show a positive correlation between the degree of trait anxiety and amygdala reactivity to fearful faces in subjects that report below-average social support, but not in those who report above average support. Related, it is also thought that the degree of social anxiety rather than trait anxiety may be more closely related to amygdala reactivity to emotional faces [23]. These factors, and other similar considerations, may explain why some, but not all, studies show a positive correlation between trait anxiety and amygdala reactivity in non-patient populations [18-21,23].

2.2. Amygdala reactivity in anxiety disorders

Hyperactivity of the amygdala in response to negatively-valenced stimuli also appears to be a common finding from a variety of clinical anxiety populations [16]. For example, individuals suffering from social anxiety disorder show heightened amygdala responses to both social and non-social highly emotive stimuli as compared to healthy control groups, with the degree of social anxiety positively correlated with amygdala reactivity [24-27]. Furthermore, activation of the amygdala by non-social stimuli has been correlated with trait anxiety in social anxiety disorder, leading to the conclusion that social anxiety disorder is characterized by a more general dysfunction in emotional processing in addition to altered processing of social stimuli and situations [26]. Importantly, reduced symptoms in a public speaking situation following either CBT or antidepressant treatment was associated with reduced amygdala reactivity [24], further suggesting a tight link between symptomology and amygdala reactivity in social anxiety disorder.

Like social anxiety disorder, a commonly replicated finding from various PTSD populations is hyperactivity of the amygdala in response to masked fearful faces or trauma-related stimuli [3,28,29]. This manifests as higher amygdala reactivity as compared to non-PTSD groups and/or a positive correlation between severity of PTSD symptoms and amygdala reactivity [28,30-33]. Furthermore, in a group of unmedicated acute PTSD subjects (1 month post trauma), the degree of PTSD symptoms also positively correlated with activity of the amygdala in response to masked fearful faces [34]. Thus, amygdala hyperactivity observed in chronic PTSD appears early in the disorder. However, it should be noted that in these same individuals, the degree of PTSD symptoms negatively correlated with activity in the amygdala in response to unmasked fearful faces [34]. This suggests amygdala hypoactivity in response to consciously-processed fearful stimuli in the early stages of PTSD, further implying a dissociation in amygdala activity in response to consciously-processed versus unconsciously-processed fearful stimuli. Interestingly, activity of the amygdala in response to fearful stimuli might not only be characteristic of PTSD, but might predict treatment outcome. Bryant et al [33] show that individuals diagnosed with PTSD that do not respond to CBT (8 one weekly sessions) show significantly greater pre-treatment amygdala activation in response to masked fearful faces as compared to those PTSD subjects who did respond to CBT, as defined by a 50% or more reduction in scores on the Clinician-Administered PTSD Scale (CAPS). Therefore, hyper-function of the amygdala might provide a useful tool for future selections of treatment options for PTSD.

Similar to PTSD and social anxiety disorder, amygdala hyperactivity as a result of highly emotional stimuli presentation or symptom provocation has been observed in specific phobia, panic disorder, and OCD [35-38]. Given the prevalence of GAD, it is surprising that few studies have assessed amygdala reactivity in GAD participants. Somewhat more surprising is that of those studies that have determined amygdala activity in response to emotive stimuli in adult GAD populations, a lack of amygdala hyperactivity has been observed [27,39,40]. This stands in contrast to findings from pediatric GAD, where hyperactivity of the amygdala is apparent in response to emotional stimuli and positively correlated with symptom severity [41,42]. However, recent findings examining amygdala function within paradigms that elicit anticipatory anxiety or emotional conflict have implicated a role for amygdala hyper-reactivity in adult GAD populations. For example, Nitschke et al. [43] report greater anticipatory amygdala activation in response to both emotional and neutral images in adult GAD subjects. Furthermore, Etkin et al [44] found that adult participants with GAD exhibited poor performance on a task that involved emotional conflict (incongruent visual emotional stimuli), accompanied by a failure of the frontal cortex to exert negative top-down control of amygdala activity (see Section 3.1 for more on top-down control of the amygdala). Therefore, amygdala hypofunction in adult GAD might be better revealed by imaging studies that create anxiogenic or conflict situations, rather than the standard presentation of fearful stimuli. While this conclusion requires direct testing, the findings that anxiogenic but not fearful stimuli reveal hypofunction of the amygdala in GAD, whereas fearful stimuli consistently elicit amygdala hyper-reactivity in other anxiety disorders (such as social anxiety disorder, PTSD and also pediatric GAD), suggests a neural dichotomy between GAD and other anxiety disorders on the anxiety to fear continuum.

In summary, there appears to be reasonable overlap across various experimental paradigms and study populations to conclude that the amygdala is reactive to fearful stimuli and anxiogenic situations, and exhibits hyper-function to emotive stimuli, anxiogenic situations and/or symptom provocation in anxiety disorders. However, which neurotransmitters and subregions of the amygdala mediate these responses if often better answered by animal studies, where spatial and neurochemical resolution is greatly improved over human imaging studies.

3. Amygdala subregions, connectivity, neurotransmission and fear/anxiety

3.1. The role of amygdala subregions in mediating fear and anxiety

As discussed above, hyper-function of the amygdala appears to be a key component of human anxiety disorders. However, the contribution of particular amygdalar subregions in the development and maintenance of this hyperactive state in humans is still being established. Only very recently have refinements in the acquisition and analysis of fMRI data allowed subregion function to be segregated effectively during emotional tasks such as avoidance learning [45] and facial expression recognition [21,46]. Similarly, effective structural identification of human amygdalar subregions and assessment of their functional connectivity using imaging techniques is still fairly new [for example, see 47-51]. Therefore, most of our understanding of causal neurochemical pathways in amygdalar circuitry related to fear and anxiety has derived from extensive studies using rodent and non-human primate models [for example, see 9,52-58].

Anatomical arrangement of the mammalian amygdala appears to have been evolutionarily conserved, with particular subregions being connected to homologous brain structures across species [as reviewed by 59]. The lateral (LA) nucleus of the amygdala is reciprocally connected with the auditory, somatosensory and visual sensory association centers in the temporal and insular cortices [59], and in rats also receives further auditory information via projections from the posterior thalamus [59,60]. The medial amygdala (MeA) is reciprocally connected with the accessory olfactory bulb and many hypothalamic and preoptic nuclei [59,61], creating a locus for assimilation of olfactory stimuli and information regarding internal hormonal state [62,63]. Information summated within the LA and MeA is then conveyed to the adjacent basal (B) and accessory basal (AB) nuclei [64], which also receive projections from the CA1 and subiculum areas of the ventral hippocampus [65-67]. The B/AB nuclei send excitatory and inhibitory projections back to the LA and MeA [64,68], creating a localized circuit that may assist in fine-tuning the filtering of sensory input into these regions [64]. Excitatory projections from this basolateral (BLA) complex target the central nucleus of the amygdala (CeA) either directly or via a series of GABAergic interneurons known as intercalated (ITC) cells located between the BLA and CeA [69], providing an effective means of gating CeA activity and output through a combination of direct excitation and feed-forward inhibition [64,70,71]. The CeA itself, principally the medial sector, sends GABAergic projections to brainstem, hypothalamic and basal forebrain regions that control expression of autonomic, hormonal and behavioral responses to emotive situations 72,73]. It should also be noted that in addition to activating the CeA, the BLA projects to the adjacent bed nucleus of the stria terminalis (BNST), which in turn targets many of the same regions as the CeA to produce similar behavioral and physiological responses [73]. The MeA is also able to regulate these responses not only via its influence on hypothalamic nuclei and brainstem targets, but by modulating activity in the BNST and CeA [61,64].

The functional connectivity between the BLA, MeA and CeA ensures that sensory and contextual information associated with emotional situations, such as fearful or anxiogenic circumstances, is channeled to effector regions to produce appropriate responses necessary for survival. The BLA and CeA, unlike the MeA, do not appear necessary for expression of unconditioned fear responses to olfactory stimuli in rodents, e.g., to novel presentation of predator odor [74-76], although the BLA does appear to play a role in responses to other types of unconditioned stimuli [77,78]. However, the functional arrangement of the BLA and CeA with other regions facilitates learning about the situation, such that appropriate reactions are maintained if cues associated with initial exposure are experienced again. The BLA in particular appears to play a crucial role in encoding positive or negative salience to relevant stimuli for future reference, as indicated by numerous studies showing that the BLA is required for fear learning and acquisition of conditioned fear responses [see 56,60]. Once fear conditioning is acquired, the CeA is necessary for expression of the conditioned response [56,60], the magnitude of which will be influenced by BLA gating of CeA activity and output. Similarly, the BLA is needed for acquisition and expression of fear extinction [79,80], which requires a subject to learn that expression of a previously conditioned fear response is no longer necessary when the conditioned stimulus no longer predicts an aversive event [57,81]. To achieve this, the BLA must integrate new sensory information (absence of the unconditioned aversive stimulus) that will result in a dampening of CeA excitation. This may result from increased BLA excitation of ITC cells during fear extinction acquisition to enhance feed-forward inhibition of the CeA [79,82,83], followed by structural remodeling within the BLA during consolidation of the extinction memory to inhibit later BLA output [79]. However, while the roles of the BLA and CeA in fear behaviors are well established, their contribution to anxiety is less clear, especially for the CeA. Animal studies suggest that changes in BLA and CeA activity can alter state anxiety [9; also see Section 3.2.]. However, most investigations have focused on the BLA with the exact role of the CeA remaining ill-defined [for example, see 84,85], although it appears that BLA to CeA circuitry can directly regulate anxiety-like behavior as measured on the elevated plus maze [EPM, 86]. This direct control is thought to result from BLA excitation of GABAergic neurons in the lateral CeA to induce feed-forward inhibition of output from the medial CeA [86], similar to that induced by BLA excitation of ITC cells during fear extinction. Thus, suppression of CeA output may be equally important for mediating expression of both fear and anxiety. Alternatively, some studies have suggested that it is BLA activation of the BNST, not of the CeA, that is responsible for mediating anxiety-like behavior as measured using light-potentiated startle responses in rodents [56,87,88]. Startle responses are also potentiated by corticotropin releasing factor (CRF) infused into the BNST [56]. This effect is presumed to result through facilitation of glutamate release from BLA afferents by CRF neurons that originate in the lateral CeA [88,89], implying that even if BNST is the principal output center for certain types of anxiety-like behaviors, the CeA may still play some modulatory role. Furthermore, the MeA has been strongly implicated in animal models of state anxiety [for example, see 90-93 and see Section 3.2], but whether its effects involve modulation of CeA activity is unknown. To direct translational research into the neurological underpinning of anxiety disorders more effectively, animal studies employing as wide a range of state anxiety paradigms as possible, along with animal models that generate trait anxiety, are required to establish the exact nature of CeA involvement and of amygdala subregion interplay in mediating anxiety-like behavior.

It is important to remember that while the amygdala can mediate fear and anxiety-like behavior, other brain regions play a major role in expression of these states, presumably by influencing activity in particular amygdalar subregions to alter the balance of output from the CeA. For example, input from the ventral hippocampus to the B/AB nuclei within the BLA is required for expression of conditioned fear responses to contextual cues in rodents and humans [60,94,95], and so receipt of this information presumably increases BLA activity, to in turn enhance CeA output in the aversive context. In rodents, the ventromedial prefrontal cortex (vmPFC) also appears to be crucial in regulating amygdalar activity, especially during fearful experiences [79]. The prelimbic (PL) subregion of the vmPFC can enhance conditioned fear expression via excitatory projections to the BLA and CeA [96-98]. In contrast, expression of conditioned fear appears to be decreased by activation of the infralimbic (IL) subregion of the vmPFC [99, but see 100]. The IL cortex is also required for effective consolidation and recall of fear extinction memories [79,98]. Both decreased conditioned fear responding and fear extinction require suppression of CeA output, which is thought to result in part via IL cortex stimulation of the series of inhibitory ITC cells that project to the CeA [71,79,96,101]. The bidirectional roles of the PL and IL cortices in regulating conditioned fear through opposing influences on CeA activity and output imply that imbalance in the influence of either cortical structure could contribute to amygdala hyperactivity seen in anxiety disorders characterized by excessive and inappropriate fear (see Table 1). This is supported by fMRI studies investigating neural correlates of impaired fear extinction in PTSD patients, who compared to healthy subjects show hyperactivity of the amygdala during extinction learning [102]. This enhanced amygdala function in PTSD patients is accompanied by greater activation of the dorsal anterior cingulate cortex (dACC, functionally equivalent to the rodent PL cortex, [3,57], which is also present during recall of the extinction memory [102]. This is in line with rodent studies demonstrating potentiated fear conditioning upon PL cortex activation [98]. However, PTSD individuals exhibit hypoactivation of the ventral portion of the vmPFC (equivalent to rodent IL cortex, [3,57]) during extinction learning and recall [102,103]. Human imaging studies also suggest that impaired regulation of amygdala activity by the ventral vmPFC may contribute to anxiety disorders characterized by hypervigilance in the absence of conditioned stimuli, such as in GAD. Specifically, the strength of the connection between the vmPFC and the amygdala, as measured using diffusion tensor imaging, predicts levels of self-reported trait anxiety, such that weaker connections are seen in more anxious individuals [104]. As mentioned earlier (Section 2.2), participants with GAD exhibited a failure of the vmPFC to exert negative top-down control of amygdala activity during a task that involved emotional conflict [44]. Further, resting state fMRI revealed that in anxious individuals, vmPFC activity was negatively correlated with amygdala activity, while a positive relationship was observed for low anxious subjects [105]. The combination of animal and human studies strongly indicates that inadequate suppression by the ventral portion of the vmPFC, most likely of the CeA, is a key factor in amygdala hyperactivity underlying the emergence of excessive fear and anxiety states.

3.2. Monoaminergic neurotransmission in the amygdala: Relation to fear and anxiety

The monoamine neurotransmitters (serotonin, dopamine and norepinephrine) have long been associated with fear and anxiety, and drugs that alter monoaminergic function are often effective across the range of anxiety disorders [8, 9, 52, 55]. Animal studies suggest a variety of anxiogenic stressors or fearful stimuli increase monoamine levels in the amygdala. To illustrate, increased serotonin (5-HT) release or increased activity of 5-HT neurons in the amygdala have been observed in response to restraint or footshock, or in association with expression of conditioned fear behavior [106-110]. Similarly, dopamine (DA) and norepinephrine (NE) levels in the amygdala are increased following restraint, handling stress, footshock or during the expression of conditioned fear behavior [107,111-118]. The source of monoamines to the amygdala arise from monoaminergic cell body regions in the brainstem. Specifically, the dorsal raphe nucleus (dRN) provides 5-HT innervation to the amygdala, while NE and DA innervation of the amygdala arise from the locus coeruleus (LC) and ventral tegmental area (VTA) respectively [55,119,120]. Regulation of monoaminergic activity in the amygdala thus can occur at the level of these brainstem cell body regions, or within the terminal regions of the amygdala.

One of the important mediators of amygdala monoaminergic activity in response to anxiogenic or fearful stimuli is CRF. A strong body of evidence implicates central CRF in mediating fear and anxiety [12,121-128], and recent clinical studies suggest an important role for CRF in anxiety disorders [129]. Like anxiogenic and fearful stimuli, central infusion of CRF or CRF receptor agonists increases 5-HT, NE and DA levels in the amygdala [130-133], and stress-induced increases in monoamine levels in the amygdala are prevented by CRF receptor antagonists [108,111]. It is thought that CRF regulation of monoaminergic activity in the amygdala occurs at the level of the monoaminergic cell bodies. The monoaminergic cell body regions receive CRF innervation from the CeA and BNST, and CRF type 1 and 2 (CRF_1 and CRF_2) receptors are localized to the dRN, LC and VTA [134-140]. Direct infusion of CRF or CRF receptor agonists into the dRN stimulates 5-HT release in the CeA or BLA [131-133]. Interestingly, CRF-induced 5-HT release in the amygdala appears to be dependent on CRF_2 receptor activation in the dRN [131,133], and CRF_2 receptors are known to increase 5-HT neuronal firing rates in the dRN [141]. Importantly, increased neuronal surface expression of CRF_2 receptors occurs in the dRN as a result of stress [142], and increased expression of CRF_2 receptors in the dRN has been observed in rat models of high anxiety [11,128,137,143]. Furthermore, CRF_2 receptor antagonists infused directly into the dRN reduce heightened anxiety-like behavior in rat models of amphetamine withdrawal or early life stress [12,128]. Combined, these findings suggest that CRF_2 receptor modulation of 5-HT activity in the amygdala may play an important role in heightened anxiety. While similar studies have not been performed to elucidate the role of CRF receptors in the LC and VTA in mediating NE and DA activity in the amygdala and anxiety states, some indirect evidence suggests an important role for CRF receptors in the LC and VTA stress responses [136,138,144]. Overall, it is clear that further investigations are needed to ascertain the role of CRF receptors in mediating NE and DA activity in the amygdala and how CRF modulation of this activity could relate to fear or anxiety.

Studies demonstrating increased monoamine activity in the amygdala in response to anxiogenic or fearful stimuli, and CRF modulation of these responses (as described above) do not allow conclusions to be made about the specific role of each monoamine in mediating anxiety or fear. Direct manipulation of monoaminergic activity within the amygdala or specific amygdala subregions, and the measurement of resultant anxiety-like or fear-related behaviors, have gone some way to providing a picture of how monoamine function in the amygdala might translate to anxiety or fear. Table 2 summarizes such studies directly manipulating 5-HT levels or 5-HT receptor activity in the amygdala. When 5-HT or 5-HT activity is decreased in the entire amygdala [145,146], a consistent increase in anxiety-like behavior is observed (Table 2). This would suggest that increased 5-HT activity in the amygdala would thus be associated with decreased anxiety, implying an anxiolytic role of 5-HT. However, this does not appear to be supported by experiments that directly manipulate 5-HT receptor activity in the amygdala with 5-HT receptor ligands (Table 2). For example, activation of postsynaptic excitatory 5-HT_2 or 5-HT_3 receptors in the amygdala decreases social interaction and increases anxiety-like behavior, whereas antagonism of 5-HT_3 receptors in particular increases social interaction and decreases anxiety-like behaviors, suggesting that 5-HT actions on postsynaptic receptors is anxiogenic (Table 2), although, see [147] for an exception to this pattern. Similarly, activation of excitatory $5HT_2$ receptors in the BLA generally increases anxiety-like behavior (Table 2), suggesting an anxiogenic role for postsynaptic 5-HT receptors in the BLA (although an exception to this is observed, [148]). In contrast, inhibitors of 5-HT_2 receptors in the MeA increase anxiety-like behavior while activation of these receptors increases social interaction and decreases anxiety behavior (Table 2). Thus like the some findings from the amygdala as a whole (Table 2), 5-HT activity in the MeA appears to play an anxiolytic role. The role of 5-HT or 5-HT receptors has not been well studied in the CeA. However, rats undergoing amphetamine withdrawal that exhibit greater anxiety-like behavior have greater 5-HT release in the CeA [12,133], suggesting a similar anxiogenic relationship between 5-HT and anxiety as for the BLA. Future work should determine whether 5-HT in the CeA reduces anxiety-like behaviors as is suggestive for the MeA, or in contrast, increases anxiety-like behaviors as appears to be the case for the BLA. Overall, the findings summarized in Table 2 suggest a dichotomy in the potential role of 5-HT in the amygdala in mediating anxiety depending on whether the entire amygdala or a specific subregion is targeted. Potential confounds in comparing the studies listed in Table 2 could be the different paradigms used to measure anxiety-like behaviors and the relative selectivity of 5-HT receptor ligands across different experiments. Future studies directly comparing the effects of 5-HT manipulations within the different amygdala subregions across several well-validated tests of anxiety-like behaviors will better elucidate the role of amygdala 5-HT in mediating anxiety.

Amygdala Subregion	Monoamine or Receptor Involvement	Behavioral Outcome	Citation
Anxiety-like Behavior			
Amygdala	Decreased 5-HT (induced by MDMA)	Increased anxiety behavior	Faria et al. [145]
Amygdala	Decreased 5-HIAA (induced by stress)	Increased anxiety behavior	Niwa et al. [146]
Amygdala	5-HT_{1A} agonist	No change in anxiety behavior	Zangrossi and Graeff [149]
Amygdala	5-$HT_{2B/2C}$ agonist	Increased anxiety behavior	Cornelio and Nunes-De-Souza [150]
Amygdala	5-HT_{3} agonist	Decreased social interaction	Higgans et al. [151]
Amygdala	5-HT_{3} agonist	Decreased anxiety behavior	Costall et al. [147]
Amygdala	5-HT_{3} antagonist	Increased social interaction	Higgans et al. [151]
Amygdala	5-HT_{3} antagonist	Decreased anxiety behavior	Costall et al. [147]
Amygdala	5-HT_{3} antagonist	Decreased anxiety behavior	Tomkins et al. [152]
BLA	5-HT_{1A} agonist	Decreased social interaction	Gonzalez et al. [153]
BLA	5-HT_{1A} agonist	No change in anxiety behavior	Gonzalez et al. [153]
BLA	5-HT_{2A} agonist	Increased anxiety behavior	Zangrossi and Graeff [149]
BLA	5-$HT_{2A/2C}$ agonist	No change in anxiety behavior	Cruz et al [148]
BLA	5-HT_{2C} agonist	Increased anxiety behavior	Vincente et al. [154]
MeA	5-HT_{2A} antagonist	Increased anxiety behavior	Zangrossi and Graeff [149]
MeA	5-HT_{2} agonist	No change in anxiety behavior	Duxon et al. [155]
MeA	5-HT_{2B} agonist	Increased social interaction	Duxon et al. [156]
MeA	5-HT_{2B} agonist	Decreased anxiety behavior	Duxon et al. [155]

Amygdala Subregion	Monoamine or Receptor Involvement	Behavioral Outcome	Citation
MeA	5-$HT_{2B/2C}$ agonist	No change in anxiety behavior	Duxon et al. [155]
Fear-related Behavior			
CeA	Increased 5-HT	Increased unconditioned freezing	Forster et al. [132]
BLA	Increased 5-HT	Decreased conditioned freezing	Inoue et al. [157]
BLA	Increased 5-HT	Decreased unconditioned tonic immobility	Leite-Panissi et al. [158]
BLA	5-HT_{1A} agonist	Decreased conditioned freezing	Li et al. [159]
BLA	5-HT_{1A} agonist	Decreased acquisition and expression of conditioned defeat	Morrison et al. [160]
BLA	5-$HT_{1A/2}$ agonist	Decreased unconditioned tonic immobility	Leite-Panissi et al. [158]

Abbreviations: 5-HIAA = 5-Hydroxyindoleacetic acid (5-HT metabolite); 5-HT = serotonin; BLA = basolateral amygdala; CeA = central nucleus of the amygdala; MDMA = 3,4-methylenedioxy-N-methylamphetamine; MeA = medial amygdala.

Table 2. The Role of Serotonin in Anxiety-Like and Fear-Related Behaviors

Determining the role of amygdala 5-HT in fear-related behavior has mainly utilized studies of freezing or immobility responses in rodents, and of 5-HT manipulation in the BLA (Table 2). From these studies, it seems clear that 5-HT in the BLA decreases the expression of unconditioned and conditioned fear responses, likely via activation of the inhibitory postsynaptic 5-HT_{1A} receptor (Table 2). Thus, it has been suggested that 5-HT in the BLA/amygdala ameliorates fear [8]. This conclusion is in contrast to the apparent role for BLA 5-HT in enhancing anxiety (Table 2), suggesting a fear versus anxiety dissociation for the role of 5-HT in the BLA. This dissociation, if upheld by more in-depth future work, could prove important information for the development of treatment strategies for the various anxiety disorders that differ in the degree of anxiety-like and fear-like symptomology (as discussed in Section 1.1).

A role for amygdala DA in anxiety has not been as well explored as for 5-HT. However, a summary of studies that have manipulated DA function in the amygdala provides a consistent picture of the role of amygdala DA in mediating anxiety in animal models (Table 3). Indirect evidence suggests that decreased DA in the amygdala leads to increased anxiety, and this is supported by direct manipulation of the CeA (Table 3). For example, decreased DA or DA receptor antagonism within the CeA all increase anxiety-like behavior (Table 3), suggesting that DA activity in the CeA is anxiolytic. This role for DA in the CeA is in direct contrast to the BLA, where converging evidence suggests that decreased DA function in the BLA decreases anxiety-like behaviors while increased DA receptor activity in the BLA increases anxiety (Table 3). Thus, DA activity in the BLA is anxiogenic, revealing an opposite role for DA activity in the CeA and BLA in mediating anxiety-like behaviors in animal models.

Amygdala Subregion	Monoamine or Receptor Involvement	Behavioral Outcome	Citation
Anxiety-like Behavior			
Amygdala	Decreased DA	Decreased rearing in open field indicative of increased anxiety behavior	Summavielle et al. [163]
CeA	Decreased DA	Decreased voluntary activity indicative of increased anxiety behavior	Izumo et al. [164]
CeA	D_1 antagonist	Increased anxiety behavior	Rezayof et al. [165]
CeA	$D_{2/3}$ antagonist	Increased anxiety behavior	de la Mora et al. [166]
BLA	DA depletion	Decreased anxiety in males but not females	Sullivan et al. [167]
BLA	D_1 agonist	Increased anxiety behavior	Banaej et al. [168]
BLA	D_2 agonist	Increased anxiety behavior	Banaej et al. [168]
BLA	D_1 antagonist	Decreased anxiety behavior	Banaej et al. [168]
BLA	D_1 antagonist	Decreased anxiety behavior	de la Mora et al. [169]
BLA	D_2 antagonist	Decreased anxiety behavior	Banaej et al. [168]
Fear-related Behavior			
Amygdala	D_2 antagonist	Decreased acquisition and retention of fear conditioning	Greba et al. [170]
CeA	D_1 agonist	Increased conditioned fear behavior	Guarraci et al. [171]
CeA	D_1 antagonist	Inhibited conditioned fear behavior	Guarraci et al. [171]
CeA	D_2 antagonist	Decreased	Guarraci et al. [172]

Amygdala Subregion	Monoamine or Receptor Involvement	Behavioral Outcome	Citation
		conditioned fear behavior	
BLA	DA depletion	Decreased fear conditioning	Seldon et al. [173]
BLA	D_1 antagonist	Inhibited acquisition of fear conditioning	Greba and Kokkinidis [174]
BLA	D_2 antagonist	Inhibited fear potentiated startle	De Oliveira et al. [175]

Abbreviations: BLA = basolateral amygdala; CeA = central nucleus of the amygdala; DA = dopamine.

Table 3. The Role of Dopamine in Anxiety-Like and Fear-Related Behaviors

In contrast, the role of DA in mediating fear-related behaviors does not appear to differ based on amygdala subregion (Table 3). Reducing DA function in the amygdala reduces or inhibits processes associated with fear conditioning, while increasing DA receptor activity increases conditioned fear (Table 3). Thus, DA in the amygdala is required for fear conditioning, and enhanced DA levels in the amygdala as elicited by fearful stimuli and conditioned cues [107,112] would thus facilitate fear conditioning. It should be noted that the studies summarized by Table 3 indicate a role for both excitatory D_1 receptors and inhibitory D_2 receptors. Dopamine D_2 receptors are localized both pre- and post-synaptically, with pre-synaptic D_2 autoreceptors limiting DA neuronal activity and DA release [161,162]. Thus, antagonism of presynaptic D_2 receptors would actually increase DA within the amygdala. Since the effects of D_2 receptor antagonism on fear-related behaviors is characteristic of reduced, not enhanced, DA function in the amygdala, it may be concluded that the results of D_2 receptor antagonism summarized by Table 3 are due to postsynaptic D_2 receptor effects. However, this conclusion requires direct testing.

Very few studies have examined the role of amygdala NE in mediating anxiety-like behavior in animal models, surprising given that anxiogenic stimuli increase NE in this region [for example, see 111,115,116] and drugs that alter NE neurotransmission are used to treat anxiety disorders [8]. There appears to be little role for NE receptors in the CeA in mediating anxiety-like behavior, although infusion of a α_1 antagonist can increase social interaction following an anxiogenic stimulus [restraint; 176; Table 4]. It is clear that more experiments are required to delineate the role of amygdala NE in mediating anxiety.

Studies determining the role of NE in fear-related behaviors have concentrated on the BLA, due to the importance of this amygdala subregion in conditioned fear responses (see Section 3.1.). The major focus of the studies summarized by Table 4 has been on the role of NE in fear conditioning and reconsolidation of fear memories in conditioned fear paradigms. Taken as a whole, findings suggest that NE in the BLA facilitates fear conditioning and fear memory, via activation of adrenergic β receptors (Table 4). Recent evidence suggests a role for α_1 receptors in the BLA in mediating fear memory, in this case, activation of α_1 receptors by NE would appear to decrease fear memory (Table 4). Thus, it is possible that NE in the

BLA could have opposing effects on reconsolidation of fear memory based on the balance of α_1 versus β receptor activity – a hypothesis that requires direct testing. The role of NE in the BLA (and β receptors in particular) in fear memory has generated interest in targeting this NE system for the treatment of anxiety disorders where enhancement in fear memory is apparent, such as PTSD [for example, see 177]. Whether NE within the BLA plays a role in other aspects of fear processing (e.g. unconditioned fear responses to non-olfactory based stimuli) or NE within other amygdala subregions mediate fear should be subjects of future investigations to fully elucidate the role of amygdala NE in fear.

Amygdala Subregion	Monoamine or Receptor Involvement	Behavioral Outcome	Citation
Anxiety-like Behavior			
CeA	α_1 antagonist	Increased social interaction	Cecchi et al. [176]
CeA	α_1 antagonist	No effect on anxiety behavior	Cecchi et al. [176]
CeA	$\beta_{1/2}$ antagonist	No effect on social interaction	Cecchi et al. [176]
CeA	$\beta_{1/2}$ antagonist	No effect on anxiety behavior	Cecchi et al. [176]
Fear-related Behavior			
BLA	Increased NE	Increased memory and retention of fear conditioning	LaLumiere et al. [178]
BLA	Decreased NE	Impaired fear conditioning	Seldon et al. [173]
BLA	Decreased NE	Impaired fear memory	Debiec and LeDoux [177]
BLA	α_1 antagonist	Increased fear memory	Lazzaro et al. [179]
BLA	$\beta_{1/2}$ antagonist	Impaired of fear memory	Debiec and LeDoux [180]
BLA	β_1 antagonist	Impaired fear memory (as enhanced by glucocorticoids)	Roozendaal et al. [181]

Abbreviations: BLA = basolateral amygdala; CeA = central nucleus of the amygdala; NE = norepinephrine.

Table 4. The Role of Norepinephrine in Anxiety-Like and Fear-Related Behaviors

In summary, it is clear that more work is required to fully understand the role of amygdala monoamines in mediating fear and anxiety. However, several patterns of interest emerge from the current literature, namely that there are distinct subregion differences in the role each monoamine plays in mediating anxiety and fear, with the one monoamine possibly playing opposing roles depending on subregion or depending on whether anxiety or fear measures are employed. Therefore, these findings suggest neurochemical dissociations between amygdala subregions and monoamines in mediating fear or anxiety.

4. The amygdala as a potential site of anxiolytic drug action

Psychopharmacological management of anxiety disorders includes the benzodiazepines, antidepressants, $5\text{-}HT_{1A}$ agonists and various "off-label" drugs such as β-blockers, mood stabilizers and antipsychotics. The mechanism by which these drugs produce anti-anxiety effects has yet to be definitively established and represents a frequently updated field of research. Because these drugs bind to target receptors throughout the brain, it is unlikely that their efficacy can be attributed to action in one particular region. However, given the role that the amygdala plays in fear and anxiety, modification of amygdala function by pharmacological agents represents a likely mechanism of action as well as a target to guide future drug development. The evidence for amygdala involvement in anxiolytic action comes from both human imaging studies as well as work in animal models.

4.1. Human imaging studies: Effects of anxiolytics on amygdala activity and emotion

Given the highly complex and subjective nature of anxiolytic drug response in humans, neuroimaging represents an invaluable tool for drug evaluation and discovery.

Benzodiazepines: Benzodiazepines exert their anxiolytic action through binding to $GABA_A$ receptors, which leads to enhanced GABA activity and a subsequent increase in inhibitory tone. Despite the long history and current prevalence of benzodiazepine use for anxiety disorders [182,183], there is a paucity of human neuroimaging studies utilizing this class of drug, especially compared to those using antidepressants. This may have to do with eclipse of benzodiazepines by antidepressants as first line agents for many anxiety disorders [182].

Various studies have utilized healthy volunteers undergoing experimental challenges in an attempt to elucidate the neurobiology underlying the anxiolytic effect of benzodiazepines. These studies have found that benzodiazepines have the ability to impair functions related to amygdala activity including fear conditioning [184-186], recognition of fearful emotional faces [187], and memory for emotional stimuli relative to neutral stimuli [188,189].

Neuroimaging work appears to support a role for the amygdala in benzodiazepine action, although this may be dependent upon the nature of the accompanying neuropsychological challenge. Specifically, lorazepam was found to decrease amygdala activation during an emotional face assessment task without modifying baseline levels of anxiety or task recognition [190]. A similar finding was found with diazepam, which decreased amygdala response to fearful faces, and also impaired fearful face recognition [191]. However, during anticipation of aversive electrical stimulation, lorazepam failed to produce changes in amygdala activity [192]. Thus, while there is support for benzodiazepine induced modulation of the amygdala during processing of threatening/emotional stimuli, further studies are needed to clarify the neural correlates of benzodiazepine-induced anxiolysis.

β-Blockers: The β-blocker propranolol has a substantial history of being utilized to reduce somatic symptoms of fear and anxiety in situations such as stage fright [193] and acute panic [194-195]. More recently, research on the role of amygdala NE and β-receptors in facilitating emotional memory formation (see Table 4 and associated text) has caused much excitement and controversy about the use of propranolol to prevent PTSD [196-198]. Thus far, initial trials have demonstrated limited efficacy [199,200]. Despite lack of success in the application of propranolol to PTSD, neuroimaging studies in healthy human subjects have confirmed the ability of propranolol to modulate amygdala activation to emotional stimuli. Propranolol was found to decrease amygdala activation to emotional faces irrespective of emotional valence [201]. Furthermore, supporting a role for the amygdala NE in the encoding and consolidation of emotional stimuli, a separate study found that propranolol was able to decrease amygdala reactivity to emotional pictures of high valence as well as decrease the subject's memory for them [202].

Selective Serotonin Re-uptake Inhibitors: Antidepressant drugs, and selective serotonin re-uptake inhibitors (SSRIs) in particular, have become first line drugs for many of the anxiety disorders [182,203]. As such, there has been comparatively more work investigating these drugs in humans using advanced imaging techniques.

Most antidepressants are unique from benzodiazepines and β-blockers in that a time lag exists between initial treatment and onset of anxiolytic effects. In line with a potential anxiogenic role of serotonin in the amygdala (see Table 2 and associated text), some patients have reported an initial exacerbation of anxiety upon acute dosing of SSRIs [203]. In studies on healthy subjects, acute dosing of the SSRI citalopram can enhance recognition of fearful faces as well as increase emotion-potentiated startle response [204-206]. These effects are reversed when citalopram treatment is continued for 7 days [207,208].

Attempts to correlate the acute versus sub-chronic effects of SSRIs with neural activation have resulted in unexpected findings. On one hand, sub-chronic citalopram treatment was found to decrease amygdala activation to unconscious fearful stimuli [209], suggesting a relationship between repeated SSRI treatment, changes in emotional processing, and decreased amygdala activity. However, acute doses of citalopram have also been found to decrease amygdala activation to fearful faces [208,210,211]. Divergent effects of acute versus sub-chronic citalopram on emotional recognition but similar effects on amygdala response could suggest that the amygdala does not play a core role in acute SSRI-induced anxiety or chronic SSRI-induced anxiolysis. However, it has been emphasized that the effects of serotonergic challenge on fear recognition and amygdala activation appear to be dependent upon the individual's baseline sensitivity to threat [212], gender [213] and genotype [214]. Thus differences in subject profiles both between and within studies could have confounded results.

Overall, it appears that pharmacotheraputics commonly used to treat anxiety disorders may modulate amygdala function. In particular, it appears that anxiolytics can reduce amygdala reactivity to highly emotive or fearful stimuli. Given that amygdala hyper-reactivity to similar stimuli is the most common finding across all anxiety disorders (with the exception of adult GAD – see Section 2.2), it is possible that the anxiolytic effects of these drugs may be in part, mediated by dampening amygdala function.

4.2. Evidence delineating effects of anxiolytic drugs on amygdala function in animal models of anxiety states

Benzodiazepines: While benzodiazepine receptors exist throughout the brain, there is a particularly high density in amygdala regions [215,216]. There is much evidence from animal models to suggest that it is the action of benzodiazepines in the amygdala that mediates their anxiolytic effect. For example, early evidence demonstrated that local amygdala infusion of benzodiazepines produces anxiolytic-like effects in conflict models of anxiety [217-220]. These effects can be reversed by systemic [217,219] or direct amygdala administration of benzodiazepine antagonists [220]. Anti-conflict effects are most apparent when the benzodiazepines are injected into the BLA, and are absent when injected into the CeA [219,220]. While anti-conflict effects of benzodiazepines have been observed in the CeA, these were with substantially higher doses [221]. Further studies suggest that the BLA and not the CeA is essential for the anxiolytic effects of benzodiazepines in the EPM [149,222,223]. However, with regards to the shock probe burying test, it appears that the CeA is responsible for benzodiazepine-induced impairment of passive avoidance [223]. Although contradictory results exist on the role of benzodiazepines in the BLA versus CeA, particularly when animals are tested on the EPM [9,84,224] have suggested that distinct benzodiazepine receptor subtypes located within subregions of the amygdala may differentially alter avoidance responses to "potential threat" (EPM and BLA) versus "discrete, unambiguous threat" (shock probe burying and CeA).

As discussed in the human studies in Section 4.1 above [184,188,189], a key aspect of benzodiazepine action may be the ability to modulate emotional memory. Here the BLA once again appears to be a main site of benzodiazepine action. Lesions of the BLA, but not the CeA, block the benzodiazepine induced deficits in inhibitory avoidance memory [225,226]. Similar impairments were seen by direct injection of benzodiazepine into the BLA and not the CeA [227]. Enhancement of memory consolidation could be induced by BLA infusion of a benzodiazepine antagonist [228]. Given that individuals with anxiety disorders may be hypervigilant to cues associated with threatening stimuli and biased to form memories regarding such stimuli [229,230], the pro-amnestic effects of benzodiazepines in the BLA may represent a putative mechanism of action.

β-Blockers: The evaluation of β-blockers (with propranolol being the prototypical agent) in animal models has revolved mainly around their utility in models of memory and fear conditioning. Within the BLA, stress hormone elicited increases in norepinephrine have been found to enhance the consolidation of emotionally relevant memories [231,232]. This appears to be particularly true with contextual fear conditioning [178] and reconsolidation of fear memory following extinction [180,197,233; Table 4]. In particular, local infusions of propranolol are able to block reconsolidation of fear [180,233]. Recently, it has been demonstrated that β-adrenoreceptor activation within the BLA decreases surface expression of $GABA_A$ receptors, and this phenomenon is necessary for the reinstatement of fear following extinction [234]. It is proposed that propranolol, through blocking the decrease in $GABA_A$ receptor surface expression, prevents fear reinstatement by maintaining feed forward inhibition from BLA interneurons and thus dampening activity of BLA projections [234]. This finding is noteworthy as it suggests that hyperactive noradrenergic activity in PTSD [235,236] may lead to reduced $GABA_A$ availability, explaining a potential mechanism for the relative ineffectiveness of benzodiazepines in PTSD populations [237,238].

Despite the action of β-blockers within the amygdala to modulate fear conditioning (see Table 4), attempts at testing propranolol in other animal models of PTSD have met with mixed results, echoing the mixed efficacy seen thus far in humans [199,200,239,240]. One such model is exposure to predator odor in rodents, which produces long lasting increases in anxiety like behavior [241-243]. The increases in anxiety like behavior following exposure to predator odor is influenced by a long lasting potentiation in BLA activity [243], supporting the role of the amygdala in mediating the consequences of fear and trauma. Propranolol administered 1 minute following exposure to predator odor to rats blocks the development of anxiogenesis in various tests, including the EPM, one week later [241]. However, when propranolol administration is delayed to 1 hour following predator odor exposure, no effects are seen when rats are subsequently tested on the EPM 30 days later [242]. These results highlight once again a potential key role of timing if propranolol is to be effectively implemented in clinical patients. Similarly, findings that propranolol seems most effective in blocking the *re*consolidation of fearful memories [233, 180, 197] (also see Table 4) suggests that future work should be aimed at establishing protocols for the integration of propranolol during exposure therapy, in which extinction and reconsolidation processes are most active. Specifically, it would seem important that propranolol not be administered shortly after exposure therapy, as this might interfere reconsolidation processes within the amygdala. On the other hand, propranolol would likely have utility when PTSD patients encounter aversive stimuli outside the context of therapy which could potentially undermine the therapeutic process and lead to reinstatement.

Selective Serotonin Re-uptake Inhibitors: Similar to human studies, animal models of anxiety-like behavior demonstrate divergent behavioral effects of acute versus chronic SSRI administration. Increased anxiety-like behavior with acute treatment of SSRIs and its reversal with chronic treatment has been found in novelty-suppressed feeding [244], EPM testing [245,246], and the social interaction test [247]. While a large percentage of studies reveal acute anxiogenic effects and chronic anxiolytic effect, there are exceptions (for review, see [248]).

Much evidence suggests that enhanced activity at $5\text{-}HT_{2C}$ within the BLA by SSRIs produces acute anxiogenic effects, while the eventual downregulation of these receptors by chronic treatment leads to eventual anxiolysis. For example, amygdala or BLA $5\text{-}HT_{2C}$ receptors have been found to produce anxiety-like responses in a variety of tests [249,250] (see Table 2). Blockade of $5\text{-}HT_{2C}$ receptors within the BLA prevents the acute anxiogenic effect of the

SSRI fluoxetine on the Vogel conflict test [251]. Systemic 5-HT_{2C} antagonism also prevents the increase in fear conditioning [252], decrease in social interaction [247,253], and escape response to airjet [254] following acute SSRI treatment. Following chronic treatment with SSRIs, 5-HT_{2C} agonists have attenuated anxiogenic effects on the exacerbation of OCD symptoms in humans [255,256], on social interaction [257] and hyperlocomotion [258], suggesting down-regulation of the ability to 5-HT_{2C} receptors in the amygdala to produce anxiogenic responses following chronic SSRI treatment. Thus, the amygdala (BLA in particular) may be an important locus of action for the long-term effects of SSRIs on anxiety.

4.3. Future potential anxiolytic targets

The literature reviewed above suggests that in part, the effects of anxiolytic drugs may be mediated by altering amygdala function – either global dampening of the amygdala by benzodiazepines, or specific actions on 5-HT and NE receptors within particular amygdala subregions. However, to improve therapeutic efficacy and reduce relapse, several aspects of amygdala pharmacology discussed above might provide useful potential anxiolytic targets in the future.

Findings suggesting down-regulation of anxiogenic 5-HT_{2C} receptors in the amygdala following chronic SSRI treatment (Section 4.2.) present a potential strategy of reducing onset latency of SSRIs as well as enhancing their effects. Specifically, blocking 5-HT_{2C} receptors at the initiation of SSRI treatment would be expected to produce a faster onset of anxiolytic action. Currently, there are no selective 5-HT_{2C} antagonists available for human use. However, atypical antipsychotics [259] as well as atypical antidepressants such as mirtazapine [260] possess 5-HT_{2C} antagonist activity. While there is evidence that antipsychotic augmentation of SSRIs may improve anxiolytic efficacy, their use has been limited by poor tolerability [for review see 261]. Although research is lacking, mirtazapine and the melatonin receptor agonist/5-HT_{2C} receptor antagonist agomelatine [262] may provide the advantage of targeting anxiogenic 5-HT_{2C} in the amygdala with less side effects.

Furthermore, the recent observation that β-adrenoreceptor activation within the BLA results in decreased of $GABA_A$ receptor surface expression necessary for fear reinstatement [234] (and see Section 4.2.) suggests that the combination of propranolol and a benzodiazepine may have unique benefit for PTSD. By blocking β-adrenoreceptors with propranolol, one might be able to enhance benzodiazepine receptor availability, and increase benzodiazepine-induced inhibition of fear circuits within the amygdala. While currently speculative, the use of propranolol to enhance benzodiazepine action in the amygdala may represent a potential creative treatment strategy in a population that is traditionally refractory to benzodiazepine treatment.

While current pharmacotherapeutic strategies for the treatment of anxiety disorders target monoamine function, this has predominantly been related to altering 5-HT or NE levels or receptor activity [8]. However, Table 3 clearly shows a role for DA in the amygdala in mediating both fear and anxiety, and the role for DA and both D_1 and D_2 receptors in acquisition and retention of conditioned fear in particular appears quite robust. Thus, reducing DA function might serve as means by which to treat anxiety disorders in which fear plays a major component. The obvious disadvantage of dopaminergic-based pharmacotheraputics is potential for major cognitive and motoric side-effects, limiting the treatment options with the currently available dopaminergic agents. Atypical antipsychotic drugs incorporate DA receptor blocking activity while avoiding many of the motoric and cognitive issues of traditional agents. There is evidence that atypical agents possess anxiolytic activity [261], but metabolic side effects make them poorly tolerated. Furthermore, because atypical antipsychotics also have high affinity for 5-HT receptors, the contribution of DA modulation to their anxiolytic effects in humans is currently unknown. One potential strategy may be the use of partial agonists to reduce DA activity in the amygdala via activation of inhibitory presynaptic D_2 autoreceptors. While non-selective for DA, the D_2 partial agonist aripiprazole has demonstrated anxiolytic efficacy similar to other atypical antipsychotic drugs [263]. In the future, more selective DA partial agonists may have additional benefit without unwanted side-effects.

Finally, CRF has been identified as an important neuropeptide in the regulation of monoaminergic activity in the amygdala in response to anxiogenic or fearful stimuli (Section 3.2). Furthermore, CRF and its receptors (CRF_1 and CRF_2) are implicated in fear and anxiety within animal models and in the development of anxiety disorders [12,121-129]. Upon the development of non-peptide CRF_1 receptor antagonists that cross the blood-brain barrier, there was great interest in the use of CRF_1 receptor antagonist in the treatment of anxiety disorders. To date, there have been limited phase II clinical trials published regarding the use of CRF_1 receptor antagonists in anxiety disorders [264]. Of those, preliminary findings suggest the CRF_1 receptor antagonist-treated groups did not differ from placebo-treated groups in anxiety symptomology in both social anxiety disorder and GAD [264]. However, it has been suggested that efficacious concentrations have not been established for the various CRF_1 receptor antagonists, and it is clear that further clinical trials are necessary. One potential promising area in the treatment of anxiety disorders may actually lie in CRF_2 receptor antagonists. As outlined in Section 3.2, CRF_2 receptors mediate 5-HT activity in the amygdala, are up-regulated in animal models of anxiety, and an antagonist of this receptor reduces heightened anxiety in rats [11,12,127,128,131,132,137). The challenge lies in developing non-peptide CRF_2 receptor antagonists that cross the blood-brain barrier, so that the efficacy of such ligands can be determined for anxiety disorders.

5. Conclusion

Human imaging studies in non-patient populations suggest amygdala activation in response to fearful stimuli, and that the magnitude of this response is positively correlated with trait anxiety. Furthermore, individuals suffering from an anxiety disorder (with the possible exception of adult GAD) show exaggerated amygdala responses to fearful or emotive stimuli, which again is positively correlated with the severity of symptoms. Moreover, reactivity of the amygdala to fearful stimuli is reduced by anxiolytic drugs in healthy subjects, and long-term pharmacotherapy or CBT reduces amygdala hyper-reactivity in anxiety disorders. Animal studies corroborate an important role for the amygdala in fear and anxiety, with specific subregions mediating acquisition and expression of fear, fear memories and anxiety, and the monoamines within each of these regions often playing a very specific role in facilitating or attenuating fear or anxiety. Both human and animal studies suggest dysfunction of the amygdala might arise in part, from inadequate top-down control by regions such as the medial prefrontal cortex, and in part, from altered neuropeptide regulation of amygdala monoaminergic systems. Overall, the amygdala plays a critical role in anxiety disorders, and understanding the function of this region in fear and anxiety states and how dysfunction of the amygdala results in anxiety disorders is critical to improving long-term treatment outcomes.

Author details

Gina L. Forster*, Andrew M. Novick, Jamie L. Scholl and Michael J. Watt
Division of Basic Biomedical Sciences, Sanford School of Medicine, University of South Dakota, Vermillion, SD, USA

Acknowledgement

This work was supported by National Institutes of Health grant R01 DA019921, and Department of Defense grants W81XWH-10-1-0925 and W81XWH-10-1-0578.

6. References

[1] Sylvers P, Lilienfeld SO, LaPrairie JL (2011) Differences between Trait Fear and Trait Anxiety: Implications for Psychopathology. Clin Psychol Rev. 31, 122-137. S0272-7358(10)00131-5 [pii] 10.1016/j.cpr.2010.08.004.

[2] McNaughton N, Corr PJ (2004) A Two-Dimensional Neuropsychology of Defense: Fear/Anxiety and Defensive Distance. Neuroscience & Biobehavioral Reviews. 28, 285-305. 10.1016/j.neubiorev.2004.03.005.

[3] Graham BM, Milad MR (2011) The Study of Fear Extinction: Implications for Anxiety Disorders. Am J Psychiatry. 168, 1255-1265. 10.1176/appi.ajp.2011.11040557 appi.ajp.2011.11040557 [pii].

[4] Ninan PT (2001) Recent Perspectives on the Diagnosis and Treatment of Generalized Anxiety Disorder. Am J Manag Care. 7, S367-376.

[5] Alexander JL, Dennerstein L, Kotz K, Richardson G (2007) Women, Anxiety and Mood: A Review of Nomenclature, Comorbidity and Epidemiology. Expert Rev Neurother. 7, S45-58.

[6] Katzman MA (2009) Current Considerations in the Treatment of Generalized Anxiety Disorder. CNS Drugs. 23, 103-120.

[7] American Psychiatric Association. Diagnostic and Statistical Manual of Mental Disorders. 4th ed. Washington, DC: American Psychiatric Association; 1994.

* Corresponding Author

[8] Inoue T, Kitaichi Y, Koyama T (2011) SSRIs and Conditioned Fear. Progress in Neuro-Psychopharmacology and Biological Psychiatry. 35, 1810-1819. 10.1016/j.pnpbp.2011.09.002.

[9] Engin E, Treit D (2008) The Effects of Intra-Cerebral Drug Infusions on Animals' Unconditioned Fear Reactions: A Systematic Review. Prog Neuropsychopharmacol Biol Psychiatry. 32, 1399-1419. 10.1016/j.pnpbp.2008.03.020.

[10] Keck ME, Sartori SB, Welt T, Müller MB, Ohl F, Holsboer F, Landgraf R, Singewald N (2005) Differences in Serotonergic Neurotransmission between Rats Displaying High or Low Anxiety/Depression-Like Behaviour: Effects of Chronic Paroxetine Treatment. J Neurochem. 92, 1170-1179. 10.1111/j.1471-4159.2004.02953.x.

[11] Lukkes JL, Mokin MV, Scholl JL, Forster GL (2009) Adult Rats Exposed to Early-Life Social Isolation Exhibit Increased Anxiety and Conditioned Fear Behavior, and Altered Hormonal Stress Responses. Horm Behav. 55, 248-256.

[12] Vuong SM, Oliver HA, Scholl JL, Oliver KM, Forster GL (2010) Increased Anxiety-Like Behavior of Rats During Amphetamine Withdrawal Is Reversed by Crf2 Receptor Antagonism. Behavioural Brain Research. 208, 278-281.

[13] Furmark T, Fischer H, Wik G, Larsson M, Fredrikson M (1997) The Amygdala and Individual Differences in Human Fear Conditioning. Neuroreport. 8, 3957-3960.

[14] Whalen PJ, Bush G, McNally RJ, Wilhelm S, McInerney SC, Jenike MA, Rauch SL (1998) The Emotional Counting Stroop Paradigm: A Functional Magnetic Resonance Imaging Probe of the Anterior Cingulate Affective Division. Biol Psychiatry. 44, 1219-1228.

[15] Liddell BJ, Brown KJ, Kemp AH, Barton MJ, Das P, Peduto A, Gordon E, Williams LM (2005) A Direct Brainstem–Amygdala–Cortical 'Alarm' System for Subliminal Signals of Fear. Neuroimage. 24, 235-243. 10.1016/j.neuroimage.2004.08.016.

[16] Etkin A,Wager TD (2007) Functional Neuroimaging of Anxiety: A Meta-Analysis of Emotional Processing in Ptsd, Social Anxiety Disorder, and Specific Phobia. Am J Psychiatry. 164, 1476-1488. 10.1176/appi.ajp.2007.07030504.

[17] Hyde LW, Gorka A, Manuck SB, Hariri AR (2011) Perceived Social Support Moderates the Link between Threat-Related Amygdala Reactivity and Trait Anxiety. Neuropsychologia. 49, 651-656. 10.1016/j.neuropsychologia.2010.08.025.

[18] Carlson JM, Greenberg T, Rubin D, Mujica-Parodi LR (2011) Feeling Anxious: Anticipatory Amygdalo-Insular Response Predicts the Feeling of Anxious Anticipation. Soc Cogn Affect Neurosci. 6, 74-81. 10.1093/scan/nsq017.

[19] Stein MB, Simmons AN, Feinstein JS, Paulus MP (2007) Increased Amygdala and Insula Activation During Emotion Processing in Anxiety-Prone Subjects. Am J Psychiatry. 164, 318-327. 10.1176/appi.ajp.164.2.318.

[20] Bishop S, Duncan J, Brett M, Lawrence AD (2004) Prefrontal Cortical Function and Anxiety: Controlling Attention to Threat-Related Stimuli. Nat Neurosci. 7, 184-188.

[21] Etkin A, Klemenhagen KC, Dudman JT, Rogan MT, Hen R, Kandel ER, Hirsch J (2004) Individual Differences in Trait Anxiety Predict the Response of the Basolateral Amygdala to Unconsciously Processed Fearful Faces. Neuron. 44, 1043-1055. 10.1016/j.neuron.2004.12.006.

[22] Dickie EW, Armony JL (2008) Amygdala Responses to Unattended Fearful Faces: Interaction between Sex and Trait Anxiety. Psychiatry Research: Neuroimaging. 162, 51-57. 10.1016/j.pscychresns.2007.08.002.

[23] Ball TM, Sullivan S, Flagan T, Hitchcock CA, Simmons A, Paulus MP, Stein MB (2012) Selective Effects of Social Anxiety, Anxiety Sensitivity, and Negative Affectivity on the Neural Bases of Emotional Face Processing. Neuroimage. 59, 1879-1887. 10.1016/j.neuroimage.2011.08.074.

[24] Furmark T, Tillfors M, Marteinsdottir I, Fischer H, Pissiota A, Langstrom B, Fredrikson M (2002) Common Changes in Cerebral Blood Flow in Patients with Social Phobia Treated with Citalopram or Cognitive-Behavioral Therapy. Arch Gen Psychiatry. 59, 425-433.

[25] Shah SG, Klumpp H, Angstadt M, Nathan PJ, Phan KL (2009) Amygdala and Insula Response to Emotional Images in Patients with Generalized Social Anxiety Disorder. Journal of Psychiatry & Neuroscience. 34, 296-302.

[26] Brühl AB, Rufer M, Delsignore A, Kaffenberger T, Jäncke L, Herwig U (2011) Neural Correlates of Altered General Emotion Processing in Social Anxiety Disorder. Brain Res. 1378, 72-83. 10.1016/j.brainres.2010.12.084.

[27] Blair K, Shaywitz J, Smith BW, Rhodes R, Geraci M, Jones M, McCaffrey D, Vythilingam M, Finger E, Mondillo K, Jacobs M, Charney DS, Blair RJ, Drevets WC, Pine DS (2008) Response to Emotional Expressions in Generalized Social Phobia and Generalized Anxiety Disorder: Evidence for Separate Disorders. Am J Psychiatry. 165, 1193-1202. 10.1176/appi.ajp.2008.07071060.

[28] Rauch SL, Shin LM, Phelps EA (2006) Neurocircuitry Models of Posttraumatic Stress Disorder and Extinction: Human Neuroimaging Research--Past, Present, and Future. Biol Psychiatry. 60, 376-382.

[29] Jovanovic T, Norrholm SD (2011) Neural Mechanisms of Impaired Fear Inhibition in Posttraumatic Stress Disorder. Frontiers in Behavioral Neuroscience. 5, 10.3389/fnbeh.2011.00044.

[30] Liberzon I, Abelson JL, Flagel SB, Raz J, Young EA (1999) Neuroendocrine and Psychophysiologic Responses in Ptsd: A Symptom Provocation Study. Neuropsychopharmacology. 21, 40-50.

[31] Shin LM, Orr SP, Carson MA, Rauch SL, Macklin ML, Lasko NB, Peters PM, Metzger LJ, Dougherty DD, Cannistraro PA, Alpert NM, Fischman AJ, Pitman RK (2004) Regional Cerebral Blood Flow in the Amygdala and Medial Prefrontal Cortex During Traumatic Imagery in Male and Female Vietnam Veterans with Ptsd. Arch Gen Psychiatry. 61, 168-176.

[32] Shin LM, Wright CI, Cannistraro PA, Wedig MM, McMullin K, Martis B, Macklin ML, Lasko NB, Cavanagh SR, Krangel TS, Orr SP, Pitman RK, Whalen PJ, Rauch SL (2005) A Functional Magnetic Resonance Imaging Study of Amygdala and Medial Prefrontal Cortex Responses to Overtly Presented Fearful Faces in Posttraumatic Stress Disorder. Arch Gen Psychiatry. 62, 273-281.

[33] Bryant RA, Felmingham K, Kemp A, Das P, Hughes G, Peduto A, Williams L (2008) Amygdala and Ventral Anterior Cingulate Activation Predicts Treatment Response to Cognitive Behaviour Therapy for Post-Traumatic Stress Disorder. Psychological Medicine. 38, 555-561. doi:10.1017/S0033291707002231.
[34] Armony JL, Corbo V, Clement MH, Brunet A (2005) Amygdala Response in Patients with Acute Ptsd to Masked and Unmasked Emotional Facial Expressions. Am J Psychiatry. 162, 1961-1963.
[35] Dilger S, Straube T, Mentzel H-J, Fitzek C, Reichenbach JR, Hecht H, Krieschel S, Gutberlet I, Miltner WHR (2003) Brain Activation to Phobia-Related Pictures in Spider Phobic Humans: An Event-Related Functional Magnetic Resonance Imaging Study. Neurosci Lett. 348, 29-32. 10.1016/s0304-3940(03)00647-5.
[36] Schienle A, Schäfer A, Walter B, Stark R, Vaitl D (2005) Brain Activation of Spider Phobics Towards Disorder-Relevant, Generally Disgust- and Fear-Inducing Pictures. Neurosci Lett. 388, 1-6. 10.1016/j.neulet.2005.06.025.
[37] van den Heuvel OA, Veltman DJ, Groenewegen HJ, Witter MP, Merkelbach J, Cath DC, van Balkom AJLM, van Oppen P, van Dyck R (2005) Disorder-Specific Neuroanatomical Correlates of Attentional Bias in Obsessive-Compulsive Disorder, Panic Disorder, and Hypochondriasis. Arch Gen Psychiatry. 62, 922-933. 10.1001/archpsyc.62.8.922.
[38] Straube T, Mentzel H-J, Miltner WHR (2006) Neural Mechanisms of Automatic and Direct Processing of Phobogenic Stimuli in Specific Phobia. Biol Psychiatry. 59, 162-170. 10.1016/j.biopsych.2005.06.013.
[39] Whalen PJ, Johnstone T, Somerville LH, Nitschke JB, Polis S, Alexander AL, Davidson RJ, Kalin NH (2008) A Functional Magnetic Resonance Imaging Predictor of Treatment Response to Venlafaxine in Generalized Anxiety Disorder. Biol Psychiatry. 63, 858-863. 10.1016/j.biopsych.2007.08.019.
[40] Palm ME, Elliott R, McKie S, Deakin JFW, Anderson IM (2011) Attenuated Responses to Emotional Expressions in Women with Generalized Anxiety Disorder. Psychological Medicine. 41, 1009-1018. doi:10.1017/S0033291710001455.
[41] McClure EB, Adler A, Monk CS, Cameron J, Smith S, Nelson EE, Leibenluft E, Ernst M, Pine DS (2007) fMRI Predictors of Treatment Outcome in Pediatric Anxiety Disorders. Psychopharmacology (Berl). 191, 97-105. 10.1007/s00213-006-0542-9.
[42] Monk CS, Telzer EH, Mogg K, Bradley BP, Mai X, Louro HM, Chen G, McClure-Tone EB, Ernst M, Pine DS (2008) Amygdala and Ventrolateral Prefrontal Cortex Activation to Masked Angry Faces in Children and Adolescents with Generalized Anxiety Disorder. Arch Gen Psychiatry. 65, 568-576. 10.1001/archpsyc.65.5.568.
[43] Nitschke JB, Sarinopoulos I, Oathes DJ, Johnstone T, Whalen PJ, Davidson RJ, Kalin NH (2009) Anticipatory Activation in the Amygdala and Anterior Cingulate in Generalized Anxiety Disorder and Prediction of Treatment Response. Am J Psychiatry. 166, 302-310. appi.ajp.2008.07101682 [pii] 10.1176/appi.ajp.2008.07101682.
[44] Etkin A, Prater KE, Hoeft F, Menon V, Schatzberg AF (2010) Failure of Anterior Cingulate Activation and Connectivity with the Amygdala During Implicit Regulation

of Emotional Processing in Generalized Anxiety Disorder. Am J Psychiatry. 167, 545-554. 10.1176/appi.ajp.2009.09070931.

[45] Prevost C, McCabe JA, Jessup RK, Bossaerts P, O'Doherty JP (2011) Differentiable Contributions of Human Amygdalar Subregions in the Computations Underlying Reward and Avoidance Learning. Eur J Neurosci. 34, 134-145. 10.1111/j.1460-9568.2011.07686.x.

[46] Boll S, Gamer M, Kalisch R, Buchel C (2011) Processing of Facial Expressions and Their Significance for the Observer in Subregions of the Human Amygdala. Neuroimage. 56, 299-306. S1053-8119(11)00160-1 [pii] 10.1016/j.neuroimage.2011.02.021.

[47] Ball T, Rahm B, Eickhoff SB, Schulze-Bonhage A, Speck O, Mutschler I (2007) Response Properties of Human Amygdala Subregions: Evidence Based on Functional MRI Combined with Probabilistic Anatomical Maps. PLoS One. 2, e307. 10.1371/journal.pone.0000307.

[48] Ball T, Derix J, Wentlandt J, Wieckhorst B, Speck O, Schulze-Bonhage A, Mutschler I (2009) Anatomical Specificity of Functional Amygdala Imaging of Responses to Stimuli with Positive and Negative Emotional Valence. J Neurosci Methods. 180, 57-70. S0165-0270(09)00144-7 [pii] 10.1016/j.jneumeth.2009.02.022.

[49] Etkin A, Prater KE, Schatzberg AF, Menon V, Greicius MD (2009) Disrupted Amygdalar Subregion Functional Connectivity and Evidence of a Compensatory Network in Generalized Anxiety Disorder. Arch Gen Psychiatry. 66, 1361-1372. 66/12/1361 [pii] 10.1001/archgenpsychiatry.2009.104.

[50] Entis JJ, Doerga P, Barrett LF, Dickerson BC (2012) A Reliable Protocol for the Manual Segmentation of the Human Amygdala and Its Subregions Using Ultra-High Resolution MRI. Neuroimage. 60, 1226-1235. S1053-8119(12)00002-X [pii] 10.1016/j.neuroimage.2011.12.073.

[51] Kim N, Kim HJ, Hwang J, Yoon SJ, Cho HB, Renshaw PF, Lyoo IK, Kim JE (2011) Amygdalar Shape Analysis Method Using Surface Contour Aligning, Spherical Mapping, and Probabilistic Subregional Segmentation. Neurosci Lett. 488, 65-69. S0304-3940(10)01446-1 [pii] 10.1016/j.neulet.2010.11.005.

[52] Millan MJ (2003) The Neurobiology and Control of Anxious States. Prog Neurobiol. 70, 83-244. S030100820300087X [pii].

[53] Kalin NH, Sheltona SE (2003) Nonhuman Primate Models to Study Anxiety, Emotion Regulation, and Psychopathology. Annals of the New York Academy of Sciences. 1008, 189-200. 10.1196/annals.1301.021.

[54] Kalin NH, Shelton SE, Davidson RJ (2004) The Role of the Central Nucleus of the Amygdala in Mediating Fear and Anxiety in the Primate. J Neurosci. 24, 5506-5515. 10.1523/JNEUROSCI.0292-04.2004 24/24/5506 [pii].

[55] Lowry CA, Johnson PL, Hay-Schmidt A, Mikkelsen J, Shekhar A (2005) Modulation of Anxiety Circuits by Serotonergic Systems. Stress. 8, 233-246.

[56] Davis M (2006) Neural Systems Involved in Fear and Anxiety Measured with Fear-Potentiated Startle. Am Psychol. 61, 741-756. 2006-21079-027 [pii] 10.1037/0003-066X.61.8.741.

[57] Milad MR, Rauch SL, Pitman RK, Quirk GJ (2006) Fear Extinction in Rats: Implications for Human Brain Imaging and Anxiety Disorders. Biol Psychol. 73, 61-71.

[58] Davis M, Antoniadis EA, Amaral DG, Winslow JT (2008) Acoustic Startle Reflex in Rhesus Monkeys: A Review. Rev Neurosci. 19, 171-185.

[59] Price JL (2003) Comparative Aspects of Amygdala Connectivity. Ann N Y Acad Sci. 985, 50-58.

[60] LeDoux JE (2000) Emotion Circuits in the Brain. Annu Rev Neurosci. 23, 155-184. 10.1146/annurev.neuro.23.1.155.

[61] Canteras NS, Simerly RB, Swanson LW (1995) Organization of Projections from the Medial Nucleus of the Amygdala: A Phal Study in the Rat. J Comp Neurol. 360, 213-245. 10.1002/cne.903600203.

[62] Newman SW (1999) The Medial Extended Amygdala in Male Reproductive Behavior a Node in the Mammalian Social Behavior Network. Annals of the New York Academy of Sciences. 877, 242-257. 10.1111/j.1749-6632.1999.tb09271.x.

[63] Herman JP, Ostrander MM, Mueller NK, Figueiredo H (2005) Limbic System Mechanisms of Stress Regulation: Hypothalamo-Pituitary-Adrenocortical Axis. Progress in Neuro-Psychopharmacology and Biological Psychiatry. 29, 1201-1213. 10.1016/j.pnpbp.2005.08.006.

[64] Pitkanen A, Savander V, LeDoux JE (1997) Organization of Intra-Amygdaloid Circuitries in the Rat: An Emerging Framework for Understanding Functions of the Amygdala. Trends Neurosci. 20, 517-523. S0166223697011259 [pii].

[65] Canteras NS, Swanson LW (1992) Projections of the Ventral Subiculum to the Amygdala, Septum, and Hypothalamus: A Phal Anterograde Tract-Tracing Study in the Rat. J Comp Neurol. 324, 180-194. 10.1002/cne.903240204.

[66] Canteras NS, Simerly RB, Swanson LW (1992) Connections of the Posterior Nucleus of the Amygdala. J Comp Neurol. 324, 143-179. 10.1002/cne.903240203.

[67] Richter-Levin G, Akirav I (2000) Amygdala-Hippocampus Dynamic Interaction in Relation to Memory. Mol Neurobiol. 22, 11-20. MN:22:1-3:011 [pii] 10.1385/MN:22:1-3:011.

[68] Savander V, Miettinen R, Ledoux JE, Pitkanen A (1997) Lateral Nucleus of the Rat Amygdala Is Reciprocally Connected with Basal and Accessory Basal Nuclei: A Light and Electron Microscopic Study. Neuroscience. 77, 767-781. S0306-4522(96)00513-1 [pii].

[69] Pare D, Smith Y (1993) The Intercalated Cell Masses Project to the Central and Medial Nuclei of the Amygdala in Cats. Neuroscience. 57, 1077-1090. 0306-4522(93)90050-P [pii].

[70] Royer S, Martina M, Pare D (1999) An Inhibitory Interface Gates Impulse Traffic between the Input and Output Stations of the Amygdala. J Neurosci. 19, 10575-10583.

[71] Pare D, Quirk GJ, Ledoux JE (2004) New Vistas on Amygdala Networks in Conditioned Fear. J Neurophysiol. 92, 1-9. 10.1152/jn.00153.2004 92/1/1 [pii].

[72] LeDoux JE, Iwata J, Cicchetti P, Reis DJ (1988) Different Projections of the Central Amygdaloid Nucleus Mediate Autonomic and Behavioral Correlates of Conditioned Fear. J Neurosci. 8, 2517-2529.

[73] Davis M, Whalen PJ (2001) The Amygdala: Vigilance and Emotion. Mol Psychiatry. 6, 13-34.
[74] Dielenberg RA, McGregor IS (2001) Defensive Behavior in Rats Towards Predatory Odors: A Review. Neuroscience & Biobehavioral Reviews. 25, 597-609. 10.1016/s0149-7634(01)00044-6.
[75] Müller M, Fendt M (2006) Temporary Inactivation of the Medial and Basolateral Amygdala Differentially Affects Tmt-Induced Fear Behavior in Rats. Behavioural Brain Research. 167, 57-62. 10.1016/j.bbr.2005.08.016.
[76] Rosen JB, Pagani JH, Rolla KL, Davis C (2008) Analysis of Behavioral Constraints and the Neuroanatomy of Fear to the Predator Odor Trimethylthiazoline: A Model for Animal Phobias. Neurosci Biobehav Rev. 32, 1267-1276. S0149-7634(08)00068-7 [pii] 10.1016/j.neubiorev.2008.05.006.
[77] Ramos C, Leite-Panissi R, Monassi R, Menescal-De-Oliveira L (1999) Role of the Amygdaloid Nuclei in the Modulation of Tonic Immobility in Guinea Pigs. Physiol Behav. 67, 717-724. S003193849900133X [pii].
[78] Macedo CE, Martinez RC, Brandao ML (2006) Conditioned and Unconditioned Fear Organized in the Inferior Colliculus Are Differentially Sensitive to Injections of Muscimol into the Basolateral Nucleus of the Amygdala. Behav Neurosci. 120, 625-631. 2006-07279-013 [pii] 10.1037/0735-7044.120.3.625.
[79] Quirk GJ, Mueller D (2008) Neural Mechanisms of Extinction Learning and Retrieval. Neuropsychopharmacology. 33, 56-72.
[80] Zimmerman JM, Maren S (2010) Nmda Receptor Antagonism in the Basolateral but Not Central Amygdala Blocks the Extinction of Pavlovian Fear Conditioning in Rats. Eur J Neurosci. 31, 1664-1670. EJN7223 [pii] 10.1111/j.1460-9568.2010.07223.x.
[81] Sotres-Bayon F, Cain CK, LeDoux JE (2006) Brain Mechanisms of Fear Extinction: Historical Perspectives on the Contribution of Prefrontal Cortex. Biol Psychiatry. 60, 329-336.
[82] Likhtik E, Popa D, Apergis-Schoute J, Fidacaro GA, Pare D (2008) Amygdala Intercalated Neurons Are Required for Expression of Fear Extinction. Nature. 454, 642-645. nature07167 [pii] 10.1038/nature07167.
[83] Amano T, Unal CT, Pare D (2010) Synaptic Correlates of Fear Extinction in the Amygdala. Nat Neurosci. 13, 489-494. nn.2499 [pii] 10.1038/nn.2499.
[84] Moreira CM, Masson S, Carvalho MC, Brandao ML (2007) Exploratory Behaviour of Rats in the Elevated Plus-Maze Is Differentially Sensitive to Inactivation of the Basolateral and Central Amygdaloid Nuclei. Brain Res Bull. 71, 466-474. S0361-9230(06)00305-4 [pii] 10.1016/j.brainresbull.2006.10.004.
[85] Zarrindast MR, Solati J, Oryan S, Parivar K (2008) Effect of Intra-Amygdala Injection of Nicotine and GABA Receptor Agents on Anxiety-Like Behaviour in Rats. Pharmacology. 82, 276-284. 000161129 [pii] 10.1159/000161129.
[86] Tye KM, Prakash R, Kim SY, Fenno LE, Grosenick L, Zarabi H, Thompson KR, Gradinaru V, Ramakrishnan C, Deisseroth K (2011) Amygdala Circuitry Mediating

Reversible and Bidirectional Control of Anxiety. Nature. 471, 358-362. nature09820 [pii] 10.1038/nature09820.

[87] Walker DL, Toufexis DJ, Davis M (2003) Role of the Bed Nucleus of the Stria Terminalis Versus the Amygdala in Fear, Stress, and Anxiety. Eur J Pharmacol. 463, 199-216. S0014299903012822 [pii].

[88] Walker DL, Miles LA, Davis M (2009) Selective Participation of the Bed Nucleus of the Stria Terminalis and Crf in Sustained Anxiety-Like Versus Phasic Fear-Like Responses. Prog Neuropsychopharmacol Biol Psychiatry. 33, 1291-1308. S0278-5846(09)00212-7 [pii] 10.1016/j.pnpbp.2009.06.022.

[89] Walker DL, Davis M (2008) Role of the Extended Amygdala in Short-Duration Versus Sustained Fear: A Tribute to Dr. Lennart Heimer. Brain Struct Funct. 213, 29-42. 10.1007/s00429-008-0183-3.

[90] Duncan GE, Knapp DJ, Breese GR (1996) Neuroanatomical Characterization of Fos Induction in Rat Behavioral Models of Anxiety. Brain Res. 713, 79-91. 0006-8993(95)01486-1 [pii].

[91] Herdade KC, Strauss CV, Zangrossi Junior H, Viana MB (2006) Effects of Medial Amygdala Inactivation on a Panic-Related Behavior. Behav Brain Res. 172, 316-323. S0166-4328(06)00292-0 [pii] 10.1016/j.bbr.2006.05.021.

[92] Troakes C, Ingram CD (2009) Anxiety Behaviour of the Male Rat on the Elevated Plus Maze: Associated Regional Increase in C-Fos mRNA Expression and Modulation by Early Maternal Separation. Stress. 12, 362-369. 906308344 [pii] 10.1080/10253890802506391.

[93] Vinkers CH, Bijlsma EY, Houtepen LC, Westphal KG, Veening JG, Groenink L, Olivier B (2010) Medial Amygdala Lesions Differentially Influence Stress Responsivity and Sensorimotor Gating in Rats. Physiol Behav. 99, 395-401. S0031-9384(09)00392-8 [pii] 10.1016/j.physbeh.2009.12.006.

[94] Marschner A, Kalisch R, Vervliet B, Vansteenwegen D, Buchel C (2008) Dissociable Roles for the Hippocampus and the Amygdala in Human Cued Versus Context Fear Conditioning. J Neurosci. 28, 9030-9036. 28/36/9030 [pii] 10.1523/JNEUROSCI.1651-08.2008.

[95] Onishi BK, Xavier GF (2010) Contextual, but Not Auditory, Fear Conditioning Is Disrupted by Neurotoxic Selective Lesion of the Basal Nucleus of Amygdala in Rats. Neurobiol Learn Mem. 93, 165-174. S1074-7427(09)00197-X [pii] 10.1016/j.nlm.2009.09.007.

[96] McDonald AJ, Mascagni F, Guo L (1996) Projections of the Medial and Lateral Prefrontal Cortices to the Amygdala: A Phaseolus Vulgaris Leucoagglutinin Study in the Rat. Neuroscience. 71, 55-75. 0306-4522(95)00417-3 [pii].

[97] Vertes RP (2004) Differential Projections of the Infralimbic and Prelimbic Cortex in the Rat. Synapse. 51, 32-58. 10.1002/syn.10279.

[98] Corcoran KA, Quirk GJ (2007) Recalling Safety: Cooperative Functions of the Ventromedial Prefrontal Cortex and the Hippocampus in Extinction. CNS Spectr. 12, 200-206.

[99] Vidal-Gonzalez I, Vidal-Gonzalez B, Rauch SL, Quirk GJ (2006) Microstimulation Reveals Opposing Influences of Prelimbic and Infralimbic Cortex on the Expression of Conditioned Fear. Learn Mem. 13, 728-733. 13/6/728 [pii] 10.1101/lm.306106.

[100] Sierra-Mercado D, Padilla-Coreano N, Quirk GJ (2011) Dissociable Roles of Prelimbic and Infralimbic Cortices, Ventral Hippocampus, and Basolateral Amygdala in the Expression and Extinction of Conditioned Fear. Neuropsychopharmacology. 36, 529-538. npp2010184 [pii] 10.1038/npp.2010.184.

[101] Li G, Amano T, Pare D, Nair SS (2011) Impact of Infralimbic Inputs on Intercalated Amygdala Neurons: A Biophysical Modeling Study. Learn Mem. 18, 226-240. 10.1101/lm.1938011 18/4/226 [pii].

[102] Milad MR, Pitman RK, Ellis CB, Gold AL, Shin LM, Lasko NB, Zeidan MA, Handwerger K, Orr SP, Rauch SL (2009) Neurobiological Basis of Failure to Recall Extinction Memory in Posttraumatic Stress Disorder. Biol Psychiatry. 66, 1075-1082. S0006-3223(09)00896-8 [pii] 10.1016/j.biopsych.2009.06.026.

[103] Rougemont-Bucking A, Linnman C, Zeffiro TA, Zeidan MA, Lebron-Milad K, Rodriguez-Romaguera J, Rauch SL, Pitman RK, Milad MR (2011) Altered Processing of Contextual Information During Fear Extinction in PTSD: An fMRI Study. CNS Neurosci Ther. 17, 227-236. 10.1111/j.1755-5949.2010.00152.x CNS152 [pii].

[104] Kim MJ, Whalen PJ (2009) The Structural Integrity of an Amygdala-Prefrontal Pathway Predicts Trait Anxiety. J Neurosci. 29, 11614-11618. 29/37/11614 [pii] 10.1523/JNEUROSCI.2335-09.2009.

[105] Kim MJ, Gee DG, Loucks RA, Davis FC, Whalen PJ (2011) Anxiety Dissociates Dorsal and Ventral Medial Prefrontal Cortex Functional Connectivity with the Amygdala at Rest. Cereb Cortex. 21, 1667-1673. bhq237 [pii] 10.1093/cercor/bhq237.

[106] Inoue T, Koyama T, Yamashita I (1993) Effect of Conditioned Fear Stress on Serotonin Metabolism in the Rat Brain. Pharmacol Biochem Behav. 44, 371-374. 0091-3057(93)90476-A [pii].

[107] Yokoyama M, Suzuki E, Sato T, Maruta S, Watanabe S, Miyaoka H (2005) Amygdalic Levels of Dopamine and Serotonin Rise Upon Exposure to Conditioned Fear Stress without Elevation of Glutamate. Neurosci Lett. 379, 37-41. S0304-3940(04)01584-8 [pii] 10.1016/j.neulet.2004.12.047.

[108] Mo B, Feng N, Renner K, Forster G (2008) Restraint Stress Increases Serotonin Release in the Central Nucleus of the Amygdala Via Activation of Corticotropin-Releasing Factor Receptors. Brain Res Bull. 76, 493-498. S0361-9230(08)00039-7 [pii] 10.1016/j.brainresbull.2008.02.011.

[109] Zanoveli JM, Carvalho MC, Cunha JM, Brandão ML (2009) Extracellular Serotonin Level in the Basolateral Nucleus of the Amygdala and Dorsal Periaqueductal Gray under Unconditioned and Conditioned Fear States: An in Vivo Microdialysis Study. Brain Res. 1294, 106-115. S0006-8993(09)01537-6 [pii] 10.1016/j.brainres.2009.07.074.

[110] Spannuth BM, Hale MW, Evans AK, Lukkes JL, Campeau S, Lowry CA (2011) Investigation of a Central Nucleus of the Amygdala/Dorsal Raphe Nucleus Serotonergic

Circuit Implicated in Fear-Potentiated Startle. Neuroscience. 179, 104-119. S0306-4522(11)00065-0 [pii] 10.1016/j.neuroscience.2011.01.042.

[111] Emoto H, Koga C, Ishii H, Yokoo H, Yoshida M, Tanaka M (1993) A CRF Antagonist Attenuates Stress-Induced Increases in NA Turnover in Extended Brain Regions in Rats. Brain Res. 627, 171-176. 0006-8993(93)90762-C [pii].

[112] Dunn AJ (1988) Stress-Related Activation of Cerebral Dopaminergic Systems. Ann N Y Acad Sci. 537, 188-205.

[113] Quirarte, GL, Galvez, R, Roozendaal B, McGaugh JL. (1998) Norepinephrine Release in the Amygdala in Response to Footshock and Opioid Peptidergic Drugs. Brain Res. 808, 134-140.

[114] Inglis FM, Moghaddam B (1999) Dopaminergic Innervation of the Amygdala Is Highly Responsive to Stress. J Neurochem. 72, 1088-1094.

[115] Morilak DA, Barrera G, Echevarria DJ, Garcia AS, Hernandez A, Ma S, Petre CO (2005) Role of Brain Norepinephrine in the Behavioral Response to Stress. Prog Neuropsychopharmacol Biol Psychiatry. 29, 1214-1224. S0278-5846(05)00270-8 [pii] 10.1016/j.pnpbp.2005.08.007.

[116] Ma S, Morilak DA (2005) Norepinephrine Release in Medial Amygdala Facilitates Activation of the Hypothalamic-Pituitary-Adrenal Axis in Response to Acute Immobilisation Stress. J Neuroendocrinol. 17, 22-28. JNE1279 [pii] 10.1111/j.1365-2826.2005.01279.x.

[117] Mitsushima D, Yamada K, Takase K, Funabashi T, Kimura F (2006) Sex Differences in the Basolateral Amygdala: The Extracellular Levels of Serotonin and Dopamine, and Their Responses to Restraint Stress in Rats. Eur J Neurosci. 24, 3245-3254. EJN5214 [pii] 10.1111/j.1460-9568.2006.05214.x.

[118] McIntyre CK, Hatfield T, McGaugh, JL (2002) Amygdala Norepinephrine Levels after Training Predict Inhibitory Avoidance Retention Performance in Rats. Eur J Neurosci. 16, 1223-1226.

[119] Carrasco GA, Van de Kar LD (2003) Neuroendocrine Pharmacology of Stress. Eur J Pharmacol. 463, 235-272.

[120] Feltenstein MW, See RE. (2008) The Neurocircuitry of Addiction: An Overview. British Journal of Pharmacology 154, 261–274.

[121] Butler PD, Weiss JM, Stout JC, Nemeroff CB (1990) Corticotropin-Releasing Factor Produces Fear-Enhancing and Behavioral Activating Effects Following Infusion into the Locus Coeruleus. J Neurosci. 10, 176-183.

[122] Basso AM, Spina M, Rivier J, Vale W, Koob GF (1999) Corticotropin-Releasing Factor Antagonist Attenuates the "Anxiogenic-Like" Effect in the Defensive Burying Paradigm but Not in the Elevated Plus-Maze Following Chronic Cocaine in Rats. Psychopharmacology (Berl). 145, 21-30.

[123] Radulovic J, Ruhmann A, Liepold T, Spiess J (1999) Modulation of Learning and Anxiety by Corticotropin-Releasing Factor (CRF) and Stress: Differential Roles of CRF Receptors 1 and 2. J Neurosci. 19, 5016-5025.

[124] Kikusui T, Takeuchi Y, Mori Y (2000) Involvement of Corticotropin-Releasing Factor in the Retrieval Process of Fear-Conditioned Ultrasonic Vocalization in Rats. Physiol Behav. 71, 323-328.

[125] Takahashi LK (2001) Role of CRF(1) and CRF(2) Receptors in Fear and Anxiety. Neurosci Biobehav Rev. 25, 627-636.

[126] Bale TL (2005) Sensitivity to Stress: Dysregulation of CRF Pathways and Disease Development. Horm Behav. 48, 1-10.

[127] Lukkes J, Vuong S, Scholl J, Oliver H, Forster G (2009) Corticotropin-Releasing Factor Receptor Antagonism within the Dorsal Raphe Nucleus Reduces Social Anxiety-Like Behavior after Early-Life Social Isolation. The Journal of Neuroscience. 29, 9955-9960. 10.1523/jneurosci.0854-09.2009.

[128] Bledsoe AC, Oliver KM, Scholl JL, Forster GL (2011) Anxiety States Induced by Post-Weaning Social Isolation Are Mediated by CRF Receptors in the Dorsal Raphe Nucleus. Brain Res Bull. 85, 117-122. 10.1016/j.brainresbull.2011.03.003.

[129] Risbrough VB, Stein MB (2006) Role of Corticotropin Releasing Factor in Anxiety Disorders: A Translational Research Perspective. Horm Behav. 50, 550-561.

[130] Matsuzaki I, Takamatsu Y, Moroji T (1989) The Effects of Intracerebroventricularly Injected Corticotropin-Releasing Factor (CRF) on the Central Nervous System: Behavioural and Biochemical Studies. Neuropeptides. 13, 147-155.

[131] Amat J, Tamblyn JP, Paul ED, Bland ST, Amat P, Foster AC, Watkins LR, Maier SF (2004) Microinjection of Urocortin 2 into the Dorsal Raphe Nucleus Activates Serotonergic Neurons and Increases Extracellular Serotonin in the Basolateral Amygdala. Neuroscience. 129, 509-519. S0306-4522(04)00718-3 [pii] 10.1016/j.neuroscience.2004.07.052.

[132] Forster GL, Feng N, Watt MJ, Korzan WJ, Mouw NJ, Summers CH, Renner KJ (2006) Corticotropin-Releasing Factor in the Dorsal Raphe Elicits Temporally Distinct Serotonergic Responses in the Limbic System in Relation to Fear Behavior. Neuroscience. 141, 1047-1055. S0306-4522(06)00490-8 [pii] 10.1016/j.neuroscience.2006.04.006.

[133] Scholl JL, Vuong SM, Forster GL (2010) Chronic Amphetamine Treatment Enhances Corticotropin-Releasing Factor-Induced Serotonin Release in the Amygdala. Eur J Pharmacol. 644, 80-87. S0014-2999(10)00705-3 [pii] 10.1016/j.ejphar.2010.07.008.

[134] Gray TS (1993) Amygdaloid CRF Pathways. Role in Autonomic, Neuroendocrine, and Behavioral Responses to Stress. Ann N Y Acad Sci. 697, 53-60.

[135] Day HE, Greenwood BN, Hammack SE, Watkins LR, Fleshner M, Maier SF,Campeau S (2004) Differential Expression of 5HT-1a, Alpha 1b Adrenergic, CRF-R1, and CFR-R2 Receptor mRNA in Serotonergic, Gamma-Aminobutyric Acidergic, and Catecholaminergic Cells of the Rat Dorsal Raphe Nucleus. J Comp Neurol. 474, 364-378.

[136] Wang B, You ZB, Rice KC, Wise RA (2007) Stress-Induced Relapse to Cocaine Seeking: Roles for the CRF(2) Receptor and CRF-Binding Protein in the Ventral Tegmental Area of the Rat. Psychopharmacology (Berl). 193, 283-294.

[137] Pringle RB, Mouw NJ, Lukkes JL, Forster GL (2008) Amphetamine Treatment Increases Corticotropin-Releasing Factor Receptors in the Dorsal Raphe Nucleus. Neurosci Res. 62, 62-65.

[138] Reyes BA, Valentino RJ, Van Bockstaele EJ (2008) Stress-Induced Intracellular Trafficking of Corticotropin-Releasing Factor Receptors in Rat Locus Coeruleus Neurons. Endocrinology. 149, 122-130.

[139] Wise RA, Morales M (2010) A Ventral Tegmental CRF–Glutamate–Dopamine Interaction in Addiction. Brain Res. 1314, 38-43. 10.1016/j.brainres.2009.09.101.

[140] Tagliaferro P, Morales M (2008) Synapses between Corticotropin-Releasing Factor-Containing Axon Terminals and Dopaminergic Neurons in the Ventral Tegmental Area Are Predominantly Glutamatergic. J Comp Neurol. 506, 616-626. 10.1002/cne.21576.

[141] Pernar L, Curtis AL, Vale WW, Rivier JE, Valentino RJ (2004) Selective Activation of Corticotropin-Releasing Factor-2 Receptors on Neurochemically Identified Neurons in the Rat Dorsal Raphe Nucleus Reveals Dual Actions. J Neurosci. 24, 1305-1311.

[142] Waselus M, Nazzaro C, Valentino RJ, Van Bockstaele EJ (2009) Stress-Induced Redistribution of Corticotropin-Releasing Factor Receptor Subtypes in the Dorsal Raphe Nucleus. Biol Psychiatry. 66, 76-83.

[143] Lukkes JL, Summers CH, Scholl JL, Renner KJ, Forster GL (2009) Early Life Social Isolation Alters Corticotropin-Releasing Factor Responses in Adult Rats. Neuroscience. 158, 845-855.

[144] Boyson C, Miguel T, Quadros I, DeBold J, Miczek K (2011) Prevention of Social Stress-Escalated Cocaine Self-Administration by CRF-R1 Antagonist in the Rat Vta. Psychopharmacology (Berl). 1-13. 10.1007/s00213-011-2266-8.

[145] Faria R, Magalhães A, Monteiro PR, Gomes-Da-Silva J, Amélia Tavares M, Summavielle T (2006) MDMA in Adolescent Male Rats: Decreased Serotonin in the Amygdala and Behavioral Effects in the Elevated Plus-Maze Test. Ann N Y Acad Sci. 1074, 643-649. 1074/1/643 [pii] 10.1196/annals.1369.062.

[146] Niwa M, Matsumoto Y, Mouri A, Ozaki N, Nabeshima T (2011) Vulnerability in Early Life to Changes in the Rearing Environment Plays a Crucial Role in the Aetiopathology of Psychiatric Disorders. Int J Neuropsychopharmacol. 14, 459-477. S1461145710001239 [pii] 10.1017/S1461145710001239.

[147] Costall B, Jones BJ, Kelly ME, Naylor RJ, Oakley NR, Onaivi ES, Tyers MB (1989) The Effects of Ondansetron (Gr38032f) in Rats and Mice Treated Subchronically with Diazepam. Pharmacol Biochem Behav. 34, 769-778.

[148] Cruz APM, Pinheiro G, Alves SH, Ferreira G, Mendes M, Faria L, et al. (2005) Behavioral effects of systemically administered MK-212 are prevented by ritanserin microinfusion into the basolateral amygdala of rats exposed to the elevated plus-maze. Psychopharmacology. 182:345–54.

[149] Zangrossi H, Graeff FG (1994) Behavioral effects of intraamygdala injections of GABA and 5-HT acting drugs in the elevated plus-maze. Braz. J Med Biol Res. 27, 2453–6.

[150] Cornelio AM, Nunes-de-Souza RL (2007) Anxiogenic-Like Effects of MCPP Microinfusions into the Amygdala (but not Dorsal or Ventral Hippocampus) in Mice Exposed to Elevated Plus-Maze. Behav Brain Res. 178, 82-89. 10.1016/j.bbr.2006.12.003.

[151] Higgins GA, Jones BJ, Oakley NR, Tyers MB (1991) Evidence that the Amygdala Is Involved in the Disinhibitory Effects of 5-HT3 Receptor Antagonists. Psychopharmacology (Berl). 104, 545-551.

[152] Tomkins DM, Costall B, Kelly ME. (1990) Release of Suppressed Behavior of rat on the Elevated X-maze by 5-HT3 Receptor Antagonists injected into the Basolateral Amygdala. J Psychopharmacol.4, 203–5.

[153] Gonzalez LE, Andrews N, File SE (1996) 5-HT1a and Benzodiazepine Receptors in the Basolateral Amygdala Modulate Anxiety in the Social Interaction Test, but Not in the Elevated Plus-Maze. Brain Res. 732, 145-153.

[154] Vicente MA, Zangrossi H (2011) Serotonin-2c Receptors in the Basolateral Nucleus of the Amygdala Mediate the Anxiogenic Effect of Acute Imipramine and Fluoxetine Administration. Int J Neuropsychopharmacol. 1-12. S1461145711000873 [pii] 10.1017/S1461145711000873.

[155] Duxon MS, Beckett SR, Baxter GS, Blackburn TP, Fone KCF. (1995). Intraamygdala Injection of the 5-HT2B Receptor Agonist BW-72386 Produces Anxiolysis on the Elevated Plus-Maze in the Rat. Br J Pharmacol 116, P331-P331.

[156] Duxon MS, Kennett GA, Lightowler S, Blackburn TP, Fone KC (1997) Activation of 5-HT2b Receptors in the Medial Amygdala Causes Anxiolysis in the Social Interaction Test in the Rat. Neuropharmacology. 36, 601-608.

[157] Inoue T, Li XB, Abekawa T, Kitaichi Y, Izumi T, Nakagawa S, Koyama T (2004) Selective Serotonin Reuptake Inhibitor Reduces Conditioned Fear through Its Effect in the Amygdala. Eur J Pharmacol. 497, 311-316. S0014 2999(04)00702-2 [pii] 10.1016/j.ejphar.2004.06.061.

[158] Leite-Panissi CR, Ferrarese AA, Terzian AL, Menescal-de-Oliveira L (2006) Serotoninergic Activation of the Basolateral Amygdala and Modulation of Tonic Immobility in Guinea Pig. Brain Res Bull. 69, 356-364. S0361-9230(06)00051-7 [pii] 10.1016/j.brainresbull.2006.02.007.

[159] Li X, Inoue T, Abekawa T, Weng S, Nakagawa S, Izumi T, Koyama T (2006) 5-Ht1a Receptor Agonist Affects Fear Conditioning through Stimulations of the Postsynaptic 5-Ht1a Receptors in the Hippocampus and Amygdala. Eur J Pharmacol. 532, 74-80. S0014-2999(05)01310-5 [pii] 10.1016/j.ejphar.2005.12.008.

[160] Morrison KE, Cooper MA (2012) A Role for 5-Ht1a Receptors in the Basolateral Amygdala in the Development of Conditioned Defeat in Syrian Hamsters. Pharmacol Biochem Behav. 100, 592-600. S0091-3057(11)00312-1 [pii] 10.1016/j.pbb.2011.09.005.

[161] Centonze D, Usiello A, Gubellini P, Pisani A, Borrelli E, Bernardi G, Calabresi P (2002) Dopamine D2 Receptor-Mediated Inhibition of Dopaminergic Neurons in Mice Lacking D2l Receptors. Neuropsychopharmacology. 27, 723-726.

[162] Rouge-Pont F, Usiello A, Benoit-Marand M, Gonon F, Piazza PV, Borrelli E (2002) Changes in Extracellular Dopamine Induced by Morphine and Cocaine: Crucial Control by D2 Receptors. J Neurosci. 22, 3293-3301.

[163] Summavielle T, Magalhães A, Castro-Vale I, de Sousa L, Tavares MA (2002) Neonatal Exposure to Cocaine: Altered Dopamine Levels in the Amygdala and Behavioral Outcomes in the Developing Rat. Ann N Y Acad Sci. 965, 515-521.

[164] Izumo N, Ishibashi Y, Ohba M, Morikawa T, Manabe T (2012) Decreased Voluntary Activity and Amygdala Levels of Serotonin and Dopamine in Ovariectomized Rats. Behav Brain Res. 227, 1-6. S0166-4328(11)00764-9 [pii] 10.1016/j.bbr.2011.10.031.

[165] Rezayof A, Hosseini SS, Zarrindast MR (2009) Effects of Morphine on Rat Behaviour in the Elevated Plus Maze: The Role of Central Amygdala Dopamine Receptors. Behav Brain Res. 202, 171-178. S0166-4328(09)00193-4 [pii] 10.1016/j.bbr.2009.03.030.

[166] de la Mora MP, Gallegos-Cari A, Crespo-Ramirez M, Marcellino D, Hansson AC, Fuxe K (2012) Distribution of Dopamine D(2)-Like Receptors in the Rat Amygdala and Their Role in the Modulation of Unconditioned Fear and Anxiety. Neuroscience. 201, 252-266. S0306-4522(11)01238-3 [pii] 10.1016/j.neuroscience.2011.10.045.

[167] Sullivan RM, Duchesne A, Hussain D, Waldron J, Laplante F (2009) Effects of Unilateral Amygdala Dopamine Depletion on Behaviour in the Elevated Plus Maze: Role of Sex, Hemisphere and Retesting. Behav Brain Res. 205, 115-122. S0166-4328(09)00440-9 [pii] 10.1016/j.bbr.2009.07.023.

[168] Bananej M, Karimi-Sori A, Zarrindast MR, Ahmadi S (2011) D1 and D2 Dopaminergic Systems in the Rat Basolateral Amygdala Are Involved in Anxiogenic-Like Effects Induced by Histamine. J Psychopharmacol. 0269881111405556 [pii] 10.1177/0269881111405556.

[169] de la Mora MP, Cardenas-Cachon L, Vazquez-Garcia M, Crespo-Ramirez M, Jacobsen K, Hoistad M, Agnati L, Fuxe K (2005) Anxiolytic Effects of Intra-Amygdaloid Injection of the D1 Antagonist SCH23390 in the Rat. Neurosci Lett. 377, 101-105. 10.1016/j.neulet.2004.11.079.

[170] Greba Q, Gifkins A, Kokkinidis L (2001) Inhibition of Amygdaloid Dopamine D2 Receptors Impairs Emotional Learning Measured with Fear-Potentiated Startle. Brain Res. 899, 218-226. S0006-8993(01)02243-0 [pii].

[171] Guarraci FA, Frohardt RJ, Kapp BS (1999) Amygdaloid D1 Dopamine Receptor Involvement in Pavlovian Fear Conditioning. Brain Res. 827, 28-40. S0006-8993(99)01291-3 [pii].

[172] Guarraci FA, Frohardt RJ, Falls WA, Kapp BS (2000) The Effects of Intra-Amygdaloid Infusions of a D2 Dopamine Receptor Antagonist on Pavlovian Fear Conditioning. Behav Neurosci. 114, 647-651.

[173] Selden NR, Everitt BJ, Jarrard LE, Robbins TW (1991) Complementary Roles for the Amygdala and Hippocampus in Aversive Conditioning to Explicit and Contextual Cues. Neuroscience. 42, 335-350. 0306-4522(91)90379-3 [pii].

[174] Greba Q, Kokkinidis L (2000) Peripheral and Intraamygdalar Administration of the Dopamine D1 Receptor Antagonist Sch 23390 Blocks Fear-Potentiated Startle but Not

Shock Reactivity or the Shock Sensitization of Acoustic Startle. Behav Neurosci. 114, 262-272.

[175] de Oliveira AR, Reimer AE, de Macedo CE, de Carvalho MC, Silva MA, Brandão ML (2011) Conditioned Fear Is Modulated by D2 Receptor Pathway Connecting the Ventral Tegmental Area and Basolateral Amygdala. Neurobiol Learn Mem. 95, 37-45. S1074-7427(10)00172-3 [pii] 10.1016/j.nlm.2010.10.005.

[176] Cecchi M, Khoshbouei H, Morilak DA (2002) Modulatory Effects of Norepinephrine, Acting on Alpha 1 Receptors in the Central Nucleus of the Amygdala, on Behavioral and Neuroendocrine Responses to Acute Immobilization Stress. Neuropharmacology. 43, 1139-1147. S0028390802002927 [pii].

[177] Debiec J, LeDoux JE (2006) Noradrenergic Signaling in the Amygdala Contributes to the Reconsolidation of Fear Memory: Treatment Implications for PTSD. Ann N Y Acad Sci. 1071, 521-524. 1071/1/521 [pii] 10.1196/annals.1364.056.

[178] LaLumiere RT, Buen TV, McGaugh JL (2003) Post-Training Intra-Basolateral Amygdala Infusions of Norepinephrine Enhance Consolidation of Memory for Contextual Fear Conditioning. J Neurosci. 23, 6754-6758. 23/17/6754 [pii].

[179] Lazzaro SC, Hou M, Cunha C, LeDoux JE, Cain CK (2010) Antagonism of Lateral Amygdala Alpha1-Adrenergic Receptors Facilitates Fear Conditioning and Long-Term Potentiation. Learn Mem. 17, 489-493. 17/10/489 [pii] 10.1101/lm.1918210.

[180] Debiec J, Ledoux JE (2004) Disruption of Reconsolidation but Not Consolidation of Auditory Fear Conditioning by Noradrenergic Blockade in the Amygdala. Neuroscience. 129, 267-272. S0306-4522(04)00745-6 [pii] 10.1016/j.neuroscience.2004.08.018.

[181] Roozendaal B, Hui GK, Hui IR, Berlau DJ, McGaugh JL, Weinberger NM (2006) Basolateral Amygdala Noradrenergic Activity Mediates Corticosterone-Induced Enhancement of Auditory Fear Conditioning. Neurobiol Learn Mem. 86, 249-255. S1074-7427(06)00032-3 [pii] 10.1016/j.nlm.2006.03.003.

[182] Cloos J-M, Ferreira V (2009) Current Use of Benzodiazepines in Anxiety Disorders. Curr Opin Psychiatry. 22, 90-95.

[183] Ravindran LN, Stein MB (2010) The Pharmacologic Treatment of Anxiety Disorders: A Review of Progress. J Clin Psychiatry. 71, 839-854.

[184] Brignell CM, Curran HV (2006) Drugs, Sweat and Fears: A Comparison of the Effects of Diazepam and Methylphenidate on Fear Conditioning. Psychopharmacol. 186, 504-516. 10.1007/s00213-006-0363-x.

[185] Hellewell JS, Guimaraes FS, Wang M, Deakin JF (1999) Comparison of Buspirone with Diazepam and Fluvoxamine on Aversive Classical Conditioning in Humans. J Psychopharmacol. 13, 122-127.

[186] Scaife JC, Hou RH, Samuels ER, Baqui F, Langley RW, Bradshaw CM, Szabadi E (2007) Diazepam-Induced Disruption of Classically-Conditioned Fear-Potentiation of Late-Latency Auditory Evoked Potentials Is Prevented by Flumazenil Given before, but Not after, CS/US Pairing. J Psychopharmacol. 21, 93-101.

[187] Zangara A, Blair RJR, Curran HV (2002) A Comparison of the Effects of a Beta-Adrenergic Blocker and a Benzodiazepine Upon the Recognition of Human Facial Expressions. Psychopharmacology (Berl). 163, 36-41.
[188] Brignell CM, Rosenthal J, Curran HV (2007) Pharmacological Manipulations of Arousal and Memory for Emotional Material: Effects of a Single Dose of Methylphenidate or Lorazepam. J Psychopharmacol. 21, 673-683. 10.1177/0269881107077351.
[189] Buchanan TW, Karafin MS, Adolphs R (2003) Selective Effects of Triazolam on Memory for Emotional, Relative to Neutral, Stimuli: Differential Effects on Gist Versus Detail. Behav Neurosci. 117, 517-525.
[190] Paulus MP, Feinstein JS, Castillo G, Simmons AN, Stein MB (2005) Dose-Dependent Decrease of Activation in Bilateral Amygdala and Insula by Lorazepam During Emotion Processing. Arch Gen Psychiatry. 62, 282-288.
[191] Del-Ben CM, Ferreira CA, Sanchez TA, Alves-Neto WC, Guapo VG, de Araujo DB, Graeff FG (2010) Effects of Diazepam on Bold Activation During the Processing of Aversive Faces. J Psychopharmacol.
[192] Schunck T, Mathis A, Erb G, Namer IJ, Demazieres A, Luthringer R (2010) Effects of Lorazepam on Brain Activity Pattern During an Anxiety Symptom Provocation Challenge. J Psychopharmacol. 24, 701-708.
[193] Brantigan CO, Brantigan TA, Joseph N (1979) The Effect of Beta Blockade on Stage Fright. A Controlled Study. Rocky Mt Med J. 76, 227-233.
[194] Heiser JF, Defrancisco D (1976) The Treatment of Pathological Panic States with Propranolol. Am J Psychiatry. 133, 1389-1394.
[195] Tyrer P (1988) Current Status of Beta-Blocking Drugs in the Treatment of Anxiety Disorders. Drugs. 36, 773-783.
[196] Bell J (2008) Propranolol, Post-Traumatic Stress Disorder and Narrative Identity. J Med Ethics. 34, e23. 10.1136/jme.2008.024752.
[197] Dębiec J, Bush DEA, LeDoux JE (2011) Noradrenergic Enhancement of Reconsolidation in the Amygdala Impairs Extinction of Conditioned Fear in Rats--a Possible Mechanism for the Persistence of Traumatic Memories in PTSD. Depress Anxiety. 28, 186-193.
[198] Fletcher S, Creamer M, Forbes D (2010) Preventing Post Traumatic Stress Disorder: Are Drugs the Answer? The Australian and New Zealand Journal of Psychiatry. 44, 1064-1071.
[199] McGhee LL, Maani CV, Garza TH, Desocio PA, Gaylord KM, Black IH (2009) The Effect of Propranolol on Posttraumatic Stress Disorder in Burned Service Members. Journal of Burn Care & Research, 30, 92-97.
[200] Stein MB, Kerridge C, Dimsdale JE, Hoyt DB (2007) Pharmacotherapy to Prevent Ptsd: Results from a Randomized Controlled Proof-of-Concept Trial in Physically Injured Patients. Journal of Traumatic Stress. 20, 923-932.
[201] Hurlemann R, Walter H, Rehme AK, Kukolja J, Santoro SC, Schmidt C, Schnell K, Musshoff F, Keysers C, Maier W, Kendrick KM, Onur OA (2010) Human Amygdala

Reactivity Is Diminished by the B-Noradrenergic Antagonist Propranolol. Psychological Medicine. 40, 1839-1848.

[202] van Stegeren AH, Goekoop R, Everaerd W, Scheltens P, Barkhof F, Kuijer JPA, Rombouts SARB (2005) Noradrenaline Mediates Amygdala Activation in Men and Women During Encoding of Emotional Material. Neuroimage. 24, 898-909.

[203] Kent JM, Coplan JD, Gorman JM (1998) Clinical Utility of the Selective Serotonin Reuptake Inhibitors in the Spectrum of Anxiety. Biol Psychiatry. 44, 812-824.

[204] Browning M, Reid C, Cowen PJ, Goodwin GM, Harmer CJ (2007) A Single Dose of Citalopram Increases Fear Recognition in Healthy Subjects. J Psychopharmacol. 21, 684-690. 10.1177/0269881106074062.

[205] Grillon C, Levenson J, Pine DS (2007) A Single Dose of the Selective Serotonin Reuptake Inhibitor Citalopram Exacerbates Anxiety in Humans: A Fear-Potentiated Startle Study. Neuropsychopharmacology. 32, 225-231.

[206] Harmer CJ, Bhagwagar Z, Perrett DI, Völlm BA, Cowen PJ, Goodwin GM (2003) Acute Ssri Administration Affects the Processing of Social Cues in Healthy Volunteers. Neuropsychopharmacology. 28, 148-152.

[207] Harmer CJ, Shelley NC, Cowen PJ, Goodwin GM (2004) Increased Positive Versus Negative Affective Perception and Memory in Healthy Volunteers Following Selective Serotonin and Norepinephrine Reuptake Inhibition. Am J Psychiatry. 161, 1256-1263.

[208] Murphy SE, Yiend J, Lester KJ, Cowen PJ, Harmer CJ (2009) Short-Term Serotonergic but Not Noradrenergic Antidepressant Administration Reduces Attentional Vigilance to Threat in Healthy Volunteers. The International Journal of Neuropsychopharmacology. 12, 169-179.

[209] Harmer CJ, Mackay CE, Reid CB, Cowen PJ, Goodwin GM (2006) Antidepressant Drug Treatment Modifies the Neural Processing of Nonconscious Threat Cues. Biol Psychiatry. 59, 816-820.

[210] Anderson IM, Del-Ben CM, McKie S, Richardson P, Williams SR, Elliott R, Deakin JFW (2007) Citalopram Modulation of Neuronal Responses to Aversive Face Emotions: A Functional MRI Study. Neuroreport. 18, 1351-1355.

[211] Del-Ben CM, Deakin JFW, McKie S, Delvai NA, Williams SR, Elliott R, Dolan M, Anderson IM (2005) The Effect of Citalopram Pretreatment on Neuronal Responses to Neuropsychological Tasks in Normal Volunteers: An fMRI Study. Neuropsychopharmacology. 30, 1724-1734.

[212] Cools R, Calder AJ, Lawrence AD, Clark L, Bullmore E, Robbins TW (2005) Individual Differences in Threat Sensitivity Predict Serotonergic Modulation of Amygdala Response to Fearful Faces. Psychopharmacology (Berl). 180, 670-679.

[213] Attenburrow MJ, Williams C, Odontiadis J, Reed A, Powell J, Cowen PJ, Harmer CJ (2003) Acute Administration of Nutritionally Sourced Tryptophan Increases Fear Recognition. Psychopharmacology (Berl). 169, 104-107. 10.1007/s00213-003-1479-x.

[214] Rhodes RA, Murthy NV, Dresner MA, Selvaraj S, Stavrakakis N, Babar S, Cowen PJ, Grasby PM (2007) Human 5-HT Transporter Availability Predicts Amygdala Reactivity in Vivo. The Journal of Neuroscience. 27, 9233-9237.

[215] Niehoff DL, Kuhar MJ (1983) Benzodiazepine Receptors: Localization in Rat Amygdala. The Journal of Neuroscience. 3, 2091-2097.
[216] Young WS, 3rd, Kuhar MJ (1980) Radiohistochemical Localization of Benzodiazepine Receptors in Rat Brain. J Pharmacol Exp Ther. 212, 337-346.
[217] Hodges H, Green S, Glenn B (1987) Evidence That the Amygdala Is Involved in Benzodiazepine and Serotonergic Effects on Punished Responding but Not on Discrimination. Psychopharmacology (Berl). 92, 491-504.
[218] Nagy J, Zámbó K, Decsi L (1979) Anti-Anxiety Action of Diazepam after Intra-Amygdaloid Application in the Rat. Neuropharmacology. 18, 573-576.
[219] Petersen EN, Braestrup C, Scheel-Krüger J (1985) Evidence That the Anticonflict Effect of Midazolam in Amygdala Is Mediated by the Specific Benzodiazepine Receptors. Neurosci Lett. 53, 285-288.
[220] Scheel-Krüger J, Petersen EN (1982) Anticonflict Effect of the Benzodiazepines Mediated by a Gabaergic Mechanism in the Amygdala. Eur J Pharmacol. 82, 115-116.
[221] Shibata K, Kataoka Y, Gomita Y, Ueki S (1982) Localization of the Site of the Anticonflict Action of Benzodiazepines in the Amygdaloid Nucleus of Rats. Brain Res. 234, 442-446.
[222] Green S, Vale AL (1992) Role of Amygdaloid Nuclei in the Anxiolytic Effects of Benzodiazepines in Rats. Behavioural Pharmacology. 3, 261-264.
[223] Pesold C, Treit D (1995) The Central and Basolateral Amygdala Differentially Mediate the Anxiolytic Effects of Benzodiazepines. Brain Res. 671, 213-221.
[224] Carvalho MC, Moreira CM, Zanoveli JM, Brandão ML (2012) Central, but Not Basolateral, Amygdala Involvement in the Anxiolytic-Like Effects of Midazolam in Rats in the Elevated Plus Maze. J Psychopharmacol. 26, 543-54.
[225] Tomaz C, Dickinson-Anson H, McGaugh JL (1992) Basolateral Amygdala Lesions Block Diazepam-Induced Anterograde Amnesia in an Inhibitory Avoidance Task. Proc Natl Acad Sci U S A. 89, 3615-3619.
[226] Tomaz C, Dickinson-Anson H, McGaugh JL, Souza-Silva MA, Viana MB, Graeff FG (1993) Localization in the Amygdala of the Amnestic Action of Diazepam on Emotional Memory. Behav Brain Res. 58, 99-105.
[227] Silva MA, Tomaz C (1995) Amnesia after Diazepam Infusion into Basolateral but Not Central Amygdala of Rattus Norvegicus. Neuropsychobiology. 32, 31-36.
[228] Da Cunha C, Roozendaal B, Vazdarjanova A, McGaugh JL (1999) Microinfusions of Flumazenil into the Basolateral but Not the Central Nucleus of the Amygdala Enhance Memory Consolidation in Rats. Neurobiology of Learning and Memory. 72, 1-7.
[229] Coles ME, Heimberg RG (2002) Memory Biases in the Anxiety Disorders: Current Status. Clin Psychol Rev. 22, 587-627.
[230] Coles ME, Turk CL, Heimberg RG (2007) Memory Bias for Threat in Generalized Anxiety Disorder: The Potential Importance of Stimulus Relevance. Cognitive Behaviour Therapy. 36, 65-73.
[231] Ferry B, McGaugh JL (2000) Role of Amygdala Norepinephrine in Mediating Stress Hormone Regulation of Memory Storage. Acta Pharmacol Sin. 21, 481-493.

[232] Ferry B, Roozendaal B, McGaugh J (1999) Role of Norepinephrine in Mediating Stress Hormone Regulation of Long-tern Memory Storage: A Critical Involvement of the Amygdala. Biol Psych. 46, 1140-1152. S0006322399001572 [pii].

[233] Berlau DJ, McGaugh JL (2006) Enhancement of Extinction Memory Consolidation: The Role of the Noradrenergic and Gabaergic Systems within the Basolateral Amygdala. Neurobiology of Learning and Memory. 86, 123-132.

[234] Lin H-C, Tseng Y-C, Mao S-C, Chen P-S, Gean P-W (2011) Gabaa Receptor Endocytosis in the Basolateral Amygdala Is Critical to the Reinstatement of Fear Memory Measured by Fear-Potentiated Startle. The Journal of Neuroscience:. 31, 8851-8861.

[235] Geracioti TD, Jr., Baker DG, Ekhator NN, West SA, Hill KK, Bruce AB, Schmidt D, Rounds-Kugler B, Yehuda R, Keck PE, Jr., Kasckow JW (2001) CSF Norepinephrine Concentrations in Posttraumatic Stress Disorder. Am J Psychiatry. 158, 1227-1230.

[236] Strawn JR, Geracioti TD, Jr. (2008) Noradrenergic Dysfunction and the Psychopharmacology of Posttraumatic Stress Disorder. Depress Anxiety. 25, 260-271.

[237] Asnis GM, Kohn SR, Henderson M, Brown NL (2004) Ssris Versus Non-Ssris in Post-Traumatic Stress Disorder: An Update with Recommendations. Drugs. 64, 383-404.

[238] Braun P, Greenberg D, Dasberg H, Lerer B (1990) Core Symptoms of Posttraumatic Stress Disorder Unimproved by Alprazolam Treatment. J Clin Psychiatry. 51, 236-238.

[239] Pitman RK, Sanders KM, Zusman RM, Healy AR, Cheema F, Lasko NB, Cahill L, Orr SP (2002) Pilot Study of Secondary Prevention of Posttraumatic Stress Disorder with Propranolol. Biol Psychiatry. 51, 189-192.

[240] Vaiva G, Ducrocq F, Jezequel K, Averland B, Lestavel P, Brunet A, Marmar CR (2003) Immediate Treatment with Propranolol Decreases Posttraumatic Stress Disorder Two Months after Trauma. Biol Psychiatry. 54, 947-949.

[241] Adamec R, Muir C, Grimes M, Pearcey K (2007) Involvement of Noradrenergic and Corticoid Receptors in the Consolidation of the Lasting Anxiogenic Effects of Predator Stress. Behav Brain Res. 179, 192-207. 10.1016/j.bbr.2007.02.001.

[242] Cohen H, Kaplan Z, Koresh O, Matar MA, Geva AB, Zohar J (2011) Early Post-Stressor Intervention with Propranolol Is Ineffective in Preventing Posttraumatic Stress Responses in an Animal Model for PTSD. European Neuropsychopharmacology. 21, 230-240.

[243] Adamec RE, Blundell J, Collins A (2001) Neural Plasticity and Stress Induced Changes in Defense in the Rat. Neurosci Biobehav Rev. 25, 721-744.

[244] Bodnoff SR, Suranyi-Cadotte B, Quirion R, Meaney MJ (1989) A Comparison of the Effects of Diazepam Versus Several Typical and Atypical Anti-Depressant Drugs in an Animal Model of Anxiety. Psychopharmacology (Berl). 97, 277-279.

[245] Griebel G, Moreau JL, Jenck F, Misslin R, Martin JR (1994) Acute and Chronic Treatment with 5-HT Reuptake Inhibitors Differentially Modulate Emotional Responses in Anxiety Models in Rodents. Psychopharmacology (Berl). 113, 463-470.

[246] Kurt M, Arik AC, Celik S (2000) The Effects of Sertraline and Fluoxetine on Anxiety in the Elevated Plus-Maze Test in Mice. Journal of Basic and Clinical Physiology and Pharmacology. 11, 173-180.

[247] Dekeyne A, Denorme B, Monneyron S, Millan MJ (2000) Citalopram Reduces Social Interaction in Rats by Activation of Serotonin (5-HT)(2c) Receptors. Neuropharmacology. 39, 1114-1117.
[248] Griebel G (1995) 5-Hydroxytryptamine-Interacting Drugs in Animal Models of Anxiety Disorders: More Than 30 Years of Research. Pharmacology & Therapeutics. 65, 319-395.
[249] Campbell BM, Merchant KM (2003) Serotonin 2c Receptors within the Basolateral Amygdala Induce Acute Fear-Like Responses in an Open-Field Environment. Brain Res. 993, 1-9.
[250] Christianson JP, Ragole T, Amat J, Greenwood BN, Strong PV, Paul ED, Fleshner M, Watkins LR, Maier SF (2010) 5-Hydroxytryptamine 2c Receptors in the Basolateral Amygdala Are Involved in the Expression of Anxiety after Uncontrollable Traumatic Stress. Biol Psychiatry. 67, 339-345.
[251] Vicente MA, Zangrossi H (2011) Serotonin-2c Receptors in the Basolateral Nucleus of the Amygdala Mediate the Anxiogenic Effect of Acute Imipramine and Fluoxetine Administration. The International Journal of Neuropsychopharmacology. 1-12.
[252] Burghardt NS, Bush DEA, McEwen BS, LeDoux JE (2007) Acute Selective Serotonin Reuptake Inhibitors Increase Conditioned Fear Expression: Blockade with a 5-HT(2c) Receptor Antagonist. Biol Psychiatry. 62, 1111-1118.
[253] Bagdy G, Graf M, Anheuer ZE, Modos EA, Kantor S (2001) Anxiety-Like Effects Induced by Acute Fluoxetine, Sertraline or M-CPP Treatment Are Reversed by Pretreatment with the 5-HT2c Receptor Antagonist Sb-242084 but not the 5-HT1a Receptor Antagonist Way-100635. Int J Neuropsychopharmacol. 4, 399-408. doi:10.1017/S1461145701002632.
[254] Salchner P, Singewald N (2006) 5-HT Receptor Subtypes Involved in the Anxiogenic-Like Action and Associated Fos Response of Acute Fluoxetine Treatment in Rats. Psychopharmacology (Berl). 185, 282-288.
[255] Hollander E, DeCaria C, Gully R, Nitescu A, Suckow RF, Gorman JM, Klein DF, Liebowitz MR (1991) Effects of Chronic Fluoxetine Treatment on Behavioral and Neuroendocrine Responses to Meta-Chlorophenylpiperazine in Obsessive-Compulsive Disorder. Psychiatry Res. 36, 1-17.
[256] Zohar J, Insel TR, Zohar-Kadouch RC, Hill JL, Murphy DL (1988) Serotonergic Responsivity in Obsessive-Compulsive Disorder. Effects of Chronic Clomipramine Treatment. Archives of General Psychiatry. 45, 167-172.
[257] Kennedy AJ, Gibson EL, O'Connell MT, Curzon G (1993) Effects of Housing, Restraint and Chronic Treatments with MCPP and Sertraline on Behavioural Responses to MCPP. Psychopharmacology (Berl). 113, 262-268.
[258] Yamauchi M, Tatebayashi T, Nagase K, Kojima M, Imanishi T (2004) Chronic Treatment with Fluvoxamine Desensitizes 5-HT2c Receptor-Mediated Hypolocomotion in Rats. Pharmacol Biochem Behav. 78, 683-689.
[259] Seeman P. (2002) Atypical antipsychotics: mechanism of action. Can J Psychiatry, 47, 27-38.

[260] de Boet T. (1996) The pharmacological profile of mirtazapine. J Clin Psychiatry. 57, 19-25.

[261] Ravindran LN, Stein MB. (2010) The pharmacologic treatment of anxiety disorders: a review of progress. J Clin Psychiatry. 71, 839-54.

[262] Rainer Q, Xia L, Guilloux JP, Gabriel C, Mocaër E, Hen R, Enhamre E, Gardier AM, David DJ. (2010) Beneficial Behavioural and Neurogenic effects of Agomelatine in a Model of Depression/Anxiety. Int J Neuropsychopharmacol. 8, 1-15.

[263] Katzman MA. (2011) Aripiprazole: a clinical review of its use for the treatment of anxiety disorders and anxiety as a comorbidity in mental illness. J Affect Disord. 128, S11-20.

[264] Kehne JH, Cain CK (2010) Therapeutic Utility of Non-Peptidic CRF1 Receptor Antagonists in Anxiety, Depression, and Stress-Related Disorders: Evidence from Animal Models. Pharmacology & Therapeutics. 128, 460-487. 10.1016/j.pharmthera.2010.08.011.

Chapter 5

The Role of Norepinephrine in Amygdala Dependent Fear Learning and Memory

Sodikdjon A. Kodirov

Additional information is available at the end of the chapter

1. Introduction

"The amygdaloid complex in the rat is very pronounced"
Gurdjian, 1928

The extensive knowledge about the significance and connexions of the amygdala with other brain regions emerged in the early XXth century (Gurdjian, 1928). Since then, the seven comprising nuclei of amygdala – *corpus amygdaloideum* in rats, have been known (Brodal 1947; Cowan et al., 1965). The presence and stereotaxic locations of all nuclei were confirmed later with more contemporary approaches (Paxinos & Franklin, 2001; Mikula et al., 2007). The additional nuclei belonging to the amygdala are established as "extended amygdala" (Fig. 1) that includes also the bed nucleus of the stria terminalis (BNST). However, the majority of studies address the lateral (LA), basolateral (BLA) and central (CeA) amygadala and their role in several emotionally driven responses in organisms. One of the latter responses is the stress and its circuit initiates in *locus coeruleus* (LC) after a release of norepinephrine (NE) by noradrenergic neurons.

Similar to other catecholamines such as epinephrine (adrenaline) and dopamine (DA), norepinephrine (noradrenaline) is released either into the circulation or locally to brain regions as a response to stress. NE subsequently also is transmitted into the amygdala. An increase in NE content within the amygdala modulates multiple physiological functions. In the amygdala the content of NE is higher than DA, but comparable to that of serotonin (Niwa et al., 2011). The noradrenergic neurons are present in the LC and amygdala. These neurons are distinguished by their positive reaction to DBH – dopamine β-hydroxylase, which enables the conversion of DA into NE. The physiological (endogenous) dynamics or pathological increase of NE occur at terminals originating from the LC (Emson et al., 1979). In individuals with a history of post-traumatic stress disorder (PTSD) the properties of the amygdala, along the hippocampus and prefrontal cortex, are affected and involve stress hormones such as cortisol and NE (for review see Bremner, 2006). Specifically, the fear-conditioning paradigm bilaterally increases the activity of the amygdala in those with symptoms of PTSD as a result of abuse. In healthy subjects, such an increase targets the left hemisphere; nevertheless, the left amygdala in the PTSD group is more active compared to the control. The upregulated activity in the amygdala correlates with increased blood flow to this region in the PTSD group.

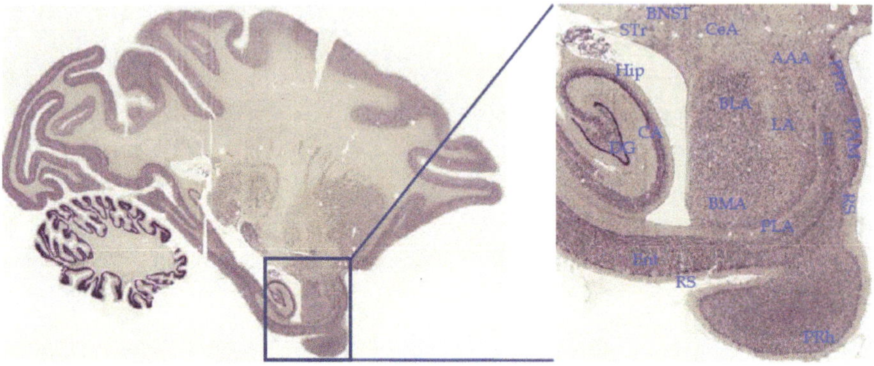

Figure 1. Amygdala of rhesus monkey *Macaca mulatta*
Left, whole brain in sagittal plane and right, amygdala and adjacent regions. AAA – anterior amygdaloid area, BLA – basolateral amygdala, BMA – basomedial amygdala, BNST – bed nucleus of the stria terminalis, CA – *cornu ammonis*, CeA – central amygdaloidal nucleus, Ent – entorhinal cortex, DG – dentate gyrus, Hip – hippocampus, LA – lateral amygdala, PRh – perirhinal cortex, PLA – paralaminar nucleus of amygdala, PMA – periamygdaloid area, PPir – prepiriform cortex, RS – rhinal sulcus, STr – stria terminalis (www.brainmaps.org and Mikula et al., 2007).

2. Emotional learning and resultant memories via amygdala

The amygdala is the main brain region responsible for emotion, at least for its intensity. Emotions, in turn, can influence memory leading to either forgetting – amnesia or stronger (compared to average) remembering – hypermnesia. The latter two events occur in anterograde or retrograde fashion.

The emotional fear response originates in the brain by the convergence (Fig. 2) of conditioned and unconditioned stimuli (CS and US), the latter can be also shown in experimental animals by employing diverse parameters depending on the area of interest (Halverson et al., 2009; Kwapis et al., 2009). A particular Pavlovian training or conditioning that has been widely used in research, enables experimental animals to associate the neutral CS with the US of a negative valence. This association results in an aversive response to the subsequently encountered CS. Fear conditioning paradigms are excellent tools for the study of neurobiological substrates of learning and memory. With regard to this, a peculiar interest has been devoted to the role of amygdala in auditory fear conditioning (LeDoux et al., 1984). The learning process in the amygdala and resultant memory undergo multiple steps involving consolidation and re-consolidation. Although the mechanisms underlying these two steps to a greater extent are controversial (Alberini, 2008). The interplay between information storage and dynamic properties of synapses are complex (Varshney et al., 2006). The consolidation of recent memories (from the previous day) are processed during sleep within the rapid eye movement (REM) phase, the latter leads to sorting of relatively earlier (then the very recent one) acquired information and its subsequent forgetting (Poe et al., 2000). Fear memory and circuits related to addiction often function synergistically (Peters et al., 2009).

The pairing paradigm that is equivalent to Pavlovian (light-food pairings) classical conditioning (Pavlov, 1927) enables the potentiated response of synapses in the amygdala also *in vitro* (Nader et al., 2000; McKernan & Shinnick-Gallagher, 1997; Rogan et al., 1997). Fear conditioning and the strength of acquired memory parallel the increased numbers of reactivated neurons (Reijmers et al., 2007) both in the LA and BLA. However, we should consider that not only the amygdala, but also the hippocampus participates in fear response and its subsequent processing (Knierim, 2003). The modulation of cognition by NE is also continuously elucidated in human subjects concurrently with established paradigm.

The neuronal excitability is a result of activities and properties of multiple ion channels including hyperpolarization-activated cyclic nucleotide gated non-selective cation (HCN or I_h) channels. It has been established that NE possesses the inverted U shaped dose response effects and targets the α2A adrenergic receptors (AR) and inhibits HCN channels (for review see Arnsten, 2007). Postsynaptic action potentials and neuronal excitability are required for the plasticity within several inputs. The neuronal excitability in turn is also prone to plasticity that indirectly involves the HCN channels (Brager & Johnston, 2007).

2.1. Clinical experiments

Cortisol and NE are considered as a main stress hormones (for literature analyses see Cahill et al., 2003). The authors reported that cortisol levels in saliva samples increases from ~3.5 to 4.2 ng/ml in response to a simple paradigm – cold pressor stress (CPS). In those subjects (control) who immersed the left forearm up to above the elbow joint level into the slightly warmer water (37–40 °C) than body temperature, the concentration of cortisol decreased to ~3 ng/ml when compared to CPS group (0–3 °C). Under these two conditions, subjects exhibited similar LTM for neutral pictures. Greater amounts of emotionally charged pictures were correctly recalled by CPS group.

Stressful events result in activation of the amygdala accompanied by increase in NE levels and surgery counts to this. Patients who underwent general anesthesia responded faster and provided correct word associations with emotionally negative cues compared to neutral ones (Gidron et al., 2002). This was the case when it concerned the old cues, however in regard to new cues the opposite effects were observed. Moreover, there was a correlation between the reaction time and spectral edge frequency (SEF) during EEG recordings. Thus, analyses revealed that patients with a SEF of lower than 9 Hz reacted slower.

It has been shown that the variation in NE levels can mimic the intensity of emotion in tested subjects (Hurlemann et al., 2005). In this study, the noradrenergic response to NE was inhibited by propranolol via blockade of β-adrenoceptors. Experimentally, the noradrenergic response was enhanced by NE reuptake inhibitor, reboxetine mesilate, a pharmaceutical that is widely used in order to reveal the resultant changes during the exposure to certain experimental paradigms. Former treatment decreased the arousal to oddball stimuli, while the latter increased it. Such outcomes were observed with both positive and negative oddball stimuli, but not with neutral ones. Moreover, the valence during all three paradigms remained unchanged. Propranolol, but not reboxetine, lowered the systolic and diastolic blood pressure. The plasma levels of these drugs at the end of recall paradigm were 20 and 75 μg/L, respectively. In fact, the plasma content depends on overall body's metabolism and prior fasting, as was shown for reboxetine (Hurlemann et al., 2007). Although, emotionally driven retrograde amnesia can occur via modulation of either NE or cortisol signaling, concurrent activation of these systems is perhaps an adequate underlying mechanism. This notion is supported by the magnitudes of recall change under negative emotion contact (E-1) for reboxetine (34 %) and synthetic cortisol (24 %), hydrocortisone, alone. The latter was increased by co-application of both (43 %). The amnesic influence was seen also on adjacent E-2 contact (22 %) and lasted 10 s. All these treatment combinations did not alter the *von Restroff* phenomenon, and the correct recall magnitudes were ~95 % for oddball stimuli.

Oral intake of yohimbine reversibly increases the content of α-amylase in human saliva (van Stegeren et al., 2010). A cortisol containing pill enhanced the endogenous cortisol level in these subjects abruptly and sustained at plateau for at least 1 h. The baseline content was documented after one week. The performance of these two groups, in terms of (better) recognition and recalling emotional pictures, when compared to neutral ones were similar. Yohimbine was ineffective while cortisol improved recognition and recall responses to both stimuli to similar extent. The combination of both agents strengthened the response to the emotional stimulus. Endogenous cortisol levels in human subjects vary greatly, and for this reason, experiments are often conducted by assigning two groups with relatively low (~5 nM) and high (~8 nM) contents (van Stegeren et al., 2007). Under placebo the magnitude of amygdalar activation in response to emotional pictures (compared to those of neutral nature) correlated well with the level of cortisol within the groups. It was suggested that the response of the amygdala underlies an increase in NE levels, since after the intake of 80 mg propranolol such correlations were absent. Additionally, propranolol increased the cortisol levels, but not to significant extent.

The cortisol concentration changes dynamically, with the highest level (~12 μg/dl) occurring during the late (REM) sleep. Oral intake of 3 g metyrapone (cortisol synthesis inhibitor) before the sleep inhibited the plasma level of cortisol during 8 h of sleep in male subjects (Wagner et al., 2005). Metyrapone increased the plasma content of NE during both learning (from ~100 to 120) and retrieval (~130 vs. 160 pg/ml) and its concentration was lower during sleep. These opposing effects of metyrapone on cortisol and NE dynamics correlate and promote the emotionally charged memory formation that occurs within the amygdala.

Emotional memories are consolidated during the slow wave sleep (SWS) and involve NE release. This was verified by intravenous infusion of α2 agonist clonidine, which inhibits NE release by the LC and decreases the retention of temporal order of emotional stories (Groch et al., 2011). Clonidine inhibited only the REM phase, which consisted of about 5% of total sleep time in tested subjects.

The NE degradation occurs by catechol-O-methyltransferase (COMT). In case of polymorphism in the COMT gene, the substitution of valine by methionine occurs at amino acid 158 (*val*^{158}*met*). In healthy subjects, the particular allele of the COMT gene is associated with emotional memory formation in the amygdala (Smolka et al., 2005). The unpleasant stimulus (pictures) was found to activate the right human amygdala as revealed by blood oxygen level-dependent (BOLD) response during fMRI scanning. The highest activity was observed in *met*^{158} homozygous individuals compared to *val*^{158} homozygous or *val/met* heterozygous.

Van Stegeren et al. (2005) confirmed that NE is a neurotransmitter involved in memories of emotional nature. Propranalol slightly increased the baseline heart rate (HR) compared to placebo group, but it significantly decreased before and after the fMRI procedure. Note that the procedure itself lowered the HR in both groups. Both groups similarly distinguished the emotional intensity of presented pictures by comparing them to prior images. The responses to gradually increased emotional intensity of pictures correlated with the pattern of activity in the amygdala. The latter activity was decreased by propranolol, but to significant extent only at intermediate intensity. In females, the amygdala exhibited about two fold less activation and higher resistance to propranolol compared to males. Male and female subjects also rated the pictures of similar intensity differently, especially former identified a greater number of images of neutral nature, while the latter rated them as emotionally intense pictures. Interestingly, propranolol did not affect the response of subjects exposed to pictures of highest emotional intensity. The overall memory performance was similar in both genders (van Stegeren et al., 2005).

2.2. Animal models

2.2.1. *In vivo studies – behavior*

The memory performance and related behaviour in rodents can be analyzed by employing multiple trainings and tests. The existing findings reflect controversial roles for NE in amygdala dependent memory.

2.2.1.1. *Studies revealing the enhancement of memory by NE*

Since moderate stress promotes memory formation and this event is accompanied by the release of NE, it is logical to expect similar effects on retention by this substance alone. The retention of memory is often manifested during the object recognition task. The overall performance depends on the duration of training, i.e. rats exploring objects for 3 min can retain memories for only one hour. By increasing the training time to 10 min, one would observe the resultant retention even after 24 h (Roozendaal et al., 2008). The latter study revealed that the NE administration into the BLA immediately after 3 min training improved the retention that lasted at least 24 h. However, the NE was effective only at lower doses up to 1 μg and declined abruptly at 3 μg. Direct exposure of BLA to propranolol resulted in impairment of retention in those rats trained during 10 min. The enhancement of fear memory by bilateral injection of NE into the BLA is reversed by prior exposure to context (Huff et al., 2005). In this regard, the latter study also provides some clarifications addressing controversial arguments in several studies. The dose response was not classical as judged by three different concentration of NE, and a clear effect was evident only at 1 μg, since at 3 μg, the freezing response – memory for fear, among tested rats declined and was not significant compared to control group. Injection of propranolol into the BLA immediately after training abolishes the enhancement of object recognition memory by corticosterone (Roozendaal et al., 2006b). The blockade of this memory via β–adrenoceptors was selective to the amygdala, since similar procedures (albeit even higher concentration of antagonist) targeting the hippocampus did not alter the discrimination index.

There are also toxins, which target noradrenergic neurons. One of them is DSP-4 [N-(2-chloroethyl)-N-ethyl-2 bromobenzylamine] with selective effects on DBH positive cells of the amygdala and LC as demonstrated 10 days after i.p. injections in adult rats (Radwanska et al., 2010). The toxicity effect on BLA neurons was more pronounced compared to LC ones. One week after the injection, animals underwent the habituation and training sessions, and active avoidance responses to US were analyzed. The majority of DSP-4 treated rats were unable to avoid the foot-shock within the 5 s consequently receiving 25 s long US. The same tendency was found also after additional seven training sessions in subsequent days and correlated with the decrease in NE neurons. The DBH positive neurons in BLA are also immunoreactive to choline acetyltransferase (ChAT). Moreover, DBH and ChAT positive terminals can also be found in close proximity, perhaps even are synaptically connected to the same neuron (Li et al., 2001).

Long lasting increase in NE level were observed in response to 0.55 mA foot-shock applied during 1 s via the floor in dark compartment of the inhibitory avoidance box (Mcintyre et al., 2002). The immediate mean release after the shock was estimated around two-fold compared to baseline. The three-fold peak increase in NE level occurred after 15 min and then gradually declined, but did not reach baseline during up to 2 h and remained at ~1.5 fold. Interestingly, the identical stimulus delivered via the grid in the bottom of the holding cage evoked a small NE release that lasted ~15 min. In some rats, the content of NE reached the highest level (~7.5 fold), and there was to some extent a correlation between the level of NE and the latency to enter the dark compartment during inhibitory avoidance (IA) test in particular animals. Rats injected i.p. with corticosterone immediately after IA training retain memories 10 fold longer (~300 vs ~30 s) compared to controls (McReynolds et al., 2010). Interestingly, this procedure resulted in a transient two-fold increase in NE level in BLA and Arc expression in the hippocampus; the latter effects were observed only in trained rats. In fractioned synaptoneurosome, the expression of PSD-95 was higher than in total homogenate from hippocampus. Direct injection of propranolol into the BLA decreased the Arc density in synaptoneurosome preparation. These results support the notion that amygdala and hippocampus may act in synergy during cognitive behavior. Note that the increase in NE levels of similar magnitude (~1.6 fold) should occur even in the absence of any drug in the amygdala after IA training, and cAMP response element-binding (CREB) antisense reduces its magnitude and duration (Canal et al., 2008). The clenbuterol administration immediately following the training improved the related memory.

One of earlier studies demonstrated that the systemic injection of epinephrine increases the NE release in the amygdaloid complex in a reversible manner (Williams et al., 1998). Its magnitude was comparable when either 0.1 or 0.3 mg/kg epinephrine were used. The authors compared these effects with those resulting after escapable foot-shock in these two groups. The 1 s foot-shock with the intensity of 0.8 mA caused only a slight NE increase in of groups, but differences appeared not to be significant. The NE increase was concluded to take place in amygdalar terminals of *nucleus tractus solitarius* (NTS) neurons. The latter was confirmed recently, since experimentally NE release could be also achieved in BNST – extended amygdala – by stimulating (60 Hz) the fibers of NTS. Such stimulation evokes higher NE release in rats intraperitoneally injected with either idazoxan (selective $\alpha 2$ adrenergic receptor antagonist) or desipramine (NE reuptake inhibitor). The evoked release is distinctly modulated by averse and pleasant stimuli (Park et al., 2011), thereby it is either increased or decreased in response to intra-oral delivery of quinine and sucrose (palatable food). Both substances affected the magnitude of NE release into the BNST to similar extent (±20 nM) with the time course of around 9 s. The content of NE metabolite, MHPG (3-methoxy-4-hydroxyphenylglycol), also changes in those areas of brain that possess noradrenergic terminals. The ratio of MHPG to NE is significantly increased within BNST when animals are fear conditioned (Onaka & Yagi, 1998).

The post-training injection of NE into the BLA enhanced the retention of contextual fear conditioning (CFC) revealed by freezing time during the Y-maze test (LaLumiere et al., 2003). The pattern of response to two different concentrations was similar when the latency of both freezing and entry into the shock arm were analyzed. The CFC could be performed also by using the straight alley test and analyzing the avoidance (latency) of rats to enter the dark shock compartment. The enhancement of retention by 1 μg NE was comparable to that in the Y-maze, but slightly less pronounced (~3 vs. 4 fold).

Finally, the improvement of the retention is also observed during antagonism of $\alpha 2$ adrenoceptors by idazoxan (Ferry & McGaugh, 2008). The effects of idazoxan differ depending on either pre- or post IA training injections. However, in both cases this selective $\alpha 2$ antagonist improves retention. Thus, idazoxan injected into the BLA 20 min prior to IA test increased the retention latency from ~120 to 180 s, which was significantly longer (~260 s) when introduced immediately after foot-shock. The dose-dependent effects of idazoxan in these two experiments were similar and the peak identically occurred at 0.3 μg demonstrating the narrow bell-shaped effects. In another group, increasing the foot-shock intensity from 0.4 to 0.5 mA resulted in prolonged retention latency to ~300 s and that was decreased by injection of agonist UK 14,304 (up to 3 ng). The subcutaneous injection of hormone corticosterone decreased the conditioned auditory-cue fear response (Roozendall et al., 2006a). The effect of corticosterone was reversed by injection of $\beta 1$-adrenoceptor antagonist atenolol (0.5 μg) into the BLA. Atenolol alone was ineffective and both agents' effects occur only when they were administered immediately after pairing of tone with the shock, but not before it.

2.2.1.2. Studies revealing the impairment of memory by NE

Most evidently, severe stress negatively impacts the memory and correlated amount of NE released during this period may exert such effects. A dramatic release of multiple neurotransmitters including NE (1200 %) is observed also after bilateral injection of antibiotic anisomycin into the amygdala. However, the latter led to amnesia (Canal et al., 2007). Interestingly, the vehicle injection increased NE levels by ~200 %. Under both conditions, the NE release was a transient event lasting ~60 and 45 min in former and latter cases. Another difference was seen in samples from anisomycin treated group that showed a rebound decrease almost to 0 % below the normalized 100 % baseline level. The baselines were not strictly stable, but to some extent identical in both groups. A rebound decrease was not observed in vehicle-injected animals, and after a transient increase, the NE levels returned to baseline values. When samples were analyzed every 45 min (vs. 15 min above), the transient increase was less pronounced in the anisomycin group, while it disappeared in the vehicle one. The rebound decrease in NE release was consistently present in anisomycin treated animals and remained at 50 % despite the prolonged experiments; baseline recovery occurred after 48 h. Amnesia by anisomycin involves the noradrenergic receptors, since either the prior injection of propranolol or subsequent administration of clenbuterol (β2 agonist) resulted in significantly lower impairment of memory in both groups of experiments. The lidocaine (Na^+ channel blocker) prevents NE release that is evoked by intra-amygdalar injection of anisomycin (Sadowski et al., 2011). The latter correlated with the reversal (to some extent) of memory impairment achieved by anisomycin. Furthermore, anisomycin attenuated c-Fos (cellular FBJ osteosarcoma oncogene) immunoreactivity (assessed by application of foot-shocks) by inhibiting the protein synthesis in BLA, and thereby providing some possible challenges for required *de novo* synthesis for long-term memory generation. The activity of c-Fos within several major nuclei of amygdala was up to 10 fold higher after 2 h of contextual fear training (Murchison et al., 2011). This increase was independent of the presence of ligand for adrenergic receptors (NE and E) as in the case of previously established $Dbh^{-/-}$ mice (see Murchison et al., 2011). Under these conditions, the lowest level of c-Fos was in the CeA. However, upon reexposure to context 1 d after conditioning the immunoreactivity was highest among tested nuclei including the LA. Moreover, in $Dbh^{-/-}$ mice both the c-Fos level and magnitude of freezing (after contextual fear conditioning) were decreased compared to $Dbh^{+/-}$ as a result of impaired memory retrieval. No differences were seen when mice were introduced to context at seven days or after that. Since in $Dbh^{-/-}$ the complete adrenergic system is disrupted, the authors used also β_1 adrenergic receptor knockout (β_1 KO) mice and obtained similar results.

Stress can be introduced to laboratory animals with paradigms closely resembling those occurring in the nature: social isolation, maternal separation or both. The combination of latter factors in mice between postnatal day 15 (P15) and P21 reduced the social interaction time by two-fold, measured during adulthood (Niwa et al., 2011). Thus, these mice were more anxious and show a decreased short-term memory (STM) compared to the control group, which is improved with antipsychotic drug clozapine. Under these conditions, the plasma level of corticosterone increased by four-fold (from ~200 to ~800 pg/ml). The NE content shows a tendency to decrease, but statistical analyses perhaps did not reveal a degree of significance contrary to that of the frontal cortex. Note that the overall level of NE in the frontal cortex was higher compared to the amygdala. Nevertheless, injection of NE into the right BLA immediately after the CFC decreases the freezing behavior in a dose-dependent manner (Berlau and McGaugh, 2006). However, this U-shaped response was narrow as judged by three logarithmic concentrations (0.3–3 μg) and show peak effects at 1 μg.

The pain perception was found to be lower in two lines of transgenic mice that lack α2A adrenergic receptors (Davies et al., 2004). One of the agonists of these receptors odexmedetomidine (i.p.) decreased the flinch threshold from 0.17 to 0.16 mA in WT mice. The odexmedetomidine in α2A AR mice did not affect the flinch response, while in D97N mice it increased the threshold (0.18 vs. 0.20 mA) that was not considered as an effect. In WT mice the freezing response was decreased, when odexmedetomidine was injected 30 min prior to fear conditioning, but not immediately after. This procedure also reduced the number of both P-CREB (phosphorylated) and c-Fos positive neurons in all three major nuclei of amygdala: LA, BLA and CeA. While the number of these two groups of neurons were comparable in LA and CeA, in BLA the content of P-CREB was five-fold and those of c-Fos two-fold.

2.2.2. *In vivo studies – electrophysiology*

Electrophysiological studies *in vivo* provided interesting results on brain structures and neurobiological processes underlying learning and memory. It was shown that amygdala modulates the LTP in *dentate gyrus* (DG) and the effects are derived selectively by LA and BLA nuclei, but not CeA (Akirav & Richter-Levin, 2002). Moreover, the effects of ipsilateral (same hemisphere) activation of two former nuclei on LTP in DG depend on timing between the two stimulations sites. The stimulation of the BLA just 30 s prior to the perforant path (PP) activation enhances LTP, while 2 h intervals decrease it. Interestingly, both effects, i.e. the enhancement and inhibition occur via two stress hormones, since the NE and corticosterone depletions by DSP-4 and metyrapone respectively reversed it. Although, also the contralateral (opposite hemisphere) priming of BLA exhibits similar effects, it was not derived by NE and corticosterone release. Note that the electrical stimulation of BLA decreases the NE release in DG (Almaguer-Melian et al., 2005).

The above-mentioned paradigm is known as DG LTP reinforcement by BLA. The injection of ~7 nM propranolol into the DG five minute prior to the BLA reinforcing paradigm decreases the LTP in DG achieved by PP stimulation (Bergado et al., 2007). The magnitudes of initial potentiation caused by PP stimulation in both groups were almost identical. Note that the control group comprises data obtained after the NaCl injections into the BLA, LC and medial septum and figure legend states that propranolol was delivered into the BLA.

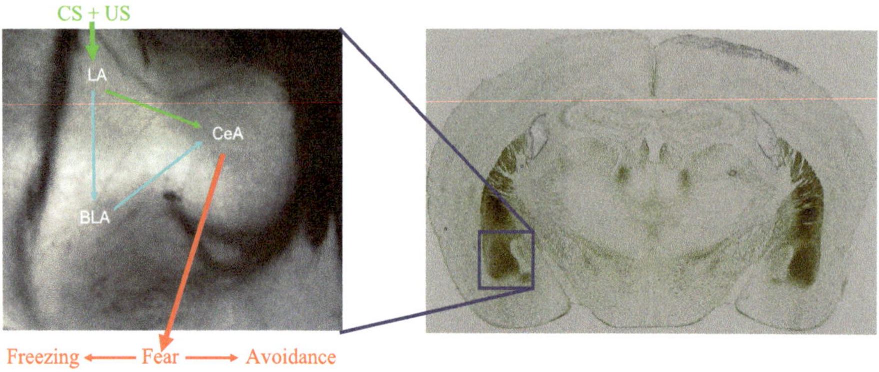

Figure 2. Amygdala and fear response pathways
Left, amygdala (in actual coronal brain slice) and its major nuclei. Right, closely matching section of brain in coronal plane (Paxinos & Franklin, 2001). LA – lateral amygdala, BLA – basolateral amygdala, CeA – central amygdaloidal nucleus. Schematic representation of fear response that originates after the convergence of conditioned and unconditioned stimuli (CS and US) into the LA.

2.2.3. In vitro studies – cellular counterpart of learning and memory in rodents

The potentiation of synaptic responses underlies the learning and memory at neuronal level.

2.2.3.1. Characteristics of LA and BLA cells involved in plasticity

Diverse cells have been observed in the amygdala, but the majority is comprised of two types. They are pyramidal and interneurons, and both are prone to plasticity (Mahanty & Sah, 1998; Tully et al., 2007). These neurons are distinguished by means of various methods; however, their electrophysiological properties could be considered a main criterion (Kodirov et al., 2009). In recent years, the attempt to recognize both types of cells by usage of biological marker – green fluorescent protein (GFP) – are starting to emerge. The interneurons in the BLA are apparently similar to other brain regions, because they express glutamate decarboxylase – 67 (GAD-67). In the BLA a single glutamatergic and three distinct GABAergic types of neurons have been distinguished (Kaneko et al., 2008). Although, this study is substantial, the characterized cell types warrant some skepticism, since in presented micrographs there are too many GFP^+ (GABAergic) cells, the soma of several neurons is pyramidal-like, and finally the size of GFP^- (glutamatergic, if those black spots are intact neurons, but not damaged ones) cells are comparable to those of GFP^+. Even during targeted recordings one would not encounter that amount of GABAergic cells in such a close proximity within the amygdala. This study is actually contrary to current dogma, since principal cells "exclusively showed regular spiking" and only about half of studied cells possess pyramidal soma. Moreover, the type-A GABAergic cells "spiked with little adaptation" and the size of their soma ranged up to 20 μm.

2.2.3.2. Plasticity in the amygdala and the role of NE

NE release can be also triggered in brain slices by excessive depolarization using higher concentrations of K^+. This procedure enables an increase (by 10-15 %) in NE content compared to basal magnitude in the amygdala (Lonart et al., 2008). Depolarization-induced NE release within the three nuclei were comparable in WT mice. In Rab3 interacting molecule 1 alpha (Rim1α) KO animals the identical approach evoked considerably lower NE release in BLA. Although in one of presented experiments, NE release from the CeA may have decreased, but the average data was not significant. The magnitude and response pattern of NE release in LA were indistinguishable from those of WT mice. Interestingly, in all these cases the peak release appeared with identical latencies of six minutes.

In control mice, NE gradually increases the frequency of spontaneous inhibitory postsynaptic currents (sIPSC) in pyramidal neurons of the BLA according to applied concentration (Braga et al., 2004). The effects of 1 μM NE was moderate, while of 10 μM high and at 100 μM excessive. Interestingly, at all tested doses the effects were completely reversible. The effects were observed also in the presence of adrenoceptor antagonists propranolol, yohimbine (α2A), CEC (α1B), and BMY 7378 (α1D). The selective α1A agonist A61603 increased both the rate and amplitude of sIPSC, and these effects were not observed in the presence of selective antagonist WB4101. NE at 10 μM had opposite effects on evoked IPSC, and note that the inhibition was not complete, but reversible and perhaps rather targeted only to those with the highest amplitude. The results became more complicated, since a blockade of $GABA_B$ receptors (although their activation was not experimentally shown) changed the effects of NE on evoked IPSC. In the stressed (immobilized and exposed to tail-shocks) group of animals, the mean frequency of sIPSC slightly decreased (3.1 *vs* 2.6 Hz). However, because of large diapason of values in individual experiments, the effects can not be considered significant. In these rats 10 μM NE was ineffective.

Contrary to data of Braga et al. (2004), NE decreased the frequency of sIPSCs in pyramidal cells of LA, but did not alter their amplitude or any parameters of miniature events and eIPSCs (Tully et al., 2007). Therefore, it was assumed that NE decreases the excitability of interneurons. However, this assumption could be evidenced by recording APs and acutely applying NE. In some of the latter neurons, NE slightly decreased the tonic GABAergic currents, while the parameters of phasic ones were not altered. The conclusion of this study needs to be defined, since indeed the release of GABA into the pyramidal neurons was affected as it is supported by selective decrease of the frequency of sIPSCs by NE.

2.2.3.3. Amygdala, placticity and fear learning

An increase in synaptic strength within the amygdalar fear circuit comprises the plasticity. Among multiple amygdaloidal nuclei, the LA has been extensively studied. The LA is modulated by excitatory afferents and involved in synaptic plasticity, i.e. the counterpart that underlies learning and memory at neuronal level. Memory formation in the LA can easily be demonstrated, since synapses can undergo LTP (Fig. 3).

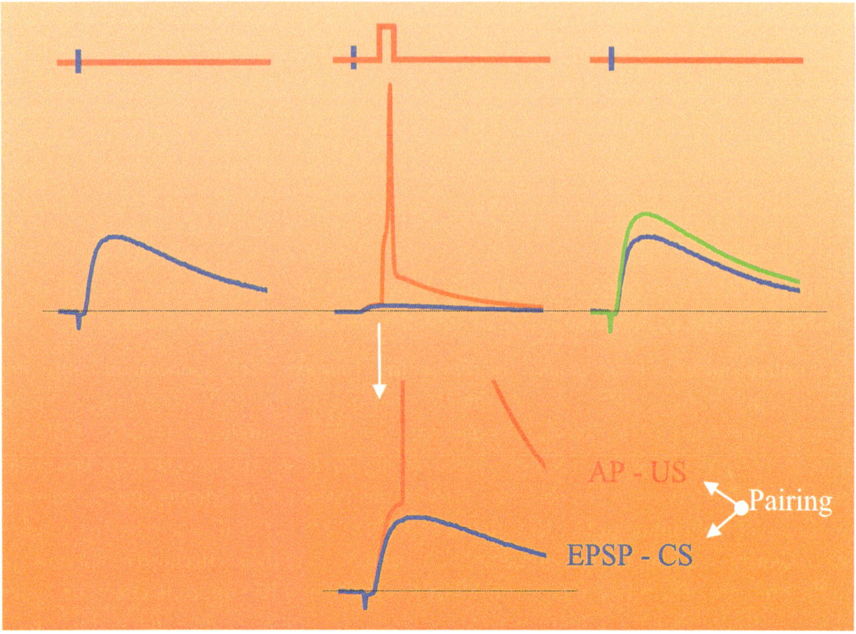

Figure 3. Induction of LTP in the LA *in vitro*
Mean baseline EPSP (blue trace) obtained in the presence of 100 μM PTX by stimulation of cortical inputs into the pyramidal neuron. Pairing of EPSPs with depolarization-induced action potentials (red) at 2 Hz led to LTP (green).

LTP has been extensively explored and its properties in the amygdala are well established (Kodirov et al., 2006; Rogan et al., 1997; Royer & Pare, 2003). In the amygdala, LTP induction can be either N-methyl-D-aspartate (NMDA) glutamate receptor dependent or independent (Mahanty & Sah, 1998; Gewirtz & Davis, 1997). Picrotoxin (PTX) facilitates the induction of LTP of excitatory postsynaptic potentials (EPSP) in the amygdala (Kodirov et al., 2006) by inhibiting the $GABA_A$ receptors. However, via the same mechanism, it can block the induction of another form of plasticity (Fink & O'Dell, 2009) known as EPSP–spike (E–S) potentiation in *cornu ammonis* 1 (CA1). Under both of these circumstances, PTX decreases the level of inhibition of the principal cells during high frequency synaptic activation. The LTP time course can be subdivided into different components and subsequent early and late phases can be distinguished (Dong et al., 2008). The early phase of LTP (E–LTP) *in vitro* corresponds to short-term memory and the late phase (L–LTP) to long-term memory *in vivo*. The impairment in L–LTP correlates with the deficit in spatial and long-term memories (Abel et al., 1997).

Thus, despite some skepticism, the best-known counterpart of learning and memory at synaptic and input levels is LTP. LTP in the amygdala occurs at both the thalamic and cortical synapses into the pyramidal neurons. Recently, the NE effects on LTP at thalamic inputs into the LA were revealed (Tully et al., 2007). Interestingly, the latter effects were seen only under physiological conditions, i.e. under undisturbed balance of excitation and inhibition. Note that under these conditions, the synapses at thalamic inputs into the LA are not prone to LTP. Therefore, NE rather enables the induction of LTP, and its effects on maintenance remains to be elucidated. Under facilitated excitatory drive, which is commonly achieved in the presence of up to 100 μM PTX, there was a tendency for enhanced LTP by NE, however, not to a significant level. Furthermore, the amplitudes of both components of glutamatergic currents remain unaltered in the presence of NE. However, two opposite effects were observed when prior to NE either α2– (yohimbine) or β–adrenoreceptors (propranolol) antagonists were applied. During the priming with yohimbine NE increased the amplitude of evoked excitatory postsynaptic currents (EPSC), while with propranolol NE decreased it. The latency was shorter and magnitude was greater in the former situation compared to the second one. Both effects were to some extent reversible after application of either yohimbine or propranolol. It has previously been shown that the NE effects vary depending on targeted influence on the latter two receptors (Ferry et al., 1999a). Therefore, perhaps just by using either yohimbine or propranolol one could observe the corresponding drug induced LTP in those experiments in the LA.

NE increased the number of evoked action potentials in pyramidal neurons of the LA. Intrinsic excitability of neurons can be attributed per se to learning and memory in *vivo* and either the ability or disability of neurons to regulate this activity results in either memory formation or its impairment (Kaczorowski & Disterhoft, 2009). The facilitated excitability of neurons by NE may contribute to the induction of LTP (if it occurs at least in part via inhibition of GABAergic or potentiation of glutamatergic neurotransmission, which can lead to increased postsynaptic depolarization during pairing with the presynaptic stimulation (Bissiere et al., 2003).

At thalamic inputs, terazosin decreased the amplitude of disynaptically induced inhibitory currents at 10 μM concentration, which did not alter the excitatory ones that were evoked in response to the first pulse (Lazzaro et al., 2010). The sequence of dysynaptic excitatory and inhibitory currents/potentials can be also evoked by stimulating the cortical inputs and adjusting the holding potential to between –30 and –40 mV (Kodirov et al., 2006). Interestingly, the amplitude of excitatory currents evoked during application of second pulse was increased by terazosin (Lazzaro et al., 2010), thus resulting in paired-pulse facilitation (PPF). Note that no PPF at both synapses was observed under control conditions, although employing the ISI of 50 ms usually results in PPF when the single pulses are applied. Interestingly, the thalamo-amygdalar synapses exhibit LTP that decay with time, but in the presence of PTX it persisted steadily at least up to 1.5 h. However, it is not clear when terazosin was applied, since the descriptions in both text and figures are contradictory. One pitfall during LTP experiments is the difficulty of comparing the potency of compounds, including NE. Nevertheless, at these inputs the LTP was more pronounced in the presence of terazosin compared to PTX. Since this compound was less effective at cortical synapses the authors conclude that the thalamic inputs are important in anxiety and $\alpha 1$ adrenoceptors play a role mostly in this pathway.

2.2.3.4. Molecular substrate of LTP

The Pavlovian paradigm also alters the expression of multiple genes in amygdala. Under control conditions, freezing response was observed in ~20 %, which was increased to ~80 % rats measured after 24 h of one trial of fear conditioning – pairing tone with foot-shock (Ploski et al., 2010). The behaviour of the rats was comparable in the next two trials. The qRT-PCR after 30 min of paradigm revealed an increase in mRNA of several genes: Arc–Activity-regulated cytoskeleton-associated protein, Egr2–Early growth response 2, Nr4a2–Nuclear receptor subfamily 4, group A, member 2, Per1–Period homolog 1 (*Drosophila*), Sat1–Spermidine/spermine Nl-acetyl transferase 1, Rnf39–Ring finger protein 39 increased. The expresion of Arc, Nr4a2, Per1 genes decreased by 90 min while those of remaining three increased. Also at 180 min two different responses were revealed. Among additional genes the highest increase at 30 min time point was revealed for Fos, although the degree of associated change is unclear (~3 fold in the graph vs. 7 fold in the table). The latter perhaps is not a reflection of data normalizations, since the magnitude of corresponding genes in the naïve group was considered either as 0 or 1, respectively. There are more molecular substrates potentially involved in LTP, and the active-zone scaffolding protein (RIM1α) is one of them (Fourcaudot et al., 2008).

We have encountered that the PPF at cortical inputs into the LA occurs less compared to other regions of the brain (Kodirov et al., 2009). A recent study demonstrates that the magnitude of PPF at these synapses decreases after a pairing paradigm from the ratio of ~2 to 1.5, at least one can estimate from representative traces (Fourcaudot et al., 2008). However, the average data is perhaps inadequately presented by subtracting the PPF of baseline from that of heterosynaptic associative LTP (LTP_{HA} – evoked by the simultaneous stimulation of cortical and thalamic inputs), thus resulting in negative paired-pulse ratios (PPR). Comparing PPF before and after the paradigm would be sufficient in order to conclude whether or not the expression of LTP is presynaptic. Moreover, it is not clear that "changes in PPR could also involve postsynaptic mechanisms" and "induction of LTP_{HA} depends on presynaptic, but not postsynaptic, NMDA receptors". The PPF ratio was reduced by 50 μM forskolin and the identical concentration rapidly (~2 min) increases the EPSP reaching within four minutes the plateau and thus induces potentiation lasting at least 20 min. Its amplitude (~150 % of baseline) was comparable with LTP triggered by the stimulation of cortical inputs. Thus, PKA and RIM1α were shown to alter the LTP_{HA}.

3. Conclusion

NE influences memory performance either via interplay between the α- and β-adrenergic receptors or by co-activation of both (Ferry et al., 1999a, b). The memory promoting effects of NE via amygdala may occur also by the activation of principal neurons in the NTS and involve epinephrine (Williams et al., 1998). Amygdala dependent fear learning involves NE as a main neurotransmitter, since the post-training intracranial injection of 1 μg NE led to amnesia in rats 24 h after passive avoidance task (Kesner & Ellis, 1983). The pathological release of catecholamine NE in mammals including humans occurs in comparable manner to invertebrates (Kodirov, 2011).

The above outlined dual effects of NE on memory (impairment and enhancement) possibly underly the distinct BLA single neuronal response, since iontophoretic injection of NE in some cells increased and others decreased the spontaneous firings *in vivo* (Buffalari & Grace, 2007). These neurons exhibit different basal frequencies of firings, ~0.1 vs. 2 Hz in former and later, respectively. The fact that these neurons could be subdivided clearly into two groups is valuable, however identifying cells with higher rate as projecting ones (even based on their antidromic response to the stimulation of entorhinal cortex), is against the properties of neurons. The projection cells should not fire high frequency APs compared to other neurons within this structure, e.g. GABAergic interneurons. Nevertheless, the experiments are precise, since the recording and 200 μM NE application was performed via the single multi-barrelled electrode at the same time. In the LA the proportion of neurons with inhibitory response to NE was higher than in the BLA, but those with excitatory ones similar. Note that NE did not alter firing of some neurons in either nuclei. Upon the termination of injection, the neurons continued to fire at baseline frequencies, therefore in the same neuron it was revealed that the NE inhibitory effects occur via $\alpha 2$ AR, since the latter was mimicked by 50 μM clonidine. The excitatory effects of NE on BLA neurons may occur via β AR (for discussions see Buffalari & Grace, 2007). Similar dual effects were observed also upon the stimulation of LC, but the baseline frequencies of two groups were only slightly apart. Although the extent of inhibition was similar after foot-shock or NE injection, the excitation was greater in the former case. The effects of NE were abrupt and those of foot-shock and LC stimulations occurred with adequate latencies.

Finally, the fear conditioning alone leads to the upregulation of ~30 genes in the LA (Ploski et al., 2010). Note that no downregulation for any genes was estimated in this study. Eventually, such results in the future could specify the role of plasticity related genes more precisely (in terms of their associations to certain neurotransmitters including NE), which then potentially could serve as a target points during diagnosis and the search for potential cure. Even in this century "how memory processing would be coded at the receptor [or gene] level remains unknown" (Ellis, 1985).

Author details

Sodikdjon A. Kodirov
Pavlov Institute of Physiology, Russian Academy of Sciences, Saint Petersburg, Russia
I. P. Pavlov Department of Physiology, State Research Institute of Experimental Medicine, Russian Academy of Medical Sciences, Saint Petersburg, Russia
Department of Molecular Physiology & Biophysics, University of Iowa, Iowa City, USA

Acknowledgement

In this instance, I would like to acknowledge contributions of authors, which I was not able to review because of either length limitations or many of them were discussed elsewhere recently. I am also grateful to Nicholas D. Leymaster and Carl J. Christel for reading this work at its final stage.

4. References

Abel T, Nguyen PV, Barad M, Deuel TAS, Kandel ER & Bourtchouladze R. 1997. Genetic demonstration of a role for PKA in the late phase of LTP and in hippocampus-based long-term memory. Cell 88:615-626.

Akirav I, Richter-Levin G. 2002. Mechanisms of amygdala modulation of hippocampal plasticity. J Neurosci 22:9912-21

Alberini CM. 2008. The role of protein synthesis during the labile phases of memory: Revisiting the skepticism. Neurobiol Learn Mem 89:234-246.

Almaguer-Melian W, Cruz-Aguado R, Riva Cde L, Kendrick KM, Frey JU, Bergado J. 2005. Effect of LTP-reinforcing paradigms on neurotransmitter release in the dentate gyrus of young and aged rats. Biochem Biophys Res Commun 327:877-83

Arnsten AF. 2007. Catecholamine and second messenger influences on prefrontal cortical networks of "representational knowledge": a rational bridge between genetics and the symptoms of mental illness. Cereb Cortex 17 Suppl 1:i6-15

Bergado JA, Frey S, Lopez J, Almaguer-Melian W, Frey JU. 2007. Cholinergic afferents to the locus coeruleus and noradrenergic afferents to the medial septum mediate LTP-reinforcement in the dentate gyrus by stimulation of the amygdala. Neurobiol Learn Mem 88:331-41

Berlau DJ, McGaugh JL. 2006. Enhancement of extinction memory consolidation: the role of the noradrenergic and GABAergic systems within the basolateral amygdala. Neurobiol Learn Mem 86:123-32

Bissiere S, Humeau Y & Luthi A. 2003. Dopamine gates LTP induction in lateral amygdala by suppressing feedforward inhibition. Nat Neurosci 6, 587-592.

Braga MF, Aroniadou-Anderjaska V, Manion ST, Hough CJ, Li H. 2004. Stress impairs α_{1A} adrenoceptor-mediated noradrenergic facilitation of GABAergic transmission in the basolateral amygdala. Neuropsychopharmacology 29:45-58

Brager DH & Johnston D. 2007. Plasticity of intrinsic excitability during long-term depression is mediated through mGluR-dependent changes in *I*h in hippocampal CA1 pyramidal neurons. J Neurosci 27:13926 –13937

Bremner JD. 2006. Traumatic stress: effects on the brain. Dialogues Clin Neurosci 8:445-61

Brodal A. 1947. The amygdaloid nucleus in the rat. J Comp Neurol 87:1-16

Buffalari DM, Grace AA. 2007. Noradrenergic modulation of basolateral amygdala neuronal activity: opposing influences of α-2 and β receptor activation. J Neurosci 27:12358-66

Cahill L, Gorski L & Le K. 2003. Enhanced human memory consolidation with post-learning stress: Interaction with the degree of arousal at encoding. Learn. Mem. 10: 270-274

Canal CE, Chang Q, Gold PE. 2007. Amnesia produced by altered release of neurotransmitters after intraamygdala injections of a protein synthesis inhibitor. Proc Natl Acad Sci U S A 104:12500-5

Canal CE, Chang Q, Gold PE. 2008. Intra-amygdala injections of CREB antisense impair inhibitory avoidance memory: role of norepinephrine and acetylcholine. Learn Mem 15:677-86

Cowan WM, Raisman G, Powell TP. 1965. The connexions of the amygdala. J Neurol Neurosurg Psychiatry 28:137-51

Davies MF, Tsui J, Flannery JA, Li X, DeLorey TM, Hoffman BB. 2004. Activation of alpha2 adrenergic receptors suppresses fear conditioning: expression of c-Fos and phosphorylated CREB in mouse amygdala. Neuropsychopharmacology 29:229-39

Dong C, Upadhya SC, Ding L, Smith TK & Hegde AN. 2008. Proteasome inhibition enhances the induction and impairs the maintenance of late-phase long-term potentiation. Learn Mem 15, 335-347.

Ellis ME. 1985. Amygdala norepinephrine involved in two separate long-term memory retrieval processes. Brain Res 342:191-5

Emson PC, Björklund A, Lindvall O, Paxinos G. 1979. Contributions of different afferent pathways to the catecholamine and 5-hydroxytryptamine-innervation of the amygdala: A neurochemical and histochemical study. Neuroscience 4:1347-57

Ferry B, McGaugh JL. 2008. Involvement of basolateral amygdala α2-adrenoceptors in modulating consolidation of inhibitory avoidance memory. Learn Mem 15:238-43

Ferry B, Roozendaal B, McGaugh JL. 1999a. Basolateral amygdala noradrenergic influences on memory storage are mediated by an interaction between β- and α1-adrenoceptors. J Neurosci 19:5119-23

Ferry B, Roozendaal B, McGaugh JL. 1999b. Involvement of α1-adrenoceptors in the basolateral amygdala in modulation of memory storage. Eur J Pharmacol 372:9-16

Fink AE & O'Dell TJ. 2009. Short trains of theta frequency stimulation enhance CA1 pyramidal neuron excitability in the absence of synaptic potentiation. J Neurosci 29, 11203-11214.

Fourcaudot E, Gambino F, Humeau Y, Casassus G, Shaban H, Poulain B, Lüthi A. 2008. cAMP/PKA signaling and RIM1α mediate presynaptic LTP in the lateral amygdala Proc Natl Acad Sci U S A 105:15130-15135

Gewirtz JC & Davis M. 1997. Second-order fear conditioning prevented by blocking NMDA receptors in amygdala. Nature 388, 471-474.

Gidron Y, Barak T, Henik A, Gurman G, Stiener O. 2002. Implicit learning of emotional information under anesthesia. Neuroreport 13:139-42

Groch S, Wilhelm I, Diekelmann S, Sayk F, Gais S, Born J. 2011. Contribution of norepinephrine to emotional memory consolidation during sleep. Psychoneuroendocrinology 36:1342-50

Gurdjian ES. 1928. The corpus striatum of the rat. Studies on the brain of the rat. No. 3. J Comp Neurol 45:249-81

Halverson HE, Hubbard EM & Freeman JH. 2009. Stimulation of the lateral geniculate, superior colliculus, or visual cortex is sufficient for eyeblink conditioning in rats. Learn Mem 16, 300-307.

Huff NC, Wright-Hardesty KJ, Higgins EA, Matus-Amat P, Rudy JW. 2005. Context pre-exposure obscures amygdala modulation of contextual-fear conditioning. Learn Mem 12:456-60

Hurlemann R, Hawellek B, Matusch A, Kolsch H, Wollersen H, et al. 2005. Noradrenergic modulation of emotion-induced forgetting and remembering. J Neurosci 25:6343-9

Hurlemann R, Matusch A, Hawellek B, Klingmuller D, Kolsch H, et al. 2007. Emotion-induced retrograde amnesia varies as a function of noradrenergic-glucocorticoid activity. Psychopharmacology (Berl) 194:261-9

Kaczorowski CC & Disterhoft JF. 2009. Memory deficits are associated with impaired ability to modulate neuronal excitability in middle-aged mice. Learn Mem 16, 362-366.

Kaneko K, Tamamaki N, Owada H, Kakizaki T, Kume N, et al. 2008. Noradrenergic excitation of a subpopulation of GABAergic cells in the basolateral amygdala via both activation of nonselective cationic conductance and suppression of resting K^+ conductance: a study using glutamate decarboxylase 67-green fluorescent protein knock-in mice. Neuroscience 157:781-97

Kesner RP, Ellis ME. 1983. Memory consolidation: brain region and neurotransmitter specificity. Neurosci Lett 39:295-300

Knierim JJ. 2003. Hippocampus and memory. Can we have our place and fear it too? Neuron 37, 372-374.

Kodirov SA. 2011. The neuronal control of cardiac functions in Molluscs. Comp Biochem Physiol A. 160: 102–116.

Kodirov SA, Jasiewicz J, Amirmahani P, Psyrakis D, Bonni K, et al. 2009. Endogenous cannabinoids trigger the depolarization-induced suppression of excitation in the lateral amygdala. Learn Mem 17:43-9

Kodirov SA, Takizawa S, Joseph J, Kandel ER, Shumyatsky GP, Bolshakov VY. 2006. Synaptically released zinc gates long-term potentiation in fear conditioning pathways. Proc Natl Acad Sci U S A 103:15218-23

Kwapis JL, Jarome TJ, Lonergan ME & Helmstetter FJ. 2009. Protein kinase Mzeta maintains fear memory in the amygdala but not in the hippocampus. Behav Neurosci 123, 844-850.

LaLumiere RT, Buen TV, McGaugh JL. 2003. Post-training intra-basolateral amygdala infusions of norepinephrine enhance consolidation of memory for contextual fear conditioning. J Neurosci 23:6754-8

Lazzaro SC, Hou M, Cunha C, LeDoux JE, Cain CK. 2010. Antagonism of lateral amygdala alpha1-adrenergic receptors facilitates fear conditioning and long-term potentiation. Learn Mem 17:489-93

LeDoux JE, Sakaguchi A, Reis DJ. 1984. Subcortical efferent projections of the medial geniculate nucleus mediate emotional responses conditioned to acoustic stimuli. J Neurosci 4:683-98.

Li R, Nishijo H, Wang Q, Uwano T, Tamura R, et al. 2001. Light and electron microscopic study of cholinergic and noradrenergic elements in the basolateral nucleus of the rat amygdala: evidence for interactions between the two systems. J Comp Neurol 439:411-25

Lonart G, Tang X, Simsek-Duran F, Machida M, Sanford LD. 2008. The role of active zone protein Rab3 interacting molecule 1 alpha in the regulation of norepinephrine release, response to novelty, and sleep. Neuroscience 154:821-31

Mahanty NK & Sah P. 1998. Calcium-permeable AMPA receptors mediate long-term potentiation in interneurons in the amygdala. Nature 394, 683-687.

McIntyre CK, Hatfield T, McGaugh JL. 2002. Amygdala norepinephrine levels after training predict inhibitory avoidance retention performance in rats. Eur J Neurosci 16:1223-6

McKernan MG & Shinnick-Gallagher P. 1997. Fear conditioning induces a lasting potentiation of synaptic currents *in vitro*. Nature 390, 607-611.

McReynolds JR, Donowho K, Abdi A, McGaugh JL, Roozendaal B, McIntyre CK. 2010. Memory-enhancing corticosterone treatment increases amygdala norepinephrine and Arc protein expression in hippocampal synaptic fractions. Neurobiol Learn Mem 93:312-21

Mikula, S., Trotts, I., Stone, J., and Jones, E.G. 2007. Internet-enabled high-resolution brain mapping and virtual microscopy. NeuroImage. 35:9-15

Murchison CF, Schutsky K, Jin SH, Thomas SA. 2011. Norepinephrine and β_1-adrenergic signaling facilitate activation of hippocampal CA1 pyramidal neurons during contextual memory retrieval. Neuroscience 181:109-16

Niwa M, Matsumoto Y, Mouri A, Ozaki N, Nabeshima T. 2011. Vulnerability in early life to changes in the rearing environment plays a crucial role in the aetiopathology of psychiatric disorders. Int J Neuropsychopharmacol 14:459-77

Onaka T, Yagi K. 1998. Role of noradrenergic projections to the bed nucleus of the stria terminalis in neuroendocrine and behavioral responses to fear-related stimuli in rats. Brain Res 788:287-93

Pavlov IP. 1927. Conditioned Reflexes. Dover, New York.

Paxinos G & Franklin KBJ. 2001. The mouse brain in stereotaxic coordinates. Academic Press.

Peters J, Kalivas PW & Quirk GJ. 2009. Extinction circuits for fear and addiction overlap in prefrontal cortex. Learn Mem 16, 279-288.

Ploski JE, Pierre VJ, Smucny J, Park K, Monsey MS, et al. 2008. The activity-regulated cytoskeletal-associated protein (Arc/Arg3.1) is required for memory consolidation of Pavlovian fear conditioning in the lateral amygdala. J Neurosci 28, 12383-95

Poe GR, Nitz DA, McNaughton BL & Barnes CA. 2000. Experience-dependent phase-reversal of hippocampal neuron firing during REM sleep. Brain Res 855, 176-180.

Radwanska K, Nikolaev E, Kaczmarek L. 2010. Central noradrenergic lesion induced by DSP-4 impairs the acquisition of avoidance reactions and prevents molecular changes in the amygdala. Neurobiol Learn Mem 94:303-11

Reijmers LG, Perkins BL, Matsuo N & Mayford M. 2007. Localization of a stable neural correlate of associative memory. Science 317, 1230-1233.

Rogan MT, Staubli UV & LeDoux JE. 1997. Fear conditioning induces associative long-term potentiation in the amygdala. Nature 390, 604-607.

Roozendaal B, Hui GK, Hui IR, Berlau DJ, McGaugh JL, Weinberger NM. 2006a. Basolateral amygdala noradrenergic activity mediates corticosterone-induced enhancement of auditory fear conditioning. Neurobiol Learn Mem 86:249-55

Roozendaal B, Okuda S, Van der Zee EA, McGaugh JL. 2006b. Glucocorticoid enhancement of memory requires arousal-induced noradrenergic activation in the basolateral amygdala. Proc Natl Acad Sci U S A 103:6741-6

Roozendaal B, Castello NA, Vedana G, Barsegyan A, McGaugh JL. 2008. Noradrenergic activation of the basolateral amygdala modulates consolidation of object recognition memory. Neurobiol Learn Mem 90:576-9

Royer S & Pare D. 2003. Conservation of total synaptic weight through balanced synaptic depression and potentiation. Nature 422, 518-522.

Sadowski RN, Canal CE, Gold PE. 2011. Lidocaine attenuates anisomycin-induced amnesia and release of norepinephrine in the amygdala. Neurobiol Learn Mem 96:136-42

Smolka MN, Schumann G, Wrase J, Grusser SM, Flor H, et al. 2005. Catechol-O-methyltransferase val158met genotype affects processing of emotional stimuli in the amygdala and prefrontal cortex. J Neurosci 25:836-42

Tully K, Li Y, Tsvetkov E, Bolshakov VY. 2007. Norepinephrine enables the induction of associative long-term potentiation at thalamo-amygdala synapses. Proc Natl Acad Sci U S A 104:14146-50

Varshney LR, Sjostrom PJ & Chklovskii DB. 2006. Optimal information storage in noisy synapses under resource constraints. Neuron 52, 409-423.

van Stegeren AH, Goekoop R, Everaerd W, Scheltens P, Barkhof F, et al. 2005. Noradrenaline mediates amygdala activation in men and women during encoding of emotional material. Neuroimage 24:898-909

van Stegeren AH, Roozendaal B, Kindt M, Wolf OT, Joels M. 2010. Interacting noradrenergic and corticosteroid systems shift human brain activation patterns during encoding. Neurobiol Learn Mem 93:56-65

van Stegeren AH, Wolf OT, Everaerd W, Scheltens P, Barkhof F, Rombouts SA. 2007. Endogenous cortisol level interacts with noradrenergic activation in the human amygdala. Neurobiol Learn Mem 87:57-66

Wagner U, Degirmenci M, Drosopoulos S, Perras B, Born J. 2005. Effects of cortisol suppression on sleep-associated consolidation of neutral and emotional memory. Biol Psychiatry 58:885-93

Williams CL, Men D, Clayton EC, Gold PE. 1998. Norepinephrine release in the amygdala after systemic injection of epinephrine or escapable footshock: contribution of the nucleus of the solitary tract. Behav Neurosci 112:1414-22

Chapter 6

Amygdala Strengthening of Cortical Memory Representations

Candice M. Chavez, James L. McGaugh
and Norman M. Weinberger

Additional information is available at the end of the chapter

1. Introduction

1.1. The basolateral amygdala and memory consolidation

Emotionally arousing experiences generally create strong, long-lasting memories [3]. Findings of many experiments using rats, as well as human subjects, indicate that arousal-induced release of adrenal hormones epinephrine and cortisol (corticosterone in rats) plays a critical role in modulating the consolidation of memories [4-6]. Systemic administration of epinephrine or corticosterone to rats shortly after training enhances memory on many kinds of learning tasks. [1, 7]. Similarly, human memory is enhanced by post-learning administration of epinephrine or stimulation that induces the release of epinephrine [8, 9]. Further, in human subjects as well as rats, administration of β-adrenoceptor antagonists block the enhancing effects of emotional arousal on memory [1, 5, 10-12].

1.2. Critical role of the basolateral amygdala in modulating memory consolidation

There is also extensive evidence from studies using rats that these adrenal stress hormones influence memory that involves noradrenergic activation of the amygdala [1, 13]. Lesions or pharmacological inactivation of the amygdala, more specifically the basolateral region (BLA), prevent the memory enhancing effects of peripherally administered epinephrine and corticosterone [14]. The release of norepinephrine (NE) within the BLA plays a critical role in modulating memory consolidation. Intra-BLA administration of β-adrenoceptor antagonists blocks epinephrine and corticosterone effects on memory [15, 16] and importantly, posttraining intra-BLA infusions of NE, as well as noradrenergic agonists, enhance memory consolidation [17-20] (Figure 1).

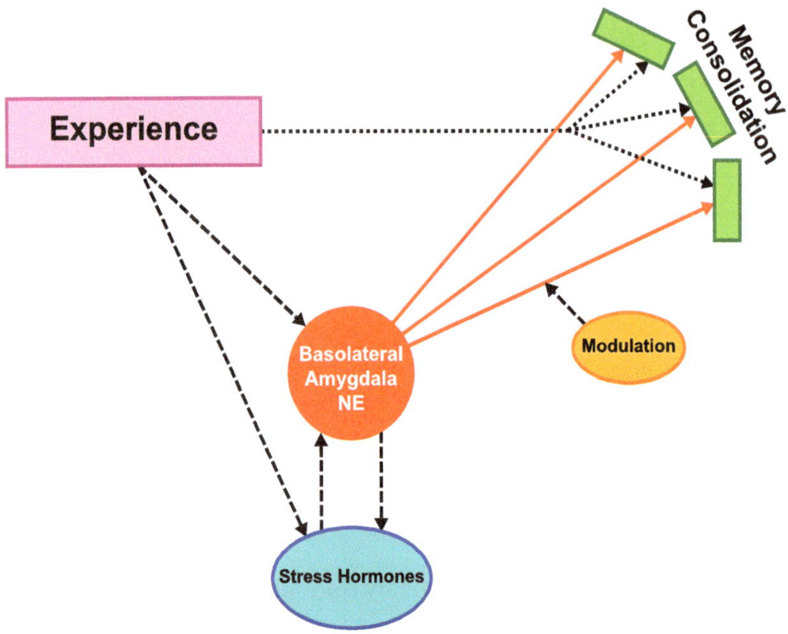

Figure 1. The BLA is activated by stress hormones released by behaviorally important experiences. Dependent upon noradrenergic actions within the BLA, memory modulation effects on experiential representations produce memory consolidation in target brain structures.

Additionally, arousal-induced training induces the release of NE within the amygdala [21] and the increase in release correlates with subsequent retention performance [22]. There is also evidence that GABAergic and opioid peptidergic drugs that enhance memory when administered post-training (e.g., picrotoxin, naloxone) enhance the release of amygdala NE and that memory impairing drugs (e.g., muscimol, β-endorphin) decrease amygdala NE release [21, 23]. Thus, GABAergic and opioid drugs act "upstream" from NE within the BLA.

Drugs affecting cholinergic functioning also influence memory consolidation when administered either systemically or intra-amygdally after training [24, 25]. However, cholinergic effects occur "downstream" from NE as blockade of β-adrenoceptors within the BLA does not prevent the memory enhancement induced by systemic intra-amygdala infusions of the muscarinic cholinergic agonist oxotremorine and intra-amygdala administration of the cholinergic antagonist atropine blocks the memory enhancement induced by NE [26, 27]. Intra-amygdala infusions of atropine also block the memory enhancing effects of systemic or intra-amygdala administration of glucocorticoid receptor agonists [28].The BLA receives a large cholinergic projection from the nucleus basalis (NB) [29]. Thus, as would be expected, in view of the evidence that acetylcholine acts downstream from NE within the amygdala in regulating memory consolidation, lesions of the NB impair memory consolidation and intra-BLA infusions of oxotremorine or the muscarinic agonist physostigmine attenuate the memory impairment [30].

1.3. BLA influences on memory for different aspects/forms of learning

It is well established that the amygdala is involved in fear-induced training using footshock [31]. However, lesions of the BLA attenuate, but do not prevent, inhibitory avoidance or contextual fear conditioning [32]. One possible interpretation of findings that post-training activation of the BLA with neuromodulatory treatments enhances inhibitory avoidance as well as contextual and cued fear conditioning might be that the stimulation simply potentiates the effects of fear. However, intra-BLA administration of NE or the cholinergic agonist oxotremorine administered following extinction, i.e. when footshock is no longer delivered, enhances extinction of contextual fear conditioning [33, 34]. These findings clearly indicate that BLA influences are not constrained to enhancing associations based on fear [1].

Findings of experiments using novel object recognition memory clearly demonstrate BLA modulation of memory that is not based on fear motivation. In one experiment [35], rats were simply placed in a box containing two identical objects (e.g., light bulbs) and allowed to investigate them. On retention tests a day later, they were replaced in the box with one of the same objects and a novel object of approximately the same size. NE infused into the BLA after the original exposure enhanced memory of the objects, as indicated by increased investigation of the novel object on the retention trial (Figure 2). Post-training activation of glucocorticoid receptors in the BLA after training also enhances novel object recognition memory and, importantly, this influence is blocked by intra-BLA infusions of an adrenoceptor antagonist [16, 36].

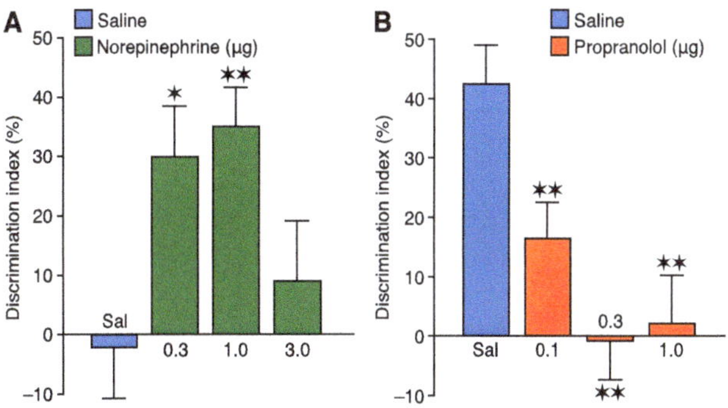

Figure 2. Noradrenergic activation of the BLA modulates consolidation of object recognition memory. (A) Enhancing effects of post-training intra-BLA infusions of norepinephrine on 24-h object recognition memory. Saline-infused controls displayed no evidence of memory of 3 min of training. The retention performance of groups given 0.3 or 1.0 µg of norepinephrine was significantly better than that of the saline controls. Data are presented as discrimination index (mean ± SEM; see main text). (B) Impairing effects of post-training intra-BLA infusions of propranolol on 24-h object recognition memory. All groups received 10 min of training. Saline infused controls displayed significant memory and propranolol produced dose-dependent impairment of memory. The performance of all three propranolol groups differed significantly from that of the saline controls. * $p < 0.05$; ** $p < 0.01$. n = 7-9 rats per group. (From [35].)

Many other learning tasks that do not employ fear motivation also have demonstrated BLA influences on memory consolidation. These include: change in reward magnitude [37], conditioned place preference [38, 39], radial maze training [40], water maze spatial and cued training [41], conditioned taste aversion [42], olfactory conditioning [43], extinction of conditioned reward [44], cortical representation of motor skill learning [45], and as discussed below, learning-induced cortical representation of auditory information [46].

1.4. BLA interactions with other brain regions in modulating memory consolidation

Each of the learning tasks mentioned above no doubt involves the selective participation of specific brain regions as well as interactions with other regions. The findings of many studies indicate that the amygdala influences memory consolidation via its extensive projections to other brain regions [47] that are involved in processing different kinds and aspects of information [7, 48]. In an early study, Packard et al. [41] investigated the effects of post-training activation (using *d*-amphetamine) of the amygdala, hippocampus or caudate nucleus on spatial and cued water maze learning. Hippocampal infusions selectively enhanced spatial learning and caudate infusions selectively enhanced cued learning. In contrast, amygdala infusions enhanced both spatial and cued learning. Importantly, infusions of lidocaine into the amygdala prior to testing did not block retention of either spatial or cued responses. These findings clearly indicated that the amygdala activation enhanced memory by activating other brain process involved in learning these tasks. Other experiments have found that lesions or inactivation of the BLA or intra-BLA infusions of β-adrenoceptor antagonists block the memory enhancing effects of post-training administration of drugs into other brain regions, including the entorhinal cortex, hippocampus and nucleus accumbens [40, 49-51].

The evidence that contextual fear conditioning involves learning both that shock is delivered and that it is delivered in a specific context [52] provided the opportunity to investigate the effects of treatments administered to different brain regions after either exposure to the context or brief shock in the context a day later [53]. Infusions of oxotremorine into the hippocampus selectively enhanced memory of contextual fear conditioning when administered after context exposure and infusions administered into the rostral anterior cingulate cortex selectively enhanced memory when administered after footshock administration. In contrast, infusions into the BLA enhanced memory of contextual fear conditioning when administered after either context exposure or footshock stimulation the following day [54]. Thus, although the hippocampus and rostral cingulate cortex were involved in processing different aspects of contextual fear conditioning (i.e., context *vs.* fear) the amygdala modulated the consolidation of memory for both kinds of information. Findings of Mcintyre et al. [55] provide additional evidence of BLA influences on hippocampal involvement in memory consolidation. Noradrenergic activation of the BLA that enhanced memory increased the expression of activity-regulated cytoskeletal protein (Arc) in the hippocampus. This immediate-early gene is known to be involved in regulating synaptic plasticity and memory consolidation [56].

Other studies have reported that electrical stimulation of the BLA enhances the development of long-term potentiation (LTP) in the hippocampus and that infusions of β-adrenoceptor antagonist into the BLA prevent this induction of LTP in the hippocampus as well as stress induced influences on LTP [57-60]. Additionally, and importantly, electrical stimulation of the BLA activates the cortex, as indicated by electroencephalogram (EEG) desynchronization. This effect appears to involve activation of the NB, as inactivation of the NB blocks the BLA-induced activation [61, 62] (Figure 3).

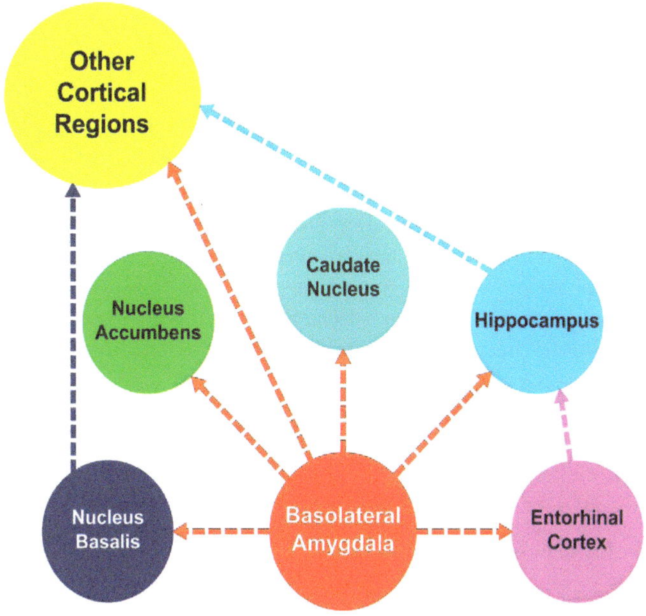

Figure 3. The Basolateral Amygdala (BLA) modulates memory representations wherever they are stored in other brain regions, with the cholinergic NB likely to play a critical role for the cerebral neocortex ("Other Cortical Regions").

There are other interactions between the BLA and the cerebral cortex. For example, stimulation of the BLA enhances cortical LTP [63]. But, how the BLA modulates memory in the cortex remains unknown. A target memory representation is needed so that its modulation by the BLA could be directly assessed. Fortunately, *specific, associatively-induced representational plasticity* in the primary auditory cortex constitutes a suitable candidate memory trace [64]. Therefore, we determined the effects of BLA activation on representational plasticity in the primary auditory cortex (A1).

2. Primary sensory cortex and memory traces

2.1. Background

It may appear strange to study memory traces in a primary sensory cortex, because the traditional assumption has been that these cortical fields function only to *analyze* stimuli in their respective modalities. This dogma was strongly promoted by the work of A.W. Campbell [65], who divided sensory cortex into "sensory" and "psychic" regions, mainly on the basis of histological considerations. "Sensory" cortex consisted of what is now known as "primary" sensory fields (auditory, A1; somatosensory, S1; visual, V1 [area 17]) while "psychic" cortex included adjacent modality-specific regions, sometimes called "sensory association" or "belt" regions (e.g., VII [areas 18 and 19]). According to Campbell, the function of "sensory" cortex was strictly the *analysis of the physical features* of sensory stimuli, e.g., sounds, touches and sights. In contrast, the function of "psychic" cortex was the *comprehension or psychological understanding* of these stimuli.

Campbell's influence has been great, as this formulation still dominates neuroscience, although now at the level of an unconscious assumption. Campbell has been regarded as bearing major responsibility for "removing psychological functions", such as learning and memory, from A1, S1 and V1 by the rare authors who have analyzed this issue [66]. Campbell's willingness to do so in the absence of compelling functional data was in keeping with the temper of the times that may itself have reflected British empiricist philosophy, particularly Locke's distinction between "primary" and "secondary" qualities of objects [67]. His idea that the basic characteristics of sensory stimuli are combined to psychologically yield the objects that give rise to them has the merit of simplicity in explaining perception, and this in turn appeals to "common sense". Thus, in an era preceding electrophysiology, when Campbell noted certain histological differences between adjacent sensory cortical areas and noted some anecdotal observations of sensory deficits following cortical damage, his leap of logic did not seem so rash.

For more than 100 years, Campbell's division of labor has remained virtually unquestioned. And thus, alone of all regions of the brain, the function of the primary sensory fields has been "known" prior to actual physiological research. Instead of trying to discover the functions of A1, S1 and V1, the goal of sensory neuroscience has been largely to determine the *mechanisms of the accepted function of sensory analysis*. Implicit in this endeavor has been the corollary assumption that cortical responses to sensory stimuli are highly consistent and accurately reflect their *physical* parameters as transduced at their respective sensory receptors. This position was apparently validated by subsequent expected findings of highly consistent evoked responses in these cortical fields (e.g. [68]). The combination of common sense, venerable belief and apparent scientific validation is very powerful.

Nonetheless, Campbell's formulation is wrong. Moreover, it has been known to be an invalid account of primary sensory cortex for more than fifty years! To begin with, the high degree of consistency of evoked responses in the primary sensory fields is true only for the preparations in which they were studied, which is the deeply anesthetized animal. However, the anesthetized brain is not the brain that has evolved. While a useful preparation, it cannot be used to validate the belief that A1, S1 and V1 perform only the analysis of the physical attributes of sensory stimuli. And even if Locke's separation of primary and secondary qualities of objects were accepted, it doesn't follow logically that they have to be carried out in primary and secondary sensory cortical fields, respectively.

More compellingly, primary sensory fields are deeply involved in the interpretation, i.e., behavioral meaning, of sensory stimuli. For example, they develop neuronal plasticity during learning. In 1956, Galambos and co-workers [69] performed a simple experiment. They presented a sound followed by a mild aversive stimulus to cats, while recording from the primary auditory cortex. The animals quickly developed conditioned responses in this simple Pavlovian conditioning study, as expected. Importantly, these workers discovered that the *amplitude of the sound elicited auditory evoked potential increased* when it acquired associative value as a predictor of the unconditioned stimulus.

This simple demonstration initiated extensive research during the subsequent thirty years, during which all necessary controls for non-associative factors were investigated and ruled out. For example, the evoked potentials might have become larger if the acoustic stimulus inadvertently became louder, which could have happened if the cats had moved closer to the loudspeaker, or if they had simply relaxed their middle-ear muscles. Direct investigation eliminated even this very subtle potential artifact [70].

Studies were extended to positive as well as aversive reinforcement, various species, more complex tasks and other forms of recording. For example, two-tone discrimination experiments, both in classical and instrumental conditioning, resulted in the same type of increased cortical response to the reinforced tone CS+ (the tone represents the conditioned stimulus, CS) and also revealed that responses to the un-reinforced tone (CS–) decreased, whether evoked potentials or cellular discharges were recorded (reviewed in [71]). Furthermore, repeated presentation of the same sound produced a decrease in response, i.e., habituation of auditory cortical processing [72, 73]. Overall, these findings indicated that auditory cortical responses "tracked" the behavioral relevance of stimuli as interactions between animals and the environment were altered: increased responses to sounds of greater importance, decreased responses to sounds of lesser importance.

2.2. Contemporary status

While these types of findings were incompatible with traditional assumptions that primary sensory cortices were sensitive only to physical stimulus parameters, they were largely ignored. This lack of interest probably was due to two factors. Within the community of learning/memory workers attention was focused on structures such as the hippocampus and amygdala. Moreover, these researchers had no reason to question the prevailing dogma because sensory cortex was viewed as the domain of sensory physiology. And within the community of sensory workers, studies of learning-induced cortical plasticity were probably seen as irrelevant, because they could shed little light on critical issues about sensory coding. Why not? Because learning/memory studies typically employ one or two different stimuli during training, e.g., a CS+ and a CS−. Such a paucity of stimulus values could not reveal how the effects of learning might modify the encoding of a stimulus dimension, such as acoustic frequency. Thus, demonstrations that learning produced increased responses in primary sensory cortex were unhelpful to sensory neurophysiology.

It is a curiosity that within neuroscience, two disciplines are concerned with the "fate" of sensory stimuli: sensory neurophysiology and learning/memory. The former seeks the coding and processing of stimuli that underlie perception; the latter seeks the transformation of stimuli into behaviorally relevant objects, usually of sufficient import to gain access to the halls of memory. Although these lines of research have developed in parallel, their basic paradigms are actually complementary. Sensory neurophysiology varies the physical parameters of stimuli while keeping constant their psychological parameters; learning/memory does the converse: it varies the psychological parameter of stimuli while keeping constant their physical parameters (Figure 4).

Discipline	Stimulus Parameters	
	Physical[a]	Psychological[b]
Sensory Physiology	Vary	Constant
Learning	Constant	Vary

[a]E.g., wavelength, kHz, dB, etc.
[b]E.g., trials to criterion, # correct responses, etc.

Figure 4. Complementarity of the disciplines of sensory neuroscience and learning/memory neuroscience. The former focuses on the coding of stimulus features from the environment (and even from the body itself) while the latter is focused on the stored representations of these stimulus features and their relation to other aspects of experience.

Such juxtaposition of paradigms suggests a new experimental synthesis: use both approaches within the same experiment to gain a more comprehensive understanding of how sensory representations may be modified during learning. Specifically, a three-phase *modus operandi* is called for: (1) perform a sensory physiology operation that determines the responses of neurons to many stimuli (e.g., different tones); this yields receptive fields which reveal how a stimulus dimension (e.g., acoustic frequency) is encoded prior to a learning experience; (2) perform a learning experiment in which subjects are trained using one of the values of the stimuli in the receptive field (e.g., tone-shock pairing); (3) repeat phase 1, thus revealing the *effects of learning on sensory coding*. In short, this approach enables the discipline of learning/memory to become relevant to the discipline of sensory physiology, and *vice-versa*. The new experimental design can reveal the extent to which a learning experience may *specifically alter stimulus representations* in the cortex. And in so doing, it provides a means for the field of learning/memory to investigate the *content* of memory, not simply the *processes* that enable the formation of memory. With an understanding of both process and content, the neurobiology of memory gains the ability to provide a comprehensive account of the "fate" of sensory events as they are transformed into behaviorally relevant objects. This unified experimental design can be further extended to shed light on the temporal dynamics of memory consolidation and storage by repeating the post-training determination of receptive fields at intervals of hours, days and weeks.

Before describing the findings, it is important to realize that determination of the effects of learning on sensory representations has the potential to greatly increase our understanding of the neural substrates of learning and memory. In contrast to most neurophysiological studies of these processes, which provide information on whether neuronal responses were increased, decreased or not changed, sensory physiology provides the ability to examine a far more comprehensive domain. Not only can it determine the *tuning specificity* of plasticity, it can also determine whether an experience has affected the *sensitivity* of the system (i.e., the *threshold* of response) and also the *selectivity* of neurons (i.e., the *bandwidth* of response).

This design was first used to study the effects of learning on frequency coding in sensory-association fields of the cat auditory cortex ("secondary" [AII] and "ventral ectosylvian" [VE]) during classical conditioning. The receptive field results showed specific changes to the frequency of the conditioned stimulus (CS), indicating that learning remodels the representation of a behaviorally relevant sensory dimension rather than facilitating responses across acoustic frequency [74]. This finding attracted little attention because, in accordance with Campbell and general assumptions, it was expected that non-primary sensory cortex would change as the psychological meaning of a stimulus changed. However, this study did demonstrate the feasibility of the new approach.

The first study of the primary auditory cortex was conducted during classical conditioning (tone–shock pairing) in the guinea pig. It revealed a heretofore unexpected type of plasticity: tuning curves (frequency receptive fields) were *shifted* to favor the representation of the frequency of the tonal conditioned stimulus. That is, responses to the CS frequency were increased while those to other frequencies decreased (Figure 5). These opposite effects were sufficiently large to often make the CS frequency the new peak of the tuning curve [75]. Thus, there is no fixed coding relationship between the physical parameters of a stimulus and the response of cells in primary sensory cortex! Hence, there is no separation between pure analysis and psychological comprehension of the meaning of a stimulus.

Subsequent studies validated and replicated such findings. For example, it might be thought that tuning shifts reflect instability and drift of cellular tuning [76]. However, investigations of both short-term (30-120 minutes [77]) and long-term stability (weeks [78]) have failed to reveal spontaneous tuning changes. Moreover, tuning shifts were directed to, not also away from, the CS frequency in several species: bat [79], guinea pig [80], rat [81] and human [82-84].

As discussed above, modulation of memory by the BLA acts on memory traces stored elsewhere [1, 7]. However, there has been no direct study of the hypothesized changes in such traces. Representational plasticity in A1 provides such an opportunity because, alone of all electrophysiological correlates of learning, it has been comprehensively studied and found to exhibit the major characteristics of associative memory itself: in addition to being associative and specific, it can be rapidly induced (five trials), consolidates (grow stronger over hours and days after brief training) and exhibits long-term retention (weeks or months). It also develops in a wide variety of tasks, for all types of reinforcement (positive brain stimulation [85]) as well as standard reward and punishment (reviewed in [2]). *In toto*, the findings suggest that receptive field re-tuning in A1 reflects the *acquired behavioral importance* of tones.

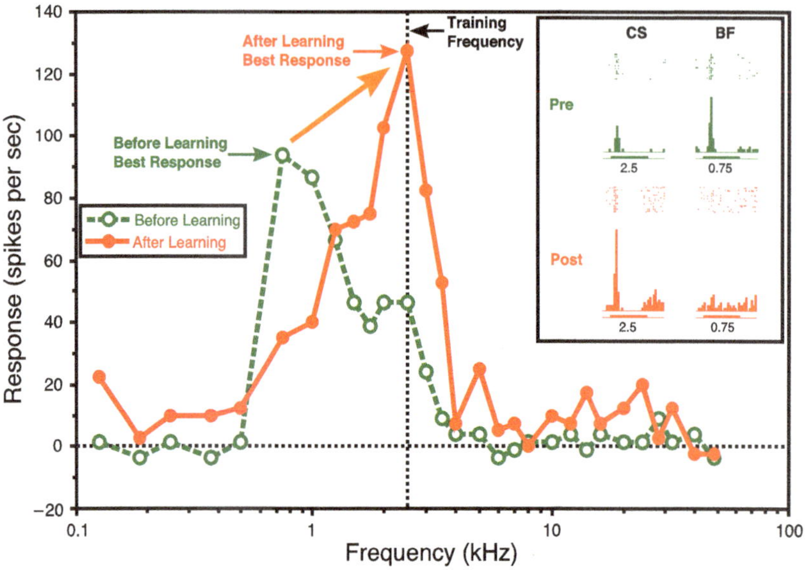

Figure 5. Associative learning is accompanied by specific shifts of neuronal tuning that favors the frequency of signal stimuli such as a CS. An example from a study of classical conditioning, of a complete shift of frequency tuning from a pre-training best frequency (BF) of 0.75 kHz to the CS frequency of 2.5 kHz after 30 trials of tone-shock pairing during which the guinea pig develops a cardiac conditioned response. Inset shows pre- and post-training post-stimulus time histograms (PSTHs) for the pre-training BF and the CS frequencies. Note the increase in response to the CS and the decreased response to the pre-training best frequency (BF, peak of the tuning curve).

The findings also suggest that the actual area of representation of the CS in the tonotopic map of A1 should be increased because such maps are basically the distribution of neuronal tuning across the cortex. A direct test of both the "importance" and "area" hypotheses was conducted by varying the relative significance of a tone that signaled the availability of water reward in differentially water deprived rats. Indeed, area expansions were found and there was a significant relationship to behavioral importance: the greater the level of importance, the greater the area of its representation [86]. Furthermore, the area of representation has been linked to the strength of memory: the greater the area of representational gain during learning, the greater the resistance to extinction, i.e., the stronger the memory [87].

Insofar as the BLA is a substrate of increased memory strength during consolidation, we hypothesized that activation of the BLA should be capable of enhancing specific memory traces, the magnitude of which appears to be a substrate of memory strength-*representational plasticity* in the *primary auditory cortex*.

3. Short-term amygdala modulation of specific sensory memory representations

To determine the capability of the BLA to facilitate cortical memory traces, we began with a study of the short-term effects of BLA stimulation on frequency receptive fields in A1. As this was a highly novel "proof of concept" investigation, we wanted to achieve maximum control over experimental procedures and animal state. Therefore, our first study was conducted in acutely prepared animals that were maintained under general anesthesia (urethane) [46]. Adult male rats (n = 16) maintained under urethane received a stimulating electrode in the BLA and an array of microelectrodes placed in the primary auditory cortex. Calibrated tones were presented to the contralateral ear as most of the input to the cortex is crossed. The EEG from A1 was continually recorded to monitor cortical state. Repeated tone presentation revealed that the frequency receptive fields were reliable and exhibited no spontaneous drift. On the basis of pre-treatment frequency tuning, we selected a tone "CS" that was not a best frequency (peak of the tuning curve), so that potential shifts of tuning could be detected. The tone (2.0 s) was paired with a 400 ms train of electrical stimulation (100 Hz) to the BLA that occurred 1 s after tone onset. This pattern simulated phasic BLA engagement during a brief "emotional" experience. All rats received a single training session of 100 trials (intertrial interval mean = 30 s).

To determine the effects of training on frequency representation, we obtained tuning curves immediately, 45 and 75 min after the training session. Insofar as prior findings had emphasized that associative learning shifts frequency tuning to favor a signal frequency [2], we calculated a "Shift Index" using the following formula:

$$SI = \frac{\text{Post BF}_{max} - \text{Pre BF}_{max}}{\text{CS} - \text{Pre BF}_{max}}$$

where BF_{max} is the tone frequency/level combination that elicited the greatest number of spikes, Pre is the average of the pre-treatment responses, and Post is the average of responses at each of the post-treatment test intervals. A positive SI indicates a shift towards the CS, while a negative SI indicates a shift away from the CS. A complete shift to the CS frequency after training would produce an SI = 1.0.

Histological analysis revealed that 11/16 rats had placements of the stimulating electrodes in the BLA. Additionally, physiological verification of functional placements was evident in that BLA stimulation in all of these animals produced electro-cortical activation ("EEG desynchronization") [62]. In contrast, five animals had stimulating placements outside of the BLA, and in none of these cases did stimulation produce cortical activation. This latter group thus constituted a control group for the anatomical specificity of modulation of sensory memory representations.

Stimulation of the BLA did induce specific tuning shifts. Figure 6 provides a particularly clear example of consolidation dynamics during a marked shift to the frequency of the signal (conditioned) stimulus. The largest response (best frequency maximum, BF_{max}) before training was at 11.3 kHz. We chose 4.0 kHz for the frequency of the CS; this was actually at the edge of the frequency receptive field. When tuning was again determined immediately after training, the BF_{max} had shifted, but only very slightly and actually away from the CS, resulting in a negligible SI score of –0.06. However, the most pronounced effect was that tuning became broader toward the CS, now extending to include this frequency. Most relevant, response to the pre-training BF_{max} decreased while responses to the CS frequency increased (Figure 6A). It is these opposing modulations of receptive fields that is particularly characteristic of associative representational plasticity, that is, the systematic reorganization of sensory memory representations (e.g. [75]).

Had recording ceased immediately after training, as is often the case in neurophysiological studies of learning, the major effects of BLA modulation would have been missed. Instead, insofar as post-training consolidation is so characteristic of memory, we sought electrophysiological consolidation. Consolidation is customarily studied as post-event temporally-graded reduced susceptibility to interference. However, reduced susceptibility actually is an indirect behavioral index of increasing strength of underlying neural mechanisms of memory. Therefore, neural bases of memory strength should themselves become stronger over time after training. As representational plasticity in the form of signal-directed tuning shifts does meet the several criteria for a memory substrate (reviewed in [2]), it would be expected to exhibit consolidation. Indeed, this predicted characteristic has been found in the case of natural memory in the form of continued increased specificity of tuning shifts over time after training [88]. Similarly, we found that the effects of BLA stimulation also produced specific neural consolidation.

Determination of tuning after a post-training silent period of 45 min revealed that the BF_{max} had shifted further, all the way *to the CS frequency*, resulting in an SI score of 1.0. Also, responses to the higher frequencies were diminished. At this point, the tuning curve was still very broad. Despite the complete shift of tuning, neural consolidation had not ceased. After an additional 30 minutes of silence, a final test revealed that the frequency receptive field had become more sharply tuned, coalescing around the CS frequency, which remained the new post-training BF_{max}. There was *no longer any response* to the pre-training BF_{max}, and the frequency receptive field had become *centered around the CS frequency*. The tuning shifts and consolidation are particularly clearly seen in difference functions, in which the pre-training tuning curve is subtracted from the post-training tuning curves (Figure 6B).

BLA stimulation produced tuning shifts across the group. Subjects with placements outside of the BLA did not show tuning shifts. This study revealed that, indeed, BLA stimulation has the capacity to reorganize the primary auditory cortex to increase the representation of an environmental stimulus. In particular, it revealed the short-term (e.g., 75 min) dynamics of BLA induced effects on cortical representations [46].

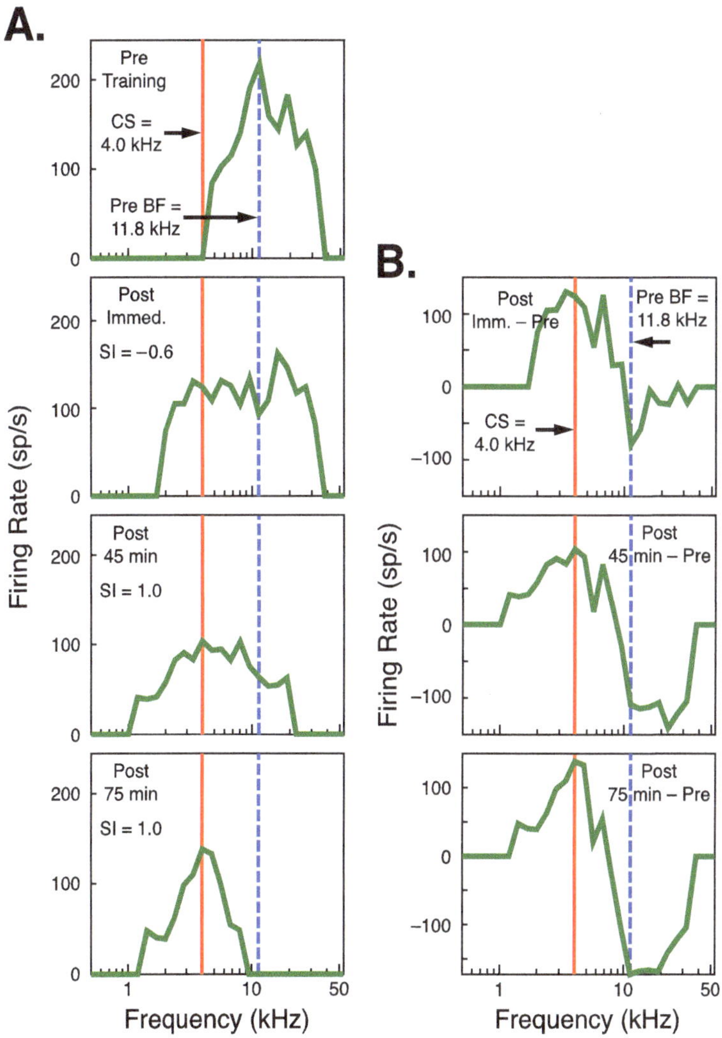

Figure 6. Pairing tone and BLA stimulation in rat under anesthesia produces specific tuning shift, including consolidation over more than an hour. (A) Top row, pre-training tuning curve with a BF_{max} that was at 11.3 kHz. The training frequency (CS) selected was 4.0 kHz. Immediately after training, there was a large decrease in responsiveness at the BF_{max} and an increase in responsiveness at the CS frequency. Tuning shifted to the CS frequency at 45 min (SI = 1.0) and the receptive field became even more sharply tuning at 75 min, while maintaining its peak at the CS frequency (SI = 1.0). (B) Difference tuning functions (pre-training subtracted from post-training data). Immediately after training, there was a maximum decrease in responsiveness to the BF_{max} and a maximum increase in response to the CS frequency. This pattern continued (*consolidated*) and grew 45 min after training and increased even more at the 75-min time period.

4. Long-term modulation of specific sensory memory representations by the BLA

The acute study in anesthetized animals clearly demonstrated that BLA activation can systematically modify *frequency tuning* in the primary auditory cortex. Moreover, the tuning shifts were directed to the CS frequency, i.e., the same type and direction of representational plasticity consistently observed during actual learning (e.g. [75, 89]). The findings constitute a "proof of concept" demonstration that the BLA can specifically enhance cortical representations of experience. However, they do not speak to two major issues. First, is the BLA capable of representational modulation in the waking animal? Second, what are the temporal dynamics of BLA modulation: are the effects transient or sufficiently enduring to promote long-term memory effects?

To address these issues, we performed an extensive series of observations on the effects of BLA activation in chronically prepared rats bearing multiple microelectrodes in A1, from whom daily recordings were obtained up to three weeks (21 days) after a single session in which a tone was paired with BLA stimulation. This constitutes a unique set of post-training neurophysiological observations, necessitated by the goal of achieving a comprehensive determination of temporal dynamics. Moreover, to determine if the effects were due to pairing per se, rather than merely BLA stimulation, we used a discrimination paradigm in which both paired tones were presented in random order. Training consisted of a single session of 60 trials of 30 trials each of a tone (2.0 s) paired with 0.2 s stimulation of the BLA (1.8 s interstimulus interval) (CS+) or tone alone (CS−). The frequency distance between the two tones was set to be relatively small (1.25 octaves), in order to require that any selective results would be obtained under rigorous circumstances.

As noted above, analysis of a primary sensory cortex provides a far more comprehensive understanding of the effects of training than even the degree of specific plasticity yields with tuning curves, as afforded in our study of short-term plasticity, which focused on modulation of frequency tuning. In the auditory system, it is possible to obtain frequency response areas (FRAs), which consist of the responses of neurons to a wide range of both frequency and intensity ("level") values. In fact, FRAs essentially circumscribe the domain of neuronal responses to pure tones. Figure 7 presents an example of such a record. Note that the effects of a treatment, whether overt learning or brain stimulation, can be determined at threshold as well as above threshold. Moreover, at and near threshold, one can determine the effects on *tuning*, which is indexed by the characteristic frequency (CF), and also the threshold itself (Th, given in decibels), and the bandwidth at selected levels above threshold (e.g., 10 and 20 dB). The absolute threshold yields the *sensitivity* of neural response while the bandwidth indicates the *selectivity* of response. Any combinations of these measures may be altered by learning, or modulated by the BLA or other brain systems. Note also that the FRA yields important data above threshold. An important marker of potential plasticity is the best frequency (BF), which is the frequency-level combination that elicits the largest neural response (BF maximum, BFx).

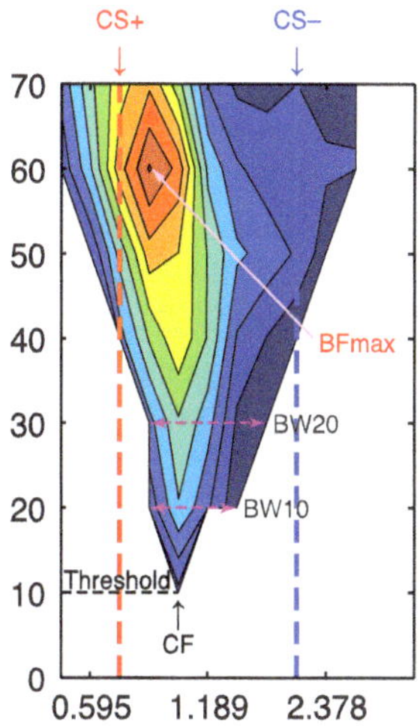

Figure 7. Frequency response area (FRA).We used a standard analysis of frequency tuning, in which cellular response is determined by random presentation of a wide range of frequency and stimulus level ("intensity") combinations. Key parameters were measured: CF (characteristic frequency, that to which the cells are most sensitive), Th (threshold, the stimulus level for the CF), BW10 and BW20 (the bandwidths 10 and 20 dB above threshold, showing degree of selectivity) and BF_{max} (best frequency maximum response in the FRA). Note that the CS+ and the CS– stimuli were set close together (1.25 octave distance) for all animals (and therefore for all recording sites) to insure that tuning shifts were highly specific.

5. Effects of BLA stimulation on specificity, sensitivity and selectivity

FRAs were obtained from several electrodes implanted in A1 of the animals, both pre-training and post-training, daily for 21 days (3 weeks). CFs (tuning at threshold) were obtained for each electrode and the mean CF was calculated for each day and averaged. First, we analyzed the results for Week 1 (7 days). Electrodes were divided into those showing an increase in the "shift index" from those showing a decrease, as follows:

$$\text{CF SI} = \frac{\text{Post CF} - \text{Pre CF}}{(\text{CS+}) - \text{Pre CF}}.$$

A value of 1.0 would indicate a tuning shift from the pre-training CF all the way to the frequency of the CS+; a value of –1.0 would signify a shift to the CS–. Data were divided into three groups: mean increase, mean decrease and mean no change. To avoid including spurious small changes in tuning, we set a criterion of SI = ± 0.1 (i.e., a shift of 10% toward the CS+). Any electrodes exhibiting a mean response of less than this value were classified as "no change", even if they exhibited much larger shifts on one or more days during the first week. Thus, our approach was conservative in order to reduce the probability of Type I errors.

A total of 55 electrodes (9 subjects) yielded reliable recordings. Of these, the majority (30) developed significant shifts toward the CS+ (increased SI mean value), 13 had no change and 12 shifted away from the CS+. However, the numbers in the three categories do not reveal the most important aspects of the data, i.e., the temporal dynamics. Shifts favoring the CS+ were evident at the first post-training test (24 h), increased over the next 2-5 days, and then were maintained for the balance of the three week recording period (Figure 8). In contrast, the less prevalent shifts away from the CS+ were transient, seen only at 24 h post-training and then diminishing toward no change during week 1, following a highly variable course thereafter.

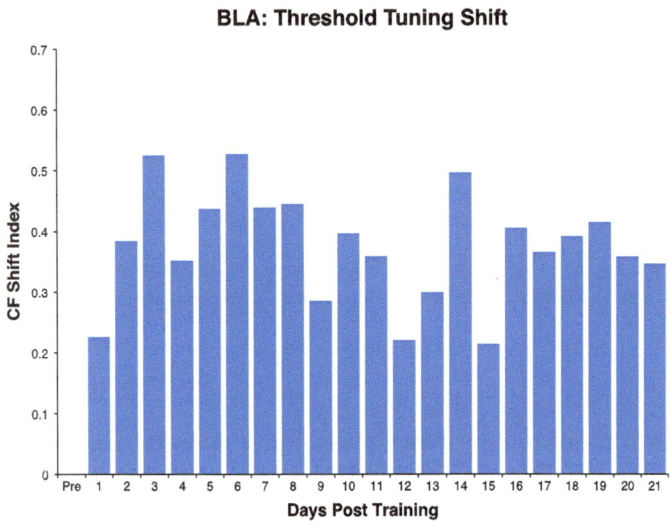

Figure 8. Tone paired with brief BLA stimulation produces tuning shifts at threshold toward the CS+ in chronically-prepared, waking rats. The tuning shift is evident on Day 1 (24 hr post-training) and consolidates (increases in magnitude) over three days. Remarkable, while declining slightly on Day 9, this specific modification of cortical representation of the CS+ was maintained for the entire recording period of three weeks. In this and subsequent figures, all values are referenced to pre-training ("Pre") during which period of several days "sham" tuning shifts were negligible.

As noted above, a marked advantage of determining the effects of modulatory processes on a primary sensory cortex is that the FRA yields information on *sensitivity* and *selectivity*. Threshold measures revealed a significant decrease in threshold of as much as 6 dB over days, restricted to neurons that had shifted toward the CS+; no changes in threshold were observed for recording sites that did not shift their tuning to favor the CS+ (Figure 9A). Bandwidth analyses showed a significant trend for a decrease in BW10 across days (Figure 9B). However, there was no significant change for BW20, which is less reflective of threshold plasticity (Figure 6C). There were no significant changes in threshold or bandwidth for recording sites that had transiently shifted away from the CS+.

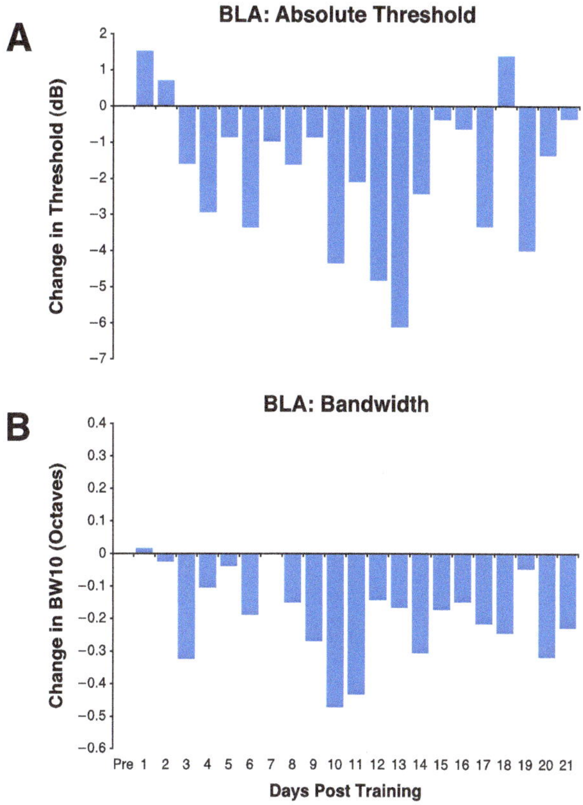

Figure 9. BLA stimulation not only shifts tuning at threshold, but also (A) lowers the absolute threshold, i.e., increased *sensitivity*. The decrease in threshold develops slowly, reaching its peak at > 6 dB on Day 13, and was still evident at the end of recording (Day 21). A 6 dB decrease in threshold constitutes a noteworthy amount of change psychophysically. (B) Also accompanying the tuning shift and reduced threshold, bandwidth at 10 dB above threshold narrowed, i.e., increased *selectivity*. Decreased BW10 was evident on Day 3 post-training, reaching its maximum on Day 10 at which time the decrease in bandwidth attained the functionally high value of 0.5 octaves. This increased selectivity was maintained at a substantial level through Day 21, the last day of recording.

6. Effects of BLA stimulation on suprathreshold responses

The maximum response in an FRA is an important index of the effects of a treatment on the representation of acoustic information. As noted, we tracked the preferred frequency of BF_{max} for three weeks post-training. A total of 50 recordings yielded reliable suprathreshold data. Of these, 18 shifted toward the CS+ significantly during week 1, and they maintained this shift for the full 3 weeks of recording (Figure 10A). Nine recording sites were classified as shifts away from the CS+, but these failed to reach significance during Week 1 or thereafter. The largest group was classified as no change (n = 23), but surprisingly these recordings did exhibit a trend of shifting over 3 weeks, albeit of a lesser magnitude (Figure 10B). Thus, the predominant effect on BF_{max} was tuning shifts toward the CS+.

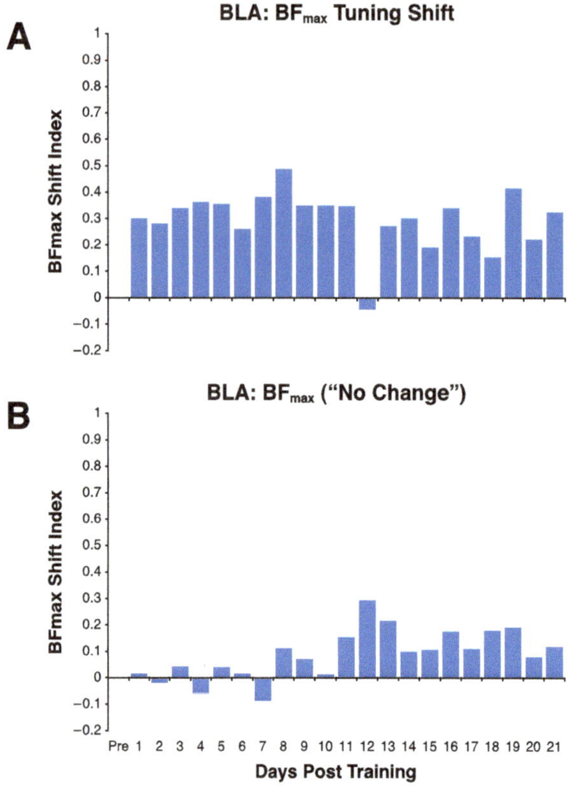

Figure 10. Suprathreshold tuning shifts induced by BLA stimulation. (A) The maximum response in the FRA (BF_{max}) is shifted when a tone is paired with BLA stimulation. In contrast to the slowing-developing shift at threshold, BF_{max} increased abruptly at the first post-training recording (Day 1) and was maintained at about that level for 3 weeks. (B) For recording sites whose mean SI during Week 1 classified them as "no change" (i.e., SI values were ≤ 0.1), there was a surprising trend of shifting toward the CS+ over three weeks.

7. Central Nucleus modulation of memory representations in the auditory cortex

The central nucleus of the amygdala (CE) has also been implicated in learning and memory [90]. However, considerable research indicates that it does not promote post-training memory consolidation, at least not to the extent to which the BLA is involved (e.g. [91–93]). To elucidate the capabilities of the CE to modulate representation in the cortex, we conducted a parallel study. Recordings were obtained from 45 sites in seven rats.

Tuning also was modified at threshold. Twenty-four sites developed post-training tuning shifts toward the CS+. Like the BLA, these developed rapidly, being clearly evident at the first recording session 24 h after training. Also like the BLA, they were maintained for three weeks (Figure 11). Recordings that exhibited either no change ($n = 10$) or shifts away from the CS+ exhibited different dynamics. The former showed a lack of tuning shifts toward or away from the CS+ while the latter exhibited a highly transient (Day 1) shift away that then returned to baseline over the balance of Week.

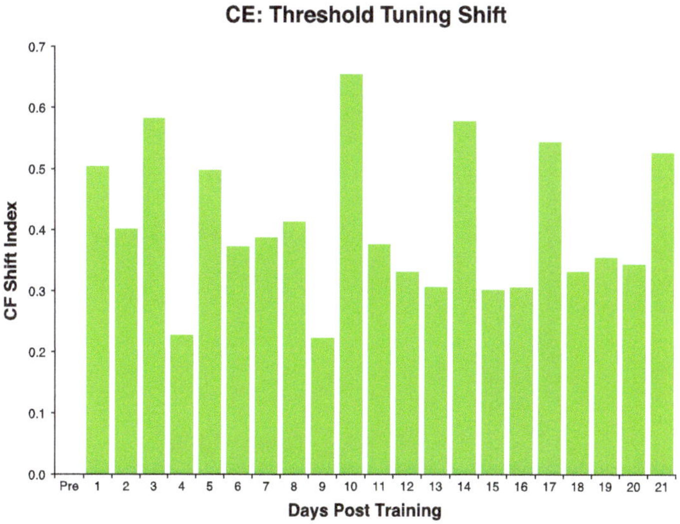

Figure 11. Stimulation of the CE, in a paradigm identical to that used with the BLA, also shifted tuning at threshold. The shift was pronounced at Day 1, thus increasing faster than the shift caused by BLA stimulation, and was maintained at a high level for the 3-week recording period.

However, in contrast to the BLA, stimulation of the CE failed to produce any significant change in threshold (Figure 12A) or bandwidth (Figure 12B) for both BW10 and BW20. Also unlike the BLA, pairing the CS+ with CE stimulation did not produce as long lasting tuning shift toward the CS+ above threshold; the BF_{max} displayed a shift that decreased before Day 21 (Figure 12C).

8. Discussion

It is now well established that the BLA can modulate memory that is stored in other brain regions (Introduction). However, the nature of exactly what is modulated has remained a mystery, largely because the presumed target memory representations had not been studied. The research reviewed in this chapter initiated a novel line of inquiry to synthesize knowledge of *processes* involved in regulating memory strength with those that underlie the *specific content* of memories. This required an approach based on the conception that sensory

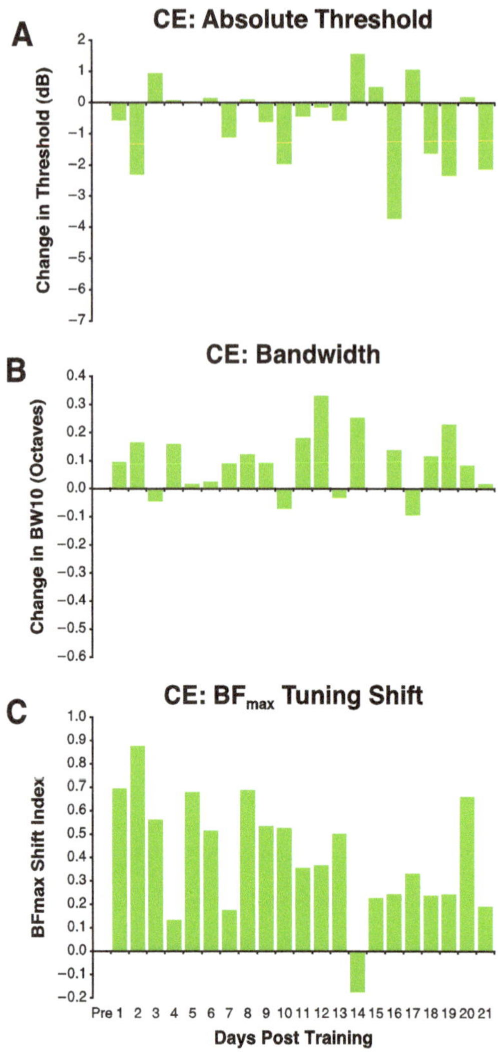

Figure 12. Stimulation of the CE (A) had no systematic effect on threshold, (B) produced a non-significant increase in BW10 and (C) did produce a BF_{max} shift toward the CS+. However, it was not maintained significantly across the 3-week recording period.

neuroscience and learning/memory neuroscience are complementary approaches to understanding how the brain processes, represents and stores experiences. Memory traces are linked to representational plasticity in the primary auditory cortex (A1) because the representations of sounds (tone frequencies) are systematically modified to emphasize stimuli that gain behavioral importance as predictors of reinforcement. Moreover, tuning shifts possess cardinal attributes of memory: they are associative, specific, rapidly formed, consolidate over hours and days and can last indefinitely [2]. Specific shifts of frequency receptive fields accomplish such increased emphasis by increasing the number of cortical neurons that respond preferentially to signal tones. Indeed, increased memory strength is encoded by an increase in the area of tonal representation in the tonotopic map of A1 [87]. Therefore, we asked whether activation of the BLA following tone presentation could specifically modulate the representation of that stimulus in the auditory cortex.

8.1. The BLA produces coordinated modulation of cortical representations

The first experiment paired a tone with stimulation of the BLA in anesthetized rats, as a "proof of concept" study [46]. This produced tuning shifts toward or even precisely to the "CS" frequency. Furthermore, tuning shifts developed over time, i.e., exhibited *neural consolidation* and were retained for the longest period tested, 75 minutes. As these attributes of receptive field plasticity are also found during natural learning [75, 88, 89], the findings support the concept that the BLA modulates specific memory representation.

Memory modulation has enduring effects on memories. Therefore, we extended this line of inquiry to chronic preparations. Rats were implanted with multiple microwires in the primary auditory cortex. They received a single session of tone either paired with BLA stimulation (CS+) or without any stimulation (CS–). We also analyzed the effects of stimulation on frequency response areas (FRAs), consisting of a matrix of responses to all frequencies and stimulus levels (intensities) to which cells responded. This comprehensive approach yielded not only potential shifts of tuning above threshold [46], but additionally cortical representations at the most sensitive region of neuronal response: tuning at threshold (characteristic frequency, CF), sensitivity (absolute threshold) and selectivity (bandwidth 10 and 20 dB above threshold). The inclusion of a CS– frequency further permitted the conclusion that any representational plasticity that emphasized the CS+ tone was attributable to the specific frequency that was followed by BLA activation.

A single session of pairing a tone with BLA stimulation produced shifted tuning toward the CS+. This shift in frequency preference is evident both at threshold (CF) and above threshold for the maximum response in the FRA (BFx). This *specificity* of tuning shifts occurs rapidly, being evident at the first post-training test 24 hours later. Most remarkably, BLA induced representational plasticity is long lasting, enduring for at least 3 weeks, the longest period tested. Additionally, BLA stimulation paired with a preceding tone increased the *sensitivity* of the primary auditory cortex, by decreasing the absolute threshold. It further increased the *selectivity* of the cortex, by decreasing the bandwidth of tuning; both of these specific changes also lasted for at least 3 weeks following the single training session. Thus, activation of the BLA produces very long-term specific modification of the cortical representation of a potentially behaviorally significant stimulus.

This representational plasticity is capable of increasing the amount of the auditory cortex that represents the CS+ while rendering the cortex more sensitive and selective to the CS+ tone. In short, the BLA is capable of increasing the number of neurons that represent an environmental stimulus while simultaneously enhancing the precision with which it is detected while rejecting similar non-reinforced stimuli by narrowing bandwidth. These changes constitute a *coordinated, mutually-supporting and comprehensive weighting* of primary sensory cortex to sounds that are likely to have been marked as behaviorally significant by the increased release of stress hormones from the adrenal glands.

Therefore, the findings of both studies support the hypothesis that the BLA strengthens memory, at least in part, by modifying sensory cortical representations of stimuli, while also increasing both their sensitivity and selectivity. The result is an increase in memory strength for behaviorally important events.

8.2. Comparison of the basolateral and central nuclei of the amygdala

A parallel study conducted by pairing tone with stimulation of the CE revealed that activation of the latter was also effective in shifting tuning toward the CS+. Furthermore, like the BLA, such representational plasticity endured for at least three weeks. However, in distinction to the BLA, stimulation of the CE was less effective. While it shifted tuning at threshold to the same extent as the BLA, it did not reduce either threshold or bandwidth. Also, above threshold, its tuning shifts had decreased by the third week post-training. In short, the CE did not produce a coordinated, long term facilitation of response to frequencies near or at the CS+. Therefore, it might not be capable of strengthening memory by a comprehensive modification of sensory cortical representations.

8.3. Possible mechanisms

The capability of the amygdala to induce specific receptive field further supports a well-investigated model of auditory cortical receptive field plasticity [94–96]. It postulates that learning-dependent tuning shifts to behaviorally significant sounds first develop in the magnocellular medial geniculate nucleus of the auditory thalamus (MGm), which then projects its plasticity to the amygdala, which in turn projects facilitated neural responses to the cholinergic NB. The latter was hypothesized to release acetylcholine (ACh) into the cortical mantle, where convergence of the activation of muscarinic receptors on cells receiving frequency specific input from the conditioned stimulus produces selective synaptic strengthening. The result would be to increase responses to the CS thereafter, shifting tuning of many cells toward or even to the CS frequency. Across the tonotopic map, the effect would be an increase in the area representing this frequency.

This model has found support in numerous studies subsequent to its formulation. For example, specific receptive field tuning shifts do develop in the MGm during auditory conditioning [97], associative plasticity in the MGm has a shorter latency than in the amygdala [98], conditioned plasticity develops in the NB before it appears in the auditory cortex [99], stimulation of the NB enhances auditory responses in A1 [100], induces specific tuning shifts in A1 [101–104] and increases the cortical representation of the paired frequency [105]. (For reviews, see [2, 106].)

The findings reviewed in this chapter provide the first test of the role of the amygdala in cortical representational plasticity. As summarized, stimulation of the BLA produces the same type of tuning shifts found during actual learning. Indeed, it goes beyond the mere demonstration of receptive field plasticity to reveal that even at threshold levels, tuning is shifted, threshold is decreased and bandwidth is narrowed. Moreover, the BLA is known to project to the NB [107, 108]. BLA stimulation also produces EEG activation in the cortex, an effect that is mediated by the NB [109], whose stimulation also produces EEG activation (e.g., [110]). These findings suggest that BLA modulation of frequency receptive fields in the auditory cortex is mediated, at least in part, via the NB.

These considerations raise the issue of whether or not the BLA actually modulates the strength of behaviorally-validated memory via its actions on sensory cortical representations which themselves have been closely linked to such memory. The following suggest that indeed the BLA may do so as an important component in the model that postulates a particular system level mechanism for the modulation of memory strength. First, tone paired with stimulation of the NB not only induces specific tuning plasticity, but also *implants actual behavioral memory* (e.g. [111-117]). Second, tone paired with NB stimulation also increases the number of neurons that become best tuned to the paired frequency [105]. Third, the number of neurons that become best tuned to a paired frequency increases directly as a function of the degree of the tone's behavioral meaning or importance [86]. Fourth, the strength of behaviorally validated memory (i.e., not merely cortical plasticity) is a function of the amount of increase of representation area for the signal stimulus in the primary auditory cortex [87]. Fifth, extinction of memory is a function of the amount of *decrease* in representational area [118]. *In toto*, these findings support the hypothesis that the brain has a memory code for the acquired behavioral significance of experiences, resulting in greater strength of memory: (a) the more important the stimulus, the greater the number of neurons that become tuned it and (b) the greater the number of tuned neurons, the stronger is the memory [87, 95].

This formulation is also concordant with the fact that lesions of the NB block the memory enhancing effect of norepinephrine injected into the BLA [119]. Nonetheless, simply because research has deeply implicated the BLA, NB and ACh in memory storage and memory modulation should not be taken to exclude many other mechanisms that may act alone or in concert with these systems. For example, noradrenergic, dopaminergic and serotonergic axons engage cholinergic cells in the NB [120] and norepinephrine excites NB neurons [121]. Cortical EEG activation and increased release of cortical ACh result from the application of histamine to the NB ([122] and [123], respectively). A gain in cortical representation of frequency can also be achieved by stimulation of the ventral tegmental area (VTA), perhaps by the release of dopamine [124].

8.4. Future directions

The findings reviewed in this chapter open up new avenues of research on memory modulation. They provide a beginning rather than a comprehensive, or even moderately complete, account. We believe that their potential importance lies in the use of primary sensory cortical representations, specifically those already strongly implicated as memory traces, as a target for achieving a far better understanding of the mechanisms of memory modulation than heretofore available. Most previous research has been focused on the *processes* that enable memory and that regulate its strength. It is now a propitious time to extend this approach to the understanding of *how memories are actually represented* in the brain, because, e.g., processes of memory modulation must target highly specific representations of experience.

Future research will need to take at least two lines of investigation. Reductionistic studies, as usual, are needed to further delineate the cellular, circuit and systems mechanisms underlying the types of BLA modulations of cortical memory representations. Such studies must include direct manipulations of BLA and related structures in the amygdala, both to up-regulate and down-regulate modulation of representations in the cortex and perhaps in subcortical structures (e.g., hippocampus, striatum). Coordinated manipulation of cortical target areas are equally needed. For example, a comprehensive accounting of the role of neuromodulators other than ACh is surely necessary. Furthermore, the role of the CE is mysterious at this early stage of research. That the CE can shift tuning at threshold as well and as for as long a time (at least 3 weeks) as the BLA was both unexpected and at this point certainly unexplained. Equally intriguing are the failures of CE stimulation to have anything more than a transient effect above threshold, and to have no effect on either absolute threshold or bandwidth.

In addition to reductionistic studies, which can begin with the findings reviewed in this chapter, is the more difficult task of synthesis, i.e., bringing together apparently diverse and unrelated reports in the pursuit of a potentially new, perhaps even paradigm shifting, conceptual framework for memory and cortex. As noted in the Introduction, the traditional concept is that primary sensory cortices are stimulus analyzers while "higher" sensory and association fields are concerned with the psychological aspects of experience. The current findings of specific amygdala modulation of basic sensory parameters within frequency response areas should render this distinction obsolete. Prior studies of learning, memory and related cognitive processes are thus augmented by the results of amygdala modulation of A1 (reviewed in [95]). Together, they call for a new conceptualization of how and where memories are stored and how they are regulated. A more holistic and integrated approach to interacting brain systems is required. There is both challenge and great opportunity.

Author details

Candice M. Chavez, James L. McGaugh and Norman M. Weinberger*
Center for the Neurobiology of Learning and Memory, and Department of Neurobiology and Behavior, University of California, Irvine, CA, USA

* Corresponding Author

Acknowledgement

This study was funded by the NIDCD Grant #DC-05592 (NMW), NIMH Grant #MH-12526 (JLM) and the APA/DPN fellowship #5-T32-MH-18882 (CMC). We are grateful to Gabriel K. Hui for preparation of the manuscript.

9. References

[1] McGaugh JL. The amygdala modulates the consolidation of memories of emotionally arousing experiences. Annual Review of Neuroscience 2004; 27: 1–28.
[2] Weinberger NM. Associative representational plasticity in the auditory cortex: A synthesis of two disciplines. Learning and Memory 2007; 14(1–2): 1–16.
[3] McGaugh JL. Memory and emotion: The making of lasting memories. New York: Columbia University Press; 2003.
[4] McGaugh JL. Involvement of hormonal and neuromodulatory systems in the regulation of memory storage. Annual Review of Neuroscience 1989; 12: 255–287.
[5] McGaugh JL. Memory — A century of consolidation. Science 2000; 287(5451): 248–251.
[6] McGaugh JL, Roozendaal B. Drug enhancement of memory consolidation: Historical perspective and neurobiological implications. Psychopharmacology 2009; 202(1–3): 3–14.
[7] McGaugh JL. Memory consolidation and the amygdala: A systems perspective. Trends in Neurosciences 2002; 25(9): 456–461.
[8] Cahill L, Alkire MT. Epinephrine enhancement of human memory consolidation: Interaction with arousal at encoding. Neurobiology of Learning and Memory 2003; 79(2): 194–198.
[9] Cahill L, Gorski L, Le K. Enhanced human memory consolidation with post-learning stress: Interaction with the degree of arousal at encoding. Learning and Memory 2003; 10(4): 270–274.
[10] Cahill L, McGaugh JL. Mechanisms of emotional arousal and lasting declarative memory. Trends in Neuroscience 1998; 21(7): 294–299.
[11] Cahill L, Prins B, Weber M, McGaugh JL. Beta-adrenergic activation and memory for emotional events. Nature 1994; 371(6499): 702–704.
[12] McGaugh JL, Roozendaal B. Role of adrenal stress hormones in forming lasting memories in the brain. Current Opinion in Neurobiology 2002; 12(2): 205–210.
[13] Roozendaal B. Glucocorticoids and the regulation of memory consolidation. Psychoneuroendocrinology 2000; 25(3): 213–238.
[14] Roozendaal B, McGaugh JL. The memory-modulatory effects of glucocorticoids depend on an intact striaterminalis. Brain Research 1996; 709(2): 243–250.
[15] Quirarte GL, Roozendaal B, McGaugh JL. Glucocorticoid enhancement of memory storage involves noradrenergic activation in the basolateral amygdala. Proceedings of the National Academy of Sciences of the United States of America 1997; 94(25): 14048–14053.
[16] Roozendaal B, Okuda S, de Quervain DJ-F, McGaugh JL. Glucocorticoids interact with emotion-induced noradrenergic activation in influencing different memory functions. Neuroscience 2006; 138(3): 901–910.

[17] Roozendaal B, Quirarte GL, McGaugh JL. Stress-activated hormonal systems and the regulation of memory storage. Annals of the New York Academy of Sciences 1997; 821: 247–258.
[18] Ferry B, McGaugh JL. Clenbuterol administration into the basolateral amygdala post-training enhances retention in an inhibitory avoidance task. Neurobiology of Learning and Memory 1999; 72(1): 8–12.
[19] Ferry B, McGaugh JL. Involvement of basolateral amygdala α_2-adrenoceptors in modulating consolidation of inhibitory avoidance memory. Learning and Memory 2008; 15(4): 238–243.
[20] Ferry B, Roozendaal B, McGaugh JL. Basolateral amygdala noradrenergic influences on memory storage are mediated by an interaction between β- and α_1-adrenoceptors. Journal of Neuroscience 1999; 19(12): 5119–5123.
[21] Quirarte GL, Galvez R, Roozendaal B, McGaugh JL. Norepinephrine release in the amygdala in response to footshock and opioid peptidergic drugs. Brain Research 1998; 808(2): 134–140.
[22] McIntyre CK, Hatfield T, McGaugh JL. Amygdala norepinephrine levels after training predict inhibitory avoidance retention performance in rats. European Journal of Neuroscience 2002; 16(7): 1223–1226.
[23] Hatfield T, Spanis C, McGaugh JL. Response of amygdalar norepinephrine to footshock and GABAergic drugs using in vivo microdialysis and HPLC. Brain Research 1999; 835(2): 340–345.
[24] Power AE, McIntyre CK, Litmanovich A, McGaugh JL. Cholinergic modulation of memory in the basolateral amygdala involves activation of both m1 and m2 receptors. Behavioural Pharmacology 2003; 14(3): 207–213.
[25] Vazdarjanova A, McGaugh JL. Basolateral amygdala is involved in modulating consolidation of memory for classical fear conditioning. Journal of Neuroscience 1999; 19(15): 6615–6622.
[26] Dalmaz C, Introini-Collison IB, McGaugh JL. Noradrenergic and cholinergic interactions in the amygdala and the modulation of memory storage. Behavioural Brain Research 1993; 58(1–2): 167–174.
[27] Introini-Collison IB, Dalmaz C, McGaugh JL. Amygdala β-noradrenergic influences on memory storage involve cholinergic activation. Neurobiology of Learning and Memory 1996; 65(1): 57–64.
[28] Power AE, Roozendaal B, McGaugh JL. Glucocorticoid enhancement of memory consolidation in the rat is blocked by muscarinic receptor antagonism in the basolateral amygdala. European Journal of Neuroscience 2000; 12(10): 3481–3487.
[29] Hecker S, Mesulam MM. Two types of cholinergic projections to the rat amygdala. Neuroscience 1994; 60(2): 383–397.
[30] Power AE, McGaugh JL. Phthalic acid amygdalopetal lesion of the nucleus basalis magnocellularis induces reversible memory deficits in rats. Neurobiology of Learning and Memory 2002; 77(3): 372–388.
[31] LeDoux JE. Emotion circuits in the brain. Annual Review of Neuroscience 2000; 23: 155–184.

[32] Vazdarjanova A, McGaugh JL. Basolateral amygdala is not critical for cognitive memory of contextual fear conditioning. Proceedings of the National Academy of Sciences of the United States of America 1998; 95(25): 15003–15007.
[33] Berlau DJ, McGaugh JL. Enhancement of extinction memory consolidation: The role of the noradrenergic and GABAergic systems within the basolateral amygdala. Neurobiology of Learning and Memory 2006; 86(2): 123–132.
[34] Boccia MM, Blake MG, Baratti CM, McGaugh JL. Involvement of the basolateral amygdala in muscarinic cholinergic modulation of extinction memory consolidation. Neurobiology of Learning and Memory 2009; 91(1): 93–97.
[35] Roozendaal B, Castello NA, Vedana G, Barsegyan A, McGaugh JL. Noradrenergic activation of the basolateral amygdala modulates consolidation of object recognition memory. Neurobiology of Learning and Memory 2008; 90(3): 576–579.
[36] Okuda S, Roozendaal B, McGaugh JL. Glucocorticoid effects on object recognition memory require training-associated emotional arousal. Proceedings of the National Academy of Sciences of the United States of America 2004; 101(3): 853–858.
[37] Salinas JA, Introini-Collison IB, Dalmaz C, McGaugh JL. Posttraining intraamygdala infusions of oxotremorine and propranolol modulate storage of memory for reductions in reward magnitude. Neurobiology of Learning and Memory 1997; 68(1): 51–59.
[38] Hsu EH, Schroeder JP, Packard MG. The amygdala mediates memory consolidation for an amphetamine conditioned place preference. Behavioural Brain Research 2002; 129(1–2): 93–100.
[39] Schroeder JP, Packard MG. Differential effects of intra-amygdala lidocaine infusion on memory consolidation and expression of a food conditioned place preference. Psychobiology 2000; 28(4): 486–491.
[40] Packard MG, Chen SA. The basolateral amygdala is a cofactor in memory enhancement produced by intrahippocampal glutamate injections. Psychobiology 1999; 27(3): 377–385.
[41] Packard MG, Cahill L, McGaugh JL. Amygdala modulation of hippocampal-dependent and caudate nucleus-dependent memory processes. Proceedings of the National Academy of Sciences of the United States of America 1994; 91(18): 8477–8481.
[42] Miranda MI, LaLumiere RT, Buen TV, Bermudez-Rattoni F, McGaugh JL. Blockade of noradrenergic receptors in the basolateral amygdala impairs taste memory. European Journal of Neuroscience 2003; 18(9): 2605–2610.
[43] Kilpatrick L, Cahill L. Modulation of memory consolidation for olfactory learning by reversible inactivation of the basolateral amygdala. Behavioral Neuroscience 2003; 117(1): 184–188.
[44] Schroeder JP, Packard MG. Systemic or intra-amygdala injections of glucose facilitate memory consolidation for extinction of drug-induced conditioned reward. European Journal of Neuroscience 2003; 17(7): 1482–1488.
[45] Bergado JA, Rojas Y, Capdevila V, González O, Almaguer-Melian W. Stimulation of the basolateral amygdala improves the acquisition of a motor skill. Restorative Neurology and Neuroscience 2006; 24(2): 115–121.
[46] Chavez CM, McGaugh JL, Weinberger NM. The basolateral amygdala modulates specific sensory memory representations in the cerebral cortex. Neurobiology of Learning and Memory 2009; 91(4): 382–392.

[47] Price JL. Comparative aspects of amygdala connectivity. Annals of the New York Academy of Sciences 2003; 985: 50–58.
[48] Labar KS. Beyond fear emotional memory mechanisms in the human brain. Current Directions in Psychological Science 2007; 16(4): 173–177.
[49] Roesler R, Roozendaal B, McGaugh JL. Basolateral amygdala lesions block the memory-enhancing effect of 8-Br-cAMP infused into the entorhinal cortex of rats after training. European Journal of Neuroscience 2002; 15(5): 905–910.
[50] Roozendaal B, McGaugh JL. Basolateral amygdala lesions block the memory-enhancing effect of glucocorticoid administration in the dorsal hippocampus of rats. European Journal of Neuroscience 1997; 9(1): 76–83.
[51] Setlow B, Roozendaal B, McGaugh JL. Involvement of a basolateral amygdala complex–nucleus accumbens pathway in glucocorticoid-induced modulation of memory consolidation. European Journal of Neuroscience 2000; 12(1): 367–375.
[52] Fanselow MS. Conditioned fear-induced opiate analgesia: A competing motivational state theory of stress analgesia. Annals of the New York Academy of Sciences 1986; 467: 40–54.
[53] Rudy JW, Barrientos RM, O'Reilly RC. Hippocampal formation supports conditioning to memory of a context. Behavioral Neuroscience 2002; 116(4): 530–538.
[54] Malin EL, McGaugh JL. Differential involvement of the hippocampus, anterior cingulate cortex, and basolateral amygdala in memory for context and footshock. Proceedings of the National Academy of Sciences of the United States of America 2006; 103(6): 1959–1963.
[55] McIntyre CK, Miyashita T, Setlow B, Marjon KD, Steward O, Guzowski JF, McGaugh JL. Memory-influencing intra-basolateral amygdala drug infusions modulate expression of Arc protein in the hippocampus. Proceedings of the National Academy of Sciences of the United States of America 2005; 102(30): 10718–10723.
[56] Guzowski JF, Lyford GL, Stevenson GD, Houston FP, McGaugh JL, Worley PF, Barnes CA. Inhibition of activity-dependent arc protein expression in the rat hippocampus impairs the maintenance of long-term potentiation and the consolidation of long-term memory. Journal of Neuroscience 2000; 20(11): 3993–4001.
[57] Akirav I, Richter-Levin G. Biphasic modulation of hippocampal plasticity by behavioral stress and basolateral amygdala stimulation in the rat. Journal of Neuroscience 1999; 19(23): 10530–10535.
[58] Akirav I, Richter-Levin G. Mechanisms of amygdala modulation of hippocampal plasticity. Journal of Neuroscience 2002; 22(22): 9912–9921.
[59] Ikegaya Y, Saito H, Abe K. High-frequency stimulation of the basolateral amygdala facilitates the induction of long-term potentiation in the dentate gyrus in vivo. Neuroscience Research 1995; 22(2): 203–207.
[60] Li Z, Richter-Levin G. Stimulus intensity-dependent modulations of hippocampal long-term potentiation by basolateral amygdala priming. Frontiers in Cellular Neuroscience 2012; 6(21): 1–9.
[61] Dringenberg HC, Saber AJ, Cahill L. Enhanced frontal cortex activation in rats by convergent amygdaloid and noxious sensory signals. NeuroReport 2001; 12(11): 2395–2398.
[62] Dringenberg HC, Vanderwolf CH. Cholinergic activation of the electrocorticogram: An amygdaloid activating system. Experimental Brain Research 1996; 108(2): 285–296.

[63] Dringenberg HC, Kuo MC, Tomaszek S. Stabilization of thalamo-cortical long-term potentiation by the amygdala: Cholinergic and transcription-dependent mechanisms. European Journal of Neuroscience 2004; 20(2): 557–565.

[64] Weinberger NM. Specific long-term memory traces in primary auditory cortex. Nature Reviews Neuroscience 2004; 5(4): 279–290.

[65] Campbell AW. Histological studies on the localisation of cerebral function. Cambridge: University Press; 1905.

[66] Diamond IT. A history of the study of the cortex: Changes in the concept of the sensory pathway. In: Kimble GA, Schlesinger K (eds.) Topics in the history of psychology, v1. Hillsdale, NJ: Lawrence Erlbaum Associates; 1985. ch8, p305–387.

[67] Locke J. An essay concerning human understanding. London: Printed by Eliz. Holt for Thomas Basset; 1690.

[68] Merzenich MM, Knight PL, Roth GL. Cochleotopic organization of primary auditory cortex in the cat. Brain Research 1973; 63: 343–346.

[69] Galambos R, Sheatz G, Vernier VG. Electrophysiological correlates of a conditioned response in cats. Science 1956; 123(3192): 376–377.

[70] Ashe JH, Cassady JM, Weinberger NM. The relationship of the cochlear microphonic potential to the acquisition of a classically conditioned pupillary dilation response. Behavioral Biology 1976; 16(1): 45–62.

[71] Weinberger NM, Diamond DM. Physiological plasticity in auditory cortex: Rapid induction by learning. Progress in Neurobiology 1987; 29(1): 1–55.

[72] Marsh JT, Worden FG. Auditory potentials during acoustic habituation: Cochlear nucleus, cerebellum and auditory cortex. Electroencephalography and Clinical Neurophysiology 1964; 17: 685–692.

[73] Westenberg IS, Weinberger NM. Evoked potential decrements in auditory cortex. II. Critical test for habituation. Electroencephalography and Clinical Neurophysiology 1976; 40(4): 356–369.

[74] Diamond DM, Weinberger NM. Classical conditioning rapidly induces specific changes in frequency receptive fields of single neurons in secondary and ventral ectosylvian auditory cortical fields. Brain Research 1986; 372(2): 357–360.

[75] Bakin JS, Weinberger NM. Classical conditioning induces CS-specific receptive field plasticity in the auditory cortex of the guinea pig. Brain Research 1990; 536(1–2): 271–286.

[76] Kisley MA, Gerstein GL. Trial-to-trial variability and state-dependent modulation of auditory-evoked responses in cortex. Journal of Neuroscience 1999; 19(23): 10451–10460.

[77] Elhilali M, Fritz JB, Chi TS, Shamma SA. Auditory cortical receptive fields: Stable entities with plastic abilities. Journal of Neuroscience 2007; 27(39): 10372–10382.

[78] Galván VV, Chen J, Weinberger NM. Long-term frequency tuning of local field potentials in the auditory cortex of the waking guinea pig. Journal of the Association for Research in Otolaryngology 2001; 2(3): 199–215.

[79] Gao E, Suga N. Experience-dependent corticofugal adjustment of midbrain frequency map in bat auditory system. Proceedings of the National Academy of Sciences of the United States of America 1998; 95(21): 12663–12670.

[80] Edeline J-M, Pham P, Weinberger NM. Rapid development of learning-induced receptive field plasticity in the auditory cortex. Behavioral Neuroscience 1993; 107(4): 539–551.

[81] Kisley MA, Gerstein GL. Daily variation and appetitive conditioning-induced plasticity of auditory cortex receptive fields. European Journal of Neuroscience 2001; 13(10): 1993–2003.
[82] Molchan SE, Sunderland T, McIntosh AR, Herscovitch P, Schreurs BG. A functional anatomical study of associative learning in humans. Proceedings of the National Academy of Sciences of the United States of America 1994; 91(17): 8122–8126.
[83] Morris JS, Friston KJ, Dolan RJ. Experience-dependent modulation of tonotopic neural responses in human auditory cortex. Proceedings of the Royal Society B, Biological Sciences 1998; 265(1397): 649–657.
[84] Schreurs BG, McIntosh AR, Bahro M, Herscovitch P, Sunderland T, Molchan SE. Lateralization and behavioral correlation of changes in regional cerebral blood flow with classical conditioning of the human eyeblink response. Journal of Neurophysiology 1997; 77(4): 2153–2163.
[85] Hui GK, Wong KL, Chavez CM, Leon MI, Robin KM, Weinberger NM. Conditioned tone control of brain reward behavior produces highly specific representational gain in the primary auditory cortex. Neurobiology of Learning and Memory 2009; 92(1): 27–34.
[86] Rutkowski RG, Weinberger NM. Encoding of learned importance of sound by magnitude of representational area in primary auditory cortex. Proceedings of the National Academy of Sciences of the United States of America 2005; 102(38): 13664–13669.
[87] Bieszczad KM, Weinberger NM. Representational gain in cortical area underlies increase of memory strength. Proceedings of the National Academy of Sciences of the United States of America 2010; 107(8): 3793–3798.
[88] Galván VV, Weinberger NM. Long-term consolidation and retention of learning-induced tuning plasticity in the auditory cortex of the guinea pig. Neurobiology of Learning and Memory 2002; 77(1): 78–108.
[89] Edeline J-M, Weinberger NM. Receptive field plasticity in the auditory cortex during frequency discrimination training: Selective retuning independent of task difficulty. Behavioral Neuroscience 1993; 107(1): 82–103.
[90] Samson RD, Duvarci S, Paré D. Synaptic plasticity in the central nucleus of the amygdala. Reviews in the Neurosciences 2005; 16(4): 287–302.
[91] C Da Cunha, B Roozendaal, A Vazdarjanova, JL McGaugh. Microinfusions of flumazenil into the basolateral but not the central nucleus of the amygdala enhance memory consolidation in rats. Neurobiology of Learning and Memory 1999; 72(1): 1–7.
[92] RT LaLumiere, LT Nguyen, JL McGaugh. Post-training intrabasolateral amygdala infusions of dopamine modulate consolidation of inhibitory avoidance memory: Involvement of noradrenergic and cholinergic systems. European Journal of Neuroscience 2004; 20(10): 2804–2810.
[93] Power AE, Vazdarjanova A, McGaugh JL. Muscarinic cholinergic influences in memory consolidation. Neurobiology of Learning and Memory 2003; 80(3): 178–193.
[94] Weinberger NM. Dynamic regulation of receptive fields and maps in the adult sensory cortex. Annual Review of Neuroscience 1995; 18: 129–158.
[95] Weinberger NM. Reconceptualizing the primary auditory cortex: Learning, memory and specific plasticity. In: Winer JA, Schreiner CE (eds.) The auditory cortex. New York: Springer; 2011. ch22, p465–491.

[96] Weinberger NM, Ashe JH, Metherate R, McKenna TM, Diamond DM, Bakin J. Retuning auditory cortex by learning: A preliminary model of receptive field plasticity. Concepts in Neuroscience 1990; 1(1): 91–132.
[97] Edeline J-M, Weinberger NM. Associative retuning in the thalamic source of input to the amygdala and auditory cortex: Receptive field plasticity in the medial division of the medial geniculate body. Behavioral Neuroscience 1992; 106(1): 81–105.
[98] Hennevin E, Maho C, Hars B. Neuronal plasticity induced by fear conditioning is expressed during paradoxical sleep: Evidence from simultaneous recordings in the lateral amygdala and the medial geniculate in rats. Behavioral Neuroscience 1998; 112(4): 839–862.
[99] Maho C, Hars B, Edeline J-M, Hennevin E. Conditioned changes in the basal forebrain: Relations with learning-induced cortical plasticity. Psychobiology 1995; 23(1): 10–25.
[100] Hars B, Maho C, Edeline J-M, Hennevin E. Basal forebrain stimulation facilitates one-evoked responses in the auditory cortex of awake rat. Neuroscience 1993; 56(1): 61–74.
[101] Bakin JS, Weinberger NM. Induction of a physiological memory in the cerebral cortex by stimulation of the nucleus basalis. Proceedings of the National Academy of Sciences of the United States of America 1996; 93(20): 11219–11224.
[102] Bjordahl TS, Dimyan MA, Weinberger NM. Induction of long-term receptive field plasticity in the auditory cortex of the waking guinea pig by stimulation of the nucleus basalis. Behavioral Neuroscience 1998; 112(3): 467–479.
[103] Dimyan MA, Weinberger NM. Basal forebrain stimulation induces discriminative receptive field plasticity in the auditory cortex. Behavioral Neuroscience 1999; 113(4): 691–702.
[104] Ma X, Suga N. Augmentation of plasticity of the central auditory system by the basal forebrain and/or somatosensory cortex. Journal of Neurophysiology 2003; 89(1): 90–103.
[105] Kilgard MP, Merzenich MM. Cortical map reorganization enabled by nucleus basalis activity. Science 1998; 279(5357): 1714–1718.
[106] Weinberger NM. The nucleus basalis and memory codes: Auditory cortical plasticity and the induction of specific, associative behavioral memory. Neurobiology of Learning and Memory 2003; 80(3): 268–284.
[107] Grove EA. Neural associations of the substantiainnominata in the rat: Afferent connections. Journal of Comparative Neurology 1988; 277(3): 315–346.
[108] Russchen FT, Amaral DG, Price JL. The afferent connections of the substantiainnominata in the monkey, *Macaca fascicularis*. Journal of Comparative Neurology 1985; 242(1): 1–27.
[109] Dringenberg HC, Vanderwolf CH. Neocortical activation: Modulation by multiple pathways acting on central cholinergic and serotonergic systems. Experimental Brain Research 1997; 116(1): 160–174.
[110] Buzsaki G, Bickford RG, Ponomareff G, Thal LJ, Mandel R, Gage FH. Nucleus basalis and thalamic control of neocortical activity in the freely moving rat. Journal of Neuroscience 1988; 8(11): 4007–4026.
[111] McLin DE 3rd, Miasnikov AA, Weinberger NM. Induction of behavioral associative memory by stimulation of the nucleus basalis. Proceedings of the National Academy of Sciences of the United States of America 2002; 99(6): 4002–4007.

[112] Miasnikov AA, Chen JC, Gross N, Poytress BS, Weinberger NM. Motivationally neutral stimulation of the nucleus basalis induces specific behavioral memory. Neurobiology of Learning and Memory 2008; 90(1): 125–137.
[113] Miasnikov AA, Chen JC, Weinberger NM. Rapid induction of specific associative behavioral memory by stimulation of the nucleus basalis in the rat. Neurobiology of Learning and Memory 2006; 86(1): 47–65.
[114] Miasnikov AA, Chen JC, Weinberger NM. Specific auditory memory induced by nucleus basalis stimulation depends on intrinsic acetylcholine. Neurobiology of Learning and Memory 2008; 90(2): 443–454.
[115] Miasnikov AA, Chen JC, Weinberger NM. Behavioral memory induced by stimulation of the nucleus basalis: Effects of contingency reversal. Neurobiology of Learning and Memory 2009; 91(3): 298–309.
[116] Miasnikov AA, Chen JC, Weinberger NM. Consolidation and long-term retention of an implanted behavioral memory. Neurobiology of Learning and Memory 2011; 95(3): 286–295.
[117] Weinberger NM, Miasnikov AA, Chen JC. The level of cholinergic nucleus basalis activation controls the specificity of auditory associative memory. Neurobiology of Learning and Memory 2006; 86(3): 270–285.
[118] Bieszczad KM, Weinberger NM. Extinction reveals that primary sensory cortex predicts reinforcement outcome. European Journal of Neuroscience 2012; 35(4): 598–613.
[119] Power AE, Thal LJ, McGaugh JL. Lesions of the nucleus basalis magnocellularis nduced by 192 IgG–saporin block memory enhancement with posttraining norepinephrine in the basolateral amygdala. Proceedings of the National Academy of Sciences of the United States of America 2002; 99(4): 2315–2319.
[120] Smiley JF, Subramanian M, Mesulam MM. Monoaminergic–cholinergic nteractions in the primate basal forebrain. Neuroscience 1999; 93(3): 817–829.
[121] Fort P, Khateb A, Pegna A, Mühlethaler M, Jones BE. Noradrenergic modulation of cholinergic nucleus basalis neurons demonstrated by in vitro pharmacological and mmunohistochemical evidence in the guinea-pig brain. European Journal of Neuroscience 1995; 7(7): 1502–1511.
[122] Dringenberg HC, Kuo MC. Histaminergic facilitation of electrocorticographic activation: Role of basal forebrain, thalamus, and neocortex. European Journal of Neuroscience 2003; 18(8): 2285–2291.
[123] Cecchi M, Passani MB, Bacciottini L, Mannaioni PF, Blandina P. Cortical acetylcholine release elicited by stimulation of histamine H1 receptors in the nucleus basalis magnocellularis: A dual-probe microdialysis study in the freely moving rat. European Journal of Neuroscience 2001; 13(1): 68–78.
[124] Bao S, Chan VT, Merzenich MM. Cortical remodelling induced by activity of ventral tegmental dopamine neurons. Nature 2001; 412(6842): 79–83.

Chapter 7

Auditory Fear Circuits in the Amygdala – Insights from Computational Models

Satish S. Nair

Additional information is available at the end of the chapter

1. Introduction

The human brain has 100 billion neurons that are constantly humming with electrical and chemical activity. These individual neurons are networked into complex local and inter-region circuits that are thought to implement functions that support life. One such circuit that is critical for survival is the fear circuit, the key elements of which are thought to include the amygdala, prefrontal cortex, and the hippocampus. Amygdala is an important site of plasticity in auditory fear conditioning and plays a key role in both the acquisition and storage of fear and extinction memories (Blair et al., 2001; LeDoux, 2000; Malkani and Rosen, 2000; Maren, 2001). The role of the amygdala in fear has been studied using fear conditioning, a training paradigm in which an organism learns to predict aversive events. Typically, a relatively neutral stimulus (conditioning stimulus, CS), such as a tone, light or an odor, is paired with an aversive one (unconditioned stimulus, US), such as a footshock. After only a few pairings, the previously neutral stimulus becomes aversive and can itself evoke an emotional reaction typically resulting in a freezing behavior. The learning processes underlying conditioning develop rapidly and the memory of this association persists for long periods of time, reflecting the biological significance of the learning experience for the organism. Even though there is consensus that the amygdala is a critical component of the mammalian fear circuit, the relevant interconnections among the amygdalar nuclei and their contributions to the acquisition and storage of fear and extinction memories are not well understood presently.

Disruption of the fear circuit is thought to underlie the pathology of post-traumatic stress and of other anxiety disorders (Corcoran and Quirk, 2007). Such disruptions are also manifested as changes in excitability of individual neurons, as well as changes in synaptic strengths between neurons in specific sub-circuits, within these areas. Increasing understanding of brain functioning due to advances in basic neuroscience techniques and imaging modalities has led to the emergence of computational modeling as an important tool for studying such changes. Progress in the areas of cellular neurophysiology and synaptic plasticity permit the development of biologically realistic computational models that more closely approximate learning, both at the membrane and network levels. *Such biologically realistic computational models have the potential to enhance our understanding of brain circuits with potential applicability to a range of phenomena from the neural basis of mental illness to the mechanism of action of drugs.*

What is a computational model? A computational model combines different types of information related to a system using mathematical equations, and then describes the system's response to prescribed inputs. In neuroscience, such computational models are typically of two types: (i) phenomenological models using connectionist (e.g., artificial neural network) and statistical schemes, and (ii) biophysical models which attempt to model the underlying biological mechanisms directly. Biophysical models are typically either at the intracellular level (e.g., gene interactions, pathways), cellular level (e.g., cell firing patterns, effect of blockers/drugs on channel conductances, etc.), or network/systems level (e.g., interconnected neurons in the fear circuit, the subject of this chapter), or may include a combination of several of these levels.

Computational modeling is a tool that has been effectively used in a variety of disciplines to integrate information related to different aspects of a problem, and to provide testable predictions. For instance, computational modeling is presently an indispensable part of the design of airplanes, e.g., Boeing 777 was claimed as being the 'first entirely computer-designed commercial aircraft' (Boeing 777, 2012). For an airplane, such a model would integrate the complex mathematical equations for air flow, engine dynamics, frame vibrations, and responses of the control surfaces, and then predict their effect on outputs such as ride quality. Computational models have now become indispensable for the airplane designer because they enable rapid and inexpensive evaluation of a variety of 'what if' scenarios, including the effect of design changes. It is argued that increased understanding of the functional organization of the brain requires integration of similar mathematical/statistical equations from molecular, cellular and network levels , something that can be facilitated by computational models (Koch and Segev, 2011). For instance, recent technical advances have resulted in a rapid accumulation of information on intracellular signaling pathways and their relationships to long-term neuronal changes (Byrne and Roberts, 2004). Computational techniques and tools are being developed to model such mechanisms with increasing accuracy and are found to be essential to generate an understanding of the underlying functions in such cases (Koch and Segev, 2001; Mauk, 2000). The term 'computational neuropharmacology' has recently been proposed for the application of computational modeling to drug development, drug discovery, and the modeling of the mechanisms of action of psychiatric drugs (Aradi and Erdi, 2006).

In this chapter, we review the preliminary insights related to the amygdalar fear circuit provided by biologically realistic computational models. Specifically, we investigate how sensory information might be associated within the amygdala, and how the various amygdalar nuclei interact to *acquire and store* both fear and extinction memories via long term potentiation and depression of synapses. The 'higher' level structures such as the prefrontal cortex and the hippocampus are known to influence the amygdala to *modulate* such memories. However, not much is known about the underlying mechanisms presently and so this modulatory effect is discussed only briefly. This is followed by a discussion of the unique insights that computational models might add to what is already known about the fear circuit, and about the potential of such models to contribute to reverse engineering the mammalian fear circuit. This ability of computational models derives from the fact that they can 'integrate' different types of information into a self-consistent and coherent portrait of how fear might be learned, and, in the process, reveal presently unknown mechanisms and interactions associated with such learning.

2. Auditory fear and the amygdala

Fear is one of the few emotions that can be observed in non-primate mammalian organisms (LeDoux, 2000). After fear conditioning, a number of physiological manifestations can be observed upon re-exposure to the conditioning stimulus, including increased autonomic arousal, increased stress hormone release, reflex potentiation, and defensive behaviors (LeDoux, 2000). Extensive studies indicate that freezing is a defensive behavior and serves as a reliable index of fear in rodents (Blanchard and Blanchard, 1972).

The mammalian circuit related to auditory fear and extinction has been studied by several researchers and, although not fully understood, consensus is emerging about the specific roles of the amygdalar nuclei in this circuit. In rodents, such studies typically use fear conditioning, which is a form of Pavlovian learning where the stimulus parameters can be regulated by the experimenter. Fear conditioning is a highly conserved form of behavior that is exhibited in both laboratory situations and in normal environments (LeDoux, 1994). Animals do not need to be food- or water-deprived to demonstrate fear conditioning.

Fear conditioning protocol. A typical auditory fear conditioning session for a rodent (see fig 1) in a cage starts with a habituation phase involving the presentation of several CS tones (e.g., 5 trials, with each trial consisting of a 2 sec 5 kHz pure tone (80 dB) + a varying 1-3 min inter-tone interval), followed by a conditioning phase where the tone is paired with shock US (e.g., 5 trials, where the tone co-terminates with a 0.5 mA, 0.5 s, foot shock). Testing is typically performed the next day using 2 CS tones. For studies that involve extinction, the paradigm continues to day 3 where pure tones are delivered during an extinction session (e.g., 30 trials with pure tones). Testing for extinction in that case takes place on day 4 (e.g., 2 trials with pure tones). Freezing, defined as the total lack of movement except for respiration, is used as the measure of learning in this task (Blanchard and Blanchard, 1972). After conditioning, a robust and long-lasting behavioral change is produced which is particularly amenable to genetic and pharmacological studies. It also affords the advantage that detailed time courses of the sequence of events that may occur after conditioning can be easily generated. Thus, fear conditioning serves as a model for elucidating the crucial electrophysiological and biochemical mechanisms underlying learning (Wehner and Radcliffe, 2004).

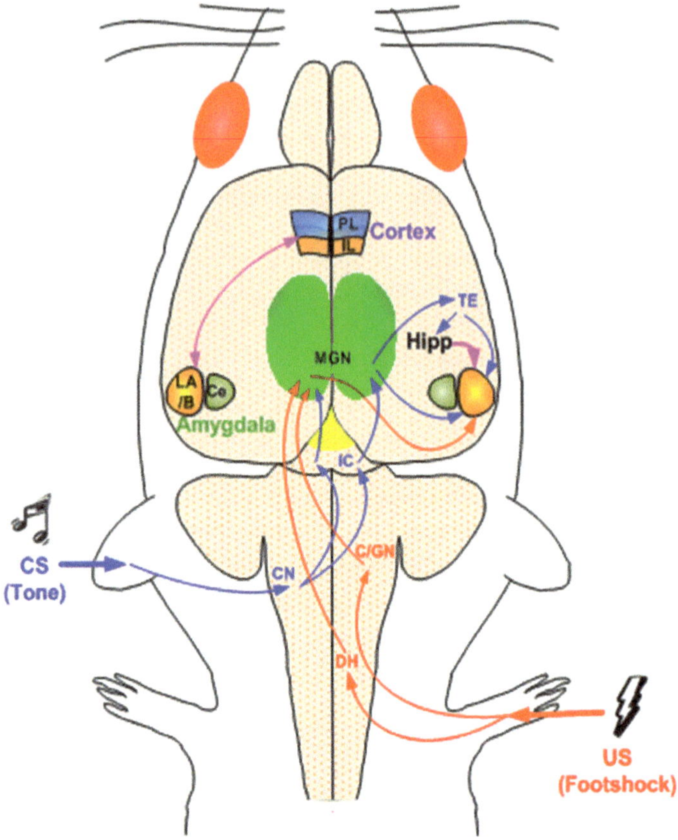

Figure 1. Pathways involved in auditory fear conditioning. The tone information is delivered to LA via the medial division of medial geniculate body (MGN) and the shock information is delivered to LA via posterior intralaminar nucleus (PIN). The tone input to LA is potentiated when tone and shock are paired. Output from the LA projects to the central nucleus (Ce) through inter-calated cells (ITC, not show in the figure) and BA neurons, eliciting a fear response. LA, lateral nucleus; BA, basal nucleus; CN, cochlear nucleus; DH, dorsal horn of spinal cord; IC, inferior colliculus; PL: prelimbic medial prefrontal cortex, IL: infralimbic medial prefrontal cortex. (adapted from figure provided by J. Kim)

Role of the amygdala. The amygdala is located within the medial temporal lobe and is recognized as being critical for Pavlovian fear learning. In their review article, Paré et al. (2004) note that identification of pathways that mediate the expression of conditioned responses by way of amygdala outputs and pathways that transmit CS information from sensory systems to the amygdala greatly increased interest in the intra-amygdaloid substrates of Pavlovian fear learning. Multiple experimental modalities including field potential response to high frequency stimulation, patch clamp recordings, single unit recordings, pharmacological manipulations and transgenic approaches all implicated the amygdala in the acquisition of learned fear. These findings have also been confirmed in humans by functional magnetic resonance imaging techniques (e.g., Buchel et al., 1998).

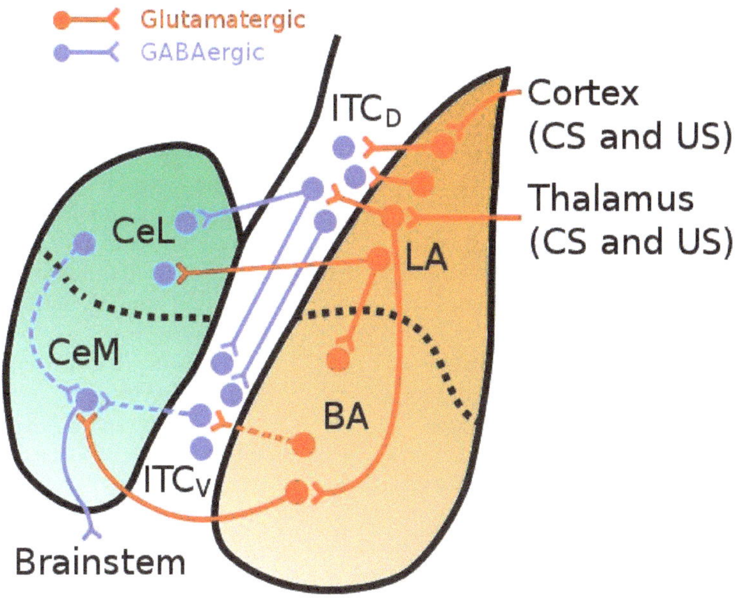

Figure 2. Amygdalar pathways relevant to auditory fear. Tone and shock information arrive at LA via thalamic and cortical routes. LA projects to BA and also to ITC$_D$ and Ce$_L$. Based on our present understanding (Amano et al., 2011), LA projects to BA, ITC$_D$ and CeL. BA fear neurons project to Ce$_M$ and BA extinction neurons project to ITC$_V$ (fear recall circuit in bold and extinction recall in dashed line type). Ce represents the amygdalar output which projects to the brainstem and other regions eliciting fear. ITC: inter-calated cells (subscripts D - dorsal, V-ventral); Ce$_L$/Ce$_M$: lateral/medial part of the central nucleus of the amygdala.

The components of the amygdala that are critical for fear conditioning are the lateral nucleus (LA), the basal nucleus (BA), intercalated cells (ITC) and the central nucleus (Ce) (Maren, 2001). Thalamic inputs conveying information about the auditory tone (conditioned stimulus, CS) and foot shock (unconditioned stimulus, US) arrive first at the lateral nucleus. LA is widely accepted to be a key site of synaptic events that contribute to fear learning (LeDoux, 1995; Paré et al., 2004; Sigurdsson et al., 2007). There are two main types of neurons within the LA and the BA: pyramidal glutamatergic projection neurons and local circuit γ-aminobutyric acid (GABA) releasing interneurons. The amygdalar nuclei LA, BA, Ce and the ITC clusters act in concert to store auditory fear and extinction memories, and these nuclei are in turn modulated by external structures such as the prefrontal cortex and hippocampus. In auditory fear conditioning, convergence of tone (conditioned stimulus, CS) and foot-shock (unconditioned stimulus, US) inputs in LA leads to potentiation of CS inputs, resulting in subsequent LA tone responses being larger (Quirk et al., 1995; Blair et al.,

2001). These increased LA responses are relayed to the Ce via BA (Amano et al., 2011), and the intercalated (ITC) cell masses (Paré et al., 2004), eliciting fear responses via successive projections to brain stem and hypothalamic sites (LeDoux, 2000). As a result, rats learn to freeze to tones CS that predict foot shock US.

In the rodent brain, estimates of the numbers of cells (unilateral) in the amygdalar nuclei are as follows: LA – 60,000; BA – 47,000; ITC – 19,000; and Ce – 37,000 (Tuunanen and Pitkanen, 2000). The principal cell to GABAergic interneuron ratio in BLA is 80:20. The amygdalar nuclei are themselves not homogeneous. LA has distinct dorsal and ventral regions which seem to store fear memories in different ways (Repa et al., 2001). Herry et al. (2008) reported three subpopulations of neurons in BA whose CS responsiveness varied with fear training and they termed these as 'fear,' 'extinction' and 'extinction-resistant' cells. Fear cells acquire CS responses as a result of fear conditioning, but lose them following extinction training; extinction cells become CS responsive only following extinction training, and extinction-resistant cells acquire CS responses during conditioning and remain CS responsive even after extinction training. Also, Amano et al. (2011) have shown that the two sub-regions within BA, the lateral part (BL), and the medial part (BM), act in concert to express fear but possess a certain amount of redundancy between themselves. Similarly, there are two different ITC cell clusters and they are thought to contribute differentially to the expression of fear and extinction memories (Royer et al., 2000; Pape and Paré, 2010). The output nucleus Ce also has distinct sub-circuits with different functions in fear learning (Coicci et al., 2010; Haubensak et al., 2010). Even with these advances in understanding, a clear portrait of how the various amygdalar nuclei interact to acquire and store fear is still lacking.

Once acquired, conditioned fear associations are not always expressed. Repeated presentation of the tone CS in the absence of the US causes conditioned fear responses to diminish rapidly, a phenomenon termed as fear extinction (Myers and Davis, 2007). The neural mechanisms of fear extinction are not well understood, and a neural analysis of extinction and inhibition is still in its infancy (Delamater, 2004; Quirk and Mueller, 2008). Some psychological theories describe extinction as an "unlearning" process due to a violation of the CS-US association established during acquisition of fear (Rescorla and Wagner, 1972). This unlearning view has been challenged by the observation that fear recovers spontaneously after extinction. An alternative theory proposes that extinction does not erase the CS-US association but instead forms a new memory that inhibits conditioned responding (Bouton and King, 1983; Quirk, 2002).

Modulation by cortical structures. Fear is thought to be expressed via projections from LA to BA, ITC and Ce (see fig 2), and expression of this fear memory has been shown to be influenced by cortical structures. For instance, although LA responds transiently to conditioned tones, the animal continues to freeze throughout the period of a 30 second tone. Quirk and colleagues investigated whether the prelimbic (PL) region of the medial prefrontal cortex (mPFC) might be involved in sustaining freezing. In a series of experiments they showed how PL was critical for the expression of fear over the duration of the tone: Pharmacological inactivation of PL was found to abolish the expression of conditioned fear (Blum et al., 2006; Corcoran and Quirk, 2007), and micro-stimulation of PL was found to augment conditioned fear (Vidal-Gonzalez et al., 2006); and, importantly, that the time course of PL tone responses parallels the time course of conditioned fear (Burgos-Robles et al., 2009). This finding is supported by studies examining neuronal activity with cFos which showed that PL activation is correlated with fear expression and extinction failure.

What are the structures that might modulate the memory of auditory fear extinction? Again, several studies by Quirk and others reveal that the infralimbic (IL) region of mPFC modulates the amygdala during recall of extinction memory: activity in IL, which is adjacent to PL, was found to facilitate recall of extinction (Quirk et al., 2006; Quirk and Mueller, 2008), and deficient IL activity results in failure to recall extinction (e.g., Milad and Quirk, 2002). Burgos-Robles et al. (2009) also noted that a higher percentage of PL neurons responded to tones in rats showing poor recall of extinction, suggesting that these rats had excessive consolidation of fear memory. This led the authors to suggest that extinction failure might be caused by excessive activity in PL, combined with deficient activity in the IL, and that recall of fear and extinction memories may depend on the optimal balance of activity between PL and IL.

What is the role of context in auditory fear? Since fear conditioning takes place in a chamber (Fig. 1b; with its own flooring, color, odor, lighting, etc. – the 'context'), the rat subsequently learns to fear not only the tone but also the context. That is, after fear conditioning, it will express fear by freezing in the trained context, even in the absence of tone. Acquisition of contextual fear may involve configural or spatial learning and many lines of evidence support hippocampal involvement in contextual fear conditioning (Anagnostaras et al., 1999). It is well established that contextual information gates behavioral response to conditioned stimuli, especially following extinction (e.g., Bouton, 2004). Contextual information is processed in the hippocampal formation (HPC), which plays a critical role in gating the response of rats to extinguished tone stimuli (Corcoran et al., 2005). The route by which the HPC exerts its effects is thought to be through the mPFC (Hobin et al., 2003; Maren and Quirk, 2004). The HPC (especially the ventral HPC) projects strongly to both PL and IL (e.g., Hoover and Vertes, 2007). This pathway has been hypothesized to serve a 'teaching' role for IL neurons, by generating Ca-dependent bursting in IL neurons. Also, it has been shown that contextual fear memories formed in the absence of the baso-lateral amygdala (BLA which includes BA and LA; Poulos et al., 2009) or the dorsal hippocampus (DH; Zelikowsky et al., 2012) do not persist across time, suggesting that both the DH and BLA are essential components of the circuitry required for a contextual fear memory to become permanent (Zelikowsky et al., 2012).

3. Modeling fear memories - A simple computational model

Computational models have been used in the field of emotional learning and memory to explain behavioral responses (e.g., Grossberg and Schmajuk, 1987). Single unit recording data were used by Armony et al. (1995) to develop an anatomically constrained thalamo-cortico-amygdala connectionist model of fear conditioning which associated tone inputs with a specific frequency (CS) with foot shock (US). The model was trained using a modified Hebbian-type learning rule and was able to reproduce data related to frequency-specific changes of the receptive fields known to exist in the auditory thalamus and amygdala. However, extinction and other related phenomena were not simulated. Balkenius and Morén (2001) proposed a neural network model for emotional conditioning focusing on the amygdala and the orbitofrontal cortex and their interaction. Amygdala was the locus of acquisition and the orbitofrontal cortex was the site for extinction learning. The model simulated basic phenomena related to emotional conditioning including acquisition, extinction, blocking, and habituation. Vlachos et al. (2011) reported a neural network model that reproduced the differential recruitment of two distinct subpopulations of basal amygdala neurons as seen in experiments. The model revealed how the two populations might encode contextual specificity of fear and extinction memories. Krasne et al. (2011) report a model of the amygdala and hippocampus where fear conditioning and extinction memories are the result of neuromodulation-controlled LTP at synapses of thalamic, cortical, and hippocampal afferents on principal cells and inhibitory interneurons of lateral and basal amygdala. The model was developed using a firing rate framework and was able to reproduce several known features of fear learning and make testable predictions. Although connectionist and reduced order models provide very useful information from a top-down systems perspective, they do not fully incorporate the neurobiological information related to individual current channels and their effect on intrinsic excitability, or related to synaptic plasticity mechanisms, and so may be not be able to shed light on the underlying mechanisms to any significant level of detail.

This chapter focuses on a class of computational models that incorporate biological realism (i.e., they include membrane channels, synapses and receptors) to more effectively model the learning brain. Such models integrate information from intracellular and cellular levels of neuroscience with the network/systems level to provide a coherent picture of the higher level functions in health and disease (e.g., behavior, symptom). Software exists presently to model systems in neuroscience at typically only one of the levels, either molecular, cellular, or network/systems level. One reason for this is the large difference in both temporal and spatial complexities between the levels. We focus largely on cellular and network level modeling in this chapter.

Computational modeling platforms at the cellular and network levels include public domain software such as NEURON (Carnevale and Hines, 2006) and GENESIS (Bower and Beeman, 2003) which are being designed for biologists, and require minimal understanding of the underlying mathematics. Figure 3 shows the hierarchical structure used for modeling. Such packages can perform simulations of models ranging from single neurons to complex networks representing brain circuits. Sources for biological information to develop such models include research articles, and databases such as CellPropDB, NeuronDB and ModelDB (http://neuron.duke.edu/). For example, Leblois et al. (2006) used a mathematical model to explain the pathology in the basal ganglia circuit with Parkinson's disease.

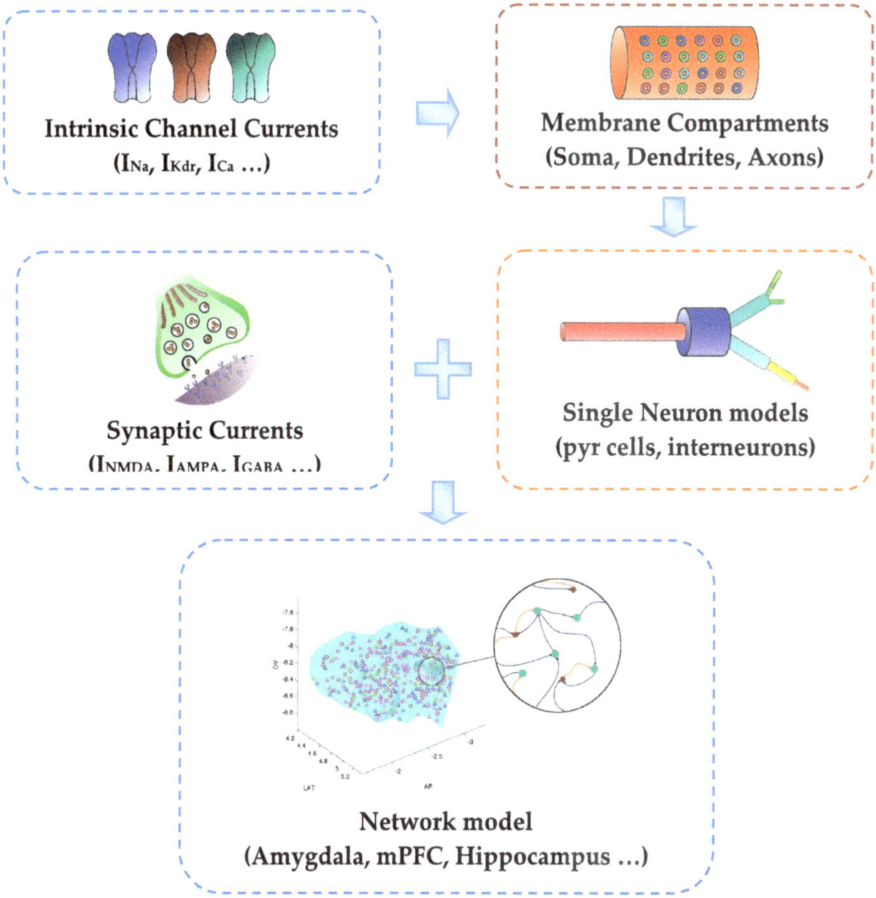

Figure 3. Elements of a biologically realistic neuronal network. The symbol 'I' represents current, e.g., I_{Na} is the sodium current. The network comprises cells (e.g., pyramidal and interneurons), which in turn consist of soma and dendrites populated with the various current channels.

Illustrative example case. Single cell models can be developed for the pyramidal cell and the interneuron using the software cited. The modeling process involves several steps where the software requires the user to define 'LEGO' blocks for the neuron, such as the soma or cell body, dendrite and axon, 'insert' into them specific suites of membrane channels, and then connect them to form networks (fig 4). Such software aim to provide an easy-to-use interface, making most of the mathematical details transparent to the user. The model parameters within all these blocks are then iteratively adjusted, within biophysical bounds, to match biological data such as resting potential, input resistance, and membrane potential responses to various current injections. After reliable single cell models are developed, they can be embedded into network models of regions and circuits.

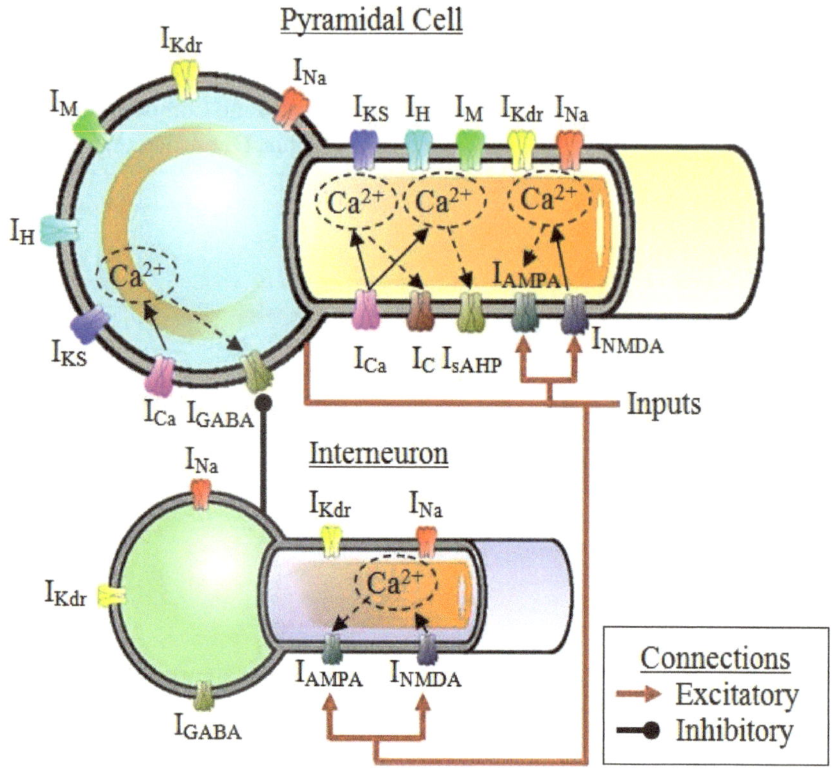

Figure 4. Two-cell model of pyramidal cell and interneuron with ionic and synaptic channels. Each cell model has soma (spherical) and dendrite (cylindrical) compartments with each having the specific current channels shown. The Ca^{2+} pools involved in the learning algorithm implemented are also depicted. Both cells receive afferent inputs (tone CS and shock US) via AMPA/NMDA synapses. In addition, the interneuron receives excitatory input from the pyramidal cell and provides feed-forward/feedback inhibition to the pyramidal cell.

Two-cell network. Figure 4 illustrates the development of a two-cell network model showing how 'memories' can be stored in the synapses (Li et al., 2008). The first step is to develop single cell models using experimental data. In this example case, we use a lateral amygdala pyramidal cell model and a lateral amygdala interneuron model. As cited, the single cell properties should match those reported in biology, including the membrane potential responses to various current injections. Once such single cell models are developed (see Li et al., 2009), they can be embedded into networks. In our simple two-cell network model, both the pyramidal cell and the interneuron received direct afferent tone/shock (CS/US) inputs via synaptic connections. The pyramidal cell was inhibited by the interneuron via a GABA-ergic synapse. The pyramidal cell, on the other hand, excited the interneuron via an excitatory AMPA (alpha-amino-3-hydroxy-5-methyl-4-isoxazolepropionic acid) synapse.

Both cells received random background inputs that represent afferent connections from other brain areas such as prefrontal cortex and hippocampus. The frequency and strength of the random inputs was adjusted to obtain pyramidal cell spontaneous firing rates of less than 1 Hz seen in LA neurons. We implemented plasticity in all the synapses using a calcium-based learning rule, and then 'trained' the model with the fear conditioning protocol used in experiments (Quirk et al., 1995). Figure 5a shows the membrane potential responses of a pyramidal cell and interneuron for a segment of the training cycle. This segment consisted of two tones (500 ms each) and two shocks (100 ms each) with the second shock occurring during the last 100 ms of the second tone. Both tone and shock excited the cells, with the shock input having a stronger effect. Due to Hebbian strengthening between tone inputs and shock inputs, the tone input to the pyramidal cell strengthens during conditioning and is maintained throughout extinction. In the interneuron, on the other hand, tone inputs strengthen during the extinction phase, due to Hebbian pairing between different sets of tone inputs. This causes inhibition of pyramidal excitation and reduction in fear behavior. Consistent with behavioral findings, the fear memory is not lost during extinction, but is suppressed by LTP-like potentiation of inhibition. This is illustrated

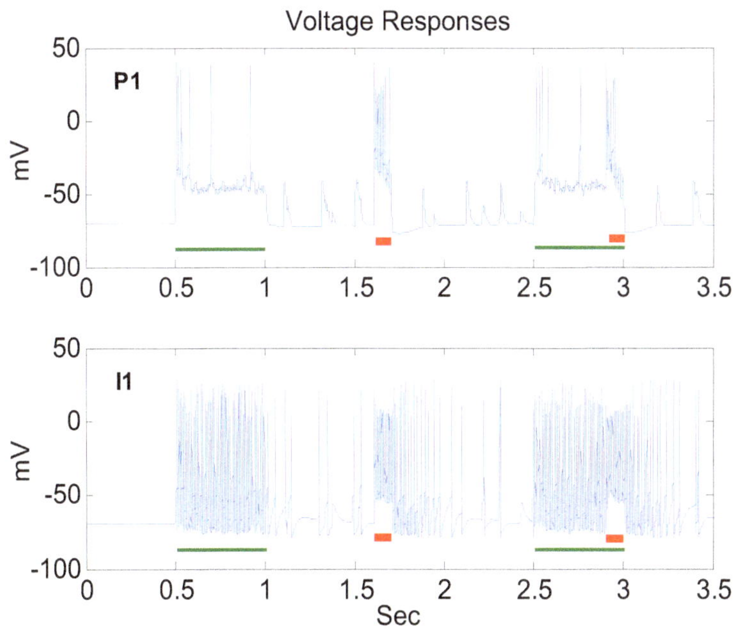

Figure 5. Response characteristics of the illustrative network model. 5a. Membrane potential responses for pyramidal cell (top panel) and interneuron (lower panel) to a segment of the training trial. In the segment the input consists of a series of two tones (green bars) and two shocks (red bars) with the second tone paired with the second shock. 5b. Schematic showing the connections between synaptic strengthening/weakening and behavior. The training protocol had four phases: SENS- unpaired tone/shock; COND – paired tone/shock; a gap with no tone or shock; and EXT – tone alone.

schematically in Fig. 5b. This unit of two cells illustrates how conditioning and extinction are learned in this network, i.e., conditioning is essentially the strengthening of the tone-pyramidal synapse which increases pyramidal cell activity, and extinction is the strengthening of tone-interneuron, interneuron-pyramidal cell and pyramidal cell-interneuron synapses, all of which decrease pyramidal cell activity. The concepts and insights illustrated by this simple two-cell network, such as potential storage sites for memory, translate directly to larger networks, as we discuss in the following.

4. Reverse engineering auditory fear circuits in the amygdala

The overall goal of the reverse engineering effort is to integrate diverse morphological and neurophysiological data into biologically realistic models of the various amygdalar nuclei (lateral nucleus, basal nucleus, intercalated cells, and the central nucleus) and then use the model to investigate how the different nuclei participate in the acquisition and extinction of auditory fear memories, and how they are modulated by cortical structures. We initiated the model development of the overall fear circuit using a bottom-up approach starting with the core unit: the lateral amygdala nucleus, LA. As the next step, we modeled the amygdala intercalated cell clusters, ITC. The LA and ITC models provided unique insights that are presently not possible to obtain via experiments.

A. Modeling the lateral amygdala (Li et al., 2009)

Motivation. LA is a key site of plasticity in auditory fear learning (Blair et al., 2001; LeDoux, 2000; Malkani and Rosen, 2000; Maren, 2001). Given the central role of LA in the acquisition and expression of fear memory, it has been proposed that this structure may be a site of inhibition in extinction (e.g., Hobin et al., 2003). The motivation of the Li et al. (2009) study was to determine how LA might acquire and store both conditioning and extinction memories related to auditory fear. After a review of the development of the model, and its validation, we discuss the unique insights provided by the model.

Single cell properties. There are two types of principal neurons within the LA: pyramidal-like glutamatergic projection neurons, and local circuit GABAergic interneurons (Faber and Sah, 2001). The electrophysiological and morphological properties of LA neurons have been characterized in a number of studies (e.g., Faber et al., 2001). Also, there are several in vitro and in vivo recordings of LA neurons during fear conditioning and extinction (e.g., Quirk et al., 1995, 1997; Repa et al., 2001).

Principal neurons in the LA exhibit a range of firing properties in response to prolonged current injection (Faber et al., 2001). Accordingly three types of pyramidal cells were modeled, types A, B, and C, where type A had strong, B had medium, and C had minimal frequency adaptation. The interneuron was modeled as a basket-type, fast-spiking, aspiny cell with each compartment containing a fast Na^+ current and a delayed rectifier K^+ current with different kinetics from those of pyramidal cells to reproduce its much shorter spike duration (Durstweitz et al., 2000). Similar to pyramidal cells, interneurons can also receive excitatory glutamatergic inputs from the thalamus and/or the cortex, and inhibitory inputs from other local interneurons. For each cell, the AMPA and the N-methyl D-aspartate (NMDA) channels were placed in the dendrite compartment, and the inhibitory $GABA_A$ channels were placed on the soma. Fig.4 provides details of typical pyramidal cell and interneuron models with the various ionic and synaptic channels.

Network model and synaptic connections. The LA network model consisted of eight pyramidal cells and two GABAergic interneurons (fig. 6) with full connectivity (Durstewitz et al., 2000; Wang, 1999). Among the eight pyramidal cells, five were type A (P1–P5), two were type B (P6 –P7), and one was type C (P8). In the network model, we were particularly interested in information processing in the dorsal sensory-receptive region of LA (LAd). Three of the pyramidal cells (P5, P7, and P8) and both the interneurons received direct tone/shock inputs; P3 received only tone input, and P1 and P4 received only shock input; and P2 and P6 received no direct afferent inputs. In this fully connected architecture, each pyramidal neuron received excitatory inputs from all other pyramidal cells as well as inhibitory inputs from the two interneurons. Both interneurons received excitatory inputs from all pyramidal cells and thus provided feedforward and feedback inhibition to pyramidal cells. Also the two interneurons inhibited each other. The synaptic delays for tone and shock inputs were set to 8 ms to represent the transmission delay between the start of tone and the arrival of information in the LA (Li et al., 1996). The synaptic delays for all intrinsic transmission were set to 2 ms.

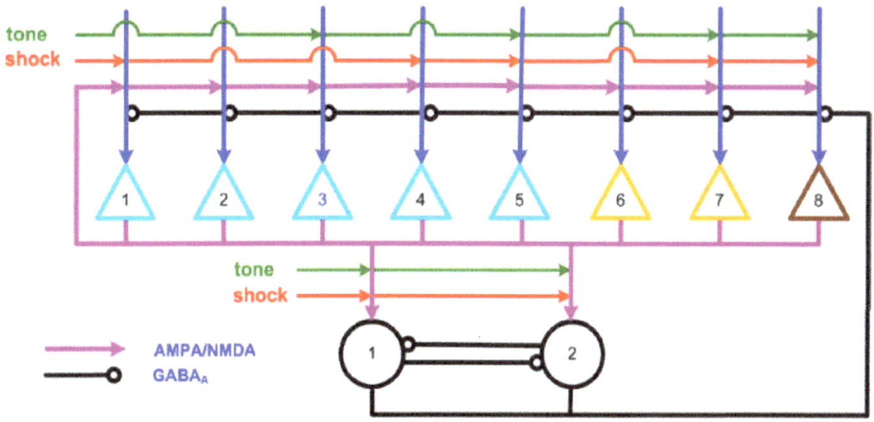

Figure 6. Biologically realistic LA network model of Li et al. (2009). Triangles 18 are pyramidal cells (5 of type A (1-5), 2 of type B (6-7), and 1 of type C (8)); circles are interneurons (1-2). Pyramidal cells excited all other pyramidal cells and interneurons, but not themselves. Interneurons inhibited one another and every pyramidal cell. Pyramidal cells 3, 5, 7, and 8, received direct tone, while pyramidal cells 1, 4, 5, 7, and 8 received direct shock input. Both interneurons received direct tone and shock inputs.

Excitatory glutamatergic AMPA synapses capable of strengthening (long term potentiation, LTP) or weakening (long term depression, LTD) with training were placed on the following synapses of each cell: (i) thalamic/cortical auditory tone synapses to pyramidal cells or interneurons, (ii) synapses between the pyramidal cells themselves, and (iii) pyramidal cell to interneuron synapses. In addition, plasticity was also modeled in GABAergic inhibitory synapses from interneurons to pyramidal cells. The occurrence of synaptic potentiation versus depression was determined by intracellular calcium levels, according to the calcium control hypothesis. Details related to the equations can be found in Li et al. (2009). Learning of conditioned fear leads to changes in synaptic strength in the neural circuitry and the magnitude and sign of these variations are unique insights that a computational model can provide.

Training protocol and background inputs. The schedule of tone and shock inputs to the model was based on in vivo studies (Quirk et al., 1995, 1997). We scaled down the timing of the auditory fear conditioning protocol by approximately two orders of magnitude so that it would be suitable for computational study. The simulation included a sensitization phase, a conditioning phase, and two extinction phases. Each tone lasted 500 ms and each shock lasted 100 ms, and the interval between two tones was 3.5 s. During the sensitization phase, 10 unpaired tones and shocks were presented to the network with the shocks occurring randomly between the tones. Following sensitization, 10 paired tones and shocks were provided in the conditioning phase with shock present during the last 100 ms of the tone. In extinction, 30 tones were delivered to the neurons without any shock (pure tones). The gap between conditioning and extinction phases was 40 s and the model was tested for spontaneous recovery after a delay of 840 s. The second extinction phase also used 30 pure tones. The entire schedule lasted 1,200 s. The specific tone and shock inputs were represented by two separate regular spike trains delivered to the AMPA/NMDA channels in the cells. The firing frequency for the tone and shock inputs was set at 200 Hz to model the summed activity of multiple inputs in vivo. The tone inputs also included noise represented by random Poisson spikes with an average frequency of 2 Hz. Given that the tone starts out as neutral and the shock as noxious, the conductance strength encoding the shock information was set much higher than that representing the tone inputs.

To achieve the low average spontaneous firing rate of ~1 Hz in the experiments modeled (Quirk et al., 1995), independent, Poisson distributed, random excitatory background inputs were delivered to all the pyramidal cells. These inputs represent unmodeled synaptic connections from other brain areas such as prefrontal cortex and hippocampus. Similar background inputs were provided to the interneurons to generate the reported spontaneous firing rates of ~8 Hz (Paré and Gaudreau, 1996). Simulations were performed on a personal computer using the software package GENESIS with the Crank-Nicholson integration method, and a time step of 10 μs.

Model validation. In addition to matching unit responses in the model to unit experimental data, the model of the 'network' should also reproduce experimentally observed behavior. Unit tone responses from the lateral amygdala of behaving animals have been reported by Quirk et al. (1995). Their main finding was that conditioning significantly increased the number of tone-elicited spikes with the greatest effects at the shortest latency following tone onset. These conditioned responses were reversed by extinction training. With tuning of the plasticity parameters in the model, the LA network model unit tone responses successfully reproduced experimental data in Quirk et al. (1995). All pyramidal neurons in the model

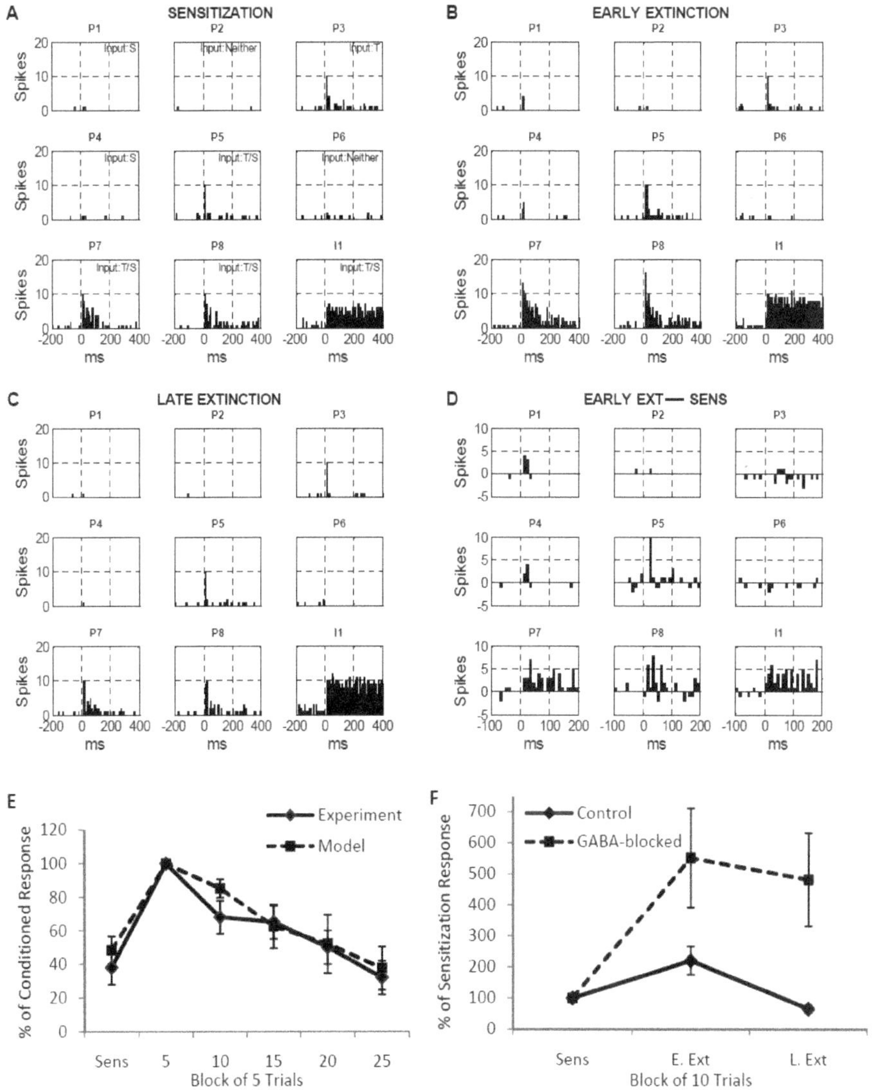

Figure 7. Comparison of the experimental data (Fig. 4, Quirk et al. 1997) and the model tone responses for the last block of 5 trials in sensitization and successive 5-trial blocks during extinction. The total spikes (0–50 ms) in each block of 5 trials were normalized to the responses in the 1st block of extinction for each cell and the mean ratio (with SE) among 4 significant conditioned pyramidal cells calculated.

showed clear frequency adaptation with the tone responses concentrated in the first 100 ms, indicating a good match with the experimental recordings. Figure 7 shows the match between experimental and model conditioned tone responses for the last block of five trials in sensitization and successive five-trial blocks during extinction. The large potentiation of the excitatory inputs onto pyramidal cells caused by conditioning, together with the potentiation of connections between several pyramidal cells leads to elevated tone responses in early extinction. As extinction progresses, increasing feedforward and feedback inhibition from the interneurons, combined with depotentiation at excitatory synapses onto pyramidal cells bring tone responses back to pre-conditioning levels or even lower. This provides an important validation for the network model. Once validated, a model can be used to provide insights into the underlying mechanisms, as described next.

Insights provided by the LA model

The Li et al. (2009) network model represents the first attempt to incorporate cellular neurophysiology and synaptic plasticity mechanisms into a biophysical model to investigate the underlying mechanisms of fear learning. The model was used to determine how the intrinsic and synaptic mechanisms interact in a network to shape unit tone responses. Computational models are unique in their ability to contribute to such insights.

How can LA can store both fear and extinction memories? After fear conditioning, the model was able to 'learn' both fear and extinction memories. In the process, the model predicted an important role for inhibition via interneurons. The model identified two possible sites for fear memory storage in LA: the tone synapses from the auditory thalamus (or cortex) onto the pyramidal cells and the synapses between pyramidal cells. Hebbian pairing indicates that the synaptic coupling between two pyramidal cells will be strengthened as long as both receive strong inputs such as shocks. In contrast, the tone synaptic weight increases only when tone and shock are paired and decreases when tone and shock are unpaired. This leads to the prediction that tone synapses only store specific tone-shock associations, while the pyr-pyr synapses are capable of storing a generalized fear memory related to the occurrence of shock, e.g., related to contextual fear conditioning. The model also showed that the pyr-pyr synapses decayed less on average in extinction compared to the tone-pyr synapses. This was because of frequency adaptation of pyramidal cells resulting in lower incidence of Hebbian weakening. Taken together, these findings suggest that the pyr-pyr synapses are well suited to encode long-term fear memory in LA neurons.

The model also suggested that the different types of principal neurons have different functional roles due to their distinct frequency adaptation characteristics (Faber et al., 2001). The cells with stronger adaptation are slower to learn fear but are able to maintain fear memory for a long time, whereas the cells with weaker adaptation learn fear faster, but also extinguish faster (Fig. 5, *A* and *B* in Li et al., 2009). This suggests that pyramidal cells with weaker adaptation are important for fear expression, whereas those with stronger adaptation are important for long-term storage of fear associations. Since about 70% of pyramidal cells in LA are strongly adapting, LA is well suited for long-term fear memory storage.

Considering extinction memory, the model suggests three possible sites of plasticity: the tone synapse at the interneuron, the inhibitory synapse from interneuron to pyramidal cell, and the excitatory synapse from pyramidal cell to interneuron. Model runs showed different decay rates of these three synapses suggesting that the first two, with large and uniform decay rates during the gap, may mediate short-term extinction memory, while the last, with smaller decay rate, could store long-term extinction memory (e.g., P1-I1 in Fig. 5C in Li et al., 2009). However, the tone-interneuron and inter-pyramidal cell synapses potentiated much larger during both extinction sessions, compared to the pyramidal-interneuron synapses.

How does the low spontaneous firing rate of pyramidal cells affect memory storage? LA cells signal fear and so it is logical that they have low spontaneous firing rates of around 1 Hz. But then, what are the implications of this low firing rate for learning? Experiments with the model revealed that the low rate of spontaneous firing in LA may act to preserve the fear memory due to decreased incidence of Hebbian weakening. The high spontaneous rates of interneurons, on the other hand, leads to a comparatively faster weakening of extinction memory stored in the interneurons synapses.

Does 'unlearning' of fear also occur with extinction? It is known that extinction involves the formation of a new and distinct memory. However, what is not clear is whether a part of the fear memory is also lost during extinction trials. Such fear memory would be stored in the tone-pyramidal synapses. Blocking NMDA receptors in experiments would prevent depotentiation of the excitatory synapses onto pyramidal cells (LTD) but at the same time it would also block potentiation of inhibitory connections. So, experiments cannot answer this question presently. A model, however, can implement selective blockade of LTD only at the tone-pyramidal and pyramidal-pyramidal synapses by preventing Ca^{2+} influx via the NMDA channels, to separate the effects of both these phenomena. To evaluate the contribution of LTD, which is independent of potentiation of inhibition, a selective blockade of LTD showed that extinction was not complete, i.e., potentiation of inhibition alone is not sufficient for complete extinction.

The LA model can be used as a test bed to investigate several other 'what if' scenarios that may be of interest but are difficult to test in experiments. Our study showed how such models are poised to complement experimental investigations by providing insights into how cellular and synaptic mechanisms contribute to implementing functions in brains. This is illustrated further by the model of intercalated cells discussed next.

B. Modeling the network of amygdala intercalated cells (Li et al., 2011)

Motivation. The amygdala intercalated cells (ITC; fig 2) are distributed along the lateral and medial parts of the basolateral amygdaloid complex. The more dorsally located ITC clusters receive glutamatergic excitatory input from LA and BA, while the medial ITC clusters receive GABAergic inhibition from the dorsal ITC clusters and excitation from BA; the medial clusters, in turn, inhibit Ce, the output station in the amygdala (Paré and Smith, 1993a,b; Royer et al., 1999; Royer et al., 2000; Jungling et al., 2008). This strategic location of the medial ITC clusters, between the sensory input (BLA) and fear output (Ce) stations of the amygdala, is thought to be critical for regulating classically conditioned fear responses (Paré et al., 2004).

It is currently believed (Paré et al., 2004; Quirk and Mueller, 2008) that extinguished conditioned stimuli activate infralimbic (IL) neurons that have glutamatergic projections to ITC cells and ITC cells in turn reduce conditioned fear responses by generating feedforward inhibition in fear output Ce neurons (Paré et al., 2004). Consistent with this, IL stimulation was found to dramatically reduce the responsiveness of Ce neurons to BLA inputs (Quirk et al., 2003). IL axons are known to target ITC cells clusters located medially (McDonald et al., 1996), and there are inhibitory connections between (Royer et al., 2000) as well as within ITC cell clusters (Geracitano et al., 2007). Additionally, three different types of short-term synaptic plasticity have been observed in inter-ITC connections (Geracitano et al., 2007), but the role of such synaptic heterogeneity is not clear. How then might IL inputs overcome the inter-ITC inhibition and reduce the responsiveness of Ce? Again, it is currently difficult to address this question experimentally, because we lack criteria to identify ITC cells on the basis of their extracellularly recorded activity. So, in order to study how inter-ITC inhibitory connections affect their responses to IL inputs, we developed a biologically realistic model of the ITC network (Fig. 8). Another objective of the Li et al. (2011) study was to examine how the peculiar electroresponsive properties of ITC cells shape their responsiveness to BLA/IL inputs. ITC cells express an unusual voltage-dependent K^+ conductance whose slow-deinactivation kinetics allow them to produce a prolonged depolarizing plateau after a transient suprathreshold depolarization (Royer et al., 2000). This enables ITC neurons to transform transient excitatory inputs into a prolonged state of increased excitability with possibly important consequences for the regulation of conditioned fear.

During prolonged auditory CSs, BLA principal neurons show rapidly adapting responses (Quirk et al., 1995, 1997; Repa et al., 2001; Herry et al., 2008), but it is not clear how such transient responses are converted into sustained behavioral output, since rats freeze throughout the duration of the tone. Also, pairing CSs with brief (300 msec) electrical IL stimulation reduces conditioned freezing in a temporally specific manner (Milad and Quirk, 2002; Milad et al., 2004), again sustaining this transient input. We used the model to test whether bistable electroresponsive properties of ITC cells allow them to transform transient BLA/IL signals into a more sustained output.

Single cell properties. Each ITC cell had two compartments representing a soma (diameter of 8 μm; length of 8 μm) and a dendrite (diameter of 5 μm; length of 200 μm). The values for the specific membrane resistance, membrane capacitance, and cytoplasmic (axial) resistivity were, respectively, R_m = 30 KΩ-cm², C_m = 1.0 μF/cm², and R_a =150 Ω-cm. The leakage reversal potential was set to -93 mV to match experimental measurements of their resting potential (–85 mV). The resulting input resistance was about 600MΩ when measured from rest, consistent with experimental observations. The ITC model contained several ionic currents including a leakage current I_L, a spike-generating sodium current I_{Na}, a potassium delayed rectifier current I_{DR}, a slow deinactivating current I_{SD}, a voltage-gated persistent muscarinic current I_M, a hyperpolarization-activated current I_H, a high-voltage activated Ca^{2+} current I_{CaL}, and a slow Ca^{2+}- dependent after-hyperpolarization current I_{sAHP}. As cited, the

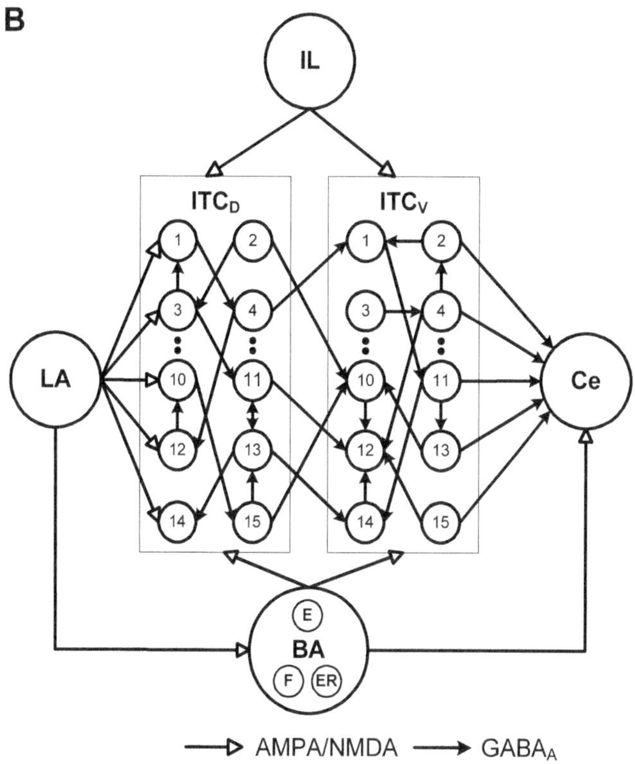

Figure 8. Structure of the model ITC network with 15 neurons each in ITC$_D$ and ITC$_V$ clusters (adapted from Li et al., 2011). For clarity and illustration purpose, the connectivity in the figure is partial and representative only. Each ITC neuron inhibits three randomly selected neurons in the same cluster. Each ITCD neuron also inhibits three randomly selected ITCV neurons (e.g., ITC$_{D2}$ inhibits ITC$_{V10}$). The network has five Ce output neurons that receive excitatory inputs from BA, and inhibitory inputs from ITC$_V$ neurons. ITC$_D$ and ITC$_V$: Neurons 1–5 facilitating output synapses; neurons 6 10 have depressing output synapses, and neurons 11–15 have constant synapses.

membrane potential and current dynamics were modeled using the standard Hodgkin-Huxley formulation (Li et al., 2011).

We modeled three different types of Ce neurons differing by their spike patterns, regular spiking, late firing, and low-threshold bursting. Each cell model had two compartments: a soma (diameter of 15 μm; length of 15 μm) and a dendrite (diameter of 5 μm; length of 300 μm), and the following currents: a leakage current I_L, a sodium current I_{Na}, a delayed rectifier I_{DR}, a muscarinic current I_M, a hyperpolarization-activated current I_H, a high-voltage-activated Ca^{2+} current I_{CaL}, and a slow Ca^{2+}-dependent after-hyperpolarization current I_{sAHP}. The late firing cell contained an additional inactivating transient K^+ current I_A known to delay the onset of the action potential (Storm 1986), while the low-threshold bursting cell included an additional low-threshold inactivating calcium current I_{CaT} .The passive membrane properties were as follows: R_m = 30 KΩ-cm^2, C_m = 1.0 μF/cm^2, and R_a =150 Ω-cm.

Network model and synaptic connections. The ITC network model (Fig. 8) had dorsal and ventral ITC modules, and a Ce module. It had 15 ITC_D and 15 ITC_V neurons, and five Ce output cells. The network received inputs from LA, BA, and IL. LA inputs projected to ITC_D, while IL inputs projected equally to ITC_D and ITC_V (McDonald et al., 1996). BA inputs also projected to both ITC_D and ITC_V clusters, but with a lower density to ITC_D neurons (Royer et al., 1999, 2000; Pape and Paré, 2010). Based on the findings of Herry et al. (2008), the BA inputs were divided into fear, extinction, and extinction-resistant (ER) groups. The extinction inputs did not project to Ce because the activation profile of extinction cells was opposite to the expression of fear (Herry et al., 2008). Instead, both fear and ER inputs projected to Ce.

ITC neurons exhibit NMDA-dependent bidirectional synaptic plasticity (Royer and Paré, 2002) and in a recent experimental study, the BA inputs to ITC cells were reported to show a three-fold potentiation during extinction training (Fig. 4 in Amano et al., 2010). Given the fact that the firing rate of LA neurons is significantly increased after conditioning (Quirk et al., 1995), it is reasonable to assume that the LA–ITC_D connection is potentiated by conditioning. Hence, we used a threefold synaptic weight (compared with the habituation state) for the LA–ITC_D synapses in the fear state and a threefold synaptic weight for the BA–ITC synapses in the extinction state. For the LA–ITC_D connection, the potentiated synapses were assumed to be partially depotentiated in the extinction state (strength reduced from 3 to 2 for AMPA synapses only, Amano et al., 2010) based on results from a previous LA network model (Li et al., 2009). The BA–Ce, ITC–ITC, and ITC–Ce synaptic weights were assumed to be fixed. However, based on experimental findings (Geracitano et al., 2007), the presynaptic release probability of the ITC–ITC and ITC–Ce synapses was modifiable, and were split equally into facilitating, depressing, and constant types. The equations and specifics related to the plasticity mechanisms can be found in Li et al. (2011).

Model runs. We determined responses of the model to a 2-sec auditory tone input (CS) during three different network states: habituation, following fear conditioning, and after extinction training. The LA and BA inputs were modeled with different degrees of spike frequency adaptation based on previous experimental data (Quirk et al., 1995, 1997; Faber et al., 2001; Herry et al., 2008) and to account for the projection from LA to BA, the firing rate of BA fear inputs was assumed to be dependent on LA inputs due to similar firing patterns across training (Quirk et al., 1995; Herry et al., 2008). The IL inputs were modeled as Poisson-distributed spike trains with a duration of 300 msec and a mean frequency of 20 Hz (Milad and Quirk, 2002). In addition, Poisson-distributed random background inputs were delivered to all ITC and Ce neurons to achieve experimentally observed spontaneous firing rates.

Model runs were performed on a personal computer using the software package GENESIS with the Crank-Nicholson integration method, and a time step of 20 msec. A simulation of 5 sec of network activity took 15 min of CPU time.

Insights provided by the network model of ITC clusters

We developed the model to investigate how the electroresponsive properties of ITC cells shape their responsiveness to BLA/IL inputs, and how IL inputs might overcome the inter-ITC inhibition after extinction training and reduce the responsiveness of Ce. The model showed that ITC neurons could transform the transient CS-related signals arising in the BLA into a persistent pattern of activity. It also showed that over a wide range of stimulation strengths, brief IL activation can overwhelm inter-ITC inhibition and reduce the activity of fear output Ce neurons. Importantly, both intrinsic properties (i.e., bistability) and variations in the short-term synaptic dynamics of ITC neurons contributed to the effectiveness of IL stimulation. Similar to the LA model case discussed earlier, the ITC model provided several insights into the functioning of this cluster of cells and how they might modulate the expression of fear and extinction memories.

Can ITC neurons help in transforming transient LA fear inputs into sustained Ce output? The model showed that despite the presence of inhibitory connections between ITC cells, transient excitatory inputs from BLA or IL were transformed by ITC cells into a sustained state of increased activity via the inactivation of I_{SD}. Although the magnitude of this persistent activity was affected by the strength of inter-ITC inhibitory connections, it remained robust for a 2.5 fold increase in inhibitory synaptic weights. This finding suggests that ITC cells express a form of short-term memory, inscribed in their intrinsic properties, allowing for persistent alterations in fear responsiveness following transient sensory signals. It was recently shown that prelimbic (PL) neurons transform transient amygdala inputs into a sustained output that drives conditioned fear responses and gates the expression of extinction (Burgos-Robles et al., 2009). Our model suggests that ITC activity could add to the role of PL in sustaining the expression of conditioned fear. While PL seems to sustain fear by increasing the excitatory drive onto Ce via BA, the present study suggests that ITC_D neurons could contribute to this sustenance by increasing their inhibition on ITC_V neurons, resulting in disinhibition of Ce. During the high fear state, strongly adaptive LA inputs were transformed into a sustained output by ITC_D neurons, leading to persistent inhibition of ITC_V cells and consequent sustained firing in Ce. Also, ITC neurons can support the expression of extinction via persistent activity in ITC_V cells. In the extinction state, LA responses diminished and the LA–ITC_D connection depotentiated, while the BA–ITC connection potentiated (Amano et al., 2010). Strongly adaptive BA inputs were then transformed into sustained firing in ITC_V cells, resulting in lowered Ce responses (see fig 8 in Li et al., 2011).

Can IL overcome inter-ITC inhibition and reduce Ce responses? The model examined the impact of a brief 300 ms IL stimulation on the responsiveness of ITC cells to strongly adaptive CS-related BLA inputs, in the high fear state. Over a wide range of strengths, IL inputs consistently caused a marked increase in the firing rate of ITC cells, which then inhibited Ce, the fear output station. Also, IL-evoked firing caused a persistent inactivation of I_{SD} in ITC neurons and this extended IL's impact beyond the 300-msec stimulation window. The model also demonstrated that IL stimulation given shortly after tone onset was most effective in reducing Ce firing, in agreement with experimental findings (Milad et al., 2004). This might be due to the fact that this timing most effectively combines the direct impact of IL in inhibiting early Ce spikes and its indirect (after IL is turned off) impact in inhibiting Ce firing subsequently, via the inactivation of the slowly de-inactivating current I_{SD}. The model also predicted that ITC neurons contacted by depressing synapses are more likely recruited by IL inputs than those contacted by facilitating or constant-type synapses.

What is the role of synaptic heterogeneity within ITC cells? Geracitano et al. (2007) have shown that the synapses within the ITC region, i.e., ITC-ITC synapses, exhibit short-term presynaptic plasticity that is distributed equally between facilitating, depressing and constant types. Their experiments also show that the ITC_V–Ce connections (fig. 8) have to be of the facilitating or constant types. Model experiments suggest that this specificity could be functionally relevant in the inhibitory control of Ce by IL inputs. The model, as expected, showed that ITC_V–Ce connections of the facilitating and constant types were more effective in inhibiting Ce output. However, for the inter-ITC connections, pure facilitating or constant synapses decrease the firing rates of both ITC_D and ITC_V neurons when IL inputs are active, resulting in elevated Ce responses. Hence, depressing inter-ITC synapses, together with inactivation of I_{SD}, would allow IL inputs to overcome the inter-ITC inhibition. These insights suggest that the specific distribution of heterogeneous short-term plasticity of the inter-ITC connections enables sufficiently high activity levels in ITC_V cells for an efficient control of fear-related Ce outputs when BA and IL neurons are active.

C. Modeling the other amygdalar nuclei, and modulation by cortical structures

The primary structures of the fear circuit, as presently understood, include the amygdala, the prefrontal cortex, and the hippocampus. These structures, in turn, are themselves composed of different sub-circuits, with different roles in auditory fear learning. The amygdala, as cited, consists of several nuclei LA, BA, Ce and the ITC clusters, all acting in concert to store auditory fear and extinction memories, and express them later via the fear output station Ce. Interestingly, these individual nuclei themselves are not homogeneous. For instance, the dorsal and ventral regions of LA participate in fear learning in different ways (Repa et al., 2001); BA has different nuclei, BL and BM, which have recently been shown to relay fear differently to Ce (Amano et al., 2011); the two different ITC cell clusters associated with the fear circuit again contribute in different ways to the expression of fear and extinction memories (Royer et al., 2000); and the output nucleus Ce has also been shown recently to have very distinct sub-circuits whose specific roles as far as influencing fear await further investigation (Coicci et al., 2010; Haubensak et al., 2010).

Amygdalar fear, in turn, is known to be modulated by mPFC (both PL and IL) and by the hippocampus, and so the expression of fear and extinction memories is also under control of these 'higher' level structures. At present, modulation of amygdalar fear by mPFC (see Burgos-Robles et al., 2009) is better understood in comparison to modulation by the hippocampus. As discussed earlier, studies related to contextual fear conditioning

(Fanselow, 2010), which involve the hippocampus, have been complicated by this lack of understanding. Hence computational models of the hippocampus and its linkages to the amygdala and mPFC in auditory fear may have to await progress in our understanding of anatomical linkages between these regions and experimental data on their interactions during the different phases of fear learning.

Opportunities and challenges. There is consensus on the critical involvement of amygdala in the fear circuit. However, it is not presently clear how the various amygdalar nuclei with different internal sub-circuits act in concert to store fear and extinction memories in a distributed manner, and what roles they play in expressing these memories (Paré et al., 2004). Neurobiological information continues to accumulate at an increasing rate, including at intracellular, cellular, circuits and behavioral levels, providing opportunities for integrating such information via 'system' level models such as the ones discussed here. Such models can then be used to address several interesting challenges related to the fear circuit: What is the distribution of tone (thalamic and cortical) and shock in the lateral amygdala? What are the different types of learning mechanisms in the amygdala (pre and post synaptic, short and long term), and what synapses do they impact? Neuromodulatory systems have been shown to play an important role in the fear circuit, but how are the receptors distributed and how do they influence intrinsic excitability and synaptic efficacy? What is the level of robustness and redundancy in storage and expression of fear and extinction memories within each structure and at the circuit level? What are the pathways for modulation of amygdalar fear by the prefrontal cortex and hippocampus (and possibly other cortical structures)?

These are important challenges that have to be addressed in order to gain an understanding of the functioning of the mammalian fear circuit. As demonstrated in the discussion above, biologically realistic models can potentially supplement experimental modalities such as patch clamp recordings, single unit recordings, pharmacological manipulations and transgenic approaches, and assist with reverse engineering the functioning of this critical circuit. They also provide tremendous opportunities for research in interdisciplinary settings with participation of neuroscientists, electrophysiologists and computational experts. For instance, similar to the insights obtained for LA and ITC clusters, such interdisciplinary research would also aid in elucidating the roles of the various sub-circuits within the other nuclei, BA and Ce. After development of the individual models of these nuclei, they can be integrated into an overall model of the amygdalar fear circuit. The level of robustness and redundancy that the circuit components and the circuit as a whole possesses (e.g., in BA as reported by Amano et al., 2011) can then be addressed effectively by such models. As cited, the role of context in fear learning is not well understood at the present time. Thus, improved neurobiological understanding of information processing within the hippocampus and of the anatomical connectivity (hippocampus to mPFC and to the amydgala) will have to precede modeling efforts related to contextual auditory fear circuits.

Limitations. Although computational modeling is increasingly used as a tool for studying complex neuronal brain circuits, some general limitations should be acknowledged. Computational models are typically designed to answer specific questions, and so consider only the relevant structures and associated functions. The size of reported model networks incorporating biological realistic cells is typically much smaller than the actual biological networks at the present time (e.g., Durstewitz et al., 2000; Morgan et al., 2007). This is compensated for presently by careful modeling including preservation of key network features and by extensive parametric studies (Morgan et al., 2007). Increasing computing speeds and specialized architectures should enable the development of larger networks directly in the near future. Lack of biological data necessitates using values for parameters such as ionic conductances from multiple brain areas, or tuning them (e.g., synaptic weights) to match behavioral output. Improved characterization of the physiology including identification of neuronal types, connectivity (including spatial constraints and axonal distributions), parameter values, and learning mechanisms will help improve the fidelity of such models. The diversity of interneurons and the networks they form in the elements of the fear circuit continue to intrigue researchers, although we are beginning to understand the functions that they might subserve, e.g., synchronization of neuronal assemblies (Bissiere et al., 2011). Also, active afferents from areas omitted in the model are typically considered as 'background' input, and better characterization of such afferents under in vivo conditions will be needed. Finally, computational research can be most effective only if the neuroscientist and electrophysiologist play an active role in the model development process, particularly in 'constraining' the model, and the computational expert is committed to an in-depth understanding of neurobiology. Notwithstanding such limitations, researchers continue to take advantage of the fact that information related to neurophysiology is accumulating at an increasing pace, and are developing very large scale biologically realistic networks (e.g., Miller, 2011; Morgan et al., 2007) to reverse engineer the functions implemented by brain circuits.

5. Summary and potential applications

There has been a surge in interest related to the role of intra-amygdaloid structures in Pavlovian fear learning. Research papers have risen from an average of 25/year in the 1980s to 200/year in the 2000s (Paré et al., 2004). Although this has resulted in an improved understanding of the underlying mechanisms, it has also highlighted the complexity of the circuit, including possible distributed storage of fear and extinction memories in the various nuclei/structures, distinct mechanism of LTP/LTD at different synapses, and recruitment of alternative pathways providing redundancy that is probably an important trait of such a critical circuit. This complexity renders the understanding of the amygdalar involvement in fear learning a bigger challenge than previously envisaged. Furthermore, modulation of the amygdala by the prefrontal cortex, hippocampus and other related regions is only beginning to be understood. Computational modeling has the potential to play an important role in our efforts to unravel this complex fear circuit.

Insights into the functioning of the sub-circuits using computational models would also be useful for studying disruptions associated with the fear circuit, leading to PTSD and anxiety disorders. For instance, studies have shown that humans with PTSD exhibit a delay in acquisition of extinction as compared to controls (Rothbaum and Davis, 2003). With the model, one can modify parameters to predict changes in the fear circuit that could be correlated with a delay in acquisition of extinction. These parameters would then point to the changes in the circuit with PTSD and provide insights into the pathology of the illness. The model could also shed light on how therapeutic approaches such as cognitive restructuring provide a new emotional significance to a negative cognition and reduce physiological arousal (Debiec et al., 2006).

Application to drug discovery research. An important future application of such models would be in identifying new pharmacological targets for therapeutic interventions (Li et al., 2008). For instance, the LA computational model predicted that three types of NMDA-glutamatergic synapses and one type of GABAergic synapse could be involved in storing fear and extinction memories. These predictions seem to be consistent with two recent experimental findings. First, a partial NMDA agonist D-cycloserine has been shown to facilitate extinction of fear conditioning in rats (Akirav et al., 2009; Walker et al., 2001). D-Cycloserine was also effective in treating social anxiety disorder and acrophobia in combination with psychotherapy (Ressler et al., 2004). The mechanism of action of D-Cycloserine and other drugs acting on the glutamatergic system can now be modeled both at receptor and cellular levels in the specific LA neurons indicated by the model. Second, NMDA receptors in the amygdala activate an intracellular signaling cascade leading to new protein synthesis. One such synthesized protein, gephyrin, clusters GABA receptors near the synapse, thereby increasing their inhibitory effect. The level of gephyrin goes down during fear conditioning, and then increases to baseline values with extinction learning (Quirk, 2002). The return to baseline level of gephyrin is associated with an increase in the surface expression of $GABA_A$ receptors, corresponding to increasing inhibitory neurotransmission in the amygdala (Harris et al., 1998). Drugs that impact these mechanisms would have a potential role for the treatment of PTSD and anxiety disorders. Finally, the cannabinoid receptor CB1 has been shown to modulate GABAergic neurons in the amygdala and facilitate extinction (Chhatwal et al., 2005). This is consistent with the model prediction that the inhibitory synapse from the interneuron to the pyramidal cell could be a site for the storage of extinction memory. With increasing availability of neurobiological information and easy-to-use software tools, such *in silico* models of brain circuits have the potential to become common place in drug discovery research.

Author details

Satish S. Nair
Department of Electrical and Computer Engineering
University of Missouri - Columbia, Columbia, MO, USA

Acknowledgement

The author is grateful to his former PhD student Guoshi Li, and to Gregory Quirk and Denis Paré for their contributions, in many ways, to the collaborative research that this review significantly draws upon. This work was supported by NIMH grant MH087755 to SSN.

6. References

Akirav I, Segev A, Montanis H, Maroun M (2009) D-Cycloserine into the BLA reverses the impairing effects of exposure to stress on the extinction of contextual fear, but not conditioned taste aversion. Learn Mem 16: 682-686.

Amano T, Unal CT, Paré D (2010) Synaptic correlates of fear extinction in the amygdala. Nat Neurosci 13: 489–494.

Amano T, Duvaci S, Popa D, and Paré D (2011) The fear circuit revisited: Contributions of basal amygdala nuclei to conditioned fear. J Neurosci 31(43): 15481-15489.

Anagnostaras SG, Maren S, Fanselow MS (1999) Temporally graded retrograde amnesia of contextual fear after hippocampal damage in rats: within-subjects examination. J Neurosci 19:1106 –1114.

Aradi I, Érdi P (2006) Computational neuropharmacology: dynamical approaches in drug discovery. Trends in Pharm Sci 27(5): 240-243.

Armony JL, Servan-Schreiber D, Cohen JD, LeDoux JE (1995) An anatomically constrained neural network model of fear conditioning. Behav Neurosci 109:246–257.

Balkenius C, Morén J (2001) Emotional learning: a computational model of the amygdala. Cybern Syst 32: 611–636, 2001.

Bissiere S, Zelikowsky M, Ponnusamy R, Jacobs NS, Blair HT, Fanselow MS (2011) Electrical synapses control hippocampal contributions to fear learning and memory. Science 331:87–91.

Blair HT, Schafe GE, Bauer EP, Rodrigues SM, and LeDoux JE (2001) Synaptic plasticity in the lateral amygdala: a cellular hypothesis of fear conditioning. Learn Mem 8: 229–242.

Blanchard DC, Blanchard RJ (1972) Innate and conditioned fear reactions to threat in rats with amygdaloid lesions. J Comp Phys Psychol 81:281–290.

Blum S, Hebert AE, Dash PK (2006) A role for the prefrontal cortex in recall of recent and remote memories. Neuroreport 17:341–344.

Boeing 777, In *Wikipedia*. Retrieved March 9, 2012, from http://en.wikipedia.org/wiki/777-200ER#777-200ER.

Bouton ME, King DA (1983) Contextual control of the extinction of conditioned fear: tests for the associative value of the context. J Exp Psychol Anim Behav Process 9:248-265.

Bouton ME. Context and behavioral processes in extinction. Learn Mem 11: 485-494, 2004.

Bower JM, Beeman D (2003) The book of GENESIS: *Exploring realistic neural models with the GEneral NEural SImulation System*, Internet Edition.

Buchel C, Morris J, Dolan RJ, and Friston KJ (1998) Brain systems mediating aversive conditioning: an event-related fMRI study. Neuron 20: 947–957.

Burgos-Robles A, Vidal-Gonzalez I, Quirk GJ (2009) Sustained conditioned responses in prelimbic prefrontal neurons are correlated with fear expression and extinction failure. J Neurosci 29: 8474–8482.

Byrne JH, Roberts JL (2004) *From Molecules to Networks – An Introduction to Cellular and Molecular Neuroscience.* Elsevier Academic Press.

Carnevale NT, Hines ML (2006) *The NEURON Book.* Cambridge, UK: Cambridge University Press.

Chhatwal JP, Myers KM, Ressler KJ, Davis M, et al. (2005) Regulation of gephyrin and $GABA_A$ receptor binding within the amygdala after fear acquisition and extinction. J Neurosci 25:502-506.

Ciocchi S, Herry C, Grenier F, Wolff SBE, Letzkus JJ, Vlachos I, Ehrlich I, Sprengel R, Deisseroth K, Stadler MB, et al. (2010) Encoding of conditioned fear in central amygdala inhibitory circuits. Nature 468:277–282.

Corcoran KA, Desmond TJ, Frey KA, Maren S (2005) Hippocampal inactivation disrupts the acquisition and contextual encoding of fear extinction. J Neurosci 25: 8978-8987.

Corcoran KA, Quirk GJ (2007) Activity in prelimbic cortex is necessary for the expression of learned, but not innate, fears. J Neurosci 27:840–844.

Corcoran KA, Quirk GJ (2007) Recalling safety: Cooperative functions of the ventromedial prefrontal cortex and the hippocampus in extinction. CNS Spect 12:200-206.

Debiec J, Doyere V, Nader K, Ledoux JE (2006) Directly reactivated, but not indirectly reactivated, memories undergo reconsolidation in the amygdale. Proc Natl Acad Sci USA 103:3428 -3433.

Durstewitz D, Seamans JK, Sejnowski TJ (2000) Dopamine-mediated stabilization of delay-period activity in a network model of prefrontal cortex. J Neurophysiol 83:1733-1750.

Faber ESL, Callister RJ, Sah P (2001) Morphological and electrophysiological properties of principal neurons in the rat lateral amygdala in vitro. J Neurophysiol 85:714-723.

Fanselow MS (2010) From contextual fear to a dynamic view of memory systems. Trends Cogn Sci 14:7–15.

Gaudreau H, Paré D (1996) Projection neurons of the lateral amygdaloid nucleus are virtually silent throughout the sleep-walking cycle. J Neurophysiol 75:1301-1305.

Geracitano R, Kaufmann WA, Szabo G, Ferraguti F, Capogna M (2007) Synaptic heterogeneity between mouse paracapsular intercalated neurons of the amygdala. J Physiol 585: 117–134.

Grossberg S, Schmajuk NA (1987) Neural dynamics of attentionally modulated Pavlovian conditioning: conditioned reinforcement, inhibition, and opponent processing. Psychobiology 15: 195–240.

Harris JA, Westbrook RF (1998) Evidence that GABA transmission mediates context-specific extinction of learned fear. Psychopharmacology 140:105-115.

Haubensak W, Kunwar PS, Cai H, Ciocchi S, Wall NR, Ponnusamy R, Biag J, Dong HW, Deisseroth K, Callaway EM, et al. (2010) Genetic dissection of an amygdala microcircuit that gates conditioned fear. Nature 468: 270–276.

Herry C, Garcia R (2002) Prefrontal cortex long-term potentiation, but not long-term depression, is associated with the maintenance of extinction of learned fear in mice. J Neurosci 22:577–583.

Herry C, Ciocchi S, Senn V, Demmou L, Muller C, Luthi A (2008) Switching on and off fear by distinct neuronal circuits. Nature 454: 600–606.

Hobin JA, Goosens KA, Maren S (2003) Context-dependent neuronal activity in the lateral amygdala represents fear memories after extinction. J Neurosci 23: 8410-8416.

Hoover WB and Vertes RP (2007) Anatomical analysis of afferent projections to the medial prefrontal cortex in the rat. Brain Struct Funct 212: 149–179.

Koch C, Segev I (2001) *Methods in Neuronal Modeling- From Ions to Networks*. The MIT Press.

Krasne FB, Fanselow MS, Zelikowsky M. Design of a neurally plausible model of fear learning (2011) Frontiers in Behavioral Neuroscience 5:41.

Leblois A, Boraud T, Meissner W, Bergman H, Hansel D (2006) Competition between feedback loops underlies pathological dynamics in the basal ganglia J Neurosci 26(13):3567-3583.

LeDoux JE (1994) Emotion, memory and the brain. Sci Am. 50-57.

LeDoux JE (1996). *The Emotional Brain: The Mysterious Underpinnings of Emotional Life*. Simon & Schuster: New York.

LeDoux JE (2000) Emotion circuits in the brain. Annu Rev Neurosci 23: 155–184.

Li G, Amano T, Paré D, Nair SS (2011) Impact of infralimbic inputs on intercalated amygdala neurons: a biophysical modeling study, Learn Mem 18:226-240.

Li G, Nair SS, Quirk GJ (2009) A biologically realistic network model of acquisition and extinction of conditioned fear associations in lateral amygdala neurons, Journal of Neurophysiology 101: 1629-1646.

Li G, Nair J, Quirk GJ, Nair SS (2008) Computational modeling – a tool for new psychiatric medication development, Psychiatric Annals, 28(4):296-304.

Malkani S and Rosen JB (200) Specific induction of early growth response gene1 in the lateral nucleus of the amygdala following contextual fear conditioning in rats. Neurosci 97: 693–702.

Maren S (2001) Neurobiology of Pavlovian fear conditioning. Annu Rev Neurosci 24: 897–931.

Maren S, Quirk GJ (2004) Neuronal signaling of fear memory. Nat Rev Neurosci 5:844-842.

Mauk MD (2000) The potential effectiveness of simulations verses phenomenological models. Nat Neurosci 23:649-711.

Milad MR, Quirk GJ (2002) Neurons in medial prefrontal cortex signal memory for fear extinction. Nature 420:70 –74.

Milad MR, Wright CL, Orr SP, Pitman RK, Quirk GJ, Rauch SL (2007) Recall of fear extinction in humans activates the ventromedial prefrontal cortex and hippocampus in concert. Biolo Psychiatry 62:446-454.

Miller G (2011) Newsmaker interview: Henry Markram - Blue Brain founder responds to critics, clarifies his goals, Science 334 (6057): 748-749

Morgan RJ, Santhakumar V, Soltesz I (2007) Modeling the dentate gyrus, Prog in Brain Res 163:639-58.

Myers KM, Davis M (2007) Mechanisms of fear extinction. Mol Psychiatry 12:120-150.

Paré D, Quirk GJ, Ledoux JE (2004) New vistas on amygdala networks in conditioned fear. J Neurophysiol 92:1-9.

Pape HC, Paré D (2010) Plastic synaptic networks of the amygdala for the acquisition, expression, and extinction of conditioned fear. Physiol Rev 90: 419–463.

Quirk GJ, Russo GK, Barron JL, Lebron K (2000) The role of ventromedial prefrontal cortex in the recovery of extinguished fear. J Neurosci 20:6225– 6231.

Quirk GJ (2002) Memory for extinction of conditioned fear is long-lasting and persists following spontaneous recovery. Learn Mem 9:402-407.

Quirk GJ, Armony JL, LeDoux JE (1997) Fear conditioning enhances different temporal components of tone-evoked spike trains in auditory cortex and lateral amygdala. Neuron 19: 613–624.

Quirk GJ, Repa C, LeDoux JE (1995) Fear conditioning enhances short-latency auditory responses of lateral amygdala neurons: parallel recordings in the freely behaving rat. Neuron 15: 1029–1039.

Quirk GJ, Garcia R, Gonzalez-Lima F (2006) Prefrontal mechanisms in extinction of conditioned fear. Biol Psychiatry 60:337-343.

Quirk GJ, Mueller D (2008) Neural mechanisms of extinction learning and retrieval. Neuropsychopharmacology 33:56–72.

Repa JC, Muller J, Apergis J, Desrochers TM, Zhou Y, LeDoux JE (2001) Two different lateral amygdala cell populations contribute to the initiation and storage of memory. Nat Neurosci 4: 724–731.

Ressler KJ , Rothbaum BO, Anderson P, Zimand E, Tannenbaum L, Hodges L, Davis M (2004) D-Cycloserine, a putative cognitive enhancer, accelerates extinction of fear in humans. Arch General Psychiatry 61:1136-44.

Rothbaum BO, Davis M (2003) Applying learning principles to the treatment of posttrauma reactions. Ann N Y Acad Sci 1008:112-121.

Royer S, Martina M, Paré D (2000) Polarized synaptic interactions between intercalated neurons of the amygdala. J Neurophysiol 83: 3509–3518.

Tunnanen and Pitkanen (2000) Do seizures cause neuronal damage in rat amygdala kindling?, Epilepsy Research, 39(2):171-176.

Vlachos I, Herry C, Luthi A, Aertsen A, Kumar A (2011) Context-dependent encoding of fear and extinction memories in a large-scale network model of the basal amygdala. PLoS Comput Biol 7(3): e1001104.

Vidal-Gonzalez I, Vidal-Gonzalez B, Rauch SL, Quirk GJ (2006) Microstimulation reveals opposing influences of prelimbic and infralimbic cortex on the expression of conditioned fear. Learn Mem 13:728 –733.

Walker DL, Ressler KJ, Lu K-T, Davis M (2002) Facilitation of conditioned fear extinction by systemic administration or intra-amygdala infusions of D-cycloserine as assessed with fear-potentiated startle in rats. J Neurosci 22:2343–2351.

Wehner JM, Radcliffe RA (2004) Current Protocols in Neuroscience 8.5C.1-8.5C.14, John Wiley & Sons, Inc.

Chapter 8

Role of Norepinephrine in Modulating Inhibitory Avoidance Memory Storage: Critical Involvement of the Basolateral Amygdala

Barbara Ferry and Gina L. Quirarte

Additional information is available at the end of the chapter

1. Introduction

The relationship between noradrenergic function, stress, and memory has long been a subject of interest. What is normally adaptive during situations of extreme physical threat, including increases in heart rate and blood pressure, increased vigilance, hyperarousal, exaggerated startle, and enhancement of memory storage are considered to be part of a response elicited in a stressful situation [1]. Indeed, emotionally arousing experiences tend to be well remembered, and studies over the past five decades have provided considerable evidence suggesting that hormones released by stressful emotional experiences play an important role in mediating the effects of emotional arousal on lasting memory. One of the brain regions involved in the stress response is the amygdala, and neuromodulatory influences occurring selectively within this structure have been widely shown to regulate memory consolidation of newly acquired information through its projections to other brain structures. This review will focus on evidence from research findings investigating the relationship between stress-elicited noradrenergic brain activation and the role of the amygdala in mediating the effects of norepinephrine (NE) on memory consolidation. Furthermore, our findings suggest that this noradrenergic activation of the amygdala or, more precisely, of the basolateral nucleus of the amygdala, serves to modulate memory storage in other brain regions.

2. Adrenergic catecholamines and stress

The locus coeruleus (LC) noradrenergic system plays an important role in the fear response and anxiety. Other brain systems are also involved in the fear response and anxiety; these include the corticotrophin-releasing factor hypothalamic-pituitary-adrenal axis system and the benzodiazepine, dopamine, opiate, and serotonergic systems. These neuropeptide and neurotransmitter systems function in a coordinated manner with NE, as reviewed elsewhere [2-4].

Diverse adaptive behavioral responses are evoked by acute exposure to a variety of stressful events. In coordination with neuroendocrine and autonomic responses induced by such events, behavioral adaptations serve to maintain homeostasis and, by enabling optimal functioning, ensure survival in the face of threat. In addition to the primary neural circuits mediating contextually specific responses, acute stress also activates other brain systems that play a modulatory role, serving to bring together the complex response of the organism to any stress. Of the systems modulated by stress, the brain noradrenergic system has been shown to be one of the most important.

The noradrenergic system originates in a relatively small number of cells located in the LC and in other cell groups in the medulla and pons that utilize NE as a neurotransmitter. Nonetheless, the extensive network of noradrenergic terminals projecting from these few cells innervates essentially the entire neural axis. This widespread and divergent anatomical organization allows this system to influence the activity of the entire nervous system under conditions of elevated noradrenergic release during stress.

Activation of the noradrenergic system alters the ''signal to noise ratio'' of responses evoked by other afferents (both excitatory and inhibitory), rather than inducing simple inhibition or excitation, thus enhancing synaptic transmission in target circuits [5]. Such modulatory effects of NE have been described in many brain circuits and have been shown to be mediated, via different transduction mechanisms, by both β and α-adrenergic receptors [6-9]. Given the anatomical organization of the central noradrenergic system, it is suggested that stimuli that activate the small population of hindbrain noradrenergic neurons result in the release of NE in many widespread target regions throughout the brain, altering the reactivity of many neural circuits mediating a variety of behavioral and physiological responses. Furthermore, the anatomical organization and potential modulatory effects of the NE system suggest that it may facilitate a number of responses evoked by other afferents. As a consequence, the observed effects of increased noradrenergic release in a particular structure will depend on the set of specific neural circuits recruited and the set of specific behavioral responses elicited by the stressful stimulus which provoked the increase in NE release.

Noradrenergic neurons are activated by specific sensory stimuli of several modalities [10, 11], suggesting that information from the external, as well as the internal, environment is transduced by a variety of sensory systems before gaining access to the noradrenergic system. Moreover, some data suggest that the strength of a stimulus in a particular context is an important factor in determining the noradrenergic response [11-13]. Both electrophysiological and neurochemical studies (i.e., in vivo microdialysis) have shown that the brain noradrenergic system is phasically and robustly activated by a diverse array of acutely stressful stimuli [14-21].

3. Adrenergic catecholamines and memory storage

Strong memories are often based on experiences that were emotionally arousing [22]. There is a large body of evidence suggesting that stress hormones released by emotional experiences play an important role in mediating the effects of emotional arousal on lasting memory. There is now extensive evidence supporting the hypothesis that the strength of long-term memories is influenced by hormonal systems activated by experience [23, 24], i.e., memory formation may involve stress-released hormones as endogenous modulators of the neurobiological processes underlying memory consolidation.

Gold and van Buskirk [25] were the first to suggest the involvement of central NE in memory. Their study showed that inhibitory avoidance (IA) training increases brain NE levels under conditions that result in good retention, suggesting an enhanced release of this neuromodulator during training. In support of this view, Haycock et al. [26] showed that intraventricular infusion of NE facilitates retention, providing further evidence for the view that central NE function modulates memory. Other studies, e.g., those of Jensen et al. [27], reported that intracerebroventricular administration of diethyldithiocarbamate (DDC), a drug that decreases central catecholamine levels, impairs IA retention when administered post-training. Furthermore, concurrent infusion of NE into the ventricles or systemic injection of NE or epinephrine blocks the retention impairment produced by peripheral administration of DDC [28-30].

Further evidence suggesting that peripherally released catecholamines may influence memory consolidation came from experiments using amphetamines. Amphetamine is known to influence the release of catecholamines from peripheral storage sites [31]. Numerous studies [e.g. 32-34] have shown that amphetamine enhances memory when administered systemically either shortly before, or shortly after training. Enhancing effects of amphetamine have been observed in a variety of tasks, such as IA, active avoidance, discriminated avoidance, and appetitive discrimination [34-36]. Moreover, the fact that amphetamine enhances memory when administered post-training supports the view that it enhances retention by influencing memory storage processes. Since amphetamine crosses the blood-brain barrier, other studies have examined whether its memory-modulating effects involve influences on peripheral or central catecholamines. Post-training systemic injection of 4-OH amphetamine (an amphetamine derivative that does not cross the blood-brain barrier) was also found to enhance IA retention, whereas central injection of amphetamine was ineffective. The effects of systemic injection of amphetamine and 4-OH amphetamine do not seem to involve peripheral sympathetic neurons, the primary source of peripheral NE, as sympathetic denervation induced by 6-hydroxydopamine hydrobromide induced 24 hours before training does not attenuate the memory-enhancing effects of either drug. In contrast, adrenal demedullation, i.e., elimination of peripheral epinephrine, blocks the effects of both amphetamine and 4-OH amphetamine on memory for active avoidance and IA training [37].

More recently, Williams et al. [38] showed that the memory-enhancing effects of systemic injection of 4-OH amphetamine are blocked by the peripherally acting β-adrenoceptor antagonist sotalol. These findings provide strong support for the view that amphetamine influences memory storage, at least in part, through effects involving the release of peripheral epinephrine from the adrenal medulla.

Systemic administration of epinephrine also enhances retention in different tasks, including IA [39], multitrial avoidance [40], a one-trial appetitive task [41], and an aversively motivated discrimination task [42]. Epinephrine is effective when given immediately after training; moderate doses produce the greatest enhancement, larger doses being less effective or even impairing retention, and the doses of epinephrine found to enhance retention produce plasma epinephrine levels comparable to those found after IA training [43].

Retention enhancement induced by epinephrine is blocked by injection of the β-adrenoceptor antagonist propranolol, a drug that readily enters the brain [41] as well as by sotalol, a β-adrenoceptor antagonist that does not enter the brain [44]. Post-training administration of β-adrenoceptor agonists that enter the brain, including dipivefrin and clenbuterol, also enhances memory consolidation, and the memory enhancement induced by dipivefrin and clenbuterol is blocked by propranolol, but not by sotalol [44]. Moreover, the memory-enhancing effect of clenbuterol is selectively blocked by centrally, but not peripherally, acting β-adrenoceptor antagonists [45]. Although the use of systemic nonspecific antiadrenergic agents has clearly implicated NE in learning and memory, the results obtained by Introini-Collison and Baratti [45] indicate that the effects of epinephrine on memory storage are initiated by activation of peripheral β-adrenoceptors, but also involve activation of β-adrenoceptors in the brain.

4. Route of stress-induced brain activation: from the LC to higher brain structures

As epinephrine does not readily cross the blood–brain barrier [46], its effects on memory consolidation appear to be initiated, at least in part, by activation of β-adrenoceptors in the periphery. This conclusion is supported by the finding that sotalol, a β-adrenoceptor antagonist that does not readily enter the brain, blocks the enhancing effects of peripherally administered epinephrine on memory [44].

A large number of studies have suggested that the effects of epinephrine on memory are most likely mediated by activation of β-adrenoceptors located on vagal afferents. For example, anatomical data have provided evidence that the dorsal and ventral branches of the vagus nerve innervate the adrenal gland [47]. In another study, Niijima [48] showed that electrical stimulation of the adrenal nerve evokes action potentials in the vagus nerve. More recently, Miyashita and Williams [49], using electrophysiological recordings of vagus nerve activity, showed that systemically administered epinephrine produces a significant increase in vagal nerve firing that is blocked by concurrent administration of the β-adrenoceptor antagonist sotalol. These data clearly show that the effects of epinephrine on the brain are mediated, at least in part, by the activation of ascending fibers of the vagus nerve and that these effects of epinephrine on vagal neural discharge are mediated through influences on peripheral β-adrenergic receptors.

Information regarding somatosensory activity, including that induced by footshock, is transmitted by ascending vagal fibers to the nucleus of the solitary tract (NTS), a brainstem structure with a high population of noradrenergic neurons [50-52]. In response to vagal nerve activation, NTS neurons influence central noradrenergic activity through direct synapses on neurons in the LC. Vagal afferents send noradrenergic projections directly and indirectly via the LC to forebrain regions [53-55], including the amygdala [56, 57]. Moreover, the finding that intra-NTS infusion of the β-adrenoceptor antagonist propranolol [58] or inactivation of the NTS with lidocaine [59] prevents epinephrine enhancement of memory provides evidence that the NTS is part of a brain stem system that, together with the LC, enables epinephrine-induced memory enhancement. Taken together, these data suggest that central noradrenergic neurons arising in the NTS mediate the effects of peripheral physiological influences on memory consolidation. This implication is supported by evidence that post-training infusion of the local anesthetic lidocaine into the NTS impairs IA retention [59]. Moreover, injection of lidocaine into the NTS blocks the memory-enhancing effects of systemic post-training injection of epinephrine [55]. Thus, the NTS appears to be an interface between peripheral adrenergic activation and brain processes regulating memory consolidation.

5. The noradrenergic system of the amygdala is involved in modulating memory storage

The amygdala is principally responsible for fear and anxiety responses to threatening environmental stimuli, including the increase in activity of the sympathetic nervous system in response to threat [60-62]. The LC densely innervates the amygdala [63, 64] and, in particular, projects to the central and basal nuclei [65-68].

Activation of the LC by electrical stimulation or administration of drugs (e.g. yohimbine) results in increased anxiety [69-72], probably as a result of the potentiation of this excitatory pathway from the LC to the amygdala. In addition to a role in anxiety, the LC projection to the amygdala may also play a role in forming and retrieving emotional memories [73, 74]. Interestingly, level of arousal, which is highly correlated with LC activity, determines the likelihood of a memory being encoded and subsequently retrieved.

Moreover, microdialysis data have shown that acute stressful immobilization induces increased NE release in the stria terminalis [15, 78], an important amygdala NE afferent, and in the medial and central nuclei of the amygdala [75-77].

Although the first evidence suggesting the involvement of the amygdala in learning and memory was published over 65 years ago [79], it is only in recent years that the amygdala has become a central focus of inquiry in studies of learning and memory. There is now extensive evidence suggesting that it is involved in the effects of attentional and reward processes [80-82] and that it may be a locus of the neural changes underlying the acquired association of cues with emotional responses, especially the somatosensitive responses elicited by fearful stimuli [83-85]. In addition, there is a strong consensus that it is involved in mediating the effects of emotional arousal on memory.

Extensive evidence indicates that the effects of peripheral epinephrine on memory are mediated by influences involving noradrenergic activation of the amygdala. For example, post-training intra-amygdala infusion of the β-adrenoceptor antagonist propranolol blocks the memory-enhancing effects of systemically administered epinephrine [86, 87] and the retention deficits induced by post-training infusion of propranolol into the amygdala are attenuated by concurrent infusion of NE [88]. Additionally, post-training infusion of NE or the β-adrenoceptor agonist clenbuterol into the amygdala induces a dose-dependent enhancement of retention [89-91] and attenuates retention deficits induced by adrenal demedullation [87]. Together, these findings strongly suggest that the amygdala mediates the effects of epinephrine on memory storage and that the effects involve activation of β-adrenergic mechanisms.

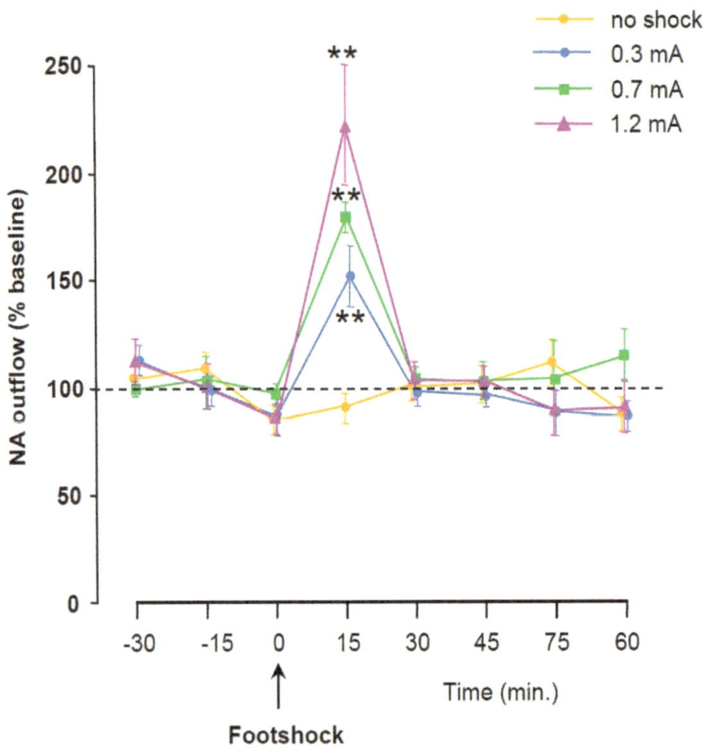

Figure 1. Effect of low- and high-intensity footshock on NE release in the amygdala assessed by in vivo microdialysis and HPLC. The data are shown as the mean (±SEM) NE levels expressed as a percentage of basal levels before footshock. **, $p < 0.01$ as compared to the no footshock group [94].

Studies using *in vivo* microdialysis and high performance liquid chromatography support these findings. The figure 1 illustrates one of the results we obtained in an experiment where a significant increase in NE levels was measured in the dialysis sample collected after exposure to footshocks of variable intensities. Other findings in our laboratory have shown that training conditions that evoke emotional arousal (e.g. footshock stimulation) or direct injection of epinephrine or corticosterone in doses that facilitate memory significantly increases NE release in the amygdala and this effect is directly related to the stimulus intensity [92-96].

Interestingly, it has been shown that the relative severity of the stressor and its physiologic impact can vary between individuals [93]. Thus, the severity of stress produced by a stimulus, whether physiologic or psychogenic, has typically been defined in terms of the magnitude of the physiological response it elicits, e.g., by measuring activation of the hormonal hypothalamic–pituitary–adrenal (HPA) stress axis or of the peripheral sympathoadrenal autonomic response system. Whereas the brief bursts of electrical activity elicited by distinct, innocuous stimuli occur over a period of 100's of milliseconds, phasic activation of noradrenergic neurotransmission by acutely stressful stimuli is much longer lasting, of the order of seconds to minutes or hours, depending on the stimulus, often outlasting the duration of the stimulus itself, and correlates temporally with peripheral physiological indicators of the stress response [77, 97].

For example, McIntyre et al. [98] examined NE release induced by IA training and, as expected on the basis of our previous studies of the effects of footshock stimulation [92, 94], found that NE levels were increased following training. However, in their study, perhaps somewhat surprisingly, the duration of the increased NE levels was greater than that previously found with footshock stimulation given without IA training [92, 94, 99]. Their findings suggest that the combination of footshock and the novel contextual information provided by training may have increased amygdala noradrenergic activation. Additionally, they showed that the extent of the increase in amygdala NE levels after training predicted the 24-h retention performance, as animals with a larger increase in NE release after training had longer retention latencies than those with smaller increases. These findings, taken together with those of studies of drug effects on NE levels, provide strong support for the hypothesis that NE release in the amygdala may play a critical role in modulating memory consolidation [100].

Studies using *in vivo* electrophysiological recordings in the cat also demonstrated that delivery of a footshock during IA training significantly increases the firing rate of lateral/basolateral amygdala neurons for 2 h following training [101]. These findings fit well with evidence that memory-modulating drugs can be effective when infused into the amygdala within hours after training [102]. Furthermore, NE release in the amygdala is potentiated by peripheral injection of epinehrine, the opiate antagonist naloxone, or amphetamine [94, 96, 103], findings consistent with evidence that intra-amygdala infusion of β-adrenoceptor antagonists blocks the effect of naloxone on memory storage [104, 105] and that opiate agonists inhibit the release of NE in other brain regions [106]. Moreover, the finding that inactivation of the NTS blocks the effects of systemic epinephrine injection on NE release in the amygdala supports the view that the noradrenergic fibers terminating in the amygdala may originate from soma in the NTS [95].

6. Different adrenoceptors in the basolateral amygdala are involved in memory storage modulation

Noradrenergic receptors on cells receiving an afferent input from the LC can be classified as α_1-, α_2-, or β-adrenoceptors. Activation of α_1-adrenoceptors by NE generally leads to excitation of the follower cells [107] and there is some evidence that β-adrenoceptors are also excitatory [108]. In contrast, activation of α_2-adrenoceptors leads to inhibition of the follower cells [107], and also of the noradrenergic neurones themselves ("autoreceptors"). The consequences of autoreceptor activation can be detected as changes in the firing rate of amygdala neurons and in the release of NE. Alpha$_2$-adrenoceptors are widely distributed in the brain [109, 110] and there are regional differences in their role in modulating NE release [111].

Several findings indicate that the memory-modulating effects of NE and other neuromodulatory and neurotransmitter systems are selectively mediated by the basolateral nucleus of the amygdala (BLA). The first series of experiments demonstrating a selective involvement of the BLA in memory storage showed that lesions of the BLA, but not of the central nucleus of the amygdala, block the memory impairment induced by systemic injection of benzodiazepines [112]. Furthermore, benzodiazepines infused into the BLA impair retention [113], whereas infusion of a benzodiazepine antagonist into the BLA enhances memory [114]. The findings of subsequent experiments suggested a selective involvement of the BLA in mediating noradrenergic influences on memory for many kinds of tasks [115, 116]. For example, Hatfield and McGaugh [117] showed that post-training infusion of NE into the BLA enhances memory for spatial learning in a water maze. In other studies, we found that infusion of the β-adrenoceptor agonist clenbuterol into the BLA enhances IA retention [119], whereas intra-BLA infusion of propranolol impairs memory of the same task [117].

Further studies demonstrated that NE in the BLA also interacts with glucocorticoids. Quirarte et al. (1997) showed that systemic injection of dexamethasone enhances IA retention when administered after training with a relative low footshock intensity and that infusion of a β1 or β2-adrenergic antagonist into the BLA, but not into the central nucleus of the amygdala, blocks the memory-enhancing effects of systemically administration of glucocorticoids (Fig. 2a). They also showed that the glucocorticoid receptor agonist RU 28362 dose-dependently increases IA retention performance when infused into the BLA and that this effect is blocked by post-training co-infusion of the β1-adrenoceptor antagonist atenolol into the BLA (Fig. 2b). These findings strongly suggest that β-adrenergic mechanisms in the BLA mediate the effects of epinephrine on memory storage and that β-adrenergic receptor activation in the BLA is required in order for glucocorticoids to modulate memory storage processes [118] (Fig. 2a and b).

Other findings indicate that α-adrenoceptors within the BLA are involved in the regulation of memory processes via an interaction with β-adrenergic mechanisms. Both α_1- and α_2-adrenoceptor subtypes are expressed at high levels in the amygdala [120, 121], though α_1-adrenoceptors predominate [122-127]. Thus, the tendency to impair IA retention that we

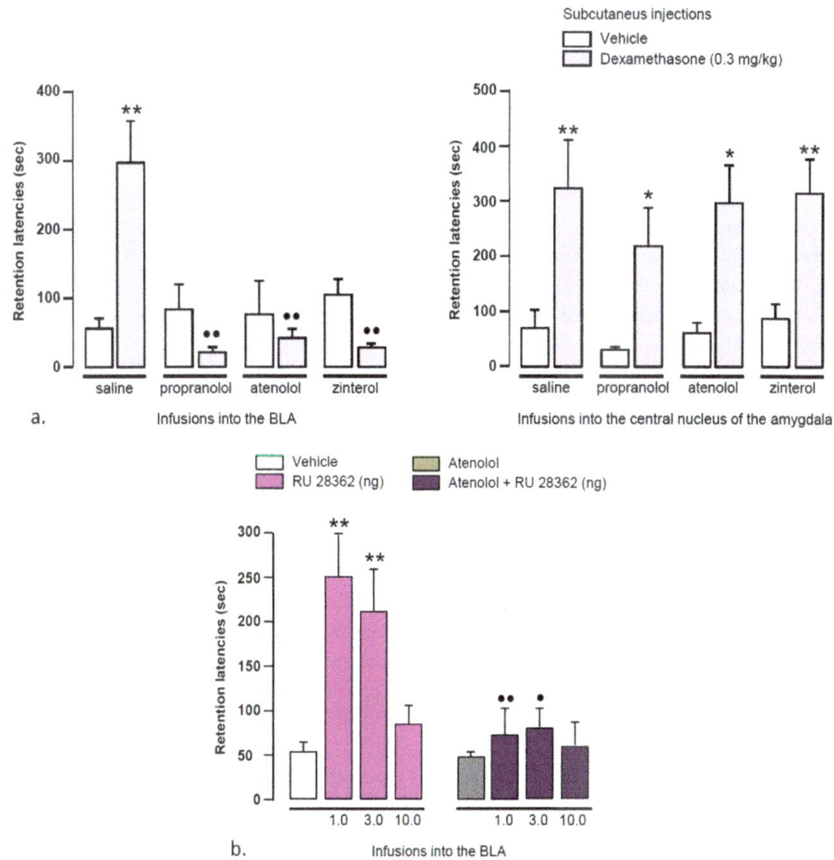

Figure 2. a. Inhibitory avoidance retention latencies of animals that received pretraining infusion of the nonspecific β-adrenergic antagonist propranolol (0.5 μg), the β_1-adrenergic antagonist atenolol (0.5 μg), or the β_2-adrenergic antagonist zinterol (0.5 μg) into the BLA or the central nucleus of the amygdala, followed by immediate post-training subcutaneous injection of dexamethasone (0.3 mg/Kg). The columns and bars show the mean (± SEM) latency in seconds. *, $p < 0.05$, **, $p < 0.01$ compared to the corresponding vehicle group; ••, $p < 0.01$ compared to the vehicle-dexamethasone group (n=8-14/group) [118].

b. Inhibitory avoidance retention latencies of animals that received concurrent administration of the glucocorticoid receptor agonist RU 28362 (1.0, 3.0, or 10 ng) and the β_1-adrenergic antagonist atenolol (0.5 μg) into the BLA. The columns and bars represent the mean (± SEM) latency in seconds. **, $p < 0.01$ compared to the vehicle group; •, $p < 0.05$; ••, $p < 0.01$ compared to the corresponding RU 28362 group (n = 9-13 per group) [118].

obtained in our series of experiments with post-training intra-BLA infusion of low doses of the nonselective α-adrenoceptor agonist phenylephrine [128] very likely resulted from a combined activation of α_1- and α_2-adrenoceptors. In order to clarify the role of each component of the α-adrenergic system in the BLA, we tested the effect of selective activation and/or blockade of these receptors in the BLA during IA training. Our results showed that post-training α_1-adrenoceptor inactivation using the selective antagonist prazosin impaired IA retention and that selective activation of α_1-adrenoceptors by infusion of a fixed concentration of the α_2-adrenoceptor antagonist yohimbine together with increasing concentrations of phenylephrine dose-dependently enhanced IA retention i.e., yohimbine reversed the tendency of phenylephrine to impair retention. Given the higher affinity of NE for α_2-adrenoceptors [151] and the fact that α_2-adrenoceptors are mostly located presynaptically [142], our results suggest that the IA memory impairing effects produced by phenylephrine alone are mainly due to presynaptic α_2-adrenoceptor activation [152]. This hypothesis is consistent with evidence that activation of presynaptic α_2-adrenoceptors blocks NE release [129 130].

The α_1-adrenergic influence on memory seems to be mediated by an interaction with β-adrenoceptors within the BLA. Indeed, intra-BLA post-training infusion of atenolol blocks the memory enhancement induced by selective activation of α_1-adrenoreceptors [128]. Moreover, we showed that intra-BLA infusion of the α_1-adrenoceptor antagonist prazosin right-shifts the dose-response effects of the β-adrenoceptor agonist clenbuterol when the two drugs are infused together into the BLA post-training [131]. These results suggest that α_1-adrenergic activity in the BLA facilitates the effects of β-adrenergic activation on memory formation. In a subsequent experiment, intra-BLA infusion of the synthetic cyclic adenosine monophosphate (cAMP) analog 8-bromo-cAMP was found to enhance retention in a manner similar to clenbuterol, but the effect induced by 8-bromo-cAMP was not affected by prazosin [131]. These findings are consistent with pharmacological evidence suggesting that β-adrenoceptors modulate memory storage by a direct coupling between Gs protein and adenylate cyclase and that α_1-adrenoceptors may act indirectly on this process by influencing the β-adrenergic-induced synthesis of cAMP [132-134].

As mentioned above, the amygdala contains α_2-adrenoceptors [125-127], which might be located on particular subsets of neurones involved in the autonomic response to stressful stimuli. In order to investigate the role of these receptors in memory for IA, we performed a series of experiments aimed at evaluating the effect of activation or blockade of these receptors in the BLA on IA retention processes. The behavioral data obtained in these experiments showed that bilateral microinfusion of the selective α_2-adrenoceptor antagonist idazoxan into the BLA immediately after training induces dose-dependent enhancement of retention performance of IA when tested 24 h later (Figure 3), whereas post-training intra-BLA infusion of the selective α_2-adrenoceptor agonist UK 14,304 induces dose-dependent impairment of retention performance (Figure 4).

These results are consistent with those of studies in which systemic injection of selective α_2-adrenergic drugs was found to disrupt and enhance consolidation of IA learning in the rat [136]. In addition, they fit with previous reports suggesting that the effects of peripheral administration of α_2-adrenergic compounds on learning and memory performance are mediated through a direct action on central NE release [136-139] and with previous results implicating amygdala α_2-adrenoceptors in footshock-based learning [140, 141]. Moreover, they clearly indicate that, in addition to involvement of α_1- and β-adrenoceptors, α_2-adrenoceptors in the BLA are involved in mediating the effects of training-induced or experimentally administered NE on memory storage [128, 131]. As pre-synaptic α_2-negative feedback is known to regulate NE release [142], including NE release in the amygdala [127, 129, 130, 140], the present findings provide additional evidence that memory consolidation is regulated by noradrenergic activation within the BLA.

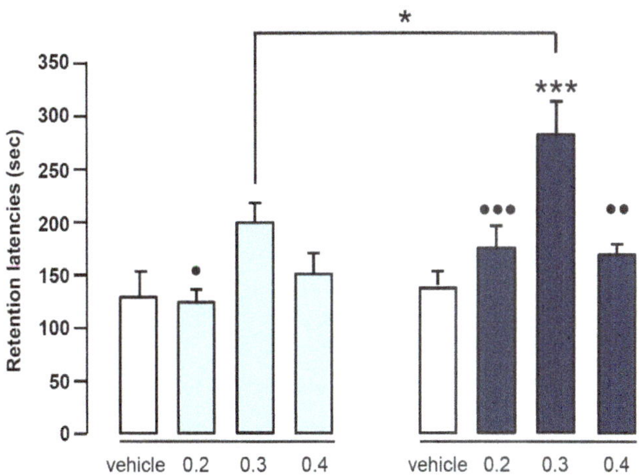

Figure 3. Effect of pre- or post-training infusion of various doses of idazoxan (a selective α_2-adrenoceptor antagonist) into the basolateral amygdala on inhibitory avoidance retention latencies. The columns and bars represent the mean ± SEM latency (in seconds) in entering the dark compartment during the retention test. The pre-training groups were infused 20 min before training, whereas the post-training groups were infused immediately after footshock administration. *, $p < 0.05$ compared to the corresponding value in the other group; ***, $P < 0.001$ compared to the vehicle-injected group; •, $p < 0.05$; ••, $p < 0.01$; •••, $p < 0.001$ compared to the value using 0.3 μg of idazoxan in the same group. n = 9–13 per group [135].

It is difficult to speculate when, and for how long, a single infusion of an adrenergic drug induces its effect on NE release, since the minimal time interval between sample collection using the microdialysis technique is about 15 min. However, the maximal effect of α_2-adrenergic drugs on NE release has been observed 30 min after infusion [143, 144]. Since the effect of α_2-adrenergic drugs on NE release in the brain and the effect of a footshock on NE release are both maximal after 30 min [98], it is likely that the effects of pre-training local injection of UK 14,304 or idazoxan into the BLA mainly results from binding to α_2-adrenergic autoreceptors, which regulate the stress-induced release of NE. The fact that retention latencies were only influenced by the highest dose of UK 14,304 [135 and Fig. 4] suggests that the pool of NE release induced by footshock within seconds or minutes after shock administration is sufficient to enable the conditioned stimulus (CS)-unconditioned stimulus (US) association. Our finding, shown in Fig. 4, that pre-training intra-BLA infusion of UK 14,304 or idazoxan induces effects on memory that are similar, but of a smaller amplitude, to those obtained in post-training groups suggests that, during IA, the α_2-adrenoceptor system in the BLA is more probably involved in very fine memory-modulated tuning control of IA consolidation, rather than in the encoding of CS-US association, as suggested previously [141]. The post-training effects are clearly consistent with the hypothesis that IA consolidation depends critically on the training-induced prolonged release of amygdala NE.

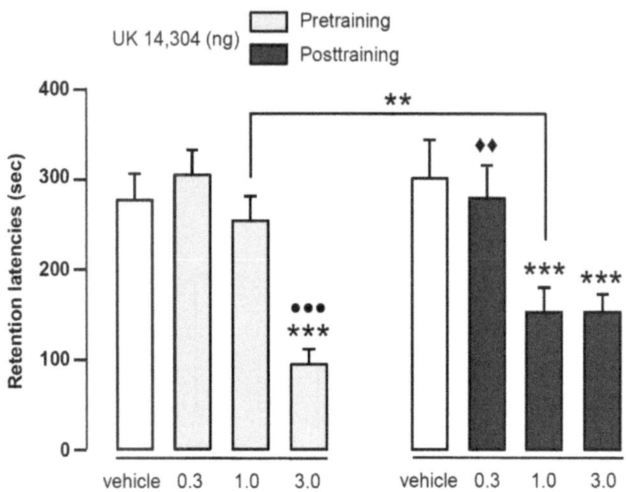

Figure 4. Effect of immediate post-training infusion of various doses of UK 14,304 (a selective α_2-adrenoceptor agonist) into the basolateral amygdala on inhibitory avoidance retention latencies. The columns and bars bars represent the mean ± SEM latency (in seconds) in entering the dark compartment during the retention test. The pre-training groups were infused 20 min before training, whereas the post-training groups were infused immediately after footshock administration. **, $p < 0.01$ compared to the corresponding value in the other group; ***, $p < 0.001$ compared to the vehicle-injected group; ●●●, $p < 0.001$ compared to the groups injected with 0.1 or 1.0 ng of UK 14,304; ♦♦, $p < 0.01$ compared to the groups injected with 1.0 or 3.0 ng of UK 14,304; $n = 9–12$ per group. [135]

In order to test this hypothesis, we investigated the effects of systemic and intra-BLA blockade or activation of α_2-adrenoceptors on the dynamics of NE in the BLA.

In the first study, anesthetized animals were microdialysed in the BLA while receiving systemic infusions of the α_2-adrenoceptor antagonist dexefaroxan or the α_2-adrenoceptor agonist UK 14,304. Results obtained in this study showed that dexefaroxan and UK 14,304 induced respectively a rapid and reversible significant increase and decrease, in NE levels in the BLA (Figure 5).

In a second study using retrodialysis, anesthetized animals received local infusion of dexefaroxan or UK 14,304 and the results showed that dexefaroxan induced a significant and reversible increase in NE levels in the BLA, whereas UK 14,304 caused a significant reduction (Figure 6).

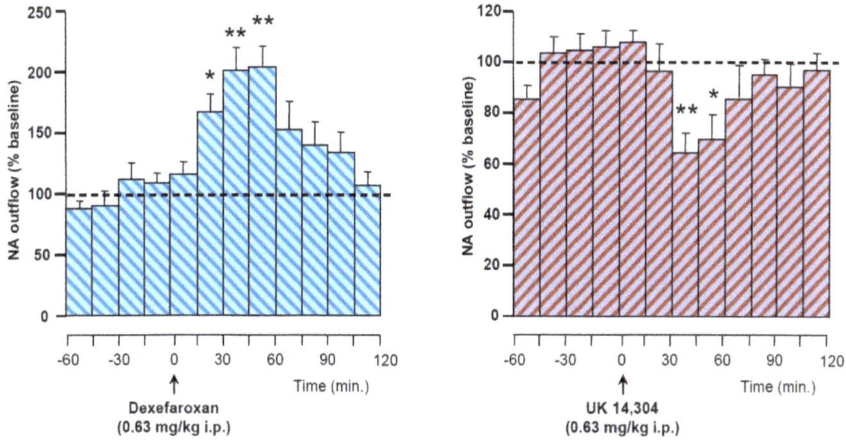

Figure 5. Effect of systemic α_2-adrenoreceptor blockade with the antagonist dexefaroxan (0.63 mg/kg) or activation with the agonist UK 14,304 (0.63 mg/kg) on NE levels in the basolateral amygdala in anesthetized animals assessed by in vivo microdialysis and HPLC. Norepinephrine levels are expressed as a mean (±SEM) value expressed as a percentage of basal levels; n = 7–9 per group. *, $p < 0.05$; **, $p < 0.01$ compared to baseline levels [145].

Our retrodialysis data indicate that drugs infused into the BLA post-training cause maximal NE release about 15 min after infusion. Moreover, this time interval has been described to be critical for the involvement of the amygdala during consolidation of IA [146, 147]. It is therefore likely that the enhancing and inhibitory effects caused, respectively, by post-training injection of idazoxan or UK 14,304 on IA retention were due to modulation of the prolonged training-induced increase in NE levels [98]. Additionally, and importantly, our findings are consistent with those of Pelletier et al. [101] showing that a single footshock increases the firing of neurons in the basolateral amygdala and that the increase peaks after 30 min, but remains high for 2 h.

In summary, our findings show that α_2-adenoreceptor-induced modulation of NE release during post-trial consolidation significantly influences IA retention performance. Providing additional evidence of the memory-modulating role of NE release in the BLA, they also suggest that α_2-adrenoceptors in the BLA are a critical component in the modulating influence of NE on IA memory consolidation and that the effect is probably due to a prolongation of the increase in training-induced levels of NE within the BLA. However, and in reference to previous results showing that NE activates three types of adrenoceptors, each involved in a different signaling pathway, a better understanding of the mechanisms by which NE in the BLA modulates the process of IA retention memory requires a detailed characterization of the signaling pathways downstream of NE binding. Indeed, NE activates β-, α_1-, and α_2-adrenoceptors, all of which are known to be metabotropic receptors. Beta-adrenoreceptors are associated with activation of the protein Gs, which activates adenylate cyclase, leading to production of cAMP, which then activates cAMP response

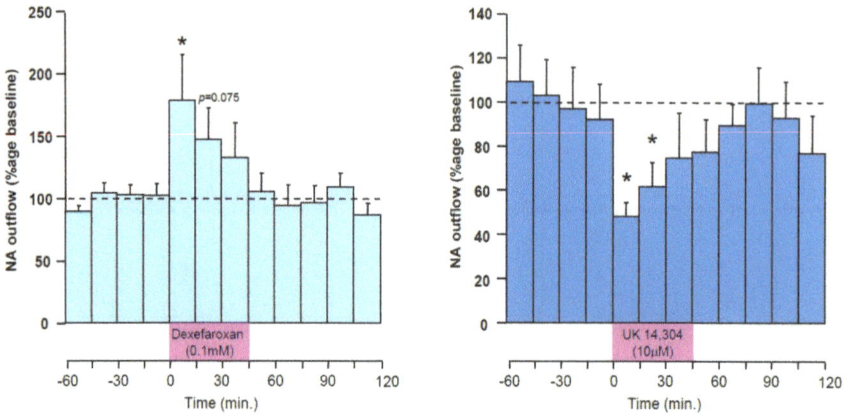

Figure 6. Effect of local α_2-adrenoreceptor blockade with the antagonist dexefaroxan or activation with the agonist UK 14,304 on norepinephrine levels in the basolateral amygdala in anesthetized animals assessed by in vivo retrodialysis and HPLC. Norepinephrine levels are expressed as the mean (±SEM) value expressed as a percentage of basal levels. n = 7-8 per group; *, $p < 0.05$ compared to baseline levels [145].

element-binding (CREB) protein. Alpha$_1$-adrenoceptors can mobilize calcium ions from intracellular stores, as well as increase calcium entry *via* voltage-gated calcium channels. Their stimulation leads to hydrolysis of membrane phospholipids *via the* G protein-mediated activation (Gq protein) of phospholipase Cβ and the resultant production of inositol triphosphate (IP3) induces α_1-adrenoceptor-elicited calcium release from intracellular stores, thereby increasing the cytosolic calcium concentration. The simultaneously produced diacylglycerol (DAG) activates protein kinase C (PKC) [148], which phosphorylates many cellular substrates, including membrane channels, pumps, and ion-exchange proteins. Alpha$_1$-adrenoceptors have also been reported to modulate other signaling pathways, resulting in increased accumulation of cAMP and cGMP, potentiation of cAMP responses elicited by the Gs-linked receptors, activation of phospholipase A2 and phospholipase D, activation of cAMP phosphodiesterase, adenosine release, and stimulation of arachidonic acid release [149]. Alpha$_2$-adrenoceptors are classically linked to Gi/o protein, with an action opposite to that of Gs, and act by inhibiting adenylate cyclase *via* a Gi protein and thereby inhibit cAMP production, while the $\beta\gamma$ subunits of Gi protein increase potassium ion conductance. Alpha$_2$-adrenoceptors also suppress voltage-activated calcium channels *via* Go protein, thus reducing the flow of extracellular calcium ions into target cells. Moreover, there is increasing evidence suggesting that α_2-adrenoceptors are linked not only to the activation of the Gi/o cascade, but also, for example, to the activation of phospholipase C (PLC) and PKC, at least in some cell types [150].

Although pharmacological data show that α_2-receptors have a higher affinity than α_1-receptors for NE and that both α_2- and α_1-receptors have a higher affinity for NE than β-receptors [151], little is known about the distribution of the three receptors subtypes within the BLA and further research is clearly needed to determine the signaling cascades initiated by the binding of NE to each of these subtypes linked to the various G proteins, which mediate the activation of specific signal transduction pathways.

A comparison of the differences and similarities between the three adrenoceptors in terms of specificity, signaling, and trafficking [152] would result in a better understanding of the dynamics of NE action on the intracellular cascade of event in the BLA leading to plastic changes underlying memory modulation of IA.

7. Conclusions

These studies indicate that adrenal stress hormones and the amygdala, especially the BLA, are involved in regulating memory consolidation. Because of its anatomical position, the amygdala is able to translate sympathetic arousal into synaptic plasticity that is distributed throughout the brain. Thus, the amygdala appears to be the core of the system involved in the physiological mechanisms promoting brain plasticity and rapid consolidation of memory for major events that drive and condition the survival of the animal. In our review, we suggest that the sympathetic response to a particular emotional or stressful event is driven along the peripheral nervous system by activating the β-adrenoceptor system on vagal afferents, which bridge the peripheral and central nervous systems by stimulating the NTS in the brainstem. As a result, adrenergic stimulation of vagal afferents that project to the NTS, induces activation of the NE system in forebrain structures either directly or indirectly via the LC onto which the NTS projects. It is therefore likely that activation of the vagal nerve will induce NE release in the amygdala through these two pathways.

The evidence that memory for various kinds of tasks is not lost when the amygdala is inactivated or lesioned [146,147,153,154] indicates that it is not the final storage site for emotionally arousing memories, but modulates memory storage in efferent brain regions [155, 156]. Indeed, several subsequent findings suggested that amygdala stimulation modulates memory consolidation and does so through influences mediated by amygdala efferents, and it has been shown that lesion of the stria terminalis, which carries both afferent and efferent projections of the amygdala, blocks the impairing effects of post-training electrical stimulation of the amygdala on memory [157]. In addition, stria terminalis lesions block the memory enhancement induced by post-training systemic injection of clenbuterol or intra-amygdala infusion of NE [89, 91]. These results strongly suggest that modulatory influences on memory involve projections from the amygdala to other brain regions. Consistent with this view, the amygdala shares extensive connections with cortical and subcortical regions implicated in memory storage processes [158-160]. Concerning this point, a large body of data shows that memory consolidation results from the direct interaction of the amygdala with many brain regions, including the nucleus accumbens [161, 162], insular cortex [163], entorhinal cortex [164, 165], rostral anterior cingulate cortex [166], and medial prefrontal cortex [167], and most extensively the hippocampus [168]. With regard to the dynamic interactions between the amygdala and limbic and temporal lobe structures in human and non-human animals, it has been suggested that emotional arousal-induced NE release in the amygdala will induce modulation of synapses in the target areas that are engaged in memory processing. Despite the growing literature on the memory-modulating role of the interaction between the amygdala and other brain regions, one must bear in mind that the present theoretical operating system is very simplistic, since memory is also modulated by the interaction between many neuromodulatory systems in the BLA. The roles of these latter interactions in memory modulation have been extensively documented and considered in recent reviews [155, 168, 169]. Very briefly, findings have shown that opioid peptides and gamma amino butyric acid both regulate NE release in the amygdala. Moreover, the acetylcholine and glutamate systems play a role in memory modulation at steps beyond the activation of β-adrenoceptors. The effects of glucocorticoids on memory consolidation are indirectly mediated by activation of the NTS and LC, both representing afferent NE projections to the amygdala, and directly by potentiating the noradrenergic signal cascade within the amygdala.

In summary, the epinephrine and NE systems, which rise, respectively from the vagus nerve and the NTS, to the amygdala, form a complicated network of critical mechanisms leading to the emergence of a memory-modulation process. Although this cannot be a complete representation, our data show that the memory-modulated role of NE is mediated differently by the various adrenergic receptors in the BLA, each of which is involved in a specific process. Eventually, through the activation of all of these systems, interacting inside and outside the amygdala, the strength of our emotional memories is determined by the weight of their emotional significance.

Author details

Barbara Ferry
Center for Research in Neuroscience, LYON (CRNL)
CNRS UMR 5292 - INSERM U 1028, University Claude Bernard, Lyon 1, France

Gina L. Quirarte
Behavioral and Cognitive Neurobiology Department, Institute of Neurobiology,
National Autonomous University of México, Campus Querétaro, Qro, México

Acknowledgement

We thank Norma Serafin for technical assistance and DGAPA-PAPIIT-UNAM (IN214111) and CONACYT 130524 for financial support.

8. References

[1] Bremner JD, Charney DS. The neurobiology of posttraumatic stress disorder: implications for treatment In: Darcourt G, Mendlewitcz J, Racagni G, Brunello N, eds.

Current Therapeutic Approaches to Panic and Other Anxiety Disorders. Monte Carlo: International Academy for Biomedical and Drug Research 1994:171-186.

[2] Bremner JD, Davis M, Southwick SM, Krystal JH, Charney DS. The Neurobiology of Posttraumatic Stress Disorder. In: Oldham JM, Riba MG, Tasman A (eds) Reviews of Psychiatry. Washington: American Psychiatric Press; 1993. p182-204.

[3] Charney DS, Deutch AY, Krystal JH, Southwick SM, Davis M. Psychobiologic mechanisms of posttraumatic stress disorder. Archives of General Psychiatry 1993;50(4):294-305.

[4] Chrousos GP, Gold PW. The concepts of stress and stress system disorders. Overview of physical and behavioral homeostasis. The Journal of the American Medical Association 1992;267(9):1244-1252.

[5] Woodward DJ, Moises HC, Waterhouse BD, Yeh HH, Cheun JE. Modulatory actions of norepinephrine on neural circuits. Advances in Experimental Medicine and Biology 1991;287:193-208.

[6] Aghajanian GK, Rogawski MA. The physiological role of α-adrenoceptors in the CNS: New concepts from single-cell studies. Trends in Pharmacological Sciences 1983;4(7):315-317.

[7] Jiang M, Griff ER, Ennis M, Zimmer LA, Shipley MT. Activation of locus coeruleus enhances the responses of olfactory bulb mitral cells to weak olfactory nerve input. The Journal of Neuroscience 1996;16(19):6319-6329.

[8] Waterhouse BD, Azizi SA, Burne RA, Woodward DJ. Modulation of rat cortical area 17 neuronal responses to moving visual stimuli during norepinephrine and serotonin microiontophoresis. Brain Research 1990;514(2):276-292.

[9] Woodward DJ, Moises HC, Waterhouse BD, Yeh HH, Cheun JE. The cerebellar norepinephrine system: Inhibition, modulation, and gating. Progress in Brain Research 1991;88:331-341.

[10] Aston-Jones G, Chiang C, Alexinsky T. Discharge of noradrenergic locus coeruleus neurons in behaving rats and monkeys suggests a role in vigilance. Progress in Brain Research 1991;88:501-520.

[11] Rasmussen K, Morilak DA, Jacobs BL. Single unit activity of locus coeruleus neurons in the freely moving cat .1. During naturalistic behaviors and in response to simple and complex stimuli. Brain Research 1986;371(2):324-334.

[12] Aston-Jones G, Rajkowski J, Cohen J. Role of locus coeruleus in attention and behavioral flexibility. Biological Psychiatry 1999;46(9):1309-1320.

[13] Aston-Jones G, Rajkowski J, Cohen J. Locus coeruleus and regulation of behavioral flexibility and attention. Progress in Brain Research 2000;126:165-182.

[14] Abercrombie ED, Jacobs BL. Single-unit response of noradrenergic neurons in the locus coeruleus of freely moving cats. I. Acutely presented stressful and nonstressful stimuli. The Journal of Neuroscience 1987;7(9):2837-2843.

[15] Cecchi M, Khoshbouei H, Javors M, Morilak DA. Modulatory effects of norepinephrine in the lateral bed nucleus of the stria terminalis on behavioral and neuroendocrine responses to acute stress. Neuroscience 2002;112(1):13-21.

[16] Morilak DA, Fornal CA, Jacobs BL. Effects of physiological manipulations on locus coeruleus neuronal activity in freely moving cats .2. Cardiovascular challenge. Brain Research 1987;422(1):24-31.
[17] Morilak DA, Fornal CA, Jacobs BL. Effects of physiological manipulations on locus coeruleus neuronal activity in freely moving cats .3. Glucoregulatory challenge. Brain Research 1987;422(1):32-39.
[18] Pacak K, Palkovits M, Kopin IJ, Goldstein DS. Stress-induced norepinephrine release in the hypothalamic paraventricular nucleus and pituitary-adrenocortical and sympathoadrenal activity: *In vivo* microdialysis studies. Frontiers in Neuroendocrinology 1995;16(2):89-150.
[19] Page ME, Akaoka H, Aston-Jones G, Valentino RJ. Bladder distention activates noradrenergic locus coeruleus neurons by an excitatory amino acid mechanism. Neuroscience 1992;51(3):555-563.
[20] Svensson TH. Peripheral, autonomic regulation of locus coeruleus noradrenergic neurons in brain: Putative implications for psychiatry and psychopharmacology. Psychopharmacology 1987;92(1):1-7.
[21] Valentino RJ, Foote SL, Page ME. The locus coeruleus as a site for integrating corticotropin-releasing factor and noradrenergic mediation of stress responses. Annals of the New York Academy of Sciences 1993;697:173-188.
[22] Christianson SV. Remembering Emotional Events: Potential Mechanisms In: Christianson SV (ed) The Handbook of Emotion and Memory: Research and Theory. Hillsdale, NJ: Lawrence Erlbaum Associates, Inc.; 1992. p307-340.
[23] Gold PE, van Buskirk RB, McGaugh JL. Effects of hormones on time-dependent memory storage processes. Progress in Brain Research 1975;42:210-211.
[24] Kety S. Brain Catecholamines, Affective States and Memory. In: McGaugh JL (ed) The Chemistry of Mood, Motivation and Memory New York Plenum Press; 1972. p65-80.
[25] Gold PE, van Buskirk RB. Posttraining brain norepinephrine concentrations: Correlation with retention performance of avoidance training and with peripheral epinephrine modulation of memory processing. Behavioral Biology 1978;23(4): 509-520.
[26] Haycock JW, Van Buskirk R, McGaugh JL. Effects of catecholaminergic drugs upon memory storage processes in mice. Behavioral Biology 1977;20(3):281-310.
[27] Jensen RA, Martinez JL, Vasquez BJ, McGaugh JL, McGuinness T, Marrujo D, et al. Amnesia produced by intraventricular administration of diethyldithiocarbamate. Society for Neuroscience; 1977; Anaheim, Cal; 1977. p. 235.
[28] McGaugh JL, Gold PE, Handwerker MI, Jensen RA, Martinez Jr JL, Meligeni JA, et al. Altering Memory by Electrical and Chemical Stimulation of the Brain In: Brazier MAB (ed) Brain Mechanisms in Memory and Learning: From the Single Neuron to Man. New York: Raven Press; 1979. p151-164.
[29] Meligeni JA, Ledergerber SA, McGaugh JL. Norepinephrine attenuation of amnesia produced by diethyldithiocarbamate. Brain Research 1978;149(1):155-164.
[30] Stein L, Belluzzi JD, Wise CD. Memory enhancement by central administration of norepinephrine. Brain Research 1975;84(2):329-335.

[31] Weiner N. Norepinephrine, Epinephrine, and the Sympathomimetic Amines. In: Gilman AG, Goodman LS, Rall TW, Murad F (eds) Goodman and Gilman's The Pharmacological Basis of Therapeutics. 7th ed. New York: MacMillan Publishing Company; 1985. p145-180.

[32] Doty BA, Doty LA. Facilitative effects of amphetamine on avoidance conditioning in relation to age and problem difficulty. Psychopharmacologia 1966;9(3):234-241.

[33] Martinez J, Joe L., Jensen RA, Messing RB, Vasquez BJ, Soumireu-Mourat B, Geddes D, et al. Central and peripheral actions of amphetamine on memory storage. Brain Research 1980;182(1):157-166.

[34] McGaugh JL. Drug facilitation of learning and memory. Annual Review of Pharmacology 1973;13:229-241.

[35] Evangelista AM, Gattoni RC, Izquierdo I. Effect of amphetamine, nicotine and hexamethonium on performance of a conditioned response during acquisition and retention trials. Pharmacology 1970;3(2):91-96.

[36] Krivanek JA, McGaugh JL. Facilitating effects of pre- and posttrial amphetamine administration on discrimination learning in mice. Inflammation Research 1969;1(2):36-42.

[37] Martinez JL, Vasquez BJ, Rigter H, Messing RB, Jensen RA, Liang KC, et al. Attenuation of amphetamine-induced enhancement of learning by adrenal demedullation. Brain Research 1980;195(2):433-443.

[38] Williams CL, Packard MG, Mcgaugh JL. Amphetamine facilitation of win-shift radial-arm maze retention: The involvement of peripheral adrenergic and central dopaminergic systems. Psychobiology 1994;22(2):141-148.

[39] Gold PE, Hankins L, Edwards RM, Chester J, McGaugh JL. Memory interference and facilitation with posttrial amygdala stimulation: effect on memory varies with footshock level. Brain Research 1975;86(23):509-513.

[40] Liang KC, Bennett C, McGaugh JL. Peripheral epinephrine modulates the effects of post-training amygdala stimulation on memory. Behavioural Brain Research 1985;15(2):93-100.

[41] Sternberg DB, Isaacs KR, Gold PE, McGaugh JL. Epinephrine facilitation of appetitive learning: Attenuation with adrenergic receptor antagonists. Behavioral and Neural Biology 1985;44(3):447-453.

[42] Introini-Collison IB, McGaugh JL. Epinephrine modulates long-term retention of an aversively motivated discrimination. Behavioral and Neural Biology 1986;45(3):358-365.

[43] McCarty R, Gold PE. Plasma catecholamines: Effects of footshock level and hormonal modulators of memory storage. Hormones and Behavior 1981;15(2):168-182.

[44] Introini-Collison I, Saghafi D, Novack GD, McGaugh JL. Memory-enhancing effects of post-training dipivefrin and epinephrine: Involvement of peripheral and central adrenergic receptors. Brain Research 1992;572(1-2):81-86.

[45] Introini-Collison IB, Baratti CM. Opioid peptidergic systems modulate the activity of β-adrenergic mechanisms during memory consolidation processes. Behavioral and Neural Biology 1986;46(2):227-241.

[46] Weil-Malherbe H, Axelrod J, Tomchick R. Blood-brain barrier for adrenaline. Science 1959;129(3357):1226-1227.

[47] Coupland RE, Parker TL, Kesse WK, Mohamed AA. The innervation of the adrenal gland. III. Vagal innervation. Journal of Anatomy 1989;163:173-181.

[48] Niijima A. Electrophysiological study on the vagal innervation of the adrenal gland in the rat. Journal of the Autonomic Nervous System 1992;41(1-2):87-92.

[49] Miyashita T, Williams CL. Epinephrine administration increases neural impulses propagated along the vagus nerve: Role of peripheral β-adrenergic receptors. Neurobiology of Learning and Memory 2006;85(2):116-124.

[50] Kalia M, Sullivan JM. Brainstem projections of sensory and motor components of the vagus nerve in the rat. The Journal of Comparative Neurology 1982;211(3):248-264.

[51] Schreurs J, Seelig T, Schulman H. β2-Adrenergic receptors on peripheral nerves. Journal of Neurochemistry 1986;46(1):294-296.

[52] Sumal KK, Blessing WW, Joh TH, Reis DJ, Pickel VM. Synaptic interaction of vagal afferents and catecholaminergic neurons in the rat nucleus tractus solitarius. Brain Research 1983;277(1):31-40.

[53] Ricardo JA, Koh ET. Anatomical evidence of direct projections from the nucleus of the solitary tract to the hypothalamus, amygdala, and other forebrain structures in the rat. Brain Research 1978;153(1):1-26.

[54] Williams CL, Jensen RA. Vagal Afferents: A Possible Mechanism for the Modulation of Memory by Peripherally Acting Agents. In: Frederickson RCA, McGaugh JL, Felten DL (eds) Peripheral Signaling of the Brain: Role in Neural- Immune Interactions, and Learning and Memory. Lewiston, NY: Hogrefe & Huber; 1991. p467-471.

[55] Williams CL, McGaugh JL. Reversible lesions of the nucleus of the solitary tract attenuate the memory-modulating effects of posttraining epinephrine. Behavioral Neuroscience 1993;107(6):955-962.

[56] Liang KC, Gold PE. Epinephrine Modulation of Memory: Amygdala Activation and Regulation of Long-Term Memory Storage. In: Gold PE, Greenough WT (eds) Memory Consolidation: Essays in Honor of James L McGaugh. Washington, DC: American Psychological Association; 2001. p165-183.

[57] Williams CL, Clayton EC. Contribution of Brainstem Structures in Modulating Memory Storage Processes. In: Gold PE, Greenough WT (eds) Memory Consolidation: Essays in Honor of James L McGaugh. Washington, DC: American Psychological Association; 2001. p141-163.

[58] Clayton EC, Williams CL. Adrenergic activation of the nucleus tractus solitarius potentiates amygdala norepinephrine release and enhances retention performance in emotionally arousing and spatial memory tasks. Behavioural Brain Research 2000;112(1-2):151-158.

[59] Williams CL, McGaugh JL. Reversible inactivation of the nucleus of the solitary tract impairs retention performance in an inhibitory avoidance task. Behavioral and Neural Biology 1992;58(3):204-210.

[60] Damasio AR. Emotion in the perspective of an integrated nervous system. Brain Research 1998;26(2-3):83-86.

[61] Kiernan JA. Barr's The Human Nervous System: An Anatomical Viewpoint. 8th ed. Baltimore: Lippincott, Williams & Wilkins; 2005.
[62] LeDoux J. Fear and the brain: where have we been, and where are we going? Biological Psychiatry 1998;44(12):1229-1238.
[63] Jones BE, Yang TZ. The efferent projections from the reticular formation and the locus coeruleus studied by anterograde and retrograde axonal transport in the rat. The Journal of Comparative Neurology 1985;242(1):56-92.
[64] Moore RY, Bloom FE. Central catecholamine neuron systems: Anatomy and physiology of the norepinephrine and epinephrine systems. Annual Review of Neuroscience 1979;2:113-168.
[65] Fallon JH, Koziell DA, Moore RY. Catecholamine innervation of the basal forebrain. II. Amygdala, suprarhinal cortex and entorhinal cortex. The Journal of Comparative Neurology 1978;180(3):509-532.
[66] Jones BE, Moore RY. Ascending projections of the locus coeruleus in the rat. II. Autoradiographic study. Brain Research 1977;127(1):25-53.
[67] Nieuwenhuys R. Chemoarchitecture of the Brain. New York: Springer-Verlag; 1985.
[68] Szymusiak R, Alam N, Steininger TL, McGinty D. Sleep-waking discharge patterns of ventrolateral preoptic/anterior hypothalamic neurons in rats. Brain Research 1998;803(1-2):178-188.
[69] Myers EA, Banihashemi L, Rinaman L. The anxiogenic drug yohimbine activates central viscerosensory circuits in rats. Journal of Comparative Neurology 2005;492(4):426-441.
[70] Redmond Jr. DE, Huang YH. New evidence for a locus coeruleus-norepinephrine connection with anxiety. Life Sciences 1979;25(26):2149-2162.
[71] Redmond Jr. DE, Huang YH, Snyder DR, Maas JW. Behavioral effects of stimulation of nucleus locus coeruleus in stump-tailed monkey Macaca arctoides. Brain Research 1976;116(3):502-510.
[72] Uhde TW, Boulenger JP, Post RM, Siever LJ, Vittone BJ, Jimerson DC, et al. Fear and anxiety: relationship to noradrenergic function. Psychopathology 1984;17 Suppl 3:8-23.
[73] Chen FJ, Sara SJ. Locus coeruleus activation by foot shock or electrical stimulation inhibits amygdala neurons. Neuroscience 2007;144(2):472-481.
[74] Sterpenich V, D'Argembeau A, Desseilles M, Balteau E, Albouy G, Vandewalle G, et al. The locus ceruleus is involved in the successful retrieval of emotional memories in humans. Journal of Neuroscience 2006;26(28):7416-7423.
[75] Cecchi M, Khoshbouei H, Morilak DA. Modulatory effects of norepinephrine, acting on alpha1 receptors in the central nucleus of the amygdala, on behavioral and neuroendocrine responses to acute immobilization stress. Neuropharmacology 2002;43(7):1139-1147.
[76] Pacák K, Palkovits M, Kvetnanský R, Fukuhara K, Armando I, Kopin IJ, Goldstein DS. Effects of single or repeated immobilization on release of norepinephrine and its metabolites in the central nucleus of the amygdala in conscious rats. Neuroendocrinology 1993; 57(4):626-33.

[77] Ma S, Morilak DA. Norepinephrine release in medial amygdala facilitates activation of the hypothalamic-pituitary-adrenal axis in response to acute immobilisation stress. Journal of Neuroendocrinology 2005;17(1):22-28.

[78] Pardon MC, Gould GG, Garcia A, Phillips L, Cook MC, Miller SA, et al. Stress reactivity of the brain noradrenergic system in three rat strains differing in their neuroendocrine and behavioral responses to stress: implications for susceptibility to stress-related neuropsychiatric disorders. Neuroscience 2002;115(1):229-242.

[79] Klüver H, Bucy PC. "Psychic blindness" and other symptoms following bilateral temporal lobectomy in Rhesus monkeys American Journal of Physiology 1937;119:352-353.

[80] Easton A, Gaffan D. Comparison of perirhinal cortex ablation and crossed unilateral lesions of the medial forebrain bundle from the inferior temporal cortex in the rhesus monkey: effects on learning and retrieval. Behavioral Neuroscience 2000;114(6):1041-1057.

[81] Everitt BJ, Cardinal RN, Hall J, Parkinson JA, Robbins TW. Differential Involvement of Amygdala Subsystems in Appetitive Conditioning and Drug Addiction. In: Aggleton JP (ed) The Amygdala: A Functional Analysis. 2nd ed. Oxford: Oxford University Press; 2000. p353-390.

[82] Gallagher M. The Amygdala and Associative Learning. In: Aggleton JP (ed) The Amygdala: A Functional Analysis. 2nd ed. Oxford: Oxford University Press; 2000. p391-423.

[83] Davis M. The Role of the Amygdala in Conditioned and Unconditioned Fear and Anxiety. In: Aggleton JP (ed) The Amygdala: A Functional Analysis. 2nd ed. Oxford: Oxford University Press; 2000. p213-287.

[84] LeDoux JE. The Amygdala and Emotion: A View Through Fear. In: Aggleton JP (ed) The Amygdala: A Functional Analysis. 2nd ed. Oxford: Oxford University Press; 2000. p289-310.

[85] Morilak DA, Barrera G, Echevarria DJ, Garcia AS, Hernandez A, Ma S, et al. Role of brain norepinephrine in the behavioral response to stress. Progress in Neuro-Psychopharmacology & Biological Psychiatry 2005;29(8):1214-1224.

[86] Liang KC, Chen LL, Huang TE. The role of amygdala norepinephrine in memory formation: Involvement in the memory enhancing effect of peripheral epinephrine. The Chinese Journal of Physiology 1995;38(2):81-91.

[87] Liang KC, Juler RG, McGaugh JL. Modulating effects of posttraining epinephrine on memory: Involvement of the amygdala noradrenergic system. Brain Research 1986;368(1):125-133.

[88] Gallagher M, Kapp BS, Musty RE, Driscoll PA. Memory formation: Evidence for a specific neurochemical system in the amygdala. Science 1977;198(4315):423-425.

[89] Introini-Collison IB, Miyazaki B, McGaugh JL. Involvement of the amygdala in the memory-enhancing effects of clenbuterol. Psychopharmacology 1991;104(4):541-544.

[90] Introini-Collison IB, Ford L, McGaugh JL. Memory impairment induced by intraamygdala β-endorphin is mediated by noradrenergic influences. Neurobiology of Learning and Memory 1995;63(2):200-205.

[91] Liang KC, McGaugh JL, Yao HY. Involvement of amygdala pathways in the influence of post-training intra-amygdala norepinephrine and peripheral epinephrine on memory storage. Brain Research 1990;508(2):225-233.
[92] Galvez R, Mesches MH, McGaugh JL. Norepinephrine release in the amygdala in response to footshock stimulation. Neurobiology of Learning and Memory 1996;66(3):253-257.
[93] McReynolds JR, Donowho K, Abdi A, McGaugh JL, Roozendaal B, McIntyre CK. Memory-enhancing corticosterone treatment increases amygdala norepinephrine and Arc protein expression in hippocampal synaptic fractions. Neurobiology of Learning and Memory 2010;93(3):312-321.
[94] Quirarte GL, Galvez R, Roozendaal B, McGaugh JL. Norepinephrine release in the amygdala in response to footshock and opioid peptidergic drugs. Brain Research 1998;808(2):134-140.
[95] Williams CL, Men D, Clayton EC, Gold PE. Norepinephrine release in the amygdala after systemic injection of epinephrine or escapable footshock: Contribution of the nucleus of the solitary tract. Behavioral Neuroscience 1998;112(6):1414-1422.
[96] Williams CL, Men DS, Clayton EC. The effects of noradrenergic activation of the nucleus tractus solitarius on memory and in potentiating norepinephrine release in the amygdala. Behavioral Neuroscience 2000;114(6):1131-1144.
[97] Jacobs BL, Abercrombie ED, Fornal CA, Levine ES, Morilak DA, Stafford IL. Single-unit and physiological analyses of brain norepinephrine function in behaving animals. Progress in Brain Research 1991;88:159-165.
[98] McIntyre CK, Hatfield T, McGaugh JL. Amygdala norepinephrine levels after training predict inhibitory avoidance retention performance in rats. European Journal of Neuroscience 2002;16(7):1223-1226.
[99] Hatfield T, Spanis C, McGaugh JL. Response of amygdalar norepinephrine to footshock and GABAergic drugs using in vivo microdialysis and HPLC. Brain Research 1999;835(2):340-345.
[100] McGaugh JL. Memory-a century of consolidation. Science 2000;287(5451):248-251.
[101] Pelletier JG, Likhtik E, Filali M, Pare D. Lasting increases in basolateral amygdala activity after emotional arousal: Implications for facilitated consolidation of emotional memories. Learning & Memory 2005;12(2):96-102.
[102] McGaugh JL, Roozendaal B. Drug enhancement of memory consolidation: historical perspective and neurobiological implications. Psychopharmacology 2009;202(1-3):3-14.
[103] Mesches MH, McGaugh JL. Effects of D-amphetamine on extracellular norepinephrine levels in the amygdala of freely moving rats as measured by in vivo microdialysis. Society for Neuroscience; 1991; New Orleans, Louisiana 1991. p. 1398.
[104] Introini-Collison IB, Nagahara AH, McGaugh JL. Memory enhancement with intra-amygdala post-training naloxone is blocked by concurrent administration of propranolol. Brain Research 1989;476(1):94-101.
[105] McGaugh JL, Introini-Collison IB, Nagahara AH. Memory-enhancing effects of posttraining naloxone: Involvement of beta-noradrenergic influences in the amygdaloid complex. Brain Research 1988;446(1):37-49.

[106] Arbilla S, Langer SZ. Morphine and beta-endorphin inhibit release of noradrenaline from cerebral cortex but not of dopamine from rat striatum. Nature 1978;271(5645):559-561.

[107] Jones BE. Activity, modulation and role of basal forebrain cholinergic neurons innervating the cerebral cortex. Progress in Brain Research 2004;145:157-169.

[108] Berridge CW, Waterhouse BD. The locus coeruleus-noradrenergic system: modulation of behavioral state and state-dependent cognitive processes. Brain Research 2003;42(1):33-84.

[109] Brown RE, Sergeeva OA, Eriksson KS, Haas HL. Convergent excitation of dorsal raphe serotonin neurons by multiple arousal systems (orexin/hypocretin, histamine and noradrenaline). The Journal of Neuroscience 2002;22(20):8850-8859.

[110] Hume SP, Lammertsma AA, Opacka-Juffry J, Ahier RG, Myers R, Cremer JE, et al. Quantification of *in vivo* binding of [^{3}H]RX 821002 in rat brain: Evaluation as a radioligand for central α_2-adrenoceptors. International Journal of Radiation Applications and Instrumentation Part B Nuclear Medicine and Biology 1992;19(8):841-849.

[111] Thomas DN, Nutt D, Holman RB. Regionally specific changes in extracellular noradrenaline following chronic idazoxan as revealed by *in vivo* microdialysis. European Journal of Pharmacology 1994;261(1-2):53-57.

[112] Tomaz C, Dickinsonanson H, Mcgaugh JL. Basolateral amygdala lesions block diazepam-induced anterograde amnesia in an inhibitory avoidance task. Proceedings of the National Academy of Sciences of the United States of America 1992;89(8):3615-3619.

[113] de Souza Silva MA, Tomaz C. Amnesia after diazepam infusion into basolateral but not central amygdala of Rattus norvegicus. Neuropsychobiology 1995;32(1):31-36.

[114] Da Cunha C, Roozendaal B, Vazdarjanova A, McGaugh JL. Microinfusions of flumazenil into the basolateral but not the central nucleus of the amygdala enhance memory consolidation in rats. Neurobiology of Learning and Memory 1999;72(1):1-7.

[115] Huff NC, Frank M, Wright-Hardesty K, Sprunger D, Matus-Amat P, Higgins E, et al. Amygdala regulation of immediate-early gene expression in the hippocampus induced by contextual fear conditioning. The Journal of Neuroscience 2006;26(5):1616-1623.

[116] LaLumiere RT, Buen TV, McGaugh JL. Post-training intra-basolateral amygdala infusions of norepinephrine enhance consolidation of memory for contextual fear conditioning. The Journal of Neuroscience 2003;23(17):6754-6758.

[117] Hatfield T, McGaugh JL. Norepinephrine infused into the basolateral amygdala posttraining enhances retention in a spatial water maze task. Neurobiology of Learning and Memory 1999;71(2):232-239.

[118] Quirarte GL, Roozendaal B, McGaugh JL. Glucocorticoid enhancement of memory storage involves noradrenergic activation in the basolateral amygdala. Proceedings of the National Academy of Sciences of the United States of America 1997;94(25):14048-14053.

[119] Ferry B, McGaugh JL. Clenbuterol administration into the basolateral amygdala post-training enhances retention in an inhibitory avoidance task. Neurobiology of Learning and Memory 1999;72(1):8-12.

[120] Unnerstall JR, Kopajtic TA, Kuhar MJ. Distribution of α_2 agonist binding-sites in the rat and human central nervous-system: Analysis of some functional, anatomic correlates of the pharmacologic effects of clonidine and related adrenergic Agents. Brain Research Reviews 1984;7(1):69-101.
[121] Zilles K, Qu M, Schleicher A. Regional distribution and heterogeneity of alpha-adrenoceptors in the rat and human central nervous system. Journal fur Hirnforschung 1993;34(2):123-132.
[122] Day HE, Campeau S, Watson SJ, Jr., Akil H. Distribution of α1a-, α1b- and α1d-adrenergic receptor mRNA in the rat brain and spinal cord. Journal of Chemical Neuroanatomy 1997;13(2):115-139.
[123] Domyancic AV, Morilak DA. Distribution of α1A adrenergic receptor mRNA in the rat brain visualized by in situ hybridization. The Journal of Comparative Neurology 1997;386(3):358-378.
[124] Papay R, Gaivin R, Jha A, McCune DF, McGrath JC, Rodrigo MC, et al. Localization of the mouse α_{1A}-adrenergic receptor (AR) in the brain: α_{1A} AR is expressed in neurons, GABAergic interneurons, and NG2 oligodendrocyte progenitors. Journal of Comparative Neurology 2006;497(2):209-222.
[125] Glass MJ, Colago EE, Pickel VM. Alpha-2A-adrenergic receptors are present on neurons in the central nucleus of the amygdala that project to the dorsal vagal complex in the rat. Synapse 2002;46(4):258-268.
[126] Rosin DL, Talley EM, Lee A, Stornetta RL, Gaylinn BD, Guyenet PG, et al. Distribution of alpha(2C)-adrenergic receptor-like immunoreactivity in the rat central nervous system. Journal of Comparative Neurology 1996;372(1):135-165.
[127] Talley EM, Rosin DL, Lee A, Guyenet PG, Lynch KR. Distribution of α(2A)-adrenergic receptor-like immunoreactivity in the rat central nervous system. Journal of Comparative Neurology 1996;372(1):111-134.
[128] Ferry B, Roozendaal B, McGaugh JL. Involvement of α1-adrenoceptors in the basolateral amygdala in modulation of memory storage. European Journal of Pharmacology 1999;372(1):9-16.
[129] Langer SZ. Presynaptic regulation of catecholamine release. Biochemical Pharmacology 1974;23(13):1793-1800.
[130] Starke K. Presynaptic Regulation of Release in the Central Nervous System. In: Paton DM (ed) The Release of Catecholamines from Adrenergic Neurons. Oxford Pergamon Press; 1979. p143-183.
[131] Ferry B, Roozendaal B, McGaugh JL. Basolateral amygdala noradrenergic influences on memory storage are mediated by an interaction between β- and α1-adrenoceptors. The Journal of Neuroscience 1999;19(12):5119-5123.
[132] Leblanc GG, Ciaranello RD. α-Noradrenergic potentiation of neurotransmitter-stimulated cAMP production in rat striatal slices. Brain Research 1984;293(1):57-65.
[133] Perkins JP, Moore MM. Characterization of adrenergic receptors mediating a rise in cyclic 3', 5'-adenosine monophosphate in rat cerebral cortex. Journal of Pharmacology and Experimental Therapeutics 1973;185(2):371-378.

[134] Schultz J, Daly JW. Accumulation of cyclic adenosine 3', 5'-monophosphate in cerebral cortical slices from rat and mouse: stimulatory effect of α- and β-adrenergic agents and adenosine. Journal of Neurochemistry 1973;21(5):1319-1326.

[135] Ferry B, McGaugh JL. Involvement of basolateral amygdala α2-adrenoceptors in modulating consolidation of inhibitory avoidance memory. Learning & Memory 2008;15(4):238-243.

[136] Chopin P, Colpaert FC, Marien M. Effects of acute and subchronic administration of dexefaroxan, an α(2)-adrenoceptor antagonist, on memory performance in young adult and aged rodents. Journal of Pharmacology and Experimental Therapeutics 2002;301(1):187-196.

[137] Abercrombie ED, Keller RW, Jr., Zigmond MJ. Characterization of hippocampal norepinephrine release as measured by microdialysis perfusion: pharmacological and behavioral studies. Neuroscience 1988;27(3):897-904.

[138] Thomas DN, Holman RB. A microdialysis study of the regulation of endogenous noradrenaline release in the rat hippocampus. Journal of Neurochemistry 1991;56(5):1741-1746.

[139] Zarrindast MR, Fazli-Tabaei S, Semnanian S, Fathollahi Y, Yahyavi SH. Effects of adrenoceptor agents on apomorphine-induced licking behavior in rats. Pharmacology Biochemistry and Behavior 2000;65(2):275-279.

[140] Fendt M, Koch M, Schnitzler HU. Amygdaloid noradrenaline is involved in the sensitization of the acoustic startle response in rats. Pharmacology, Biochemistry, and Behavior 1994;48(2):307-314.

[141] Schulz B, Fendt M, Schnitzler HU. Clonidine injections into the lateral nucleus of the amygdala block acquisition and expression of fear-potentiated startle. European Journal of Neuroscience 2002;15(1):151-157.

[142] Starke K. Presynaptic autoreceptors in the third decade: focus on alpha2-adrenoceptors. Journal of Neurochemistry 2001;78(4):685-693.

[143] Mateo Y, Meana JJ. Determination of the somatodendritic alpha2-adrenoceptor subtype located in rat locus coeruleus that modulates cortical noradrenaline release in vivo. European Journal of Pharmacology 1999;379(1):53-57.

[144] Van Gaalen M, Kawahara H, Kawahara Y, Westerink BHC. The locus coeruleus noradrenergic system in the rat brain studied by dual-probe microdialysis. Brain Research 1997;763(1):56-62.

[145] Ferry B, Chaussabel M, Lazarus C, Cassel JC. Alpha2-autoreceptors modulate norepinephrine release in the basolateral amygdala: A mechanism involved in inhibitory avoidance consolidation in the rat? Society for Neuroscience; 2010; San Diego, CA; 2010. p. 407.412.

[146] Bevilaqua LR, Ardenghi PG, Schroder N, Bromberg E, Schmitz PK, Schaeffer E, et al. Drugs acting upon the cyclic adenosine monophosphate/protein kinase A signalling pathway modulate memory consolidation when given late after training into rat hippocampus but not amygdala. Behavioural Pharmacology 1997;8(4):331-338.

[147] Izquierdo I, Quillfeldt JA, Zanatta MS, Quevedo J, Schaeffer E, Schmitz PK, et al. Sequential role of hippocampus and amygdala, entorhinal cortex and parietal cortex in

formation and retrieval of memory for inhibitory avoidance in rats. European Journal of Neuroscience 1997;9(4):786-793.

[148] Tanaka C, Nishizuka Y. The protein kinase C family for neuronal signaling. Annual Review of Neuroscience 1994;17:551–567.

[149] Jiao X, Gonzalez-Cabrera PJ, Xiao L, Bradley ME, Abel PW, Jeffries WB. Tonic inhibitory role for cAMP in alpha(1a)-adrenergic receptor coupling to extracellular signal-regulated kinases 1/2. Journal of Pharmacology and Experimental Therapeutics 2002;303:247–256

[150] Carr DB, Andrews GD, Glen WB, Lavin A. alpha2-Noradrenergic receptors activation enhances excitability and synaptic integration in rat prefrontal cortex pyramidal neurons via inhibition of HCN currents. Journal of Physiology 2007;584:437–450.

[151] Arnsten AF. Through the looking glass: differential noradenergic modulation of prefrontal cortical function. Neural Plasticity. 2000;7:133–146.

[152] Marzo A , Bai J, Otani, S. Neuroplasticity Regulation by Noradrenaline in Mammalian Brain. Current Neuropharmacology 2009;7(4):286-295.

[153] Parent MB, Avila E, McGaugh JL. Footshock facilitates the expression of aversively motivated memory in rats given post-training amygdala basolateral complex lesions. Brain Research 1995;676(2):235-244.

[154] Parent MB, West M, McGaugh JL. Memory of rats with amygdala lesions induced 30 days after footshock-motivated escape training reflects degree of original training. Behavioral Neuroscience 1994;108(6):1080-1087.

[155] McGaugh JL. The amygdala modulates the consolidation of memories of emotionally arousing experiences. Annual Review of Neuroscience 2004;27:1-28.

[156] McGaugh JL, Cahill L, Roozendaal B. Involvement of the amygdala in memory storage: Interaction with other brain systems. Proceedings of the National Academy of Sciences of the United States of America 1996;93(24):13508-13514.

[157] Liang KC, McGaugh JL. Lesions of the stria terminalis attenuate the enhancing effect of post-training epinephrine on retention of an inhibitory avoidance response. Behavioural Brain Research 1983;9(1):49-58.

[158] McDonald AJ. Topographical organization of amygdaloid projections to the caudatoputamen, nucleus accumbens, and related striatal-like areas of the rat brain. Neuroscience 1991;44(1):15-33.

[159] McDonald AJ. Organization of amygdaloid projections to the prefrontal cortex and associated striatum in the rat. Neuroscience 1991;44(1):1-14.

[160] Petrovich GD, Canteras NS, Swanson LW. Combinatorial amygdalar inputs to hippocampal domains and hypothalamic behavior systems. Brain Research Reviews 2001;38(1-2):247-289.

[161] LaLumiere RT, Nawar EM, McGaugh JL. Modulation of memory consolidation by the basolateral amygdala or nucleus accumbens shell requires concurrent dopamine receptor activation in both brain regions. Learning & Memory 2005;12(3):296-301.

[162] Setlow B, Roozendaal B, McGaugh JL. Involvement of a basolateral amygdala complex-nucleus accumbens pathway in glucocorticoid-induced modulation of memory consolidation. European Journal of Neuroscience 2000;12(1):367-375.

[163] Miranda MI, McGaugh JL. Enhancement of Inhibitory avoidance and conditioned taste aversion memory with insular cortex infusions of 8-Br-cAMP: Involvement of the basolateral amygdala. Learning & Memory 2004;11(3):312-317.
[164] Ferry B, Wirth S, Di Scala G. Functional interaction between entorhinal cortex and basolateral amygdala during trace conditioning of odor aversion in the rat. Behavioral Neuroscience 1999;113(1):118-125.
[165] Roesler R, Roozendaal B, McGaugh JL. Basolateral amygdala lesions block the memory-enhancing effect of 8-Br-cAMP infused into the entorhinal cortex of rats after training. European Journal of Neuroscience 2002;15(5):905-910.
[166] Malin EL, Ibrahim DY, Tu JW, McGaugh JL. Involvement of the rostral anterior cingulate cortex in consolidation of inhibitory avoidance memory: interaction with the basolateral amygdala. Neurobiology of Learning and Memory 2007;87(2):295-302.
[167] Roozendaal B, McReynolds JR, McGaugh JL. The basolateral amygdala interacts with the medial prefrontal cortex in regulating glucocorticoid effects on working memory impairment. The Journal of Neuroscience 2004;24(6):1385-1392.
[168] Roozendaal B, McGaugh JL. Memory modulation. Behavioral Neuroscience 2011;125(6):797-824.
[169] McIntyre CK, McGaugh JL, Williams CL. Interacting brain systems modulate memory consolidation. Neuroscience and Biobehavioral Reviews 2011;doi:10.1016/j.neubiorev.2011.11.001.

Chapter 9

The Insular Cortex and the Amygdala: Shared Functions and Interactions

Rodrigo Moraga-Amaro and Jimmy Stehberg

Additional information is available at the end of the chapter

1. Introduction

The Insular Cortex (IC) is a portion of the cerebral cortex folded deep within the lateral sulcus – in rodents surrounding the rhinal fissure - between the temporal and frontal lobes. The IC was first described by J.C. Reil in 1809 [1], after whom it received the name "the island of Reil". Historically, the IC has been mentioned with several names, including "the central lobe", "the fifth lobe", "intersylvian convolutions" and "intralobular gyri" (reviewed in [2]).

The most accepted subdivisions of the IC are the three regions described by Cecheto and Saper (1987) [3], based on the cytoarchitecture of its layers within the ventrodorsal plane. These include (1) the agranular insular cortex (AI) which surrounds the rhinal fissure and lacks a granular layer, (2) the dysgranular insular cortex (DI) which is located just dorsal to the rhinal fissure and contains a diffuse granular layer, and (3) the granular insular cortex (GI), situated just ventral to the secondary somatosensory cortex with a clear granular layer [3]. Each subdivision is believed to process particular sensory information. For example, the AI is believed to participate in nociceptive [4-6] and autonomic processing [3], the DI plays a role in gustatory processing [7, 8] and the GI has an important role in modulating visceral function [3].

In the rostrocaudal plane, subdivisions of the IC are still controversial. Several studies suggest at least two regions - one posterior and the other rostral. Within the rostral, two more subdivisions are usually described: the posterior rostral (sometimes called "central") and the anterior rostral.

In rodents, particularly in the rat, the IC runs along the rostral half of the rhinal fissure. There is, to date, no consensus on the exact location of the border between the IC and the perirhinal cortex, which runs along the caudal half of the rhinal fissure. The rostral end of the IC corresponds to 2 mm of the anterior rostral portion, which runs roughly anterior to the bregma – anterior to the genu of the corpus callosum. It is mostly agranular and usually subdivided into 2 strips: dorsal and ventral [9].

This anterior area is connected with the lateral frontal cortices and the motor thalamic nuclei [10] and receives projections mainly from the ventral part of the medial mediodorsal (MD), the parafascicular and central medial (CM) nuclei of the thalamus [11, 12], as well as with the motor-related amygdala regions [10], the locus coeruleus and the nucleus raphe magnus [4].

Posterior to this rostral agranular area is the central or posterior rostral portion, which includes the 3 main dorsoventral subdivisions described above [3].

The rat granular area is connected to the paraventricular [13], the visceral thalamic nucleus (the parvicellular division of the ventroposterior lateral nucleus of the thalamus, VPLpc; [3, 11]), the gustatory thalamic nucleus (the parvicellular part of the ventroposterior medial nucleus of the thalamus, VPMpc;[10]), the reticular nucleus [14], the sustantia innominata [15], the ventromedial parts of somatosensory thalamic nucleus (the ventroposterior medial thalamic nucleus; VPM, [10]), the posterior thalamic complex (Po), and the central medial nucleus (CM) of the thalamus [10, 16] as well as the medial parabrachial nucleus of the mesencephalon (PBN) and the nucleus of the solitary tract (NTS) [17-19]. Connections with the lateral hypothalamic area and the visceromotor regions in the brainstem including the vago-solitary complex have also been reported [17, 20, 21]. Cortically, it is connected with the primary somatosensory cortex (SI) and the secondary somatosensory cortex (SII), the infralimbic cortex [22], the caudate-putamen, the amygdala [23-27] and the bed nucleus of the stria terminalis (BNST, [19]).

The dysgranular area is connected to the paraventricular [13] and the gustatory thalamus (VPMpc; [3, 10, 28, 29]), the medial PBN, the rostral NTS [19, 21] reticular nucleus of the thalamus [30], the somatosensory secondary (SII; [23]), the basolateral and central nuclei of the amygdala [23, 29, 31], the BST [20] and the lateral hypothalamic area [29].

The more posterior part, which extends caudally from roughly 2 mm posterior to bregma [23], has been suggested to be involved in somatosensory functions, including pain [16, 32]. For a simplified scheme of IC connections, see **Fig. 1**.

2. Functions of the insular cortex

Following the reports on intraoperative recordings made by Penfield and colleagues showing that the IC is a viscerosensory and visceromotor region [33, 34], the old James–Lange theory of emotions was revived. The James–Lange theory of emotions states that "bodily changes follow directly the perception of the exciting fact… our feeling of the same changes as they occur is the emotion… we feel sorry because we cry… afraid because we tremble" [35]. In other words, our nervous system responds to emotional experiences with physiological changes (e.g., a rise in the heart rate and dryness of the mouth), primarily mediated by the autonomic system (e.g., sympathetic responses) and the hypothalamus-pituitary-adrenal axis. Emotions are the feelings that result from these physiological changes. Thus, the insula appears as a possible site where such autonomic responses and general bodily states are represented cortically at any given time.

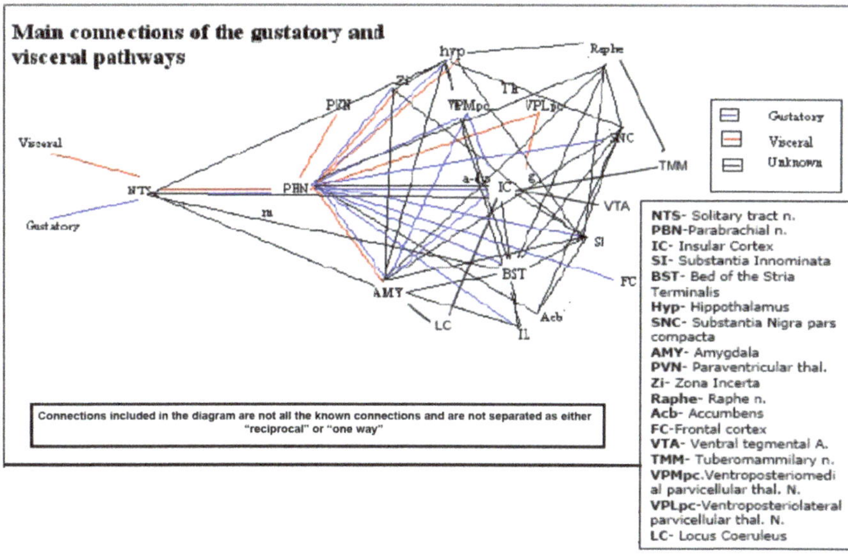

Figure 1. Anatomical connections of taste and visceral areas of the insular corex

Damasio's somatic marker hypothesis suggests that such ever changing representations of bodily states are required for decision making [36], stored in the insula and other somatosensitive areas [36-39] and triggered by the amygdala or prefrontal cortex (as primary or secondary inducers, [39]). Thus, congruent with both the James-Lange theory of emotions and Damasio's somatic marker hypothesis, the IC is believed to be the brain site where the representations of bodily states are created in response to emotional stimuli and which mediates interoceptive awareness and the subjective experience of feelings [38].

Support for this notion comes from a large number of recent studies in humans, monkeys and rodents, recently reviewed in [40]. Such studies include anatomical, electrophysiological, lesion, pharmacological and imaging studies, as well as operatory stimulation techniques which have yielded plausible roles for the IC in dozens of different functions. Several studies indicate that the IC is involved in taste processing [7, 8, 28, 41], viscerosensory information processing [3, 20, 26, 38, 42, 43], temperature and pain perception [44, 45], olfaction [46] auditory processing [47-49], somatosensory perception [49, 50], drug craving [51], motor tasks [52] and post-stroke motor-recovery functions [53].

Studies in humans have suggested a role for the IC in the ability to feel our own heartbeat [54, 55], negative emotional states including pain [56], social exclusion [57] positive emotional states [58, 59], empathy [60, 61], cognitive control tasks [62] and speech [62, 63-66]. All the above functions may have as a common denominator the IC as a possible correlate of awareness [66], while others have suggested that the role of the IC may be to respond to the perceived salience, novelty or unexpectedness of sensory events mediated by the representation of bodily reactions [67].

In spite of the fact that complex cognitive functions, speech and self awareness are associated with humans and non-measurable in rodents, when IC functional maps of rats and humans are compared, the similarities are striking. In fact, the rat and human insular cortices have common functional areas - as shown in Figure 2 - which suggests a degree of convergence in overall IC functions (compiled from: Rat IC [7, 16, 23, 32, 45, 46, 68-70]; Human IC [71-75]).

Insular dysfunction or hypofunction has also been associated with neurological disorders, such as frontotemporal dementia [76] and spatial neglect [77, 78], as well as with common neuropsychiatric disorders [79] such as schizophrenia [80, 81], depression [82, 83], autism [54, 84], eating disorders [85], anxiety [86, 87], Parkinson´s disease [88, 89] and addiction [90].

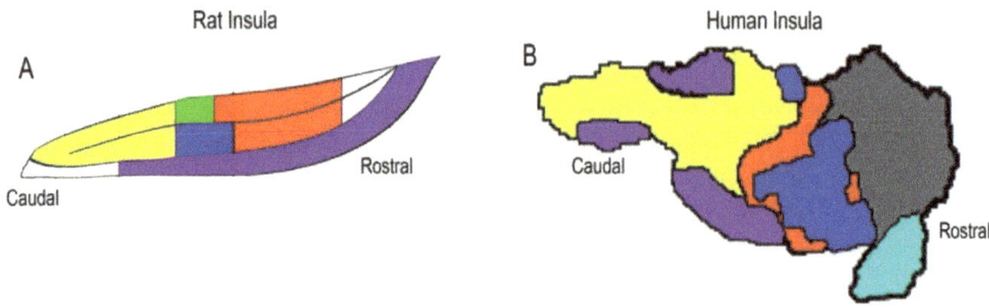

Figure 2. Functional organization of the rat (a) and the human (b) Insular Cortex. Green represents auditory related functions. Yellow represents somatosensory related functions. Purple represents pain associated functions. Red represents cardiac related functions. Blue represents taste related functions. Grey represents cognitive functions and Cyan represents social related functions.
Auditory (green), somatosensory (yellow), pain (purple), cardiovascular (red), taste (blue), cognitive (grey) and social (cyan) representations are shown within the insula.

3. The primary viscerosensory cortex within the insular cortex

Visceral sensory information reaches the IC from the lateral parabrachial nucleus, the nucleus of the solitary tract [18, 19, 21, 91] and the visceral thalamus (VPLpc) [68]. Although a clear map of the viscerosensory area of the IC is still missing, areas within both the dysgranular and granular cortices have been identified as viscerosensory responsive [3, 10, 19, 92-94]. In Cechetto and Saper (1987) [3], a viscerosensory area within the Insular cortex was reported while exploring from 2.0 mm anterior to 0.5 mm posterior to the crossing of the anterior commissure (around the bregma) in rats. They found the majority of the baroreceptor-responsive units between +1.00 and -0.5 mm. Yasui and colleagues [27] explored the rat left insula between 3 mm anterior to 1 mm posterior to bregma and found viscerosensory responsive neurons to aggregate 0.5 mm around the anterior commissure. Zhang and Oppenheimer [94] found responsive cells throughout the rat insular cortex, as far rostral as +2.0 mm and as posterior as -1.5 mm from the bregma, with rightward predominance. In contrast, Shi and Casell (1998) found responsive cells throughout the rat insular cortex, but with leftward predominance [10, 23].

Unlike the visceromotor infralimbic cortex, the IC is usually considered viscerosensory [42, 95, 96]. However, extensive evidence suggests that the IC may have direct motor functions. This idea is supported by major efferent projections from the IC to autonomic brain centres, including the lateral hypothalamic area, the parabrachial nucleus [20], the vago-solitary complex, the nucleus of the solitary tract [17, 21] and the central nucleus of the amygdala [24-27, 97, 98]. Yasui and colleagues [27] reported that intrainsular microstimulation of the rostral part of the DI-GI induced increased arterial pressure and tachycardia, while stimulation of the caudal part produced a reduction of arterial pressure and bradycardia. Other studies have reported that electrical stimulation of the IC in mammals (including humans, non-human primates, cats, dogs and rodents) elicits changes in blood pressure, heart rate and respiratory frequency, respiratory arrest, gastric and bowel motility, gastric and abdominal sensations, nausea and vomiting [34, 49, 98-105]. There is evidence suggesting that this effect is direct where identified visceral insular efferents are linked to the autonomic effects of insular electrical stimulation [106], while it has also been reported that the IC is the main projection site of the cardiovascular depressor sites of the lateral hypothalamic area [107].

The lateralization seen in electrophysiological studies has also been described after stroke models using middle cerebral artery occlusion (MCAO). Right MCAO-damage to the insula and adjacent frontoparietal cortex in rats, significantly increased blood pressure, renal sympathetic nerve activity and plasma norepinephrine levels was compared with left MCAO and controls [69, 108].

4. Taste–related behaviours

The rat, like all other mammals, displays an innate fear for novel tastes (neophobia, [109]). This spontaneous behaviour limits the consumption of novel food until the rat's brain assesses its gastrointestinal effects. Provided that the tastant does not become associated with toxicosis, the consumption will increase on subsequent exposures to that same taste (attenuation of neophobia, i.e., familiarity). If, however, the consumption of the novel tastant results in visceral malaise, robust aversion specific to that tastant develops (conditioned taste aversion - CTA). This is one of the most robust paradigms used to study learning and is called conditioned taste aversion (CTA) [110, 111]. In the laboratory, a malaise-inducing agent - usually LiCl i.p. - is used to induce transient malaise in controlled CTA training. After a single exposure to a novel taste (conditioned stimulus - CS) and the subsequent injection of LiCl (unconditioned stimulus - US), the animal associates the malaise with the taste and acquires an aversion to it.

In the case that the malaise follows the consumption of a familiar taste, the animal has to relearn that the familiar harmless taste is now associated with a malaise. This involves a process known as latent inhibition (LI - the decreased potency of a pre-exposed CS to be associated with an US) and produces, behaviourally, a lower aversion on a subsequent CTA to that taste [112-114].

A CTA memory can last for months if un-retrieved [115], but after repetitive exposures of the taste in the absence of the negative reinforcer, the animal relearns rapidly that the taste is not noxious and the memory is extinguished (experimental extinction [115-117]).

5. The gustatory system in the rat

Gustatory information arrives from taste buds to the rostral pole of the nucleus of the solitary tract (NTS) from cranial nerves VII, IX and X [118]. From the NTS, both taste and viscerosensory neurons project to the parabrachial nucleus in the pons (PBN) [118, 119]. Gustatory neurons arrive mainly to the medial PBN (mPBN) [120-122] and visceral neurons to the lateral part (latPBN) [3, 18, 118], with some overlap [123].

The PBN has been shown to be essential for the perception and learning of tastes (reviewed in [123]). Lesions on either the medial or lateral parts of the nucleus disrupt taste preference [120, 124], selective neophobia [125, 126], sodium appetite [127, 128] and CTA [121, 126-130].

From the mPBN the gustatory responsive neurons project to the gustatory thalamus (the VPMpc [3, 131]) and later reach the IC [3, 67, 132]. However, in contrast to other sensory systems (except olfaction) where sensory input reaches the thalamus before getting to the cortex, the gustatory system shows a direct connection between the mPBN and the IC that bypasses the thalamus [21]. The role of each of these connections remains unknown. Besides the PBN and the IC, the VPMpc sends and receives projections from the reticular nucleus of the thalamus [30] and from the amygdala [133], although the cells from the VPMpc that project to the amygdala are different to those that project to the IC [31]. There is still no consensus to date over the role of the VPMpc-IC or the VPMpc-amygdala pathways.

Lesion studies have not been able to shed light into the functions of the VPMpc. Some studies have reported that VPMpc-lesioned animals retain a normal concentration response to preferred and non-preferred tastes [134-137] but may have disrupted [137], impaired [127, 130] or else have no effects on CTA [134, 135, 138, 139]. Current views suggest a role in comparing novel and familiar tastes [140] in more complex gustatory learning tasks or in attention to gustatory function [135, 136, 141].

6. The primary taste cortex within the insular cortex

The gustatory area within the IC is localized in the dysgranular insular cortex [21, 29], roughly between the rhinal fissure and the medial cerebral artery (MCA) - an area that has also been identified in the rat as taste-responsive using intrinsic signal imaging [141] and electrophysiological recordings [7, 28, 69, 140, 142-144].

7. Role of the IC in taste function

Lesions of the IC produce no perceptual deficits [145, 146] or effects on taste discrimination to preferred tastes [146, 147]. Moreover, recent evidence suggests that IC lesions after CTA lead to the original preference of the taste [148], which implies that IC may not have a role in modulating the original taste preference.

Taste neophobia corresponds to the reluctance to try a novel food. IC lesions induce a consistent decrease in taste neophobia when the novel taste is presented in a familiar environment [146, 148-152]. As most studies so far have focused on taste memory, pharmacological interventions into the IC are performed only after taste presentation and very few - if any - pharmacological studies have investigated the neurotransmitters involved in taste neophobia per se.

When it comes to the role of the IC in taste familiarity, reports show an interesting duality. IC lesions appear to produce no effects on animals' capacity to attain taste familiarity [151], but several reports document a role for the IC in taste familiarity learning as a result of pharmacological manipulations [153, 154], showing that taste familiarity requires cholinergic activity in the IC [155, 156] but that it is independent of NMDA and AMPA channel activity [157-160]. Perhaps this dichotomy can be explained either by compensation from other areas after IC lesions or, given the role of neophobia discussed above, it is possible that IC output per se may modulate familiarity. In the last case, lacking a neophobic/novelty output may not affect familiarity, but altering such output pharmacologically may affect a familiarity trace processed elsewhere, possibly at the PBN.

8. Conditioned taste aversion

A large number of studies using transient pharmacological manipulations of the gustatory IC have shown that the IC has a role in CTA to novel tastes [117, 161], familiar tastes (also known as latent inhibition) [155, 162] and the extinction of CTA [115, 117]. Interestingly, IC lesions only partially affect CTA acquisition [145, 146, 148, 149, 163] but, when performed after CTA learning, IC lesions completely disrupt CTA memory retention [143, 145, 146, 164, 165] leading to the original preference for the taste [148]. This suggests that when an intact IC is present, it is not only involved in CTA acquisition and consolidation, but it may even be the site where CTA memories are stored (or else the capacity to retrieve them). The partial impairments seen when IC lesions are performed before CTA, on the other hand, suggest that such a seemingly crucial role for the IC in CTA can be compensated for when lacking IC. The area that can compensate for the lack of IC remains unidentified, although subcortical structures - including the PBN - have been proposed [166]. How can the IC be the site of memory acquisition and retention and yet be compensated almost completely? It is possible that the IC is part of a complex network of areas involved in aversive taste learning. A role for the amygdala in CTA acquisition (as will be discussed below), the redundancy seen in the direct PBN-IC, the PBN-VPMpc-IC and the PBN-amygdala-IC connections explained above, the possibility of attaining compensation from the olfactory system for the lack of taste proper and the possibility that IC lesions may induce unspecific taste aversion responses such as generalization, are some of the various possible hypotheses that have not been tested to date but which may explain this compensation.

When an animal with an intact IC is CTA trained, CTA memories (or the capacity to retrieve them) are stored in the IC. This role in storage appears to be non-time-dependent [146], unlike hippocampal-dependent learning systems where hippocampal involvement in memory retention lasts for a limited time only [167-171].

Determining whether IC lesions after CTA induce CTA retention deficits or a loss of the capacity to retrieve the memory is difficult to assess. Support for the idea that CTA memories are stored in the IC come from a complete lack of spontaneous recovery in several pharmacological and lesion studies, whereas support for the idea that the IC is involved in retention but not the storage of CTA memory comes from studies by Bermudez-Rattoni and colleagues, showing that foetal implants into the IC can recover the capacity to retrieve previously acquired CTA [172-173].

It must be kept in mind that the perception of flavour requires an interaction between smell and taste [174]. IC lesions have also been shown to impair both CTA learning and taste-potentiated odour aversion (POA) learning, suggesting that the IC may also have a role in the integration of odours, tastes and illness [147].

Congruent with animal studies showing a role for the IC in taste function and taste-odour integration, reports from humans show that electrical microstimulation of the gustatory IC induces changes in gustatory function [175, 176] as well as different olfactory sensations [34].

In conclusion, the IC is not involved in taste perception or basic discrimination. The fact that IC lesions after CTA render complete amnesia implies that an intact IC is crucial for CTA memory retention or retrieval. Pharmacological manipulations affecting CTA memory consolidation, reconsolidation, extinction and latent inhibition, suggest that the IC is also involved in CTA acquisition.

The evidence that IC lesions disrupt taste neophobia leading to the original preference of the taste but have no effect on taste familiarity, together with the fact that pharmacological manipulations of the IC affect familiarity and memory extinction, suggest a role for the IC in novelty and novelty-induced taste rejection. In fact, the IC has been suggested to be involved in reactions to the novelty and associative salience exclusive to taste stimuli [149].

A role for the IC in taste saliency and novelty is congruent with the majority of human studies reported for different IC functions, where a common denominator could be a role in the perceived salience, novelty or unexpectedness of sensory events mediated by the representation of bodily reactions [67], which could lead to self-awareness. In this sense, assuming that the output of the IC will eventually be turned into emotion, it is possible that the visceral and gustatory areas within the IC - together with other IC regions - create a bodily representation of taste perception, odour, autonomic responses, pain and somatosensory activation, visual and auditory stimulation, all of which are integrated to determine the salience of a given combination of sensory inputs and autonomic responses relevant to creating an emotion. One must keep in mind that at any given time a huge amount of sensory information flows to the cortex (visual, auditory, tactile, pain, proprioception, taste and smell) together with a huge amount of information from autonomic functions, most of which change constantly to maintain body homeostasis. Thus, the bodily representation required for an emotion needs to be filtered out to only the most salient, novel and relevant information.

9. The insula-amygdala network

Anatomically, the IC and the amygdala are closely connected, both directly and through their main outputs and inputs (see figure 1). There are massive reciprocal connections between the insular cortex and the amygdala [10, 23, 29, 177, 178] to all amygdalar subdivisions [179]. The ventral agranular insular area projects preferentially to the medial extended amygdala, while the viscerosensory and somatosensory portions of the insular cortex project preferentially to the central extended amygdala [180]. Furthermore, the amygdaloid projections from the posterior insular cortex appear to be organized in a feedforward parallel fashion targeting all levels of the intra-amygdaloid connections linking the lateral, basolateral and central nuclei [10, 23]. It must be noted that the PBN-insular cortex projections pass across the central nucleus of the amygdala [21]. Interestingly, Shi and Cassel (1998) [23] reported that cortical connections from the somatosensory secondary cortex to the IC may convey somatosensory information to the amygdala [23] and relay shock information to the BLA during fear conditioning [181].

All other main areas that are connected to the IC have reciprocal connections to the amygdala. The VPMpc projects to the amygdala [31, 132, 182] although the cells from the VPMpc that project to the amygdala are different from those that project to the IC [31]. The BNST also projects to the amygdala [20, 183], the LHA [20] and the PBN [18].

Within the PBN, the latPBN sends dense afferents to the central nucleus of the Amygdala (CeA) and more sparse afferents to the basolateral nucleus (BLA) and the lateral area (LAA), whilst the mPBN projects more densely to the BLA and LAA, but more scarcely to the CeA [18]. The lateral part of the BNST also receives inputs from the PBN and, from there, the BNST axons join those coming from the PBN and project together to the amygdala [18].

Other PBN subnuclei also project to both the IC and the amygdala. The externo-lateral PBN (elPBN) receives both gustatory and visceral inputs and projects with a calcitonin-gene related peptide (CGRP) into the insular cortex ([184] and to the amygdala ([27, 185]). CGRP microinjections into the amygdala induce fear-like behaviour in absence of aversive stimuli [186] as well as with increased heart rate and arterial pressure [187].

10. The role of the amygdala in taste function

The BLA has a crucial modulatory role in almost all memory tasks that include an emotion-arousing component. For Pavlovian fear conditioning, the BLA is not only the site where memory consolidation takes place but is also the site of long-term memory storage (for a review, see [188, 189]). As for other learning tasks, such as inhibitory avoidance or CTA, the BLA is not the site of memory storage but rather it modulates the memory consolidation of those memories stored in other brain regions (for reviews, see [190-192].

Dunn and Everitt (1988) [149] reported that BLA - but not CeA - lesions impair CTA. Furthermore, BLA lesions may impair taste neophobia [150] and arousal-induced taste neophobia, as well as passive avoidance [149]. Pharmacological BLA manipulations suggest a modulatory role in CTA after novel taste presentation, during visceral malaise and its association with the taste [193-197].

BLA stimulation affects IC neuronal responses [8] whereas BLA tetanic stimulation induces long-term potentiation in the ipsilateral IC [157, 158, 198]. Interestingly, induction of this long-term potentiation in the BLA–IC projection before CTA training enhances memory retention [199].

Other studies have suggested that CTA memory acquisition in the IC requires an intact BLA [200] and combined IC and BLA reversible or permanent lesions induce stronger CTA impairment than IC or BLA lesions alone [130, 193, 201-203].

Lesions in the BLA and LAA impair CTA moderately, but the combination of lesions of the VPMpc and the amygdala completely disrupts CTA [130, 204] and neophobia and induces weight loss [204]. Lesions of the amygdala have also been shown to produce the faster extinction of odour-taste (saccharin) association learning [205]. Moreover, transient pharmacological manipulations of the amygdala have been shown to impair CTA [140, 192, 206-208] and suggest that CTA consolidation depends upon protein synthesis and requires CREB and cfos activation in the CeA [192, 206, 207], whereas extinction depends upon protein synthesis in the BLA [192]. Interestingly, neither amygdalar nucleus is involved in CTA memory reconsolidation [140, 208], which probably suggests that the amygdala is involved in CTA acquisition but not in CTA memory storage.

Interactions of the amygdala with other brain regions have also been shown to be necessary for CTA. One study reported that lesions in the basal forebrain that deplete the neocortical innervation of acetylcholine (ACh), paired with lesions of the BLA, completely disrupt CTA, while each by itself may only impair learning [203, 209].

The amygdala has been well established as subserving fear and other emotional responses (reviewed in [188]). Together with other frontal cortical areas, it constitutes a major part of the so-called limbic system. Thus, it is possible that the role of the amygdala in taste function could be linked to the emotional and hedonic valence of gustatory stimuli in response to the salient bodily representation provided by the IC.

11. Other amygdalar functions shared by the IC

Ample evidence suggests that the amygdala can modulate memory consolidation in different memory systems through its many efferent projections to other brain regions [210]. Several reports show that the amygdala is involved in hippocampus-dependent (spatial or contextual) learning paradigms [211]. The basolateral complex of the amygdala (BLA; consisting of the lateral, basal and accessory basal nuclei) is critical for mediating the effects of stress on memory in several types of learning [212]. BLA also interacts with the IC in regulating taste neophobia [151, 20, 213] and, as mentioned earlier, CTA.

Interestingly, the IC has also been reported to be involved in the memory consolidation of inhibitory avoidance [214] and object recognition memory [215] - both learning systems that have been shown to be modulated by the amygdala [216, 217]. As stated at the beginning of this chapter, in humans insula activation has been correlated to processing threats and seeing emotional images in patients with anxiety disorders [218, 219], contextual fear conditioning [220], negative emotional states, including pain [56, 221], and positive emotions [58, 59]. Interestingly, all of the above conditions have also been reported to activate the amygdala [220-224]. As such, does the IC have shared functions with the amygdala? Do they interact?

12. Insular cortex and amygdala interactions

For learning and memory, extensive evidence suggests that the amygdala interacts with other brain regions, including the BNST, the nucleus basalis, the hippocampus and the entorhinal cortex (reviewed in [190, 225]).

In CTA, studies have shown that learning is modulated by interactions between the amygdala and the IC. Ferreira and colleagues (2005) showed that the glutamatergic activation of the amygdala enhances CTA, an effect that can be blocked by the glutamatergic blockage of the IC [226].

Interactions between the insular cortex and the amygdala have been hinted at in some human studies [227]. In one of these, the over-activation of both areas was reported in patients with anxiety disorder [219], while in another study the ventral agranular frontoinsula was shown to co-activate with the amygdala in social–emotional paradigms [38, 45, 52, 228].

As we have discussed before, IC activity has been correlated with several functions that also recruit amygdala activity. The fact that IC stimulation elicits cardiovascular responses is also not unique for the IC. In fact, electrical stimulation of the amygdala induces stress-related responses, including tachycardia and elevated arterial pressure as well as renal, intestine and skin vasoconstriction [229], while the stimulation of the CeA produces bradycardia, dilation of the pupils and movements of the mouth and tongue [230]. Furthermore, a study using single cell recordings of the amygdala in the cat reported that 46% of cells responded to carotid sinus nerve stimulation and that half of them responded to selective baroreceptor or chemoreceptor activation [231].

Other electrophysiological recordings have also shown that amygdala neurons respond to cardiovascular challenges. Cechetto and colleagues reported that over 23% of all recorded amygdala neurons responded to chemoreceptor activation and 16% to baroreceptor activation in cats [232]. In a different study, a cardiovascular pressure stimulus elicited predominantly inhibitory responses in one-half of amygdalar neurons. Most neurons in the central and basal nuclei responded to carotid chemoreceptor activation with excitation. Moreover, when testing responses to external sensory stimulation, 33% of recorded neurons responded to visual stimulation, 55% to acoustic, 39% to tactile and 59% to olfactory stimuli. Two-thirds of the neurons responded to more than one external sensory stimulus, demonstrating a convergence of sensory processing on single amygdalar neurons. Also, and as expected, 86% of recoded neurons responded to behavioural arousal [233].

So far, evidence seems to indicate that the IC and the amygdala share an enormous number of functions and properties. Although the idea that the IC is involved in creating bodily representations that are used by the amygdala to produce the correct emotional response is attractive, there is to date no real evidence that can distinguish the roles of either area.

Nevertheless, if we were to accept this model, where the role of the IC is to create and convey a bodily representation to the amygdala, which would be used to modulate and coordinate an emotional response to the stimulus, both the IC and the amygdala would be expected to receive direct autonomic and sensory information and to elicit cardiovascular responses. As such, the IC projections to the amygdala, together with the cortical connections from the somatosensory secondary cortex to the IC that convey somatosensory information to the amygdala [23], would relay the salient autonomic and sensory information needed to create an emotional response.

The mode and timing of the IC-amygdala interaction remains elusive and has not been the subject of much research. In an fMRI study in cats, depressor cardiovascular challenges produced a decline of signal-intensity in the right insula and increased signal intensity in the amygdala [234]. By way of contrast, Williams and colleagues reported using fMRI in humans such that the initial perception of fearful faces induced, first, increased activity in the insula, then a greater engagement of the medial prefrontal cortex and, finally, activity in the left amygdala [235]. Does the IC-Amygdala interaction imply synergic activation? Or does it imply inhibition? Is the IC expected to be activated before the amygdala? According to the data so far, the presence of massive feedforward excitatory projections and the electrophysiological studies commented on throughout this chapter suggest reciprocal excitatory connections. Furthermore, according to the IC´s bodily representation-amygdala´s emotional response model, IC activation should precede that of the amygdala. To date, there is no conclusive evidence as to how this interaction takes place. Nevertheless, it is clear that in order to understand emotions we need to comprehend how the two of its major participants interact.

Author details

Rodrigo Moraga-Amaro
Laboratorio de Neurobiología, Facultad de Ciencias Biológicas y Medicina, Universidad Andres Bello, Santiago, Chile

Jimmy Stehberg
Laboratorio de Neurobiología, Facultad de Ciencias Biológicas y Medicina, Universidad Andres Bello, Santiago, Chile
Centro de Investigaciones Biomédicas, Universidad Andrés Bello, Santiago, Chile

Acknowledgement

This chapter was supported by the Grant UNAB DI-02-11/N

13. References

[1] Reil J (1809) Die sylvische Grube. Arch. physiol. (Halle) 9: 195-208.
[2] Augustine J (1985) The insular lobe in primates including humans. Neurol. Res. 7: 2-10.

[3] Cechetto D, Saper C (1987) Evidence for a viscerotopic sensory representation in the cortex and thalamus in the rat. J. comp. neurol. 262: 27-45.

[4] Jasmin L, Rabkin S, Granato A, Boudah A, Ohara P (2003) Analgesia and hyperalgesia from GABA-mediated modulation of the cerebral cortex. Nature 424: 316–320.

[5] Burkey A, Carstens E, Wenniger J, Tang J, Jasmin L (1996) An opioidergic cortical antinociception triggering site in the agranular insular cortex of the rat that contributes to morphine antinociception. J. neurosci. 16: 6612–6623.

[6] Burkey A, Carstens E, Jasmin L (1999) Dopamine reuptake inhibition in the rostral agranular insular cortex produces antinociception. J. neurosci. 19: 4169–4179.

[7] Yamamoto T, Takahashi T, Kawamura Y (1981) Access to the cerebral cortex of extra-lingual taste inputs in the rat. Neurosci. lett. 24: 129-132.

[8] Yamamoto T, Yuyama N, Kato T, Kawamura Y (1984) Gustatory responses of cortical neurons in rats. I. Response characteristics. Neurophysiol. 51: 616-635.

[9] Krettek J, Price J (1978) Amygdaloid projections to subcortical structures within the basal forebrain and brainstem in the rat and cat. J. comp. neurol. 178: 225-254.

[10] Shi C, Cassell M (1998) Cortical, thalamic, and amygdaloid connections of the anterior and posterior insular cortices. J. comp. neurol. 399: 440-468.

[11] Groenewegen H (1988) Organization of the afferent connections of the mediodorsal thalamic nucleus in the rat, related to the mediodorsal-prefrontal topography. Neuroscience 24: 379-431.

[12] Ray J, Price J (1992) The organization of the thalamocortical connections of the mediodorsal thalamic nucleus in the rat, related to the ventral forebrain-prefrontal cortex topography. J. comp. neurol. 323: 167-197.

[13] Moga M, Weis R, Moore R (1995) Efferent projections of the paraventricular thalamic nucleus in the rat. J. comp. neurol. 359: 221-238.

[14] Stehberg J, Acuña-Goycolea C, Ceric F, Torrealba F (2001) The visceral sector of the thalamic reticular nucleus in the rat. Neuroscience 106: 745-755.

[15] Grove E (1988) Efferent connections of the substantia innominata in the rat. J. comp. neurol. 277: 347-364.

[16] Gauriau C, Bernard J (2004) Posterior triangular thalamic neurons convey nociceptive messages to the secondary somatosensory and insular cortices in the rat. J. neurosci. 24: 752-761.

[17] Shipley M (1982) Insular cortex projection to the nucleus of the solitary tract and brainstem visceromotor regions in the mouse. Brain res. bull. 8: 139-148.

[18] Saper C, Loewy A (1980) Efferent connections of the parabrachial nucleus in the rat. Brain res. 197: 291-317.

[19] Cechetto D, Saper C (1990) Role of the cerebral cortex in autonomic functions. In: Central Regulation of Autonomic Functions, edited by A. D. Loewy and K. M. Spyer. New York: Oxford Univ. pp. 208–223.

[20] Saper C (1982) Convergence of autonomic and limbic connections in the insular cortex of the rat. J comp. neurol. 210: 163-73.

[21] Shipley M, Sanders M (1982) Special senses are really special: evidence for a reciprocal, bilateral pathway between insular cortex and nucleus parabrachialis. Brain res. bull. 8: 493-501.

[22] Hurley K, Herbert H, Moga M, Saper C (1991) Efferent projections of the infralimbic cortex of the rat. J. comp. neurol. 308: 249-276.

[23] Shi C, Cassell M (1998) Cascade projections from somatosensory cortex to the rat basolateral amygdala via the parietal insular cortex. J. comp. neurol. 399: 469-491.

[24] van der Kooy D, McGinty J, Koda L, Gerfen C, Bloom F (1982) Visceral cortex: a direct connection from prefrontal cortex to the solitary nucleus in rat. Neurosci. lett. 33: 123-127.

[25] van der Kooy D, Koda L, McGinty J, Gerfen C, Bloom F (1984) The organization of projections from the cortex, amygdala, and hypothalamus to the nucleus of the solitary tract in rat. J. comp. neurol. 224: 1-24.

[26] Yasui Y, Itoh K, Mitani A, Takada M, Mizuno N (1985) Cerebral cortical projections to the reticular regions around the trigeminal motor nucleus in the cat. J. comp. neurol. 241: 348-356.

[27] Yasui Y, Breder C, Saper C, Cechetto D (1991) Autonomic responses and efferent pathways from the insular cortex in the rat, J. comp. neurol. 303: 355–374.

[28] Kosar E, Grill H, Norgren R (1986) Gustatory cortex in the rat. I. Physiological properties and cytoarchitecture. Brain res. 379: 329-341.

[29] Allen G, Saper C, Hurley K, Cechetto D (1991) Organization of visceral and limbic connections in the insular cortex of the rat. J. comp. neurol. 311: 1-16.

[30] Hayama T, Hashimoto K, Ogawa H (1994) Anatomical location of a taste-related region in the thalamic reticular nucleus in rats. Neurosci. res. 18: 291-299.

[31] Nakashima M, Uemura M, Yasui K, Ozaki H, Tabata S, Taen A (2000) An anterograde and retrograde tract-tracing study on the projections from the thalamic gustatory area in the rat: distribution of neurons projecting to the insular cortex and amygdaloid complex. Neurosci. res. 36: 297-309.

[32] Rodgers K, Benison A, Klein A, Barth D (2008) Auditory, somatosensory, and multisensory insular cortex in the rat. Cereb. cortex 18: 2941-2951.

[33] Penfield W, Rasmussen T (1950) The cerebral cortex of man. A clinical study of localization of function. New York: Macmillan.

[34] Penfield W, Faulk M Jr (1955) The insula; further observations on its function. Brain 78: 445–470.

[35] Ellsworth P (1994) William James and Emotion: Is a Century of Fame Worth a Century of Misunderstanding? Psychol. Rev. 101: 222-229.

[36] Damasio, A R (1994). Descartes' error: Emotion, reason, and the human brain. New York: Grosset/Putnam.

[37] Craig A (2002) How do you feel? Interoception: the sense of the physiological condition of the body. Nat. rev. neurosci. 3: 655–666.

[38] Critchley H (2005) Neural mechanisms of autonomic, affective, and cognitive integration. J. comp. neurol. 493: 154–166.

[39] Bechara A, Damasio A R (2005) The somatic marker hypothesis: A neural theory of economic decision. Games and Economic Behavior 52: 336–372.
[40] Nieuwenhuys R (2012) The insular cortex: a review. Prog. brain res. 195: 123-163.
[41] Krushel L, van der Kooy D (1988) Visceral cortex: integration of the mucosal senses with limbic information in the rat agranular insular cortex. J. comp. neurol. 270: 39-54.
[42] Yaxley S, Rolls E, Sienkiewicz Z (1990) Gustatory responses of single neurons in the insula of the macaque monkey. J. neurophysiol. 63: 689–700.
[43] Saper C (2002) The central autonomic nervous system: conscious visceral perception and autonomic pattern generation. Annu. rev. neurosci. 25: 433–469.
[44] Biemond A (1956) The conduction of pain above the level of the thalamus opticus. AMA Arch. neurol. psychiatry 75: 231-244.
[45] Ostrowsky K, Magnin M, Ryvlin P, Isnard J, Guenot M, Mauguiere F (2002) Representation of pain and somatic sensation in the human insula: A study of responses to direct electrical cortical stimulation. Cereb. cortex 12: 376-385.
[46] Kurth F, Zilles K, Fox P, Laird A, Eickhoff S (2010) A link between the systems: functional differentiation and integration within the human insula revealed by meta-analysis. Brain struct. funct. 214: 519-534.
[47] Bieser A (1998) Processing of twitter-call fundamental frequencies in insula and auditory cortex of squirrel monkeys. Exp. brain res. 122: 139–148.
[48] Bamiou D, Musiek E, Luxon, L (2003) The insula (Island of Reil) and its role in auditory processing. Literature review. Brain res. brain res. rev. 42: 143–154.
[49] Kimura A, Imbe H, Donishi T (2010) Efferent connections of an auditory area in the caudal insular cortex of the rat: anatomical nodes for cortical streams of auditory processing and cross-modal sensory interactions. Neuroscience 166: 1140-1157.
[50] Stephani C, Fernandez-Baca Vaca G, Maciunas R, Koubeissi M, Luders H (2011) Functional neuroanatomy of the insular lobe. Brain struct. func. 216: 137–149.
[51] Contreras M, Ceric F, Torrealba F (2007) Inactivation of the interoceptive insula disrupts drug craving and malaise induced by lithium. Science 318: 655-658.
[52] Mutschler I, Wieckhorst B, Kowalevski S, Derix J, Wentlandt J, Schulze-Bonhage A, Ball T (2009) Functional organization of the human anterior insular cortex. Neurosci. lett. 457: 66–70.
[53] Weiller C, Chollet F, Friston K, Wise R, Frackowiak R (1992) Functional reorganization of the brain in recovery from striatocapsular infarction in man. Ann. neurol. 31: 463–472.
[54] Di Martino A, Ross K, Uddin L, Sklar A, Castellanos F, Milham M (2009) Functional brain correlates of social and nonsocial processes in autism spectrum disorders: an activation likelihood estimation meta-analysis. Biol. psychiatry 65: 63–74.
[55] Xue G, Lu Z, Levin I, Bechara A (2010) The impact of prior risk experiences on subsequent risky decision-making: the role of the insula. Neuroimage 50: 709-16.
[56] Peyron R, Laurent B, Garcia-Larrea L (2000) Functional imaging of brain responses to pain. A review, meta-analysis. Neurophysiol. clin. 30: 263–288.
[57] Eisenberger N, Lieberman M, Williams K (2003) Does rejection hurt? An FMRI study of social exclusion. Science 302: 290–292

[58] Bartels A, Zeki S (2004) The neural correlates of maternal and romantic love. Neuroimage 21: 1155–1166.
[59] Jabbi M, Swart M, Keysers C (2007) Empathy for positive and negative emotions in the gustatory cortex. Neuroimage 34: 1744– 1753
[60] de Vignemont F, Singer T (2006) The empathic brain: how, when and why? Trends cogn. sci. 10: 435-441.
[61] Sterzer P, Stadler C, Poustka F, Kleinschmidt A (2007) A structural neural deficit in adolescents with conduct disorder and its association with lack of empathy. NeuroImage 37: 335–342.
[62] Cole M, Schneider W (2007) The cognitive control network: Integrated cortical regions with dissociable functions. NeuroImage 37: 343–360.
[63] Afif A, Minotti L, Kahane P, Hoffmann D (2010) Anatomofunctional organization of the insular cortex: A study using intracerebral electrical stimulation in epileptic patients. Epilepsia 51: 2305–2315.
[64] Ackermann H, Riecker A (2004) The contribution of the insula to motor aspects of speech production: a review and a hypothesis. Brain lang. 89: 320–328.
[65] Dronkers N (1996) A new brain region for coordinating speech articulation. Nature 384: 159-161.
[66] Craig A (2009) How do you feel—now? The anterior insula and human awareness. Nat. rev. neurosci. 10: 59–70
[67] Sterzer P, Kleinschmidt A (2010) Anterior insula activations in perceptual paradigms: often observed but barely understood. Brain struct. funct. 214: 611-622.
[68] Zhang Z, Oppenheimer S (2000) Baroreceptive and somatosensory convergent thalamic neurons project to the posterior insular cortex in the rat. Brain res. 861: 241-256.
[69] Ogawa H, Ito S, Murayama N, Hasegawa K (1990) Taste area in granular and dysgranular insular cortices in the rat identified by stimulation of the entire oral cavity. Neurosci. res. 9: 196-201.
[70] Butcher K, Hachinski V, Wilson J, Guiraudon C, Cechetto D (1993) Cardiac and sympathetic effects of middle cerebral artery occlusion in the spontaneously hypertensive rat. Brain res. 621: 79–86.
[71] Cechetto D, Shoemaker J (2009) Functional neuroanatomy of autonomic regulation. Neuroimage 47: 795-803.
[72] Henderson L, Rubin T, Macefield V (2011) Within-limb somatotopic representation of acute muscle pain in the human contralateral dorsal posterior insula. Hum. brain mapp. 32: 1592-1601.
[73] Kinomura S, Kawashima R, Yamada K, Ono S, Itoh M, Yoshioka S, Yamaguchi T, Matsui H, Miyazawa H, Itoh H (1994) Functional anatomy of taste perception in the human brain studied with positron emission tomography. Brain res. 659: 263–266.
[74] Mazzola L, Isnard J, Peyron R, Guénot M, Mauguière F (2009) Somatotopic organization of pain responses to direct electrical stimulation of the human insular cortex. Pain 146: 99-104.
[75] Small D (20120) Taste representation in the human insula. Brain struct. funct. 214: 551-561.

[76] Seeley W (2010) Anterior insula degeneration in frontotemporal dementia. Brain struct. funct. 214: 465-475.
[77] Karnath H, Fruhmann-Berger M, Kuker W, Rorden C (2004) The anatomy of spatial neglect based on voxelwise statistical analysis: a study of 140 patients. Cereb. cort. 14: 1164–1172.
[78] Manes F, Paradiso S, Springer J, Lamberty G, Robinson R (1999) Neglect after right insular cortex infarction. Stroke 30: 946–948.
[79] Nagai M, Kishi K, Kato S (2007) Insular cortex and neuropsychiatric disorders: a review of recent literature. Eur. psychiatry 22: 387–394.
[80] Fornito A, Yucel M, Patti J, Wood S, Pantelis C (2009) Mapping grey matter reductions in schizophrenia: an anatomical likelihood estimation analysis of voxel-based morphometry studies. Schizophr. res. 1081: 104–113.
[81] Wylie K, Tregellas J (2010) The role of the insula in schizophrenia. Schizophr. res. 123: 93-104.
[82] Schlund M, Verduzco G, Cataldo M, Hoehn-Saric R (2012) Generalized anxiety modulates frontal and limbic activation in major depression. Behav. brain funct. 9; 8:8.
[83] Koenigs M, Grafman J (2009) The functional neuroanatomy of depression: distinct roles for ventromedial and dorsolateral prefrontal cortex. Behav. brain res. 201: 239-243.
[84] Uddin L, Menon V (2009) The anterior insula in autism: underconnected and under-examined. Neurosci. biobehav. rev. 33: 1198–1203.
[85] Schienle A, Schafer A, Hermann A, Vaitl D (2009) Binge-eating disorder: reward sensitivity and brain activation to images of food. Biol. psychiatry 65: 654–661.
[86] Rotge J, Guehl D, Dilharreguy B, Cuny E, Tignol J, Bioulac B, Allard M, Burbaud P, Aouizerate B (2008) Provocation of obsessive-compulsive symptoms: a quantitative voxel-based meta-analysis of functional neuroimaging studies. J. psychiatry neurosci. 33: 405–412.
[87] Paulus M, Stein M (2006) An insular view of anxiety. Biol. psychiatry 60: 383-387.
[88] Tops M (2006) Are the insular cortex and cortisol implicated in Parkinsonian features? Parkinsonism relat. disord. 12: 467-471.
[89] Kaasinen V, Aalto S, Någren K, Rinne J (2004) Insular dopamine D2 receptors and novelty seeking personality in Parkinson's disease. Mov. disord. 19: 1348-1351.
[90] Naqvi N, Bechara A (2009) The hidden island of addiction: the insula. Trends neurosci. 32: 56–67.
[91] Norgren R, Wolf G (1975) Projections of thalamic gustatory and lingual areas in the rat. Brain res. 92: 123-129.
[92] Bagaev V, Aleksandrov V (2006) Visceral-related area in the rat insular cortex. Auton. neurosci. 125: 16-21.
[93] King A, Menon R, Hachinski V, Cechetto D (1999) Human forebrain activation by visceral stimuli. J. comp. neurol. 413: 572-582.
[94] Zhang Z, Oppenheimer S (1997) Characterization, distribution and lateralization of baroreceptor-related neurons in the rat insular cortex. Brain res. 760: 243-250.

[95] Hurley-Gius K, Neafsey E (1986) The medial frontal cortex and gastric motility: microstimulation results and their possible significance for the overall pattern of organization of rat frontal and parietal cortex. Brain res. 365: 241-248.

[96] Ongür D, Price J (2000) The organization of networks within the orbital and medial prefrontal cortex of rats, monkeys and humans. Cereb. cortex 10: 206-219.

[97] Ross D, Glick S (1981) Lateralized effects of bilateral frontal cortex lesions in rats. Brain res. 210: 379-382.

[98] Ruggiero D, Mraovitch S, Granata A, Anwar M, Reis D (1987) A role of insular cortex in cardiovascular function. J comp. neurol. 257: 189-207.

[99] Kaada B (1951) Somato-motor, autonomic and electrocorticographic responses to electrical stimulation of rhinencephalic and other structures in primates, cat, and dog; a study of responses from the limbic, subcallosal, orbito-insular, piriform and temporal cortex, hippocampus-fornix and amygdala. Acta physiol. Scand. suppl. 24: 1-262.

[100] Hoffman B, Rasmussen T (1953) Stimulation studies of insular cortex of Macaca mulatta. J. neurophysiol. 16: 343-351.

[101] von Euler U, Folkow B (1958) The effect of stimulation of autonomic areas in the cerebral cortex upon the adrenaline and noradrenaline secretion from the adrenal gland in the cat. Acta physiol. scand. 42: 313-320.

[102] Delgado J (1960) Circulatory effects of cortical stimulation. Physiol. Rev. suppl. 4: 146-178.

[103] Hoff E, Kell J Jr, Carrol M Jr (1963) Effects of cortical stimulation and lesions on cardiovascular function. Physiol. rev. 43: 68-114.

[104] Hall A, Moossa A, Skinner D (1977) Effect of 50% distal small bowel resection on gastric emptying in Rhesus monkeys. Ann. surg. 185: 214-218.

[105] Oppenheimer S (2006) Cerebrogenic cardiac arrhythmias: Cortical lateralization and clinical significance. Clin. aut. res. 16: 6–11.

[106] Cechetto D, Chen S (1990) Subcortical sites mediating sympathetic responses from insular cortex in rats. Am. j. physiol. 258: R245-255.

[107] Allen G, Cechetto D (1993) Functional and anatomical organization of cardiovascular pressor and depressor sites in the lateral hypothalamic area. II. Ascending projections. J. comp. neurol. 330: 421-438.

[108] Cechetto D, Wilson J, Smith K, Silver M, Hachinski V (1989) Autonomic and myocardial changes in middle cerebral artery stroke models in the rat. Brain res. 502: 296–305.

[109] Reilly S, Trifunovic R (1999) Gustatory thalamus lesions eliminate successive negative contrast in rats. Behav. neurosci. 113: 1242-1248.

[110] Bures J, Bermudez-Rattoni F, Yamamoto T (1998) Conditioned Taste Aversion. Oxford Psychology Series N#31. Oxford University Press.

[111] Welzl H, D'Adamo P, Lipp H (2001) Conditioned taste aversion as a learning and memory paradigm. Behav. brain res. 125: 205-213.

[112] Lubow R (1973) Latent inhibition. Psychol. bull. 79: 398-407.

[113] Weiss K, Brown B (1974) Latent inhibition: a review and a new hypothesis. Acta neurobiol. exp. (Wars). 34: 301-316.

[114] De la Casa G, Lubow R (1995) Latent inhibition in conditioned taste aversion: the roles of stimulus frequency and duration and the amount of fluid ingested during preexposure. Neurobiol. learn. mem. 64: 125-132.

[115] Berman D, Hazvi S, Stehberg J, Bahar A, Dudai Y (2003) Conflicting processes in the extinction of conditioned taste aversion: behavioral and molecular aspects of latency, apparent stagnation, and spontaneous recovery. Learn. mem. 10: 16-25.

[116] Rescorla R (1973) Effect of US habituation following conditioning. J comp. physiol. psychol. 82: 137-143.

[117] Berman D, Dudai Y (2001) Memory extinction, learning anew, and learning the new: dissociations in the molecular machinery of learning in cortex. Science 291: 2417-2419.

[118] Norgren R (1978) Projections from the nucleus of the solitary tract in the rat. Neuroscience 3: 207-218.

[119] Di Lorenzo P, Monroe S (1997) Transfer of information about taste from the nucleus of the solitary tract to the parabrachial nucleus of the pons. Brain res. 763: 167-181.

[120] Norgren R, Pfaffmann C (1975) The pontine taste area in the rat. Brain res. 91: 99-117.

[121] Reilly S, Grigson P, Norgren R (1993) Parabrachial nucleus lesions and conditioned taste aversion: evidence supporting an associative deficit. Behav. neurosci. 107: 1005-1017.

[122] Grigson P, Reilly S, Scalera G, Norgren R (1998) The parabrachial nucleus is essential for acquisition of a conditioned odor aversion in rats. Behav. neurosci. 112: 1104-1113.

[123] Hermann G, Rogers R (1985) Convergence of vagal and gustatory afferent input within the parabrachial nucleus of the rat. J. auton. nerv. syst. 13: 1-17.

[124] Reilly S (1999) The parabrachial nucleus and conditioned taste aversion. Brain res. bull. 48: 239-254.

[125] Reilly S, Trifunovic R (2000) Lateral parabrachial nucleus lesions in the rat: long-and short-duration gustatory preference tests. Brain res. bull. 51: 177-186.

[126] Corey D, Walton A, Wiener N (1978) Development of carbohydrate preference during water rationing: a specific hunger? Physiol. behav. 20: 547-552.

[127] Reilly S, Trifunovic R (2001) Lateral parabrachial nucleus lesions in the rat: neophobia and conditioned taste aversion. Brain res. bull. 55: 359-366.

[128] Flynn F, Grill H, Schulkin J, Norgren R. (1991a) Central gustatory lesions: II. Effects on sodium appetite, taste aversion learning, and feeding behaviors. behav. neurosci. 105: 944-954.

[129] Flynn F, Grill H, Schwartz G, Norgren R (1991b) Central gustatory lesions: I. Preference and taste reactivity tests. Behav. neurosci. 105: 933-943.

[130] Yamamoto T, Fujimoto Y, Shimura T, Sakai N (1995) Conditioned taste aversion in rats with excitotoxic brain lesions. Neurosci. res. 22: 31-49.

[131] Bester H, Bourgeais L, Villanueva L. Besson, M, Bernard F (1999) Differential projections to the intralaminar and gustatory thalamus from the parabrachial area: A PHA-L study in the rat. J. comp. neurol. 405: 421–449.

[132] Norgren R, Leonard C (1973) Ascending central gustatory pathways. J. comp. neurol. 150: 217-237.

[133] Yasui Y, Itoh K, Mizuno N (1984) Projections from the parvocellular part of the posteromedial ventral nucleus of the thalamus to the lateral amygdaloid nucleus in the cat. Brain res. 292: 151-155.

[134] Scalera G, Grigson P, Norgren R (1997) Gustatory functions, sodium appetite, and conditioned taste aversion survive excitotoxic lesions of the thalamic taste area. Behav. neurosci. 111: 633-645.

[135] Reilly S, Pritchard T (1996) Gustatory thalamus lesions in the rat: II. Aversive and appetitive taste conditioning. Behav. neurosci. 110: 746-759.

[136] Reilly S, Pritchard T (1997) Gustatory Thalamus Lesions in the Rat: III. Simultaneous Contrast and Autoshaping. Physiol. behav. 62: 1355–1363.

[137] Lasiter P (1985) Thalamocortical relations in taste aversion learning: II. Involvement of the medial ventrobasal thalamic complex in taste aversion learning. Behav. neurosci. 99: 477-495.

[138] Reilly S, Bornovalova M, Dengler C, Trifunovic R (2003) Effects of excitotoxic lesions of the gustatory thalamus on latent inhibition and blocking of conditioned taste aversion in rats. Brain res. bull. 62: 117–128.

[139] Grigson P, Lyuboslavsky P, Tanase D (2000) Bilateral lesions of the gustatory thalamus disrupt morphine- but not LiCl-induced intake suppression in rats: evidence against the conditioned taste aversion hypothesis. Brain res. 858: 327–337.

[140] Bahar A, Dudai Y, Ahissar E (2004) Neural signature of taste familiarity in the gustatory cortex of the freely behaving rat. J. neurophysiol. 92: 3298-3308.

[141] Reilly S, Bornovalova M, Trifunovic R (2004) Excitotoxic lesions of the gustatory thalamus spare simultaneous contrast effects but eliminate anticipatory negative contrast: evidence against a memory deficit. Behav. neurosci. 118: 365-376.

[142] Accolla R, Bathellier B, Petersen C, Carleton A (2007) Differential spatial representation of taste modalities in the rat gustatory cortex. J. neurosci. 27: 1396-1404

[143] Yamamoto T, Matsuo R, Kawamura Y (1980) Localization of cortical gustatory area in rats and its role in taste discrimination. J. neurophysiol. 44:440-455.

[144] Yamamoto T, Yuyama N, Kato T, Kawamura Y (1985) Gustatory responses of cortical neurons in rats. III. Neural and behavioral measures compared. J. neurophysiol. 53: 1370-1386.

[145] Kiefer S, Orr M (1992) Taste avoidance, but not aversion, learning in rats lacking gustatory cortex. Behav. neurosci. 106: 140-146.

[146] Stehberg J, Simon F (2011) Involvement of the insular cortex in retention of conditioned taste aversion is not time dependent. Neurobiol. learn. mem. 95: 14-8.

[147] Lasiter P, Deems D, Oetting R, Garcia J (1985) Taste discriminations in rats lacking anterior insular gustatory neocortex. Physiol. behav. 35: 277-285.

[148] Stehberg J, Moraga-Amaro R, Simon F (2011) The role of the insular cortex in taste function. Neurobiol. learn. mem. 96: 130-135.

[149] Dunn L, Everitt B (1988) Double dissociations of the effects of amygdala and insular cortex lesions on conditioned taste aversion, passive avoidance, and neophobia in the rat using the excitotoxin ibotenic acid. Behav. neurosci. 102: 3-23.

[150] Lin J, Roman C, St. Andre J, Reilly S (2009) Taste, olfactory and trigeminal neophobia in rats with forebrain lesions. Brain res. 1251: 195–203.
[151] Roman C, Reilly S (2007) Effects of insular cortex lesions on conditioned taste aversion and latent inhibition in the rat. Eur J. neurosci. 26: 2627-2632.
[152] Roman C, Lin J, Reilly S (2009) Conditioned taste aversion and latent inhibition following extensive taste preexposure in rats with insular cortex lesions. Brain res. 1259: 68-73.
[153] Gutierrez R, Rodriguez-Ortiz C, De La Cruz V, Nunez-Jaramillo L, Bermudez-Rattoni F (2003) Cholinergic dependence of taste memory formation: evidence of two distinct processes. Neurobiol. learn. mem. 80: 323-331.
[154] Figueroa-Guzmán Y, Kuo J, Reilly S (2006) NMDA receptor antagonist MK-801 infused into the insular cortex prevents the attenuation of gustatory neophobia in rats. Brain res. 1114: 183-186.
[155] Naor C, Dudai Y (1996) Transient impairment of cholinergic function in the rat insular cortex disrupts the encoding of taste in conditioned taste aversion. Behav. brain res. 79: 61-67.
[156] Gutierrez R, Tellez L, Bermudez-Rattoni F (2003) Blockade of cortical muscarinic but not NMDA receptors prevents a novel taste from becoming familiar. Eur. j. neurosci. 17: 1556-1562.
[157] Escobar M, Alcocer I, Chao V (1998) The NMDA receptor antagonist CPP impairs conditioned taste aversion and insular cortex long-term potentiation in vivo. Brain res. 812: 246-251.
[158] Escobar M, Alcocer I, Bermudez-Rattoni F (2002) In vivo effects of intracortical administration of NMDA and metabotropic glutamate receptors antagonists on neocortical long-term potentiation and conditioned taste aversion. Behav. brain res. 129: 101-106.
[159] Gutierrez R, De la Cruz V, Rodriguez-Ortiz C, Bermudez-Rattoni F (2004) Perirhinal cortex muscarinic receptor blockade impairs taste recognition memory formation. Learn. mem. 11: 95-101.
[160] Jimenez B, Tapia R (2004) Biochemical modulation of NMDA receptors: role in conditioned taste aversion. Neurochem. res. 29: 161-168.
[161] Berman D, Hazvi S, Neduva V, Dudai Y (2000) The role of identified neurotransmitter systems in the response of insular cortex to unfamiliar taste: activation of ERK1-2 and formation of a memory trace. J. neurosci. 20: 7017-7023.
[162] Rosenblum K, Meiri N, Dudai Y (1993) Taste memory: the role of protein synthesis in gustatory cortex. Behav. neural. biol. 59: 49-56.
[163] Bermudez-Rattoni F, McGaugh J (1991) Insular cortex and amygdala lesions differentially affect acquisition on inhibitory avoidance and conditioned taste aversion. Brain res. 549: 165-170.
[164] Braun J, Kiefer S, Ouellet J (1981) Research note psychic ageusia in rats lacking gustatory neocortex. Exp. neurol. 72: 711-716.

[165] Kiefer S, Leach L, Braun J (1984) Taste agnosia following gustatory neocortex ablation: dissociation from odor and generality across taste qualities. Behav. neurosci. 98: 590-608.

[166] Yamamoto T, Shimura T, Sako N, Yasoshima Y, Sakai N (1994) Neural substrates for conditioned taste aversion in the rat. Behavioural brain research 65(2): 123–137.

[167] Scoville W, Milner B (1957) Loss of recent memory after bilateral hippocampal lesions. J. neurol. neurosurg. psychiatry 20: 11 – 21.

[168] Zola-Morgan S, Squire L (1990) The primate hippocampal formation: evidence for a time-limited role in memory storage. Science 250: 288-290.

[169] Kim J, Fanselow M (1992) Modality-specific retrograde amnesia of fear. Science 256: 675-677.

[170] Squire L, Alvarez P (1995) Retrograde amnesia and memory consolidation: a neurobiological perspective, Curr. opin. neurobiol. 5: 169– 177.

[171] Takehara K, Kawahara S, Takatsuki K, Kirino Y (2002) Time-limited role of the hippocampus in the memory for trace eyeblink conditioning in mice. Brain res. 951: 183-190.

[172] Escobar M L, Russell R W, Booth R A, Bermúdez-Rattoni F. (1994). Accelerating behavioral recovery after cortical lesions. I. Homotopic implants plus NGF. Behav. neural. biol. 61: 73-80.

[173] Ormsby C E, Ramírez-Amaya V, Bermúdez-Rattoni F (1998) Long-term memory retrieval deficits of learned taste aversions are ameliorated by cortical fetal brain implants. Behav. neurosci. 112: 172-182.

[174] Sherperd G (2006) Smell images and the flavor system in the human brain. Nature 444: 316-321.

[175] Bagshaw M, Pribram K (1953) Cortical organization in gustation (Macaca mulatta). J. neurophysiol. 16: 499–508.

[176] Sudakov K, MacLean P, Reeves A, Marino R (1971) Unit study of exteroceptive inputs to claustrocortex in awake, sitting, squirrel monkey. Brain res. 28: 19–34.

[177] McDonald A, Jackson T (1987) Amygdaloid connections with posterior insular and temporal cortical areas in the rat. J. comp. neurol. 262: 59-77.

[178] Sripanidkulchai K, Sripanidkulchai B, Wyss J (1984) The cortical projection of the basolateral amygdaloid nucleus in the rat: a retrograde fluorescent dye study. J. comp. neurol. 229: 419-431.

[179] Ottersen O (1982) Connections of the amygdala of the rat. IV: Corticoamygdaloid and intraamygdaloid connections as studied with axonal transport of horseradish peroxidase. J. comp. neurol. 205: 30-48.

[180] McDonald A, Shammah-Lagnado S, Shi C, Davis M (1999) Cortical afferents to the extended amygdala. Ann. N. Y. acad. sci. 877: 309-338.

[181] Shi C, Davis M (1999) Pain pathways involved in fear conditioning measured with fear-potentiated startle: lesion studies. J. neurosci. 19: 420-430.

[182] Yasui Y, Itoh K, Sugimoto T, Kaneko T, Mizuno N (1987) Thalamocortical and thalamo-amygdaloid projections from the parvicellular division of the posteromedial ventral nucleus in the cat. J. comp. neurol. 257: 253-268.

[183] Fulwiler C, Saper C (1984). Subnuclear Organization of the Efferent Connections of the Parabrachial Nucleus in the rat. Brain res. rev. 7: 229-259.

[184] Yasui Y, Saper C, Cechetto D (1989) Calcitonin gene-related peptide immunoreactivity in the visceral sensory cortex, thalamus, and related pathways in the rat. J. comp. neurol. 290: 487-501.

[185] Schwaber J, Sternini C, Brecha N, Rogers W, Card J (1988) Neurons containing calcitonin gene-related peptide in the parabrachial nucleus project to the central nucleus of the amygdala. J. comp. neurol. 270: 416-26, 398-9.

[186] Kocorowski L, Helmstetter F (2001) Calcitonin gene-related peptide released within the amygdala is involved in Pavlovian auditory fear conditioning. Neurobiol. learn. mem. 75: 149-163.

[187] Nguyen K, Sills M, Jacobowitz D (1986) Cardiovascular effects produced by microinjection of calcitonin gene-related peptide into the rat central amygdaloid nucleus. Peptides 7: 337-339.

[188] LeDoux J (2000) Emotion circuits in the brain. Annu. rev. neurosci. 23: 155-184.

[189] LeDoux J (2003) The emotional brain, fear, and the amygdala. Cell mol. neurobiol. 23: 727-738.

[190] McGaugh J (2002) Memory consolidation and the amygdala: a systems perspective. Trends neurosci. 25: 456.

[191] McGaugh J, McIntyre C, Power A (2002) Amygdala modulation of memory consolidation: interaction with other brain systems. Neurobiol. learn. mem. 78: 539-552.

[192] Bahar A, Samuel A, Hazvi S, Dudai Y (2003) The amygdalar circuit that acquires taste aversion memory differs from the circuit that extinguishes it. Eur. j. neurosci. 17: 1527–1530.

[193] Gallo M, Roldan G, Bures J (1992) Differential involvement of gustatory insular cortex and amygdala in the acquisition and retrieval of conditioned taste aversion in rats. Behav. brain res. 52: 91–97.

[194] Roldan G, Bures J (1994) Tetrodotoxin blockade of amygdala overlapping with poisoning impairs acquisition of conditioned taste aversion in rats. Behav. brain res. 65: 213–219.

[195] Yasoshima Y, Yamamoto T (1997) Rat gustatory memory requires protein kinase C activity in the amygdala and cortical gustatory area. Neuroreport 8: 1363–1367.

[196] Yasoshima Y, Morimoto T, Yamamoto T (2000) Different disruptive effects on the acquisition and expression of conditioned taste aversion by blockades of amygdalar ionotropic and metabotropic glutamatergic receptor subtypes in rats. Brain res. 869: 15–24.

[197] Miranda M, Ferreira G, Ramirez-Lugo L, Bermudez-Rattoni F (2003) Role of cholinergic system on the construction of memories: taste memory encoding. Neurobiol. learn. mem. 80: 211-222.

[198] Jones M, French P, Bliss T, Rosenblum K (1999) Molecular mechanisms of long-term potentiation in the insular cortex in vivo. J. neurosci. 19: RC36.

[199] Escobar M, Bermúdez-Rattoni F (2000) Long-term potentiation in the insular cortex enhances conditioned taste aversion retention. Brain res. 852: 208-212.

[200] Miranda M, McGaugh J (2004) Enhancement of inhibitory avoidance and conditioned taste aversion memory with insular cortex infusions of 8-Br-cAMP: involvement of the basolateral amygdala. Learn. mem. 11: 312-317.

[201] Buresová O (1978) Neocortico-amygdalar interaction in the conditioned taste aversion in rats. Act. nerv. super (Praha). 20: 224-230.

[202] Bielavska E, Roldan G (1996) Ipsilateral connections between the gustatory cortex, amygdala and parabrachial nucleus are necessary for acquisition and retrieval of conditioned taste aversion in rats. Behav. brain res. 81: 25-31.

[203] Gutierrez H, Gutierrez R, Silva-Gandarias R, Estrada J, Miranda M I, Bermudez-Rattoni F (1999) Differential effects of 192IgG-saporin and NMDA-induced lesions into the basal forebrain on cholinergic activity and taste aversion memory formation. Brain res. 834: 136-141.

[204] Rollins B, Stines S, McGuire H, King B (2001) Effects of amygdala lesions on body weight, conditioned taste aversion, and neophobia. Physiol. behav. 72: 735-742.

[205] Sakai N, Yamamoto T (2001) Effects of excitotoxic brain lesions on taste-mediated odor learning in the rat. Neurobiol. learn. mem. 75: 128-139

[206] Lamprecht R, Dudai Y (1996) Transient expression of c-Fos in rat amygdala during training is required for encoding conditioned taste aversion memory. Learn. mem. 3: 31-41.

[207] Lamprecht R, Hazvi S, Dudai Y (1997) cAMP response element-binding protein in the amygdala is required for long- but not short-term conditioned taste aversion memory. J. neurosci. 17: 8443-8450.

[208] Bahar A, Dorfman N, Dudai Y (2004) Amygdalar circuits required for either consolidation or extinction of taste aversion memory are not required for reconsolidation. Eur j. neurosci. 19: 1115-1118.

[209] Gutierrez H, Gutierrez R, Ramirez-Trejo L, Silva Gandarias R, Ormsby C, Miranda M, Bermudez-Rattoni F (1999) Redundant basal forebrain modulation in taste aversion memory formation. J. neurosci. 19: 7661-7669.

[210] Phelps E, LeDoux J (2005) Contributions of the amygdala to emotion processing: from animal models to human behavior. Neuron 48: 175-187.

[211] Roozendaal B, Nguyen B, Power A, McGaugh J (1999) Basolateral amygdala noradrenergic influence enables enhancement of memory consolidation induced by hippocampal glucocorticoid receptor activation. Proc. Natl. Acad. Sci. USA. 96: 11642-11647.

[212] McGaugh J (2004) The amygdala modulates the consolidation of memories of emotionally arousing experiences. Annu. rev. neurosci. 27: 1-28.

[213] Roozendaal B, Cools A (1994) Influence of the noradrenergic state of the nucleus accumbens in basolateral amygdala mediated changes in neophobia of rats. Behav. neurosci. 108: 1107-1118.

[214] Fornari R, Wichmann R, Atucha E, Desprez T, Eggens-Meijer E, Roozendaal B (2012) Involvement of the insular cortex in regulating glucocorticoid effects on memory consolidation of inhibitory avoidance training. Front behav. neurosci. 6: 10.

[215] Bermudez-Rattoni F, Okuda S, Roozendaal B, McGaugh J (2005) Insular cortex is involved in consolidation of object recognition memory. Learn. mem. 12: 447-449.
[216] Roozendaal B, Portillo-Marquez G, McGaugh J (1996) Basolateral amygdala lesions block glucocorticoid-induced modulation of memory for spatial learning. Behav. neurosci. 110: 1074-1083.
[217] Roozendaal B, Schelling G, McGaugh J (2008) Corticotropin-releasing factor in the basolateral amygdala enhances memory consolidation via an interaction with the beta-adrenoceptor-cAMP pathway: dependence on glucocorticoid receptor activation. J. neurosci. 28: 6642-6651.
[218] Klumpp H, Angstadt M, Phan K (2012) Insula reactivity and connectivity to anterior cingulate cortex when processing threat in generalized social anxiety disorder. Biol. psychol. 89: 273-276.
[219] Shah S, Klumpp H, Angstadt M, Nathan P, Phan K (2009) Amygdala and insula response to emotional images in patients with generalized social anxiety disorder. J. psychiatry neurosci. 34: 296-302.
[220] Alvarez R, Biggs A, Chen G, Pine D, Grillon C (2008) Contextual fear conditioning in humans: cortical-hippocampal and amygdala contributions. J. neurosci. 28: 6211-6219.
[221] Duerden E, Albanese M (2012) Localization of pain-related brain activation: A meta-analysis of neuroimaging data. Hum Brain Mapp. 2011 Dec 1. doi: 10.1002/hbm.21416.
[222] Miskovic V, Schmidt L (2012) Early information processing biases in social anxiety. Cogn. emot. 26: 176-185.
[223] Schneider F, Grodd W, Weiss U, Klose U, Mayer K, Nägele T, Gur R (1997) Functional MRI reveals left amygdala activation during emotion. Psychiatry res. 76: 75-82.
[224] Phan K, Wager T, Taylor S, Liberzon I (2002) Functional neuroanatomy of emotion: a meta-analysis of emotion activation studies in PET and fMRI. Neuroimage 16:331-348.
[225] McGaugh JL. (2004). The amygdala modulates the consolidation of memories of emotionally arousing experiences. Annu. rev. neurosci. 27: 1-28.
[226] Ferreira G, Miranda M, De la Cruz V, Rodríguez-Ortiz C, Bermúdez-Rattoni F (2005) Basolateral amygdala glutamatergic activation enhances taste aversion through NMDA receptor activation in the insular cortex. Eur. j. neurosci. 22: 2596-2604.
[227] Stein M, Simmons A, Feinstein J, Paulus M (2007) Increased amygdala and insular activation during emotion processing in anxiety-prone subjects. Am. j. Psychiatry 164: 318-327.
[228] Singer T, Critchley H, Preuschoff K (2009) A common role of insula in feelings, empathy and uncertainty. Trends cogn. sci. 13: 334–340.
[229] Timms R (1981) A study of the amygdaloid defence reaction showing the value of althesin anaesthesia in studies of the functions of the fore-brain in cats. Plugers arch. 391: 49- 56
[230] Applegate C, Kapp B, Underwood M, McNall C (1983) Autonomic and somatomotor effects of amygdala central N. stimulation in awake rabbits. Physiol. behav. 31: 353-360.
[231] Schütze I, Knuepfer M, Eismann A, Stumpf H, Stock G (1987) Sensory input to single neurons in the amygdala of the cat. Exp. neurol. 97: 499-515.

[232] Cechetto D, Calaresu F (1984) Units in the amygdala responding to activation of carotid baro- and chemoreceptors. Am. j. physiol. 246: R832-836.

[233] Knuepfer M, Eismann A, Schütze I, Stumpf H, Stock G (1995) Responses of single neurons in amygdala to interoceptive and exteroceptive stimuli in conscious cats. Am. j. physiol. 268: 666-675.

[234] Henderson L, Richard C, Macey P, Runquist M, Yu P, Galons J, Harper R (2004) Functional magnetic resonance signal changes in neural structures to baroreceptor reflex activation. J. appl. physiol. 96: 693-703.

[235] Williams L, Brown K, Das P, Boucsein W, Sokolov E, Brammer M, Olivieri G, Peduto A, Gordon E (2004) The dynamics of cortico-amygdala and autonomic activity over the experimental time course of fear perception. Brain res. cogn. brain res. 21: 114-123

Chapter 10

Amygdalar Models of Neurological and Neuropsychiatric Disorders

Trevor H. Gilbert

Additional information is available at the end of the chapter

1. Introduction

A basic underlying propensity of the central nervous system is the capacity to change. Neuroplasticity refers to the adaptive capacity of the brain to undergo alteration of structural organization and functioning in response to environmental change [1]. While this appears to be a very useful process, potential extremes of such plasticity can result in various forms of neurological and neuropsychiatric anomalies. Therefore, it appears that the same mechanisms that are important in adaptive activity, like learning and memory, can provide the basis for abnormal discharge. This being the case, how is it that the normal healthy brain becomes transformed into an abnormal brain? Neuroscientists use animal models to help them uncover the underlying neural mechanisms.

While animal research has revealed extensive information on the cellular, synaptic, and pathological mechanisms of neurological and neuropsychiatric processes, many unanswered questions remain. For instance, there is no neuropsychiatric disorder that is adequately understood from the level of clinical manifestations to the underlying cellular and molecular mechanisms. Because of the ethical barriers to using humans and the inherent limitations of using excised human tissue, inquiry into neurological and neuropsychiatric disorders has necessarily relied upon experimental models. For example, *in vivo* animal models have been indispensable for the testing of anticonvulsant drugs, for determining some of the basic mechanisms of seizure expression, and for determining changes in functional and morphological properties [2-4].

Animal models have been, and will continue to be invaluable for: 1) modeling the clinical condition, 2) determining the basic mechanisms underlying the genesis and progression of the disease, and 3) screening potential pharmacological agents. While an ideal model would possess properties identical to all aspects of the particular human condition, this is most likely unattainable. The characteristics of a valuable model should possess a substantial degree of similarity to, at least some aspect, of the disorder of interest [5,6]. Accordingly, a good animal model should be able to provide new understanding into the disorder it models and respond in a reproducible and predictable manner. For example, the kindling model, depending on the animal species, possesses many of these characteristics and is an excellent model for certain clinical disorders, their underlying mechanisms, and as a screening tool for newer pharmacological agents [3,4].

An understanding of the brain circuitry that underlies normal and adaptive behaviors provides a foundation for clarifying the pathology and pathophysiology of psychiatric disorders. The key structures and pathways associated with abnormal behaviors have been framed through a weighty historical record of anatomical observations. Neuroscience has been gradually unveiling the neural networks that subserve the functional domains of motivation, emotion, and cognition, central tenets to psychiatry. The convergence of findings from the multiplicity of research methods and techniques across both animal and human studies has provided the neurocircuitry framework pertinent to neurological and neuropsychiatric diseases.

A brain structure that receives substantial scientific interest today is the amygdala. The amygdalae are a group of nuclei located deep within the medial temporal lobe of the brain [7]. It has a wide range of connections with other brain regions, allowing it to participate in a wide variety of behavioral functions. Considered to be part of the limbic system, the amygdala performs an important role in the processing and memory of emotional reactions. Structural and functional changes within the amygdala are associated with a broad range of psychiatric conditions in humans, such as anxiety disorders [8], depression [9], schizophrenia [10], and autism [11].

This chapter will review the various experimental models employed to gain insight into the underlying mechanisms of key neurological and neuropsychiatric disease states, with a focus on the amygdalae. In particular, this chapter will examine models of brain plasticity, models of epilepsy, fear and anxiety, affective disorders, neurodevelopmental disorders, and neurodegenerative disorders.

2. The amygdala

The amygdaloid complex is a large subcortical structure located in the rostromedial part of the temporal lobe in front of the hippocampus and underneath the uncus of the parahippocampal gyrus (i.e., entorhinal cortex). Some of the most prominent pathways to the amygdaloid complex come from cortical areas in the temporal and frontal lobes. Its components are morphologically and histochemically heterogenous, as are its functions and connections with other brain regions [12]. The amygdala has close interconnections with both cortical and subcortical areas. The cortical areas include temporal (perirhinal and entorhinal), frontal, insular, and cingulate association areas and the subcortical areas include brainstem, hypothalamus, thalamus, hippocampus, and claustrum [12,13].

The many components of the amygdaloid complex can be grouped into three principal divisions: the basolateral, cortical, and centromedial nuclear groups. The largest part of the amygdala is the basolateral nuclear group. It is closely related to many cortical areas in the prefrontal, temporal, insular, and occipital regions and is reciprocally connected to them. The basolateral amygdala projects to the striatum and also has close relations with the thalamus. The cortical, or olfactory, amygdala receives olfactory input directly from the olfactory bulb and indirectly from the olfactory cortex. The olfactory amygdala in turn projects to the centromedial amygdala and the hypothalamus. The centromedial amygdala receives direct input from the cerebral cortex, but is largely restricted to fibers from the hippocampal formation, insula, and orbitofrontal cortex. Because the amygdala is a bidirectional pathway that can relay information between association cortices and subcortical structures it is in an optimal position to simultaneously influence excitability of numerous brain regions at any given time [12,13].

3. Kindling as a model of brain plasticity

An excellent model for investigating brain mechanisms associated with neurological and neuropsychiatric disorders is kindling. It was Graham Goddard who first acknowledged the potential importance of repeated stimulation to the brain as a useful scientific tool. Goddard observed that some of his rats began to develop seizures, even with invariant stimulation [14]. He and his colleagues studied the phenomenon in more detail [15,16] and subsequently referred to the development of stimulation-induced convulsions as "kindling," analogous to starting a fire with an initially benign stimulus [14]. The original kindling work identified the amygdala as a critical site due to its reliable and rapid kindling progression. Although subsequent research has revealed other salient sites, the amygdala is the most frequently targeted structure for kindling studies due to its proximal connections with both cortical and subcortical areas.

In its original description, kindling refers to the progressive development of epileptiform activity and associated behavioural convulsions in response to low-intensity electrical stimulation of the brain [15,16]. Kindling is generally considered to be the best available model of temporal lobe epilepsy and is particularly well suited for experimental study because precise control can be implemented over experimental conditions [17]. Progression of behavioural and electrographic activity is gradual enough to allow for particular manipulation at various phases of the kindling process [18,19]. There are several significant characteristics that support kindling's validity as a clinical model, especially for epilepsy. For example, the EEG patterns are similar between the experimental and human conditions, the anticonvulsant pharmacology is similar, and the cognitive and behavioural abnormalities associated with each condition are also similar [17,20]. These characteristics, along with kindling as a model of epilepsy, will be described in more detail below.

Although most kindling investigations have utilized rats, kindling has been described in many other animals, including amphibians, reptiles, mice, gerbils, cats, monkeys, baboons [21], and guinea-pigs [3,4,22,23]. It would be surprising to find a phenomenon that bridges vertebrates, including amphibians, reptiles, and mammals that would not include humans. Indeed, it has also been reported that a human has been kindled [24]. This highlights the applicability of the animal model for humans. Although kindling was originally defined as resulting from electrical stimulation, it now collectively refers to the eventual development of persistent brain activity following repeated exposure to a stimulus - this can be in the form of stimulus trains (electrical activity) or chemical agents. Although kindling is usually employed as an experimental model of human temporal lobe epilepsy, kindling in its simplest dimension is a model of neural plasticity [14]. In particular, the realization that persistent changes in brain function occur in response to an invariant stimulus has led many researchers to believe that such mechanisms may be similar to those underlying learning [16,25].

4. Kindling as a model of neuropsychiatric illness

As mentioned, kindling is commonly used as a model of epilepsy, but many researchers suggest that kindling shows a number of attributes that are similar to neuropsychiatric disorders. In particular, kindling is useful in understanding the long-term and developing patterns of non-seizure related disorders [26]. Kindling is associated with a progressive increase in behavioural and physiological responsivity and a decrease in threshold for an event (e.g., a seizure) and can eventually result in a spontaneous event (i.e., spontaneous seizure). Because the seizure is used as a convenient endpoint for behavioural and physiological responsivity, it is believed that the kindling model can be used to understand the progression of various neuropsychiatric disorders [27]. The justification is as follows. The disorders are initially expressed with minor behavioural and physiological changes, to more complete symptomatology, and then finally to the spontaneous elicitation of the disorder.

As mentioned previously, the amygdala is a bidirectional pathway that can relay information between association cortices and subcortical structures, and is therefore optimally positioned to simultaneously influence the excitability of numerous brain regions at any given time. It has become increasingly perceptible that structural and functional changes in the amygdala, and associated limbic circuitry, are linked to a variety of clinical conditions in humans. It is highly conceivable that the amygdala has been connected to various neuropsychiatric and neurodevelopmental disorders more than any other brain region.

The recurrent nature of many neuropsychiatric disorders has been documented for nearly as long as the disorders have been investigated [28]. Although it should not be surprising that there are many variations within patients, the general course of untreated illnesses tends to be predictable. There is a characterization of a diminished healthy period between episodes, and a transition from induced events (e.g., personal losses and stressors) to those periods that occur more spontaneously. Perhaps the best illustration of this is seen in bipolar disorder – minor episodes give way to major episodes. In the beginning there are isolated and intermittent events to more continuous rhythmical events, and then to the rapid cycling variety [29]. In context of the kindling model, the course of the illness is progressive in that there is threshold lowering, and a movement from triggered episodes to spontaneous episodes. Stated in a theoretical framework, kindling provides a model for conceptualizing physiological and behavioural abnormalities that progress in severity in response to the same inducing stimulus over time.

In panic disorders, it is apparent that some patients progress from highly intermittent attacks that are precipitated by a cue, to those that begin to occur more frequently and spontaneously. In addition, some patients become increasingly more paralyzed by agoraphobia, which may increase to the point of complete incapacitation. In the case of cocaine-related panic attacks, some individuals with a history of anxiety-free episodes with repeated administration can suddenly experience a full-blown panic attack. Furthermore, it appears that some users can display panic attacks in the absence of continued drug administration [30]. Again, it is kindling's progressive feature with a threshold lowering and the move from induced to spontaneous events, that models panic disorder.

In obsessive compulsive disorder (OCD), initial obsessions and compulsions often increase in severity and lead to incapacitation. This progressive nature can be modeled by kindling. In post-traumatic stress disorder (PTSD), individuals who have experienced prior traumatic events also appear more likely to suffer from PTSD upon repeated exposure to trauma [31,32]. Additionally, it appears that repeated inducing events result in more severe and long-lasting consequences than isolated events. It appears that there may be a progression in the emergence of flashbacks, which are initially triggered by cues linked to the original event and occur more spontaneously. The decreases in threshold observed in kindling may model greater episode recurrence in this disorder.

Kindling has also been used to study emotionality [33]. It has been shown that the kindling in rats [34] and cats [35] can result in enhanced reactivity and aggressive behaviour. Other more enduring behavioural changes that have also been reported following limbic kindling have included diminished predatory attack behaviour in cats [36] and decreased ability to learn passive avoidance in rats [37]. More recently, it has been reported that repeatedly inducing seizures in the amygdala of rats can produce various changes in emotional responding, particularly those involving fear and anxiety [38].

It may be argued that these neuropsychiatric phenomena are perhaps only analogous, and not homologous, to kindling. However, because of many phenomenological similarities, kindling may be pertinent to the understanding of the long-term and progressive nature of such disorders.

5. Epilepsy

The epilepsies comprise a diverse collection of disorders that affect approximately 1% of the general population [39]. Epilepsy is a chronic brain disorder, characterized by recurrent seizures due to excessive discharge of neurons, with a spectrum of severity ranging from mild and benign to severe and intractable. Epilepsy involves a temporary electrical disturbance in the brain that can produce effects ranging from momentary loss of consciousness to full-blown generalized seizures that involve involuntary jerking of the muscles. The various epilepsies affect an estimated 40-50 million people worldwide, signifying that epilepsy is a serious neurological disorder and a significant health problem in our society. Much of our understanding about epilepsy has come from research on animals.

Although research has revealed much information about the cellular and synaptic mechanisms of seizures and epileptogenesis, many unanswered questions remain. Animal models have been and will likely continue to be invaluable for determining the underlying mechanisms of the genesis, expression, and propagation of seizures, as well as for the screening of new anticonvulsant drugs (ACDs). The identification of new ACDs remains the most obvious and important avenue for therapeutic advancement. Because all new ACDs are tested on animal models, it seems prudent to test these new drugs on appropriate seizure models so as not to discard a potentially valuable drug because it was inadvertently tested in an unsuitable model. Accordingly, an important consideration in ACD development is the choice of an appropriate animal model for in vivo drug testing [3,4].

Experimental testing of novel ACDs requires animal models that are predictive in anticonvulsant efficacy against specific seizure types and in terms of adverse or toxic effects at anticonvulsant doses. Models that mimic the symptoms, natural history, etiology, and response to therapy of human seizures are crucial. The most commonly used animal models are the maximal electroshock (MES) test and the pentylenetetrazol (PTZ) seizure test. While both these models are thought to represent valid models for generalized tonic-clonic (grand mal) seizures and generalized absence (petit mal) seizures, respectively [40], they are not valid models for partial seizures. Unfortunately the anticonvulsant activity of common ACDs in these models are not effective against partial seizures, the most common type of all epileptic seizures. Therefore, valid models of partial seizures should be used to test the anticonvulsant efficacy against partial epileptic activity [3,4,41].

As introduced previously, kindling is generally considered to be the best available model of human partial epilepsy, and is particularly convenient for experimental study because precise control can be implemented over experimental conditions. The progression of behavioural and electrographic activity is gradual enough to allow for specific manipulations at various phases of the kindling process. There are several significant characteristics that support kindling's validity as a model for partial epilepsy: (1) the EEG patterns of hippocampal and amygdala kindled seizures are similar to human complex partial seizures; (2) the behaviour associated with initial and later seizures is similar to those of human complex partial (limbic or temporal lobe) seizures; (3) the anticonvulsant pharmacology of kindled and human partial seizures are markedly similar; (4) the occurrence of heterogenous interictal spike transients are common to the kindling model and human partial epilepsy; (5) the occurrence of spontaneous seizures in kindled animals; (6) kindling can be produced in subhuman primates and kindling-like effects have also been observed in humans; and (7) cognitive and behavioural abnormalities have been reported to occur in kindled animals and in human epileptics [17,20].

Although amygdalar kindling is widely used in rat models, its application to guinea-pig models provides a unique vehicle. With its important interconnections, relative ease of anatomical location, and reliable epileptiform correlates, the amygdala remains an important target for study. With repeated stimulation, guinea-pigs show some initial growth of the electrographic indices and behavioural seizures. However, unlike rats, guinea-pigs become arrested at partial and complex partial seizures and do not progress to fully generalized convulsions during regular single-site kindling [22,23]. This suggests that guinea-pig kindling may be a better model for human complex partial epilepsy because the majority of humans with complex partial epilepsy also do not progress to fully generalized convulsions. Furthermore, guinea-pig seizures mimic human seizure behaviour and have a similar EEG pattern for both ictal and interictal events [3,4].

Because guinea-pig kindling shares many characteristics with human partial epilepsy it will most likely continue to develop as an excellent model of the disorder. Seizures kindled in guinea-pigs echo that of human seizure expression, have a similar EEG pattern, display more severe seizures when multiple foci are present, and share a close correspondence in anticonvulsant pharmacology. Moreover, guinea-pigs slowly manifest seizures and become arrested at partial seizures, a consistent observation associated with many species of primates [42], including humans [20].

The guinea-pig with its sustained period of partial epileptic activity provides certain advantages over rats and mice as a model system for human partial epilepsy. There is a striking correlation between drugs effective against guinea-pig kindled seizures and drugs effective against partial seizures in humans. This correlation strengthens the validity of guinea-pig kindling as a model of the human condition, as it seems unlikely that a drug that is ineffective against guinea-pig kindled partial seizures will be efficacious against partial seizures in humans. Accordingly, examining the efficacy of experimental drugs in this model would seem to be a beneficial step before undertaking expensive human clinical trials. However, if examination of secondarily generalized seizures was of primary interest, then rat kindling would be the preferential model due to their speedy seizure progression and development of tonic-clonic seizures.

Future pharmacological studies should be implemented in the guinea-pig model of partial epilepsy to determine the effectiveness of other existing and newer ACDs to further elucidate the value of this model for the screening of prospective ACDs. Such studies should extend detailed acute and chronic pharmacokinetic analysis to the test drugs in an attempt to understand the drug's absorption and elimination parameters. Concurrent objective behavioural assessment should also be carried out to determine potential adverse effects of the drugs. While general observation of the animal's behaviour is important, objective quantitative tests allow for greater inter-observer reliability and are potentially more sensitive to the behavioural impairment of an ACD. Administration of an ACD requires the optimal balance between the anticonvulsant effect and the level of behavioural toxicity. Ideally, the more efficacious drugs will have powerful anticonvulsant actions in the absence of behavioural impairment. Thus, the sedation and ataxic effects of the test drug need to be assessed over multiple doses. It is only with a more in depth inquiry into the underlying mechanisms of epilepsy that will prove to be useful in human therapeutic approaches.

6. Anxiety disorders

Anxiety is chronic fear that persists in the absence of any direct threat, and is a common psychological correlate of stress. When anxiety becomes so disruptive that it interrupts normal functioning, it may manifest as an anxiety disorder. Anxiety disorders are the most prevalent of all psychiatric disorders, in that about 17% of people suffer from an anxiety disorder at some point in their lives [43,44].

The amygdala is known to play an important role in normal fear conditioning and is implicated in the pathophysiology of anxiety disorders. The amygdala may also be a target for the beneficial effects of cognitive-behavioral and medication treatments for anxiety disorders [45]. Animal models have played an important role in the study of anxiety, and in the assessment of anxiolytic properties of new psychotherapeutics. Such models typically involve animal defensive behaviors, with the assumption that defensive behaviors are motivated by fear, where fear and anxiety are identical states. Common models anxiety in animals include the elevated-plus maze test, defensive burying, and risk assessment [46].

In the elevated-plus maze test, rats are placed within a four-armed maze that is raised above the floor. Two of the arms have sides, and two do not have sides. The measure of anxiety is the proportion of time spent in the enclosed arms versus the time spent in the exposed arms. In the defensive-burying test, rats are exposed to a shock apparatus housed at one end of a test chamber. Anxiety is measured by the amount of time rats spend spraying bedding material towards the source of the shock. In the risk-assessment test, rats are briefly exposed to the presence of a cat. They quickly flee to their burrows and freeze, and then engage in a variety of risk–assessment behaviors (e.g., cautiously exploring the surface) before their normal behavior returns. Anxiety is measured by the amount of time that the rat spends in both freezing and in risk assessment behaviors. Note that these anxiety models have generally been validated by observation of anxiety reduction through the use of benzodiazepines versus non-anxiolytic drugs [47].

A primary technique for investigating the mechanisms underlying emotional associative learning is Pavlovian conditioning. Studies investigating the neural mechanisms of fear conditioning across species indicate that the amygdala has a critical function in the acquisition, storage, and expression of conditioned fear [48]. Further, research suggests that interaction between the amygdala, the ventromedial prefrontal cortex and the hippocampus supports the acquisition, storage, retrieval, and contextual modulation of fear extinction.

Neuroimaging research has helped to advance neurobiological models of anxiety disorders. In individuals with PTSD, research suggests altered emotion neurocircuitry. Emotion activation studies in these individuals have shown hyperactivation in emotion-related regions, including the amygdala and insula, and hypoactivation in emotion-regulation regions, including the medial prefrontal cortex and anterior cingulate cortex. Increased connectivity between the amygdala and insula may suggest enhanced anticipation of negative events [49].

7. Neurodevelopmental disorders

The amygdala has been implicated in a range of neurodevelopmental disorders. Like our entire nervous system, it seems that the amygdala is sensitive to threshold variances. Amygdalar dysregulation can result in perceptual changes related to environmental danger and sociality, and thereby result in dysfunctional anxiety. Across a range of studies investigating neurodevelopmental disorders, there is evidence of amygdala dysregulation from postmortem studies, structural MRI analyses, and functional MRI [50].

Schizophrenia is a disorder characterized by deteriorating ability to function in everyday life, and includes some combination of hallucinations, delusions, thought disorder, movement disorder, and inappropriate emotional expression. It attacks about 1% of individuals of all races and cultural groups, typically beginning in adolescence or early adult [43,51].

Given the substantial contribution of genetic factors to many disease conditions, an obvious way of developing animal models would be insertion of human disease–associated alleles into mice. Indeed, genetic animal models developed from highly penetrant human mutations seem like suitable candidates [52]. However, caution is required as work is ongoing to identify which of the genes, or deleted genes, are responsible for the relevant behavioral abnormalities in mouse models. While such genetic animal models made with variants of small effect may demonstrate interesting neurobiological properties, perhaps it is still too early to accept these models as mirroring the etiology of the disease [46].

Animal models of maternal infection, or environmental models, have been widely employed to look at immune involvement in schizophrenia. For example, prenatal viral infection has been used to induce behavioral and neural abnormalities [53], such as the expression of immune-related molecules (cytokines) in the brain and cerebral spinal fluid. Perhaps this represents a permanent state of brain immune dysregulation which begins during early development. Although such results related to immune involvement encourage novel therapeutic immune interventions, the role of viral infection in schizophrenia remains unclear.

Other experimental attempts have used pharmacological manipulations or lesions to produce symptoms of schizophrenia. The efficacy of dopamine receptor antagonist drugs in treating positive symptoms of schizophrenia gave rise to the deep-rooted dopamine hypothesis. Subsequently, the observation that NMDA (n-methyl-d-aspartate) glutamate receptor antagonists (e.g., phencyclidine, ketamine) produce psychotic symptoms and cognitive disturbances redolent of schizophrenia gave rise to the glutamate hypothesis [54]. Consequently, diverse animal models have been based on manipulations of these principal transmitter systems, although the putative dopaminergic or glutamatergic abnormalities in schizophrenia have not been indubitably established [55].

On the basis of evidence obtained from in vivo brain imaging, postmortem, and rodent studies, it seems likely that amygdalocortical circuitry has an important function in the pathophysiology of schizophrenia. Projections of the basolateral amygdala may be of particular importance to the induction of abnormal circuitry in schizophrenia, as their ingrowth during late adolescence and early adulthood may help to trigger the onset of illness in susceptible individuals [56]. Ultimately then, it seems that abnormalities in limbic lobe components may contribute to a dysfunctional regulation of affective responses in schizophrenics.

Autism is a complex debilitating neurodevelopmental disorder, which involves a wide range of problematic behaviours including deficits in language, deficits in perceptual and motor development, defective reality testing, and an inability to function in social situations [43].

The amygdala has long been a site of intense interest in the search for neuropathology in the brains of people with autism, given its role in modulating anxiety levels and social behavior. Schumann et al. [50] conducted a study where autistic adults showed a decrease in neurons in the amygdala compared to control groups. It appears that the amygdala undergoes an abnormal pattern of postnatal development that includes unusual enlargement, followed by a reduction of amygdala size, or decreased neurons, into adulthood.

Howard et al. [57] found that individuals with high-functioning autism demonstrated neuropsychological profiles characteristic of the effects of amygdala damage such as, impairment in the recognition of facial expressions of fear, perception of eye-gaze direction, and recognition memory for faces. They used MRI analysis techniques to show that the same individuals also demonstrated abnormalities of medial temporal lobe brain structure, notably bilaterally enlarged amygdala volumes, perhaps reflecting incomplete neuronal pruning in early development. These results suggest that developmental malformation of the amygdala may underlie the social-cognitive impairments characteristic of autism.

Other studies have reported that amygdala lesions in isolation are not sufficient for producing autistic symptoms. Instead, it may be abnormal connectivity between the amygdala and other structures that contributes to autistic symptoms at a network level [58]. Dziobek et al. [59] used imaging techniques to measure fusiform gyrus cortical thickness and to measure amygdala volumes, and suggest that dysfunction of the amygdalafusiform system might represent a crucial pathophysiological mechanism of autism.

With recent findings linking multiple genes to autism spectrum disorders, novel rodent mutants with deletions, truncations, and/or overexpression of these candidate genes have been developed and studied both behaviorally and biologically. As the diagnostic criteria for autism are behavioural, phenotyping these mouse models requires behavioural assays with high relevance to each category of the diagnostic symptoms. These include tests for social interaction, communication and repetitive behaviours to test hypotheses about the causes of autism. Such mouse models hold great promise as tools for discovering effective treatments for components of autism spectrum disorders [60].

8. Mood disorders

Although there a continuum of mood disorders has been identified, the best documented ones are depression and mania. The primary symptoms of major depression are prolonged feelings of worthlessness and guilt, disruption of normal eating habits, sleep disturbances, a general slowing of behavior, and frequent thoughts of suicide. Mania is the polar opposite from depression, and is characterized by excessive euphoria. The affected person is typically hyperactive and often formulates grandiose plans. The periods of mania often fluctuate into states of depression and back again into mania. This condition is referred to as bipolar disorder (BD). There is a high incidence of affective disorders in Western societies, with about 5% of the population suffering from major depression, and 1-2% suffering from bipolar disorder [51,61].

Several chronic stress procedures have been employed in various animal models [46]. Typically, chronic mild or chronic unpredictable stress involves subjecting normal rodents to a series of repeated physical stresses (e.g., restraint, foot shock, cold temperature) over a period of weeks. The animals show signs of anhedonia (e.g., reduced sucrose preference), which can be reversed by chronic administration of antidepressant medications. Further, repeated stress results in hyperexcitability in the basolateral amygdala in rodents [62], suggesting a mechanism that might produce pathological amygdala activity in depression.

Chronic social defeat stress involves subjecting rodents to repeated cycles of social subordination, after which the rodents show a range of depression symptom (e.g., anhedonia, social withdrawal) which can be reversed by chronic antidepressants [63]. It appears that chronic social defeat also induces a metabolic syndrome in mice characterized by weight gain, and insulin and leptin resistance, a finding that is consistent with homeostatic abnormalities observed in human depression [64].

Another model of depression is based on early life stress. Maternal separation in rat pups induces life-long behavioral and neuroendocrine abnormalities in the pups, some of which can be reversed by antidepressant medications [65]. In addition, it was recently found that prolonged exposure (weeks to months) of adult rodents to social isolation induces anhedonia, which can also be treated effectively with chronic antidepressant medication [66].

Patients with mood disorders manifest abnormalities of morphology in several medial prefrontal network and limbic structures. A large body of human data from functional and structural imaging, as well as analysis of lesions and histological material indicates that this system is centrally involved in mood disorders. Neural models of depression suggest that dysfunction within the medial network and related limbic structures underlie the disturbances in emotional behavior and other cognitive aspects of the major depressive syndrome [62].

The most often used model of mania involves treating normal rodents with psychostimulants (e.g., cocaine or amphetamine). The repeated administration of the drugs causes sensitization of the acute locomotor-activating effects of the drugs, which in turn can be reduced by lithium or valproate, two chief treatments for human bipolar disorder [67]. Although these are intriguing findings, caution with this model is warranted. It remains unclear that the molecular and cellular changes associated with psychostimulant-induced sensitization have direct equivalence with the pathophysiology of bipolar disorder.

As mentioned previously, chronic stress is known to induce hyperactivation of amygdala, enhancing amygdala-dependent unlearned fear, fear conditioning, and aggression. Similarly, many of the symptoms experienced by patients with bipolar disorder appear to be associated with abnormalities in emotional processing, and an enlargement of the amygdala has been described as a prominent abnormality in BD. Abnormal age related increases in the amygdala volume have been found in bipolar adolescents. In addition to structural changes in this circuitry, functional neuroimaging studies indicate increased activity in the amygdala during acute mood episodes [68].

Other imaging studies have looked at changes in amygdalar regulation in BD. Bechdolf et al. [69] investigated adolescents and young adults with BD prior to the onset of first episode mania. They found that amygdala and insula volume reductions are present prior to the onset of first episode mania, a reduction consistent with the amygdala's central role in emotion processing, such as associating stimuli with emotional responses, enhancing memory consolidation and influencing perception of stimuli. Another study found increased amygdalar activation in BD patients, suggesting an exaggerated response to negative emotional stimuli [70].

9. Neurodegenerative diseases

Alzheimer's disease (AD) is a devastating degenerative brain disorder related to aging that first appears as progressive memory loss and later develops into generalized dementia. About 10% of the general population over the age of 65 suffers from the disease, and the proportion is about 35% in those over 85 [43].

AD brains are characterized by the presence of amyloid plaques and neurofibrillary tangles. Plaques are clumps of scar tissue composed of degenerating neurons and amyloid protein, and the tangles are knots of protein in the cytoplasm. Although plaques and tangles are observed throughout the cerebral cortex, they are most prevalent in medial temporal lobe structures such as the amygdala, entorhinal cortex, and hippocampus [71]. The amygdala of AD patients shows significant shrinkage, distortion and loss of neurons as well as extensive gliosis [72,73]. Additionally, the extent of the amygdalar atrophy correlates positively with the degree of emotional memory impairment [71].

Knafo et al. [74] describes the neuropathological changes in the amygdala and alterations in emotional memory of transgenic AD mouse models. They suggest that the morphological changes found in the neurons of the lateral nucleus of the amygdala may contribute to the impaired auditory fear conditioning observed in this model. Further, they note that AD patients also show marked impaired fear conditioning, indicating that deficits in nondeclarative memory is common to both AD patients and the transgenic mice. It seems then that the behavioral features detected in this AD model are similar to those found in AD.

Parkinson's disease (PD) is a disorder of the motor system correlated with the loss of dopamine in the brain and characterized by tremors, muscular rigidity, and reduction in voluntary movement. Parkinson's disease is a movement disorder of middle and old age that affects about .5% of the population [61]. PD is associated with widespread neuronal degeneration and the presence of cortical and brainstem Lewy bodies (clumps of proteins).

Bouchard et al. [75] bolstered evidence for a linkage between PD and volumetric decreases in limbic system structures. Through MR imaging, they found specific and predictable correlations between the age and sex of a PD patient and the degree of volumetric loss in the hippocampus and amygdala.

Freichel et al. [76] used a transgenic mouse model to assess the behavioral and structural implications of mutant α-synuclein (αSYN) expression, a neuronal protein. αSYN inclusions constitute the hallmark lesions of a number of neurodegenerative diseases, including PD and dementia with Lewy bodies. Using fear conditioning, active avoidance, and water-maze tests, they assessed transgenic mice across a 12 month span for cognitive impairment and possible dementia. The mice showed α-synucleinopathy in several brain regions, including the central nucleus of the amygdala, which is involved in cognitive behavior of mice, and is susceptible to αSYN pathology in human patients.

In a clinico-pathological study looking at postmortem PD brains, Kalaitzakis et al. [77] assessed the correlation between various presentations of PD and specific anatomical and pathological correlates, including αSYN, tau, and amyloid deposits in regions associated with cognition. They found that the amygdala is specifically burdened with αSYN in cases of PD with dementia and also was strongly associated with visual hallucinations. These findings support the literature on the phenomenology of hallucinations in neurodegenerative diseases and the link between such hallucinations and irregularities in the limbic system.

Huntington's disease (HD) is a rare degenerative disease of the central nervous system that affects about .01% of the population. Huntington's disease is a progressive motor disorder of middle to old age, has a strong genetic basis, and is associated with severe dementia [61].

The last 10 years or so have seen a significant generation of various transgenic models of HD. In particular, a rat model exhibits prominent cellular accumulation of huntingtin, a pathological hallmark of HD, in addition to exhibiting ongoing emotional changes [78]. It appears that this model will be valuable in interpreting various psychiatric aspects of HD.

Further, Faure et al. [79] describe emotional blunting and hypersensitivity to negative emotional situations in symptomatic transgenic HD, and suggest that some of these symptoms may be related to amygdala dysfunction. In particular, they propose that functional alteration in brain circuits, with a possible deficit in frontal control, such as shrinkage of the central nucleus of the amygdala, may be responsible for these emotional disorders.

10. Discussion

Animal research has uncovered considerable information on the cellular and synaptic mechanisms of neurological and neuropsychiatric processes, however, many questions remain. Unfortunately there is no neuropsychiatric disorder that is effectively understood from the level of clinical manifestations to the underlying cellular and molecular mechanisms. Given the ethical and practical limitations to human experimental biology and neuropsychiatry, animal models will almost certainly be a necessary aspect of progress.

The development of valid and effective animal models for neurological and neuropsychiatric disorders represents a significant challenge. However, despite these challenges, model systems are necessary for understanding disease pathophysiology in order to allow for the development of appropriate treatments. A good animal model should be able to provide new understanding into the disorder it models and respond in a reproducible and predictable manner. Other practical characteristics of the model that must be taken into account include cost, ease of maintenance, genetic uniformity, and amenability to behavioural testing.

Neuroscience has focused significant attention to the amygdala, unmasking its structure, function, and physiological mechanisms, across both animals and humans. It has become more and more evident that structural and functional changes in the amygdala are associated with a wide variety of clinical conditions in humans. Perhaps more than any other brain region, the amygdala has been linked to numerous neuropsychiatric, neurodevelopmental, and neurological disorders, and therefore a potential target for therapeutics to alleviate associated symptoms. The amygdala is an integral part of a neural system that evolved early in order to detect environment dangers and modulate subsequent responses, a role which can profoundly influence human behavior. Notwithstanding this systematic progress, much remains unknown, but the foundational knowledge obtained has provided a solid grounding in which to build upon in future work.

Author details

Trevor H. Gilbert
Centre for Psychology, Faculty of Humanities & Social Sciences, Athabasca University, Canada

Acknowledgement

The author wishes to acknowledge the excellent research contributions of Jenna Hildebrandt, Johanna MacDonell, and Rory St. Clair.

11. References

[1] Shaw C, McEachern J (2001) Toward a theory of neuroplasticity. London, England: Psychology Press.
[2] Fisher RS (1989) Animal models of the epilepsies. Brain Research Reviews. 14: 245-278.
[3] Gilbert TH, Bharadia V, Teskey GC (2001) Conventional anticonvulsant drugs in the guinea-pig kindling model of partial seizures: effects of acute phenytoin. Exp. Brain Res. 140: 469-478.
[4] Gilbert TH, Teskey GC (2007) Effects of conventional anticonvulsant drugs during repeated administration in amygdala-kindled guinea-pigs. Exp. Brain Res. 178: 115-125.
[5] Nestler EJ, Hyman SE (2010) Animal models of neuropsychiatric disorders. Nature Neuroscience. 13: 1161–1169.
[6] Fernando AB, Robbins TW (2011) Animal models of neuropsychiatric disorders. Annu. Rev. Clin. Psychol. 7: 39–61.
[7] LeDoux JE (2000) Emotion circuits in the brain. Annu Rev Neurosci. 23: 155–184.
[8] Rauch SL, Shin LM, Wright CI (2003) Neuroimaging studies of amygdala function in anxiety disorders. Ann NY Acad Sci. 985: 389-410.
[9] Price, JL, Drevets, WC (2010) Neurocircuitry of mood disorders. Neuropsychopharmacology Reviews. 35: 192–216.
[10] Benes F (2010) Amygdalocortical circuitry in schizophrenia: From circuits to molecules. Neuropsychopharmacology Reviews. 35: 239–257.

[11] Dziobek I, Bahnemann M, Convit A, Heekeren HR (2010) The role of the fusiform-amygdala system in the pathophysiology of autism. Arch Gen Psychiatry. 67(4): 397-405.
[12] Amaral DG, Price JL, Pitkanen A, Carmichael ST (1992) Anatomical organization of the primate amygdaloid complex. In: Aggleton JP (ed) The Amygdala: Neurobiological Aspects of Emotion, Memory, and Mental Dysfunction. Wiley-Liss Inc., New York, pp1-66.
[13] Kandel ER, Schwartz JH, Jessell TM (2000) Principles of neural science (4th ed). Appleton & Lange, New Jersey.
[14] Corcoran ME (1988) Characteristics and mechanisms of kindling. In: Kalivas P, Barnes C (eds) Sensitization of the Nervous System. The Telford Press, Caldwell, NJ, pp 81-116.
[15] Goddard GV (1967) Development of epileptic seizures through brain stimulation at low intensity. Nature. 214: 1020-1021.
[16] Goddard GV, McIntyre DC, Leetch CK (1969) A permanent change in brain function resulting from daily electrical stimulation. Experimental Neurology. 25: 295-330.
[17] Sato M, Racine RJ, McIntyre DC (1990) Kindling: basic mechanisms and clinical validity. Electroencephalography and Clinical Neurophysiology. 76: 459-472.
[18] Racine RJ (1972a) Modification of seizure activity by electrical stimulation: I. After-discharge threshold. Electroencephalography and Clinical Neurophysiology. 32: 269-279.
[19] Racine RJ (1972b) Modification of seizure activity by electrical stimulation: II. Motor seizure. Electroencephalography and Clinical Neurophysiology. 32: 281-294.
[20] Engel J (1998) The syndrome of mesial temporal lobe epilepsy: a role for kindling. In: Corcoran ME, Moshe SL (eds) Kindling 5. Plenum Press, New York, pp 469-484.
[21] McNamara JO (1984) Kindling: an animal model of complex partial epilepsy. Ann Neurol. 16 (suppl): S72-S76.
[22] Teskey GC, Thiessen EJ, Gilbert TH (1999) Alternate-site kindling in the guinea-pig results in accelerated seizure progression and generalization. Epilepsy Research. 34: 151-159.
[23] Teskey GC, Valentine PA, Sainsbury RS, Trepel C (1995) Evolution of afterdischarge and seizure characteristics during electrical kindling of the guinea pig. Brain Research. 672: 137-147.
[24] Sramka M, Sedlak P, Nadvornik P (1977) Observation of kindling phenomenon in treatment of pain by stimulation in thalamus. In: Sweet WH, Obdor S, Martin-Rodriguez JG (eds) Neurological Treatment in Psychiatry, Pain and Epilepsy, University Park Press, Baltimore, MD, pp 651-654.
[25] Cain DP (1989) Long-term potentiation and kindling: how similar are the mechanisms? Trends in Neuroscience. 12: 6-10.
[26] Bolwig TG (1989) New possibilities in neuropsychiatry. Ugeskr Laeger. 151(21):1339-1343.
[27] Post RM, Weiss SR (1998) Sensitization and kindling phenomena in mood, anxiety, and obsessive-compulsive disorders: the role of serotonergic mechanisms in illness progression. Biol Psychiatry. 44(3):193-206.
[28] Shepherd M (1998) Emil Kraepelin and modern psychiatry. Kaohsiung J Med Sci. 14(7): 395-404.
[29] Julien RM (2001) A Primer of Drug Action (9th ed). Worth Publishers.

[30] Post RM, Weiss SR, Pert A (1987) The role of context and conditioning in behavioral sensitization to cocaine. Psychopharmacol Bull. 23(3): 425-9.

[31] Post RM, Weiss SR, Smith M, Rosen J, Frye M (1995) Stress, conditioning, and the temporal aspects of affective disorders. Ann N Y Acad Sci. 771: 677-96.

[32] Post RM, Weiss SR, Smith M, Li H, McCann U (1997) Kindling versus quenching. Implications for the evolution and treatment of posttraumatic stress disorder. Ann N Y Acad Sci. 821: 285-95.

[33] Adamec R (1990) Kindling, anxiety and limbic epilepsy: Human and animal perspectives. In: Wada JA (ed) Kindling 4. Raven Press, New York, pp 329-341.

[34] Mucha RF, Pinel JPJ (1977) Postseizure inhibition of kindled seizures. Experimental Neurology. 54: 266-282.

[35] Wada JA, Sato, M, Wake A, Green JR, Troupin AS (1976) Prophylactic effects of phenytoin, phenobarbital, and carbamazepine examined in kindling cat preparations. Archives of Neurology. 33(6): 426 434.

[36] Adamec R (1975) Behavioral and epileptic determinants of predatory attack behavior in cat. Canadian Journal of Neurological Science. 2: 457-467.

[37] Boast CA, McIntyre D (1977) Bilateral kindled amygdala foci and inhibitory avoidance behavior in rats: a functional lesion effect. Physiology and Behavior. 18: 25-28.

[38] Kalynchuk LE, Pinel JP, Treit D, Kippin TE (1997) Changes in emotional behavior produced by long term amygdala kindling in rats. Biological Psychiatry. 1(4): 438 451.

[39] Wiebe S (2000) Seizure control as an indicator of therapeutic usefulness. Canadian Journal of Neurological Sciences. 27(1): S97-105.

[40] Löscher W (1998) New visions in the pharmacology of anticonvulsion. European Journal of Pharmacology. 342: 1-13.

[41] Löscher W, Schmidt D (1994) Strategies in antiepileptic drug development: is rational drug design superior to random drug screening and structural variation? Epilepsy Research. 17: 95-134.

[42] Wada JA (1998) Genetic predisposition and kindling susceptibility in primates. In: Corcoran ME, Moshe SL (eds) Kindling 5. Plenum Press, New York, pp 1-14.

[43] Kolb B, Whishaw IQ (2009) Fundamentals of human neuropsychology (6th ed). Worth Publishers, New York.

[44] Shin LM, Liberzon I (2010) The neurocircuitry of fear, stress, and anxiety disorders. Neuropsychopharmacology Reviews. 35:169–191.

[45] Rauch SL, Shin LM, Wright CI (2003) Neuroimaging studies of amygdala function in anxiety disorders. Ann NY Acad Sci. 985: 389-410.

[46] Nestler EJ, Hyman SE (2010) Animal models of neuropsychiatric disorders. Nature Neuroscience. 13: 1161–1169.

[47] Davis M, Walker DL, Miles L, Grillon C (2010) Phasic vs sustained fear in rats and humans: role of the extended amygdala in fear vs anxiety. Neuropsychopharmacology Reviews. 35: 105–135.

[48] Hartley CA, Phelps EA (2010) Changing fear: the neurocircuitry of emotion regulation. Neuropsychopharmacology Reviews 35: 136–146.

[49] Sripada RK, King AP, Garfinkel SN, Wang X, Sripada CS, Welsh RC, Liberzon I (2012) Altered resting-state amygdala functional connectivity in men with posttraumatic stress disorder. J Psychiatry Neurosci. 37(2): 1-9.
[50] Schumann CM, Bauman MD, Amaral DG (2011) Abnormal structure or function of the amygdala is a common component of neurodevelopmental disorders. Neuropsychologia. 49(4): 745–759.
[51] Kandel ER, Schwartz JH, Jessell TM (2000) Principles of neural science (4th ed). Appleton & Lange, New Jersey.
[52] Karayiorgou M, Simon TJ, Gogos JA (2010) 22q11.2 microdeletions: linking DNA structural variation to brain dysfunction and schizophrenia. Nat. Rev. Neurosci. 11: 402–416.
[53] Patterson PH (2009) Immune involvement in schizophrenia and autism: etiology, pathology and animal models. Behav. Brain Res. 204: 313–321.
[54] Bickel S, Javitt D (2009) Neurophysiological and neurochemical animal models of schizophrenia:Focus on glutamate. Behav. Brain Res. 204: 352–362.
[55] Seillier A, Giuffrida A (2009) Evaluation of NMDA receptor models of schizophrenia: Divergences in the behavioral effects of sub-chronic PCP and MK-801. Behav. Brain Res. 204: 410–415.
[56] Benes F (2010) Amygdalocortical circuitry in schizophrenia: From circuits to molecules. Neuropsychopharmacology Reviews. 35: 239–257.
[57] Howard MA, Cowell PE, Boucher J, Broks P, Mayes A, Farrant A, Roberts N (2000) Convergent neuroanatomical and behavioural evidence of an amygdala hypothesis of autism. NeuroReport. 11(13): 2931-2935.
[58] Paul LK, Corsello C, Tranel D, Adolphs R (2010) Does bilateral damage to the human amygdala produce autistic symptoms? J Neurodevelop Disord. 2: 165-173.
[59] Dziobek I, Bahnemann M, Convit A, Heekeren HR (2010) The role of the fusiform-amygdala system in the pathophysiology of autism. Arch Gen Psychiatry. 67(4): 397-405.
[60] Silverman JL, Yang M, Lord C, Crawley JN (2010) Behavioural phenotyping assays for mouse models of autism. Nature Reviews Neuroscience. 11: 490-502.
[61] Butcher JN, Mineka S, Hooley JM (2007) Abnormal psychology (13th ed). Boston: Pearson Education, Inc.
[62] Price, JL, Drevets, WC (2010) Neurocircuitry of mood disorders. Neuropsychopharmacology Reviews. 35: 192–216.
[63] Krishnan V et al (2007) Molecular adaptations underlying susceptibility and resistance to social defeat in brain reward regions. Cell. 131: 391–404.
[64] Chuang JC et al (2010) A b3-adrenergic-leptin-melanocortin circuit regulates behavioral and metabolic changes induced by chronic stress. Biol. Psychiatry. 67: 1075–1082.
[65] Meaney MJ (2001) Maternal care, gene expression and the transmission of individual differences in stress reactivity across generations. Annu. Rev. Neurosci. 24: 1161–1192.
[66] Wallace DL, Han MH, Graham DL, Green TA, Vialou V, Iñiguez SD, Cao JL, Kirk A, Chakravarty S, Kumar A, Krishnan V, Neve RL, Cooper DC, Bolaños CA, Barrot M, McClung CA, Nestler EJ (2009) CREB regulation of nucleus accumbens excitability mediates social isolation–induced behavioral deficits. Nat. Neurosci. 12: 200–209.

[67] Einat H, Manji HK (2006) Cellular plasticity cascades: genes-to-behavior pathways in animal models of bipolar disorder. Biol. Psychiatry. 59: 1160–1171.

[68] Kapczinskia F, Vietab E, Andreazzaf AC, Freye BN, Gomesa FA, Tramontinaa J, Annaf MKS, Grassi-Oliveirag R, Post RM (2008) Allostatic load in bipolar disorder: implications for pathophysiology and treatment. Neuroscience and Biobehavioral Reviews. 32: 675–692.

[69] Bechdolf A, Wood SJ, Nelson B, Velakoulis D, Yücel M, Takahashi T, Yung AR, Berk M, Wong MT, Pantelis C, McGorry PD (2012) Amygdala and insula volumes prior to illness onset in bipolar disorder: a magnetic resonance imaging study. Psychiatry Research: Neuroimaging. 201(1): 34-39.

[70] Hulvershorn LA, Karne H, Gunn AD, Hartwick SL, Wang Y, Hummer TA, Anad A (2011) Neural activation during facial emotion processing in unmedicated bipolar depression, euthymia, and mania. Biological Psychiatry. 71(7): 603-610.

[71] Mori E, Ikeda M, Hirono N, Kitagaki H, Imamura T, Shimomura T (1999) Amygdalar volume and emotional memory in Alzheimer's disease. Am J Psychiatry. 156: 216-222.

[72] Herzog AG, Kemper TL (1980) Amygdaloid changes in aging and dementia. Arch Neurol. 37: 625-629.

[73] Vereecken THLG, Vogels OJM, Nieuwenhuys R (1994) Neuron loss and shrinkage in the amygdala in Alzheimer's disease. Neurobiology of Aging. 15: 45-54.

[74] Knafo S, Venero C, Merino-Serrais P, Fernaud-Espinosa I, Gonzalez-Soriano J, Ferrer I, Santpere G, DeFelipe J (2009) Morphological alterations to neurons of the amygdala and impaired fear conditioning in a transgenic mouse model of Alzheimer's disease. Journal of pathology. 219: 41-51.

[75] Bouchard TP, Malykhin N, Martin WRW, Hanstock CC, Emery DJ, Fisher NJ, Camicioli RM (2008) Age and dementia-associated atrophy predominates in the hippocampal head and amygdala in parkinson's disease. Neurobiology of Aging. 29(7): 1027-1039.

[76] Freichel C, Neumann M, Ballard T, Müller V, Woolley M, Ozmen L, Kahle PJ (2007) Age-dependent cognitive decline and amygdala pathology in alpha-synuclein transgenic mice. Neurobiology of Aging. 28(9): 1421.

[77] Kalaitzakis ME, Christian LM, Moran LB, Graeber MB, Pearce RKB, Gentleman SM (2009) Dementia and visual hallucinations associated with limbic pathology in Parkinson's disease. Parkinsonism and Related Disorders. 15(3): 196-204.

[78] Petrasch-Parwez E, Nguyen HP, Löbbecke-Schumacher M, Habbes HW, Wieczorek S, Riess O, Andres KH, Dermietzel R, Von Hörsten S (2007) Cellular and subcellular localization of Huntingtin aggregates in the brain of a rat transgenic for Huntington disease. J Comp Neurol. 501: 716-30.

[79] Faure A, Höhn S, Von Hörsten S, Delatour B, Raber K, Le Blanc P, Desvignes N, Doyère V, El Massioui N (2011) Altered emotional and motivational processing in the transgenic rat model for Huntington´s disease. Neurobiol Learn Mem. 95: 92-101.

Chapter 11

Amygdala and Taste Learning

Andrés Molero Chamizo

Additional information is available at the end of the chapter

1. Introduction

The amygdala is a particular forebrain structure which is widely involved in many cognitive processes, such as attention and emotional learning, among others. The amygdala is part of the limbic system, which is critical for survival. In rats, it is located bilaterally in the medial temporal lobes, and its nuclei are similar to those of primates [1, 2]. In mammals, the amygdala is involved in the expression of many behaviours, such as fear responses, reproduction, aggressiveness and social behaviour and also in physiological processes such as modulation of the neuroendocrine and autonomic systems and homeostasis [3]. The amygdala consists of several nuclei that form a complex network of information processing. The three main nuclei of this structure are the medial, the central and the basolateral nucleus. These nuclei have complex connections with other structures; therefore it is thought that the activity of the amygdala is relevant in the modulation of some types of learning and memory [4]. In particular, the amygdala appears to participate in several complex processes underlying taste learning [5-11].

This chapter will summarize the most relevant data from animal models involving the amygdala in three complex processes underlying associative learning using a taste stimulus. The first section will aim to describe the role of the amygdala in the acquisition of the conditioned taste aversion (CTA) learning, a particular conditioning in which the subject learns to associate a novel taste stimulus with a successive visceral discomfort. The second section will review the data evidencing the role of the amygdala in the latent inhibition process of CTA that is obtained when the taste stimulus is presented to the subject several times prior to conditioning. Finally, we will discuss recent research that suggests that the participation of some cortical and subcortical structures (including the amygdala) in the influence of several contextual stimuli (such as the spatial context or time of day in the sleep/wake cycle) on the acquisition of CTA and latent inhibition of CTA. With this we hope to highlight some of the possible mechanisms of taste learning in which the different amygdaloid nuclei seem to have a specific function.

2. Amygdala and conditioned taste aversion learning

This section will review the studies that implicate the amygdala in taste learning processes [12]. First, a brief description of the phenomenon of CTA will be provided. Then we will analyse the research that points to the amygdala and its nuclei as part of the brain mechanisms of CTA.

2.1. Description of the conditioned taste aversion paradigm

Conditioned taste aversion learning is a particular conditioning paradigm which exists for the subject to associate the consumption of a new taste with a visceral disease that occurs after. Since a delay usually separates the presentation of the taste from the visceral disease, it is suggested that the learning results from the association between the memory trace of that taste and the disease [13]. The CTA learning is vital for numerous species because the learned aversion could reduce the probability of re-experiencing the toxic effects of a harmful substance. Even though this is a conditioning process, it has some special features when compared to most other forms of associative learning. Taste aversion learning is a paradigm widely used in animal research exploring the brain mechanisms of learning and memory [14]. Therefore, we will describe the taste aversion learning paradigm, which was mainly shown in animals. In humans, CTA has also been studied to a much lesser extent than in animals. For example, taste aversion learning has been examined in humans in order to understand the neurobiology of eating behaviour. Studies using positron emission tomography (PET) have shown that the amygdala and orbitofrontal cortex are activated when processing an aversive taste stimuli [15, 16]. Recent research with functional magnetic resonance imaging (fMRI) in humans has confirmed the involvement of the orbitofrontal cortex, anterior cingulated cortex, insular cortex and amygdala in processing highly aversive flavours [17]. Since the amygdala also seems to be involved in conditioned taste aversion in humans, it is possible that the acquisition of this learning requires biological mechanisms that are common in different species of vertebrates [18]. Moreover, because the food aversion associated with chemotherapy treatment is similar to the experimentally induced taste aversion [19], the CTA paradigm has helped to develop different strategies for dealing with the taste aversion that occurs in patients being treated with chemotherapy [20].

A crucial role in food selection processes is the ability to learn taste aversions [21]. This is particularly relevant for omnivorous species. The discrimination process between edible and harmful, or even potentially deadly, substances starts from the gustatory sensory information. This information stimulates a biological mechanism of precaution against new flavours, which facilitates the evaluation of the consequences of the ingestion of novel substances [22] and subsequently promotes the acquisition of conditioned taste aversions or preferences [8]. The initial response of caution is accompanied by a lower consumption of the novel substances. This phenomenon is called neophobia. If the sensory characteristics of the novel substance are associated with negative visceral consequences (such as poisoning), the animal will then acquire an aversion to that particular taste [23]. If the intake is associated with a positive visceral consequence (as in the case of an energetic food), or non-aversive, the new flavour will be recognized as being safe. Evolution has resulted in the development of neural mechanisms of attention, motivation, learning and memory that allow such identification of edible substances to be made.

Conditioned taste aversion paradigm exhibits three important features of associative learning; each feature exists separately in other classical conditioning paradigms. First, CTA can be acquired with a single pairing between the taste and the visceral discomfort [6, 13, 22-25]. Second, conditioned taste aversion is an example of a biological predisposition to associate certain stimuli more easily. For example, the taste-illness association occurs more easily than sound-disease or odour-disease associations [26]. The third characteristic of CTA learning refers to the delay that separates the presentation of the taste and visceral stimuli, or absence of temporal contiguity. The association between a new taste (the conditioned stimulus -CS-) and visceral consequences following its ingestion (the unconditioned stimulus -US-) results in a subsequent aversion to that taste, even though a delay of minutes or even hours (far superior to that seen in any other type of associative learning) is used. This unusual property of CTA to resist to a long inter-stimulus delay is related to the physiological processes of digestion. Indeed, in physiological conditioning, a delay always separates the ingestion from a potential poisoning. This delay is necessary for the completion of gastric digestion which results in the transport of nutrients through the gastrointestinal system and the gradual absorption of the products of digestion. Consequently, the association between gustatory and visceral stimuli must comply with this temporal requirement [27].

The experimental procedure used to induce conditioned taste aversion is a tool that has been used for decades in research into learning and the biological substrates of learning and memory [6, 11, 13, 14, 24, and 28]. In the laboratory, the procedure involves water deprivation with limited access to a daily amount of water, or water limited to a restricted time period within the day (usually 15 minutes). Once the daily amount of water consumed is stabilized, the animals receive the presentation of a new taste (representing the conditioned stimulus, generally a saccharin solution dissolved in water at 1%) during the conditioning session. The consumption of this taste is followed twenty or thirty minutes later by a gastrointestinal distress (representing the unconditioned stimulus, generally induced by an intraperitoneal injection of lithium chloride (LiCl), although some other aversive agents [29-36] have been used to induce aversion). Forty eight hours after conditioning, CTA tests can be used to detect the strength of the aversion to the CS previously paired with the malaise [37]. The reduction in the consumption of the CS after learning indicates more than a conditioned avoidance response. In fact, the learned aversion to taste really involves a change in the incentive properties of that stimulus, with its hedonic value becoming repulsive [38]. This learning is easily reproduced in the laboratory, and has proven to be a relevant paradigm for discovering important aspects of the neurobiological substrate involved in associative learning and memory. The following section will describe the findings that appear implicate the amygdala in the acquisition of this kind of learning.

2.2. Amygdaloid nuclei and acquisition of CTA

Conditioned taste aversion learning depends on a complex neural circuit that includes brainstem areas, as well as subcortical and cortical mechanisms [8, 11, 39, and 40]. Lesion studies have provided important information about the different structures and regions of the brain involved in the acquisition of taste aversion [10, 18, 41, 42-44]. The processing of sensory information necessary for the acquisition of a taste aversion involves multiple systems. The taste system detects information from the lingual papillae and palate via the cranial facial nerve (VII), glossopharyngeal (IX) and vagus (X) [8]. The visceral sensory system receives information via the vagus nerve and area postrema of the brainstem [45]. The information from both sensory systems are transported separately to the primary relay brainstem nuclei (nucleus of the solitary tract) and secondary relay (parabrachial nucleus), as well as to brain structures involved in processing visceral and taste, such as the thalamus, the insular cortex and the amygdala [46]. The processing of taste qualities [47] and subsequent association with the visceral effects of toxicity [48-50] requires complex neuroanatomical relationships in which the amygdala seems to be involved [51].

The amygdala and other cortical and subcortical areas are related to the brainstem associative processes necessary for taste aversion conditioning [41, 52-57]. In reference [52], the blockade of protein synthesis or beta-adrenergic receptors in the central amygdala blocks acquisition but not extinction of CTA. The same procedure in the basolateral amygdala blocks extinction but not acquisition of this learning. The authors of this research argue that the neural circuit that makes the acquisition of taste aversion memory possible and the extinction of the aversion requires the activity of the amygdala. However, the involvement of the amygdala and other structures in the associative processes of CTA has been studied by examining protein synthesis associated with learning. In one research it has been observed that the long-term aversive taste memory requires protein degradation in the insular cortex and the amygdala [56]. The selective involvement of the amygdala in CTA has also been analysed in other ways in animal models. There are studies of receptor expression during taste aversion learning [58, 59], studies of the c-Fos expression [60] and other genes [61] in the amygdala, studies of receptors blockade of the amygdala [62] and numerous studies using brain lesions [63], all in the CTA paradigm. For example, possible changes of the leptin receptor expression in the basolateral amygdala in relation to CTA acquisition have been analyzed [59]. Leptin receptor mRNA in the brain was analyzed by *in situ* hybridization and the expression of this receptor was assessed by immunohistochemistry method. Both measures were significantly higher after the formation of CTA. The authors concluded that the amygdaloid leptin receptor is involved in neuronal communication for CTA formation. Other studies [62] have also implicated other amygdaloid receptors in CTA, particularly the noradrenergic receptors. The researchers administered selective bilateral microinfusions of the beta-adrenergic antagonist propranolol into the basolateral amygdala immediately before intraperitoneal LiCl injections. This procedure disrupted CTA memory and the authors proposed that the basolateral amygdala is a critical structure in modulating the consolidation of taste memory. Genetic studies have confirmed the relation between amygdala and CTA. In this regard, studies have recently identified some specific genes in the amygdala (associated with neuropeptides, G protein-coupled receptors, ion channels, kinases and phosphatases) that contribute to CTA acquisition [61].

Regarding the lesion procedure; the studies that describe a lesion in the amygdala have not been decisive so far as they have shown a weak effect on taste learning or even no effect at all. However, electrolytic lesions of amygdala were shown to attenuate or disrupting CTA [64, 65] and also been shown to affect the neophobia phenomenon [65, 66]. Taken together with other studies that reported a selective involvement of the basolateral nucleus in CTA [67], it has been suggested that the effect of the basolateral injury on CTA is due to an alteration of the proper appreciation of the gustatory signal novelty, which could have affected the subsequent expression of taste aversion [63,68]. Subsequent studies have confirmed this hypothesis by reporting a selective effect on CTA [69] or a dual effect on neophobia and taste aversion [70] after basolateral nucleus lesion.

Moreover, electrolytic lesioning of the basolateral nucleus of the amygdala did not induce any effect on the formation of taste aversion in different studies [71-73]. Some authors have argued that the involvement of the basolateral amygdala in CTA is indirectly mediated by its interactions with the nucleus of the solitary tract [74] or the insular cortex [71, 72] therefore showing that the electrolytic lesions indirectly affects the acquisition of taste aversion. Nevertheless, other brain manipulation tools and neurophysiological techniques have also implicated the basolateral nucleus of the amygdala in the acquisition of CTA learning [51, 75-80]. In other studies [51] it has been found that specific neurons in basolateral amygdala respond to convergent taste stimulus and unconditioned stimulus information during CTA. The authors used a procedure of analysis of temporal gene transcription by fluorescence *in situ* hybridization in order to locate these populations of neurons. In [77], it was shown that CTA memory needs protein synthesis in the basolateral amygdala, and in [79] it has been proposed that the basolateral amygdala interacts with the insular cortex to modulate the memory consolidation because the infusions of the beta-adrenergic antagonist propranolol administered into this nucleus blocked the enhancing effects on CTA of a muscarinic agonist infused into the insular cortex.

The local injection of excitotoxic agents (such as NMDA or ibotenic acid) induces a more selective lesion in the cell bodies of the target structure. Although the excitotoxic lesioning of the amygdala has not always resulted in deterioration of CTA [71, 81, 82], the excitotoxic lesions of the basolateral amygdala often reproduce the effects obtained with electrolytic lesion on CTA [10, 44, 50, 83-86]. In contrast, the excitotoxic lesion of the central amygdala does not affect the formation of taste aversion [44, 83, 84, and 87]. The possible role of the central nucleus of the amygdala in CTA seems to be related to the processing of visceral information. For example, immunohistochemistry has found increased levels of a specific protein kinase associated with the memory of CTA in the cells of the central nucleus of the amygdala after injection of a high dose of LiCl-induced visceral malaise (US) [88]. A local microinjection of an inhibitor of this kinase into this nucleus decreased the strength of the CTA as well as the levels of this protein in the central amygdala. The authors of this study proposed that the intracellular levels of this protein kinase in the central amygdala are critical to process the visceral information in CTA. Therefore, it seems that the amygdaloid nucleus, which is involved in the acquisition of CTA, is the basolateral nucleus. In this regard, an unpublished study conducted in our laboratory has shown that excitotoxic lesions of the basolateral amygdala decreases taste aversion but does not disrupt the learning. In this study we performed bilateral excitotoxic lesions in the basolateral nucleus of the amygdala by local injection of NMDA and compared these animals' learning with two control groups. One was sham-lesioned in the amygdala and one with a lesion in the hippocampus, a structure not involved in CTA. The results showed a learning impairment in the case of animals with a basolateral lesion, compared with both control sham- and hippocampus-lesioned groups (see Figure 1).

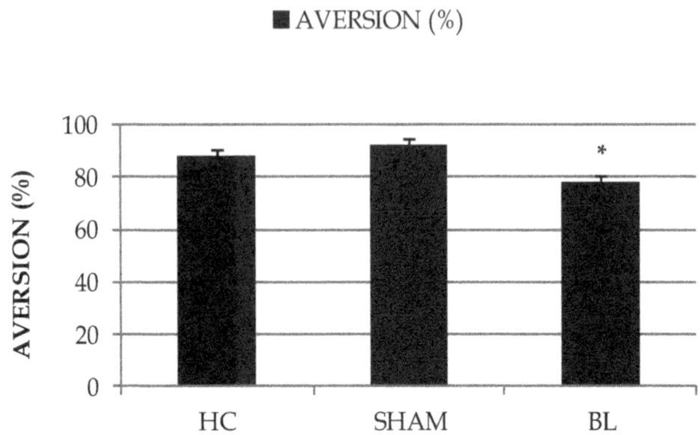

Figure 1. Percentage of taste aversion to saccharin in animals with lesion in the hippocampus (HC) or the basolateral amygdala (BL), as well as in the sham group. The percentage was calculated as a ratio between the saccharin consumed the day of acquisition of learning / saccharin consumed the day of acquisition of learning + saccharin consumed the testing day [X100].

Figures 2 and 3 show stained brain sections of a sham-lesioned animal and an animal with excitotoxic lesion in the basolateral amygdala induced by local injection of NMDA.

These results suggest that the basolateral amygdala is part of the brain circuitry of CTA, but is not a necessary structure for this learning. In other studies, the inactivation of the basolateral amygdala has not disrupted the CTA [89], or has impaired the learning but did not prevent its acquisition [7]. Therefore, our study, which used excitotoxic lesions, is consistent with the hypothesis that the formation of taste aversion does not require the integrity of the amygdala, although it does seem to be an important structure in the modulation of CTA [41] since the selective lesion of the basolateral amygdala reduces, but does not prevent, the learning. The reversible lesion studies also suggest that the amygdala, or any of its nuclei, is involved in the neural mechanism responsible for CTA learning. For example, the inactivation of the amygdala using local microinfusions of tetrodotoxin (TTX) has confirmed the involvement of this structure in the acquisition and recovery of CTA [7, 90].

In summary, the evidence indicates that the amygdala is part of the neurobiology of taste aversion learning [51, 63, and 91]. Although the exact mechanism is unknown, the data suggest that anatomical and functional relationships between amygdala and insular cortex are necessary for the correct acquisition of conditioned aversion [79, 92]. Research also indicates that the projections from the amygdala to the hypothalamus [93,94] and, in particular, to the brainstem nuclei involved in taste aversion learning [46,74,95-99] also play a significant role in this kind of conditioning.

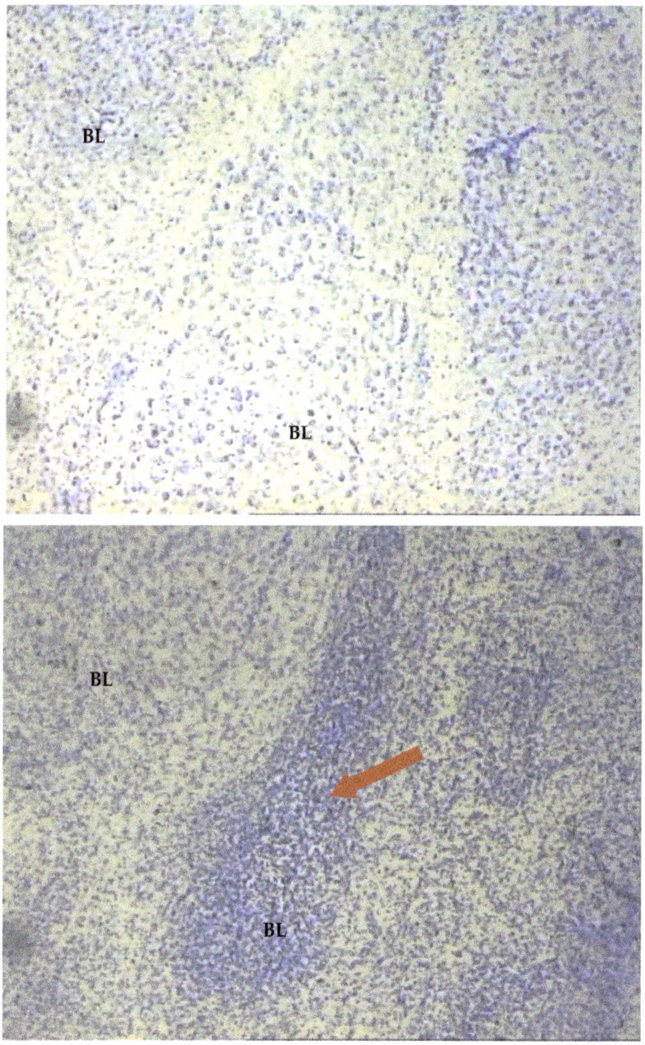

Figure 2. Section of the brain of a sham animal (above) and an animal with excitotoxic lesion in the basolateral (BL) amygdala (below). The arrow indicates the reaction of the microglia in this nucleus of the amygdala induced by the neurotoxin, compared with sham animal (image amplified 40x).

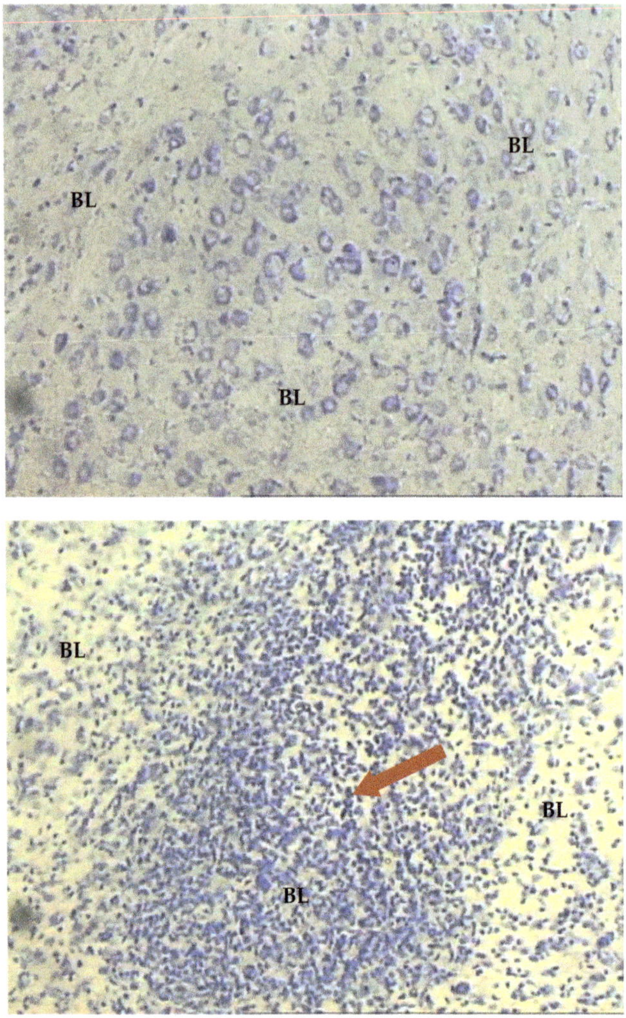

Figure 3. Detail amplified 100x of the sections of the Figure 2.

3. Latent inhibition and amygdala

Latent inhibition refers to a reduction in the conditioned aversion to a stimulus that has been previously pre-exposed without reinforcement. This phenomenon is easily reproduced in the laboratory and is demonstrated by presenting a stimulus several times (for example a sweet solution), which will subsequently be paired with a visceral malaise during one acquisition session. The latent inhibition response results in an absence, or a significant decrease, in the aversive response to the conditioned stimulus during the test session. In the following sections we will describe the phenomenon of latent inhibition in the CTA paradigm, and then review the studies implicating the involvement of the amygdala in the mechanisms underlying this learning.

3.1. Latent inhibition of taste aversion learning

The effect of latent inhibition has been demonstrated consistently in CTA learning [100-105]. Non-reinforced pre-exposure to a particular taste reduces the magnitude of CTA when this taste is subsequently associated with gastrointestinal discomfort. The experimentally obtained latent inhibition (LI) results in a higher aversion to the taste not experienced before the acquisition, in comparison to the aversion to the taste that has been pre-exposed. This reduction in the conditioned response is comparable to that obtained by pre-exposure in conventional experiments of classical conditioning [101,104].

Several cortical areas and subcortical structures have been specifically involved in the neural mechanisms that support latent inhibition depending on the learning paradigm used. For example, latent inhibition of the CTA, the fear conditioning and the cued fear conditioning, the eye blink response and some appetitive conditioning [106-114]. Some of the structures and systems involved in latent inhibition are the hippocampus, the mesolimbic dopaminergic pathway, the entorhinal cortex and the nigrostriatal dopaminergic pathway [115]. In addition, the nuclei of the amygdala have also been studied in relation to latent inhibition in several learning paradigms, although in CTA the results do not confirm the involvement of any of these nuclei in this phenomenon [110].

3.2. Amygdala and latent inhibition of taste aversion learning

According to [113], a complex neural circuit involving the connection of the medial prefrontal cortex, the striatum and the amygdala with the nucleus accumbens, is involved in the phenomenon of latent inhibition. The specific role of each component of the circuit could explain the discrepancy between the results obtained with lesions. For example, [114] has reported that electrolytic lesioning of the basolateral amygdala leaves latent inhibition intact in a conditioned emotional response procedure. In contrast, in [116] it was observed that excitotoxic lesioning of the basolateral amygdala interferes with the effect of pre-exposure to a light-food pairing in a reinforcer devaluation procedure. Furthermore, in an appetitive conditioning task it was found that the lesions in the basolateral amygdala disrupted the latent inhibition [117]. The authors of this research concluded that the connections between the basolateral amygdala and the entorhinal cortex are crucial in the formation of latent inhibition. Molecular biology has also provided extensive information that suggests the involvement of the amygdala in latent inhibition depends on NMDA receptors. Blockade of these receptors in the basolateral amygdala by selective antagonists prevents the expression of latent inhibition in a fear conditioning task [118]. Moreover, it has been found that excitotoxic lesioning of the central amygdala does not affect the latent inhibition in a Pavlovian appetitive conditioning task [119] or a reinforcer-devaluation procedure [116]. Nevertheless, [120] observed an intense production of c-Fos protein in central amygdala neurons (which is associated with intense cellular activity), which correlated with the decrease in the conditioned response to a familiar stimulus. Therefore, although the real function of the amygdala in latent inhibition is still being researched, the data appear to suggest some involvement of the basolateral amygdala in this learning. These findings also seem to confirm that the regions involved in the brain circuit that support the latent inhibition process may be different, depending on the type of conditioning used.

Experiments on latent inhibition in CTA have not yet permitted us to define the neural mechanisms supporting the learning processes of this paradigm, although CTA is probably the paradigm that has provided the most documented information about the neurobiology of latent inhibition. The hippocampal lesion studies have attempted to demonstrate the involvement of this structure in latent inhibition but the results have not been decisive. For example, in reference to [121] it has been observed, by computer simulations, that depending on the behavioural protocol (particularly the total time of pre-exposure), the perception of novelty after hippocampal lesion could be larger, equal to, or smaller compared to the novelty in control animals. In contrast, the striatum has been clearly involved in latent inhibition of taste aversion learning [111, 122]. Regarding the amygdala; lesions of the basolateral nucleus have also not shown detrimental effects on latent inhibition of conditioned taste aversion [123]. In latent inhibition of CTA, the dopaminergic system of the basolateral amygdala has also been examined and has shown that dopamine in this nucleus does not appear to modulate the latent inhibition but rather the phenomenon of prepulse inhibition [110].

In order to test the involvement of the amygdala or the hippocampus in latent inhibition of CTA, we tested the effect of bilateral excitotoxic lesions of both structures in this paradigm. The results of this study showed that neither lesion of the amygdala (mainly located in the basolateral nucleus) nor hippocampus affected latent inhibition of CTA (see Figure 4).

Figures 5 and 6 show stained animal brain sections with excitotoxic lesion in the hippocampus or the basolateral amygdala, respectively, induced by local injection of NMDA.

Taken together, the results of this study indicate that the expression of latent inhibition in taste aversion learning paradigm does not require the participation of the hippocampus or amygdala.

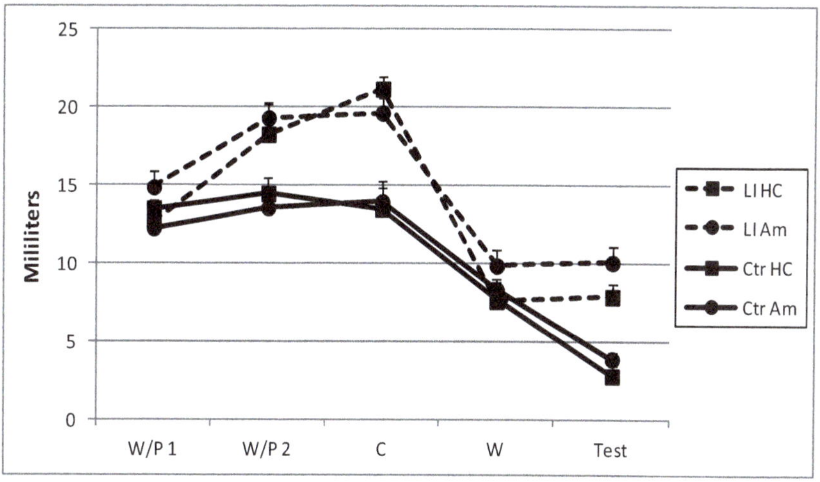

Figure 4. Representation of the average quantity of fluid in milliliters ingested by each of the groups (latent inhibition -LI- and control -Ctr-, with lesion in hippocampus -HC- or amygdala -Am-) over the days (W/P = water vs. pre-exposure to saccharin -CS-; C = conditioning; W = recovery with water; Test).

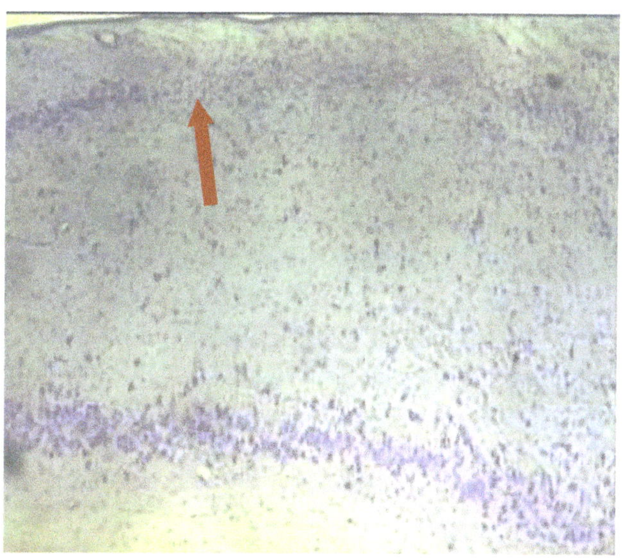

Figure 5. Section of the brain of an animal with excitotoxic lesion in the hippocampus. The arrow indicates the neurodegeneration of the CA1 hippocampal region induced by the neurotoxin (image amplified 40x).

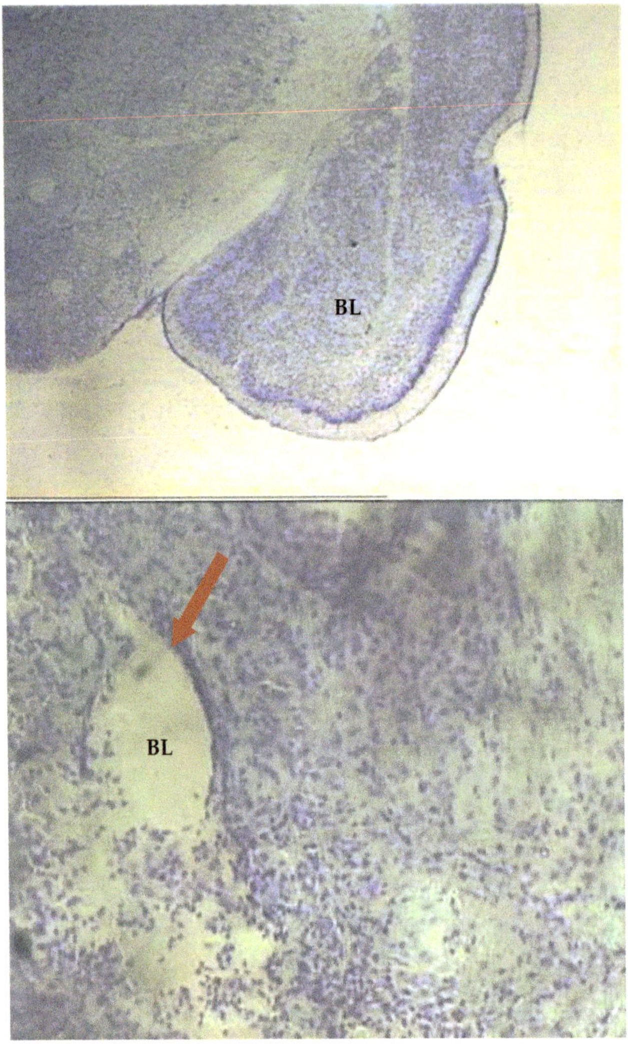

Figure 6. Section of the brain of an animal with lesion in the basolateral nucleus (BL) of the amygdala (above). Below, the arrow indicates the neuronal loss induced by NMDA in the basolateral amygdala (image amplified 40x).

4. Context, taste learning and amygdala

Contextual cues can modulate the conditioned response in numerous paradigms of learning. The brain mechanisms supporting this contextual effect on learning are not fully known.

The research indicates that the hippocampus and the amygdala participate in a different way in the context-learning relation, depending on the contextual cues and the behavioural paradigm used. The following sections will review the effects of context on learning and describe the involvement of the amygdala and hippocampus in the contextual modulation process of taste learning.

4.1. Effects of context on taste learning

Different contextual cues, both physical and interoceptive, can influence the processes that lead to associative learning [124-126]. The most explored contextual cue is the spatial context, represented by the physical characteristics of the experimental box [124,127]. For example, latent inhibition of fear conditioning [128] and latent inhibition of CTA are sensitive to the effects of a change in spatial context [101, 129, and 130]. Similarly, taste aversion learning [131] and its extinction [132] are also sensitive to the spatial context of learning. However, the influence of temporal context in associative processes is also a good model for understanding the mechanisms of learning and memory [133]. Regarding the modulating effect of time of day, we have shown in our laboratory that the time of day in the sleep/wake cycle acts as a contextual cue and modulates latent inhibition of taste aversion learning [134] and CTA retrieval [135].

The neurobiological processes underlying contextual effects on associative learning may vary depending on the characteristics of the contextual cues involved and the learning paradigm used. In this sense, the hippocampus and the amygdala appear to be specifically involved in the contextual effects on conditioning, depending on the type of learning paradigm. The hippocampus seems to be involved in memory processes and contextual learning [136], mainly in the paradigm of fear conditioning and in spatial tasks, such as the Morris water-maze [137-139]. Some reports also suggest that the amygdala is part of the brain mechanism that allows the context to influence fear conditioning [140-142] and place conditioning [143]. The amygdala appears to be an important structure involved in the effects of context on other forms of associative learning, for example, on conditioned potentiation of eating [144]. The next section will evaluate the role of the amygdala and hippocampus in the modulating effects of context on taste learning.

4.2. The limbic system and the effect of context on CTA

The spatial context dependency of the latent inhibition phenomenon appears to involve the activity of the hippocampus [120,121,145,146]. Temporal context dependency also seems to be mediated by the hippocampus in the paradigm of latent inhibition of taste aversion learning [147], as well as in CTA [14]. However, no studies have reported the role of the amygdala in the temporal modulation of taste learning [134,135]. It is possible that the amygdala is involved in CTA selectively but not in the phenomenon of latent inhibition in this paradigm, nor in the contextual dependency of this phenomenon. This possibility can be contrasted with the apparent involvement of the hippocampus in the contextual effects on latent inhibition of CTA [147], but not in taste aversion learning. To elucidate this differential involvement of both structures, we have performed some experiments aimed at evaluating the effect of a change in temporal context between pre-exposure and conditioning in animals with bilateral excitotoxic lesion in the amygdala or the hippocampus. These groups were further divided into two subgroups, one consisting of animals pre-exposed to the taste (CS) and conditioned at the same time of day (groups "same") and the other one pre-exposed and conditioned at different times of day (groups "different").

Figure 7 shows the consumption of animals throughout the behaviour procedure. All groups were pre-exposed and conditioned in different temporal contexts (groups "different") consumed significantly less (except the group with hippocampal lesion) that the "same" groups in test days. Therefore, a change in the time of day between pre-exposure and conditioning disrupted the latent inhibition learning of CTA. Nevertheless, the group with lesion in the hippocampus did not show this temporal context specificity, and the consumption of these animals after conditioning was similar to that of the "same" groups.

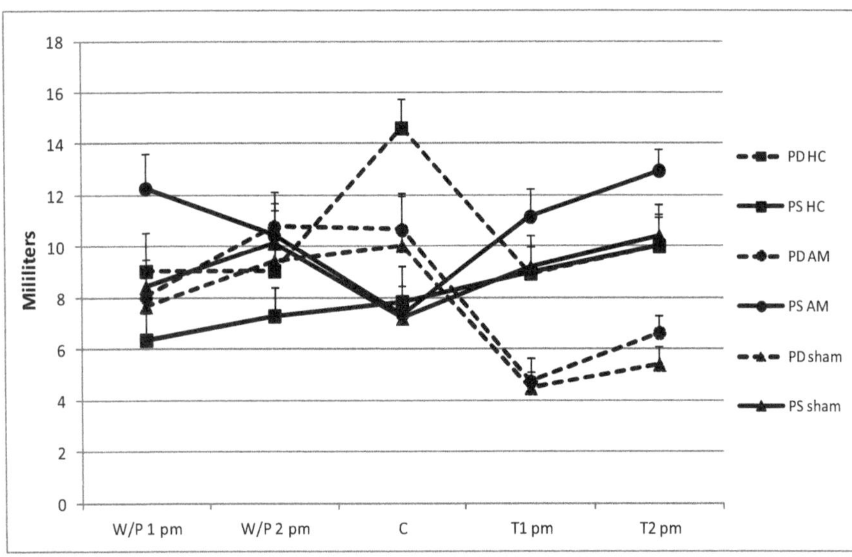

Figure 7. Representation of the average quantity of fluid in millilitres ingested by each of the groups (pre-exposed different -PD- and pre-exposed same -PS-, with lesion in hippocampus -HC- or amygdala -Am-, and pre-exposed different -PD- and pre-exposed same -PS- sham groups) over the days (W/P 1-2 pm = water vs. pre-exposure to saccharin in the evening session; C = conditioning in the morning - different- or evening -same- sessions; T1-2 pm= tests 1 and 2 in the evening session).

Figures 8 and 9 show stained brain sections of animals with NMDA-induced excitotoxic lesion in the hippocampus or the basolateral amygdala, respectively, compared with sections of sham animals.

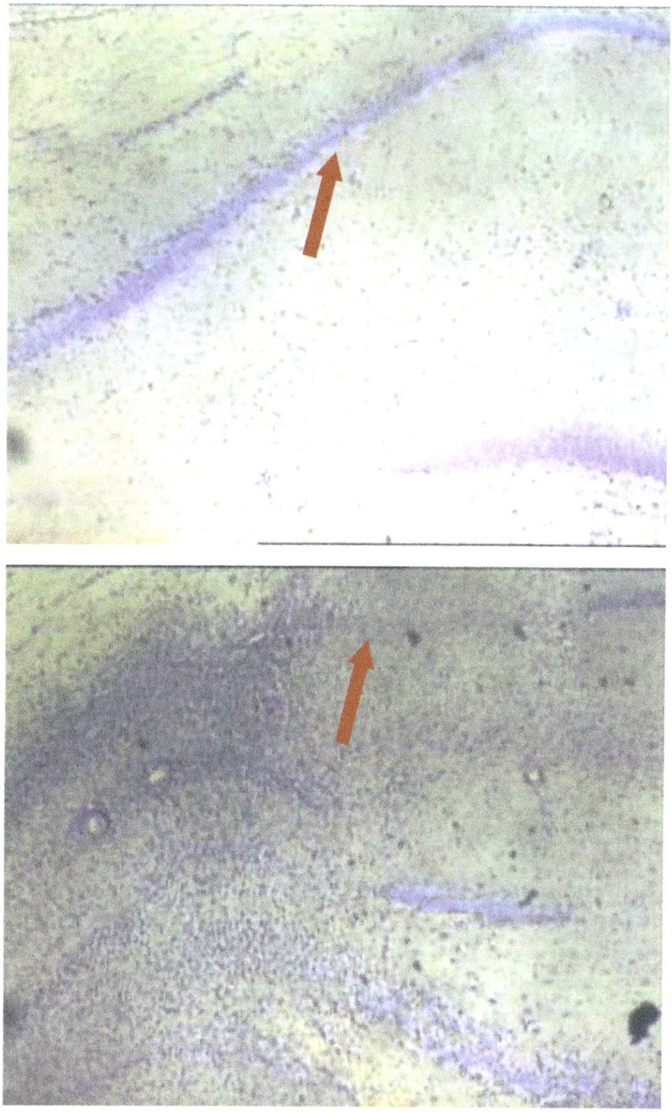

Figure 8. Section of the brain of an animal with sham lesion in the hippocampus (above). The arrow indicates intact cells of the CA1 hippocampal region. The bottom panel shows a section of the brain of an animal with hippocampal lesion. The arrow shows the destruction of the cells of the CA1 hippocampal region induced by the neurotoxin (images amplified 40x).

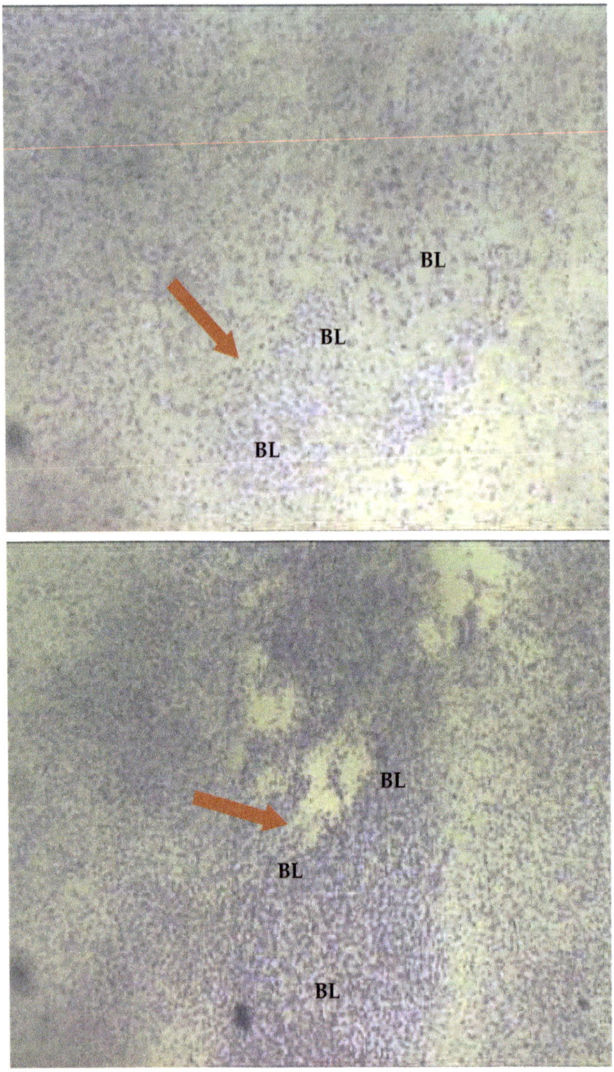

Figure 9. Section of the brain of an animal with a sham lesion in the basolateral (BL) amygdala (above). The arrow indicates intact cells of this nucleus. The bottom panel shows a section of the brain of an animal with lesion in the basolateral (BL) amygdala. The arrow shows the destruction of the cells of this amygdaloid nucleus induced by the neurotoxin (images amplified 40x).

In summary, our studies have shown that the hippocampus is necessary for the temporal specificity of latent inhibition of taste aversion learning, but not the amygdala. Subsequent studies performed in our laboratory have shown that the lesion in the hippocampus does not affect the phenomenon of latent inhibition in the CTA paradigm, confirming the selective function of this structure on the effects of a change of context on the phenomenon of latent inhibition of taste aversion learning. On the contrary, the amygdala is involved selectively in the acquisition of taste aversion, but not in the complex phenomena of latent inhibition and contextual modulation of taste learning.

5. Conclusions

The amygdala is a limbic structure involved in various processes of associative learning. Specifically, research has shown that the amygdala is part of the brain mechanism of taste aversion learning [11, 24, 41, 67, and 75]. Its role in aversive taste memory, however, is not entirely clear. Apparently, the taste memory trace requires the activity of the insular cortex [148]. The association between gustatory and visceral stimuli takes place in the brainstem [11, 41, 44, 60], although the consolidation of the memory of the association certainly seems to imply other structures such as the insular cortex or the amygdala [149]. The functional connections between the insular cortex and amygdala [92], and between the visceral processing nuclei and the amygdala [88], mean it is possible that the involvement of this structure or any of its nuclei in CTA is limited to a modulatory function, either of the sensory processing or the association between stimuli and its recovery [67]. This could explain the data obtained in some studies that shows amygdaloid lesion or its inactivation does not disrupt learning. In our study, excitotoxic lesion altered the acquisition of CTA but did not prevent learning, which may suggest that the amygdala regulates the associative process or the associative memory retrieval once established. Amygdaloid activation observed in different studies in the CTA paradigm [58, 59, and 61] is consistent with this proposal and supports the idea that the amygdala is an active structure in the acquisition of CTA but is not necessary to establish the association between stimuli or for the recovery of the association. The modulatory effects of the amygdala on learning and memory have also been described in studies of working memory and memory consolidation and extinction [150], consolidation of emotional memory [151], sensory memory representations in the cortex [152], acquisition of avoidance reactions [153], and CTA [149], among others.

The different effects on the magnitude of aversion resulting from the manipulation of the amygdala can be attributed to the particular mediation of the neophobia phenomenon in taste aversion, as well as the specific technique and procedure used. Nevertheless, in general, lesioning or inactivation of the amygdala does not prevent the CTA but reduces the magnitude of taste aversion. It seems, as described above, that the amygdala is a structure relevant for the correct acquisition of taste aversion. In this respect, our studies have shown that the excitotoxic lesioning of the amygdala does not eliminate CTA learning but decreases the acquired aversion. However, studies into the involvement of the amygdala in taste learning complex phenomena suggest that this structure is not decisive for the acquisition of latent inhibition of taste aversion learning [123], nor has its participation in the effects of spatial or temporal context on this phenomenon been demonstrated. Our experimental data support the hypothesis that the amygdala is selectively involved in the acquisition of taste aversion but not in the phenomenon of latent inhibition of taste aversion learning, nor in the contextual dependence of this phenomenon. In contrast, another structure of the limbic system, the hippocampus, does not seem to be involved in conditioned taste aversion nor in latent inhibition of this learning [121]. However, our experiments have shown that the contextual dependency of latent inhibition of taste aversion learning requires the integrity of the hippocampus [147], even when this structure is not necessary for the acquisition of latent inhibition in taste aversion learning paradigm. These findings demonstrate the differential functions of the amygdala and hippocampus in taste learning.

Author details

Andrés Molero Chamizo
University of Huelva, Spain

Acknowledgement

This work was supported by the University of Huelva. We are grateful to the University of Granada for the collaboration in conducting the experiments described. For helpful comments on earlier drafts of the manuscript, we also thank Jason Lauder and G. Nathzidy Rivera.

6. References

[1] Amaral DG., Price JL., Pitkänen A., Carmichael ST. Anatomical organization of the primate amygdaloid complex. In: Aggleton JP. (ed.) The Amygdala: Neurobiological Aspects of Emotion, Memory, and Mental Dysfunction. New York: Wiley-Liss, Inc.; 1992. p1-66.

[2] de Olmos JS. The amygdala. In: Paxinos G. (ed.) The Human Nervous System. New York: Academic Press; 1990. p583-710.

[3] Aggleton JP., editor. The amygdala: neurobiological aspects of emotion, memory and mental dysfunction. New York: Wiley-Liss, Inc.; 1992.

[4] Medina L, Bupesh M, Abellán A. Contribution of genoarchitecture to understanding forebrain evolution and development, with particular emphasis on the amygdala. Brain, Behavior and Evolution 2011; 78(3): 216-36.

[5] Bermúdez-Rattoni F. Molecular mechanisms of taste-recognition memory. Nature Reviews Neuroscience 2004; 5(3): 209–17.

[6] Gallo M, Ballesteros MA, Molero A, Morón I. Taste aversion learning as a tool for the study of hippocampal and non-hippocampal brain memory circuits regulating diet selection. Nutritional Neuroscience 1999; 2(5): 277-302.

[7] Roldán G, Bures J. Tetrodotoxin blockade of amygdala overlapping with poisoning impairs acquisition of conditioned taste aversion in rats. Behavioral Brain Research 1994; 65(2): 213-19.

[8] Scott TR. Learning through the taste system. Frontiers in Systems Neuroscience 2011; 5(87): 1-6.

[9] Tucci S, Rada P, Hernandez L. Role of glutamate in the amygdala and lateral hypothalamus in conditioned taste aversion. Brain Research 1998; 813(1): 44-9.

[10] Yamamoto T. Neural mechanism of taste aversion learning. Neuroscience Research 1993; 16(3): 181-5.

[11] Yamamoto T, Ueji K. Brain mechanisms of flavor learning. Frontiers in Systems Neuroscience 2011; 5(76): 1-7.

[12] Yamamoto T. Neural substrates for the processing of cognitive and affective aspects of taste in the brain. Archives of Histology and Cytology 2006; 69(4): 243-55.

[13] Bures J. The CTA paradigm: terminology, methods, and conventions. In: Bures J, Bermúdez-Rattoni F, Yamamoto T. (ed.) Conditioned taste aversion: Memory of a Special Kind. New York: Oxford University Press; 1998. p14-25.

[14] Gámiz F, Gallo M. Taste learning and memory: a window on the study of brain aging. Frontiers in Systems Neuroscience 2011; 5(91): 1-6.

[15] Zald DH, Lee JT, Fluegel KW, Pardo JV. Aversive gustatory stimulation activates limbic circuits in humans. Brain 1998; 121(6): 1143-54.

[16] Zald DH, Hagen MC, Pardo JV. Neural correlates of tasting concentrated quinine and sugar solutions. Journal of Neurophysiology 2002; 87(2): 1068-75.

[17] Sarinopoulos I, Dixon GE, Short SJ, Davidson RJ, Nitschke JB. Brain mechanisms of expectation associated with insula and amygdala response to aversive taste: implications for placebo. Brain, Behavior, and Immunity 2006; 20(2): 120-32.

[18] Bernstein IL. Taste aversion learning: a contemporary perspective. Nutrition 1999; 15(3): 229-34.

[19] Walker EA. Animal models. Advances in Experimental Medicine and Biology 2010; 678: 138-46.

[20] Jacobsen PB, Bovbjerg DH, Schwartz MD, Andrykowski MA, Futterman AD, Gilewski T, et al. Formation of food aversions in cancer patients receiving repeated infusions of chemotherapy. Behaviour Research and Therapy 1993; 31(8): 739-48.

[21] Manabe Y, Fushiki T. Aversive sensation in the brain after eating unpalatable food. Journal of Nutritional Science and Vitaminology 2002; 48(2): 81-8.

[22] Bures J, Buresova O, Krivanek J. Brain and Behavior. Paradigms for research in neural mechanisms. Oxford: John Wiley & Sons; 1988.

[23] García J, Kimmeldorf DJ, Koelling RA. Conditioned aversion to saccharin resulting from exposure to gamma radiation. Science 1955; 122(3160): 157-8.

[24] Bures J. Ethology, physiological psychology, and neurobiology of CTA. In: Bures J, Bermúdez-Rattoni F, Yamamoto T. (ed.) Conditioned taste aversion: Memory of a Special Kind. New York: Oxford University Press; 1998. p1-10.

[25] Scalera G. Effects of conditioned food aversions on nutritional behavior in humans. Nutritional Neuroscience 2002; 5(3): 159-88.

[26] García J, Koelling RA. Relation of cue to consequence in avoiding learning. Psychonomic Science 1966; 4: 123-4.
[27] Kalat JW, Rozin P. "Learned safety" as a mechanism in long-delay taste-aversion learning in rats. Journal of Comparative Physiological Psychology 1973; 83(2): 198-207.
[28] Spector AC, Breslin P, Grill HJ. Taste reactivity as a dependent measure of the rapid formation of conditioned taste aversion: a tool for the neural analysis of taste-visceral associations. Behavioral Neuroscience 1988; 102(6): 942-52.
[29] Ballesteros MA, Gallo M. Bilateral tetrodotoxin blockade of the rat vestibular nuclei substitutes the natural unconditioned stimulus in taste aversion learning. Neuroscience Letters 2000; 279(3): 161-4.
[30] Eccles S, Kim EM, O'Hare E. Granisetron attenuates exercise-induced conditioned taste aversion in the rat. Appetite 2005; 44(3): 325-8.
[31] Guitton MJ, Dudai Y. Anxiety-like state associates with taste to produce conditioned taste aversion. Biological Psychiatry 2004; 56(11): 901-4.
[32] Masaki T, Nakajima S. Further evidence for conditioned taste aversion induced by forced swimming. Physiology and Behavior 2005; 84(1): 9-15.
[33] Revillo, DA, Spear NE, Arias C. Ontogenetic differences in sensitivity to LiCl- and amphetamine-induced taste avoidance in preweanling rats. Chemical Senses 2011; 36(6): 565-77.
[34] St. John SJ, Pour L, Boughter JD. Phenylthiocarbamide produces conditioned taste aversion in mice. Chemical Senses 2005; 30(5): 377-82.
[35] Traverso LM, Ruiz G, De la Casa LG. MK-801 induces a low intensity conditioned taste aversion. Pharmacology Biochemistry and Behavior 2012; 100(3): 645-51.
[36] Vidal J, Chamizo VD. The conditioned stimulus elicits taste aversion but not sickness behavior in conditioned mice. Neuroimmunomodulation 2010; 17(5): 325-32.
[37] Batsell WR, Best M. One bottle too many? Method of testing determines the detection of overshadowing and retention of taste aversions. Animal Learning & Behavior 1993; 21(2): 154-8.
[38] Ossenkopp KP, Eckel LA. Toxin-induced conditioned changes in taste reactivity and the role of the chemosensitive area postrema. Neuroscience and Biobehavioral Reviews 1995; 19(1): 99-108.
[39] Yamamoto T, Shimura T, Sakai N, Ozaki N. Representation of hedonics and quality of taste stimuli in the parabrachial nucleus of the rat. Physiology and Behavior 1994; 56(6): 1197-202.
[40] Yamamoto T, Shimura T, Sako N, Yasoshima Y, Sakai N. Neural substrates for conditioned taste aversion in the rat. Behavioural Brain Research 1994; 65(2): 123-37.
[41] Bermúdez-Rattoni F, Yamamoto T. Neuroanatomy of CTA: lesions studies. In: Bures J, Bermúdez-Rattoni F, Yamamoto T. (ed.) Conditioned taste aversion: Memory of a Special Kind. New York: Oxford University Press; 1998. p28-44.
[42] Spector AC. Gustatory function in the parabrachial nuclei: implications from lesion studies in rats. Reviews in Neurosciences 1995; 6(2): 143-75.

[43] Yamamoto T. A neural model for taste aversion learning. In: Kurihara K, Suzuki N. (ed.) Olfaction and taste, XI. Tokyo: Springer-Verlag; 1994. p471-4.
[44] Yamamoto T, Fujimoto Y, Shimura T, Sakai N. Conditioned taste aversion in rats with excitotoxic brain lesions. Neuroscience Research 1995; 22(1): 31-49.
[45] Cameron OG. Visceral brain-body information transfer. Neuroimage 2009; 47(3): 787-94.
[46] Spray KJ, Bernstein IL. Afferent and efferent connections of the parvicellular subdivision of iNTS: defining a circuit involved in taste aversion learning. Behavioural Brain Research 2004; 154(1): 85-97.
[47] Houpt TA. Molecular neurobiology of ingestive behavior. Nutrition 2000; 16(10): 827-36.
[48] Coil JD, Rogers RC, García J, Novin D. Conditioned taste aversion: vagal and circulatory mediation of the toxic unconditioned stimulus. Behavioral Biology 1978; 24(4): 509-19.
[49] García J, Hankins WG, Rusiniak KW. Behavioral regulation of the milieu interne in man and rat. Science 1974; 185(4154): 824-31.
[50] Sakai N, Yamamoto T. Possible routes of visceral information in the rat brain in formation of conditioned taste aversion. Neuroscience Research 1999; 35(1): 53-61.
[51] Barot SK, Kyono Y, Clark EW, Bernstein IL. Visualizing stimulus convergence in amygdala neurons during associative learning. Proceedings of the National Academy of Sciences of USA 2008; 105(52): 20959-63.
[52] Bahar A, Samuel A, Hazvi S, Dudai Y. The amygdalar circuit that acquires taste aversion memory differs from the circuit that extinguishes it. European Journal of Neuroscience 2003; 17(7): 1527-30.
[53] Bahar A, Dorfman N, Dudai Y. Amygdalar circuits required for either consolidation or extinction of taste aversion memory are not required for reconsolidation. European Journal of Neuroscience 2004; 19(4): 1115-8.
[54] Ma L, Wang DD, Zhang TY, Yu H, Wang Y, Huang SH, et al. Region-specific involvement of BDNF secretion and synthesis in conditioned taste aversion memory formation. The Journal of Neuroscience 2011; 31(6): 2079–90.
[55] McGaugh JL, Introini-Collison IB, Cahill L, Munsoo K, Liang KC. Involvement of the Amygdala in Neuromodulatory influences on Memory Storage. In: Aggleton JP. (ed.) The Amygdala: Neurobiological Aspects of Emotion, Memory, and Mental Dysfunction. New York: Wiley-Liss, Inc.; 1992. p431-51.
[56] Rodriguez-Ortiz CJ, Balderas I, Saucedo-Alquicira F, Cruz-Castañeda P, Bermudez-Rattoni F. Long-term aversive taste memory requires insular and amygdala protein degradation. Neurobiology of Learning & Memory 2011; 95(3): 311-5.
[57] Welzl H, D'Adamo P, Lipp HP. Conditioned taste aversion as a learning and memory paradigm. Behavioral Brain Research 2001; 125(1-2): 205-13.
[58] Ge H, Chiesa R, Pena de Ortiz S. Hzf-3 expression in the amygdala after establishment of conditioned aversion. Neuroscience 2003; 120(1): 1-4.

[59] Han Z, Yan JQ, Luo GG, Liu Y, Wang YL. Leptin receptor expression in the basolateral nucleus of amygdala of conditioned taste aversion rats. World Journal of Gastroenterology 2003; 9(5): 1034-7.

[60] Yamamoto T, Shimura T, Sako N, Sakay N. c-fos immunohistochemical study on brainstem mechanisms of conditioned taste aversion in the rat. Abstracts of the Fourth IBRO Congress at Kyoto 1995; 393.

[61] Panguluri SK, Kuwabara N, Kang Y, Cooper N, Lundy RF. Conditioned taste aversion dependent regulation of amygdala gene expression. Physiology & Behavior 2012; 105(4): 996-1006.

[62] Miranda MI, LaLumiere RT, Bue TV, Bermúdez-Rattoni F, McGaug JL. Blockade of noradrenergic receptors in the basolateral amygdala impairs taste memory. European Journal of Neuroscience 2003; 18(9): 2605-10.

[63] Reilly S, Bornovalova MA. Conditioned taste aversion and amygdala lesions in the rat: a critical review. Neuroscience & Biobehavioral Reviews 2005; 29(7): 1067-88.

[64] Buresova O. Neocortico-amygdalar interaction in the conditioned taste aversion in rats. Activitas Nervosa Superior 1978; 20(3): 224-30.

[65] Nachman M, Ashe JH. Effects of basolateral amydala lesions on neophobia, learned taste aversions, and sodium appetite in rats. Journal of Comparative and Physiological Psychology 1974; 87(4): 622-43.

[66] Kesner RP, Berman RF, Tardif R. Place and taste aversion learning: role of basal forebrain, parietal cortex and amygdala. Brain Research Bulletin 1992; 29(3-4): 345-53.

[67] Yasoshima Y, Yamamoto T, Kobayashi K. Amygdala-dependent mechanisms underlying memory retrieval of conditioned taste aversion. Chemical Senses 2005; 30(1): 158-9.

[68] Aggleton JP, Petrides M, Iversen SD. Differential effects of amygdaloid lesions on conditioned taste aversion learning by rats. Physiology and Behavior 1981; 27(3): 397-400.

[69] Kolakowska L, Larue-Achagiotis C, Le Magnen ET. Effets comparés de la lésion du noyau latéral de l'amygdale sur la néophobie et l'aversion gustative conditionnée chez la rat. Physiology and Behavior 1984; 32(4): 647-51.

[70] Rollins BL, Stines SG, McGuire HB, King BM. Effects of amygdala lesions on body weight, conditioned taste aversion, and neophobia. Physiology and Behavior 2001; 72(5): 735-42.

[71] Dunn LT, Everitt BJ. Double dissociations of the effects of the amygdala and insular cortex lesions on conditioned taste aversion, passive avoidance and neophobia in the rat using the excitotoxin ibotenic acid. Behavioral Neuroscience 1988; 102(1): 3-23.

[72] Fitgerald RE, Burton MJ. Effects of small basolateral amygdala lesions on ingestion in the rat. Physiology and Behavior 1981; 27(3): 431-7.

[73] Galaverna OG, Seeley RJ, Berridge KC, Grill HJ, Epstein AN, Schulkin J. Lesions of the central nucleus of the amygdala. I: Effects on taste reactivity, taste aversion learning and sodium appetite. Behavioral Brain Research 1993; 59(1-2): 11-7.

[74] Schafe GE, Bernstein IL. Forebrain contribution to the induction of a brainstem correlate of conditioned taste aversion: I. The amygdala. Brain Research 1996; 741(1-2): 109-16.
[75] Bermúdez-Rattoni F, Ramírez-Lugo L, Gutiérrez R, Miranda MI. Molecular signals into the insular cortex and amygdala during aversive gustatory memory formation. Cellular and Molecular Neurobiology 2004; 24(1): 25-36.
[76] Escobar ML, Alcocer I, Chao V. The NMDA receptor antagonist CPP impairs conditioned taste aversion and insular cortex long-term potentiation in vivo. Brain Research 1998; 812(1-2): 246-51.
[77] Josselyn SA, Kida S, Silva AJ. Inducible repression of CREB function disrupts amygdale-dependent memory. Neurobiology of Learning & Memory 2004; 82(2): 159-63.
[78] Lamprecht R, Hazvi S, Dudai Y. cAMP response element-binding protein in the amygdala is required for long-but not short-term conditioned taste aversion memory. Journal of Neuroscience 1997; 17(21): 8443-50.
[79] Miranda MI, McGaugh JL. Enhancement of inhibitory avoidance and conditioned taste aversion memory with insular cortex infusions of 8-Br-cAMP: involvement of the basolateral amygdala. Learning and Memory 2004; 11(3): 312-7.
[80] Pennanen L, Welzl H, D'Adamo P, Nitsch RM, Gotz J. Accelerated extinction of conditioned taste aversion in P301L tau transgenic mice. Neurobiology of Disease 2004; 15(3): 500-9.
[81] Bermúdez-Rattoni F, McGaugh JL. Insular cortex and amygdala lesions differentially affect acquisition of inhibitory avoidance and conditioned taste aversion. Brain Research 1991; 549(1): 165-70.
[82] Pacheco-López G, Niemi MB, Kou W, Härting M, Fandrey J, Schedlowski M. Neural substrates for behaviorally conditioned immunosuppression in the rat. The Journal of Neuroscience 2005; 25(9): 2330-7.
[83] Dwyer DM. Lesions of the basolateral, but not central, amygdala impair flavour-taste learning based on fructose or quinine reinforcers. Behavioral Brain Research 2011; 220(2): 349-53.
[84] Morris R, Frey S, Kasambira T, Petrides M. Ibotenic acid lesions of the basolateral, but not the central, amygdala interfere with conditioned taste aversion: Evidence from a combined behavioral and anatomical tract-tracing investigation. Behavioral Neuroscience 1999; 113(2): 291-302.
[85] Schafe GE, Thiele TE, Bernstein IL. Conditioning method dramatically alters the role of amygdala in taste aversion learning. Learning and Memory 1998; 5(6): 481-92.
[86] Wilkins EE, Bernstein IL. Conditioning method determines patterns of c-fos expression following novel taste-illness pairing. Behavioural Brain Research 2006; 169(1): 93-7.
[87] Touzani K, Taghzouti K, Velley L. Increase of the aversive value of taste stimuli following ibotenic acid lesion of the central amygdaloid nucleus in the rat. Behavioral Brain Research 1997; 88(2): 133-42.

[88] Kwon B, Houpt TA. Mitogen-activated protein kinase in the amygdala plays a critical role in lithium chloride-induced taste aversion learning. Neurobiology of Learning & Memory 2012; 97(1): 132-9.
[89] Ferry B, Sandner G, Di Scala G. Neuroanatomical and functional specificity of the basolateral amygdaloid nucleus in taste-potentiate odor aversion. Neurobiology of Learning & Memory 1995; 64(2): 169-80.
[90] Gallo M, Roldán G, Bures J. Differential involvement of gustatory insular cortex and amygdala in the acquisition and retrieval of conditioned taste aversion in rats. Behavioral Brain Research 1992; 52(1): 91-7.
[91] Yamamoto T, Fujimoto Y. Brain mechanisms of taste aversion learning in the rat. Brain Research Bulletin 1991; 27(3-4): 403-8.
[92] Yamamoto T, Azuma S, Kawamura Y. Functional relations between the cortical gustatory area and the amygdala: electrophysiological and behavioral studies in rats. Experimental Brain Research 1984; 56(1): 23-31.
[93] Bernardis LL, Bellinger LL. The lateral hypothalamic area revisited: ingestive behavior. Neuroscience & Biobehavioral Reviews 1996; 20(2): 189-287.
[94] Lundy RF, Norgren R. Activity in the hypothalamus, amygdala, and cortex generates bilateral and convergent modulation of pontine gustatory neurons. Journal of Neurophysiology 2004; 91(3): 1143-57.
[95] Bielavska E, Roldan G. Ipsilateral connections between the gustatory cortex, amygdala and parabrachial nucleus are necessary for acquisition and retrieval of conditioned taste aversion in rats. Behavioural Brain Research 1996; 81(1-2): 25-31.
[96] Gallo M, Bures J. Acquisition of conditioned taste aversion in rats is mediated by ipsilateral interaction of cortical and mesencephalic mechanisms. Neuroscience Letters 1991; 133(2): 187-90.
[97] Schafe GE, Fitts DA, Thiele TE, LeDoux JE, Bernstein IL. The induction of c-Fos in the NTS after taste aversion learning is not correlated with measures of conditioned fear. Behavioral Neuroscience 2000; 114(1): 99-106.
[98] Tokita K, Karádi Z, Shimura T, Yamamoto T. Centrifugal inputs modulate taste aversion learning associated parabrachial neuronal activities. Journal of Neurophysiology 2004; 92(1): 265-79.
[99] Yamamoto T. Central mechanisms of roles of taste in reward and eating. Acta Physiologica Hungarica 2008; 95(2): 165-86.
[100] Hall G. Perceptual and associative learning. Oxford: Clarendon Press; 1991.
[101] Hall G, Channell S. Context specificity of latent inhibition in taste aversion learning. Quarterly Journal of Experimental Psychology 1986; 38(2): 121-39.
[102] Klamer D, Pålsson E, Wass C, Archer T, Engel JA, Svensson L. Antagonism of the nitric oxide synthase inhibitor, L-NAME, of the effects of phencyclidine on latent inhibition in taste aversion conditioning. Behavioural Brain Research 2005; 161(1): 60-8.
[103] Lubow RE. Latent inhibition. Psychological Bulletin 1973; 79(6): 398-407.

[104] Lubow RE. Latent inhibition and conditioned theory. Cambridge: Cambridge University Press; 1989.
[105] Traverso LM, Ruiz G, De la Casa LG. Latent inhibition disruption by MK-801 in a conditioned taste-aversion paradigm. Neurobiology of Learning & Memory 2003; 80(2): 140-6.
[106] Reilly S, Bornovalova M, Dengler C, Trifunovic R. Effects of excitotoxic lesions of the gustatory thalamus on latent inhibition and blocking of conditioned taste aversion in rats. Brain Research Bulletin 2003; 62(2): 117-28.
[107] Roman C, Lin JY, Reilly S. Conditioned taste aversion and latent inhibition following extensive taste preexposure in rats with insular cortex lesions. Brain Research 2009; 1259: 68-73.
[108] Schmajuk NA, Lam YW, Christiansen BA. Latent inhibition of the rat eyeblink response: effect of hippocampal aspiration lesions. Physiology Behavioural 1994; 55(3): 597-601.
[109] Schmajuk NA, Lam YW, Gray JA. Latent inhibition: a neural network approach. Journal of Experimental Psychology: Animal Behavior Processes 1996; 22(3): 321-49.
[110] Stevenson CW, Gratton A. Role of basolateral amygdala dopamine in modulating prepulse inhibition and latent inhibition in the rat. Psychopharmacology 2004; 176(2): 139-45.
[111] Turgeon SM, Reichstein DA. Decreased striatal c-Fos accompanies latent inhibition in a conditioned taste aversion paradigm. Brain Research 2002; 924(1): 120-3.
[112] Weiner I, Feldon J. Phencyclidine does not disrupt latent inhibition in rats: implications for animal models of schizophrenia. Pharmacology and Biochemistry of Behavior 1992; 42(4): 625-31.
[113] Weiner I, Feldon J. The switching model of latent inhibition: an update of neural substrates. Behavioural Brain Research 1997; 88(1): 11-25.
[114] Weiner I, Tarrasch R, Feldon J. Basolateral amygdala lesions do not disrupt latent inhibition (LI). Behavioral Brain Research 1995; 72(1-2): 73-81.
[115] Schmajuk NA, Cox L, Gray JA. Nucleus accumbens, entorhinal cortex and latent inhibition: a neural network model. Behavioural Brain Research 2001; 118(2): 123-41.
[116] Hatfield T, Han JS, Conley M, Gallagher M, Holland P. Neurotoxic lesions of basolateral, but not central, amygdala interfere with Pavlovian second-order conditioning and reinforcer devaluation effects. Journal of Neuroscience 1996; 16(16): 5256-65.
[117] Coutureau E, Blundell JP, Killcross S. Basolateral amygdala lesions disrupt latent inhibition in rats. Brain Research Bulletin 2001; 56(1): 49-53.
[118] Schauz C, Koch M. Blockade of NMDA receptors in the amygdala prevents latent inhibition of fear-conditioning. Learning and Memory 2000; 7(6): 393-9.
[119] Holland PC, Gallagher M. Amygdala central nucleus lesions disrupt increments, but not decrements, in conditioned stimulus processing. Behavioral Neuroscience 1993; 107(2): 246-53.

[120] Radulovic J, Kammermeier J, Spiess J. Relationship between fos production and classical fear conditioning: effects of novelty, latent inhibition, and unconditioned stimulus preexposure. The Journal of Neuroscience 1998; 18(18): 7452-61.

[121] Buhusi CV, Gray JA, Schmajuk NA. Perplexing effects of hippocampal lesions on latent inhibition: a neural network solution. Behavioural Neuroscience 1998; 112(2): 316-51.

[122] Ellenbroek BA, Knobbout DA, Cools AR. The role of mesolimbic and nigrostriatal dopamine in latent inhibition as measured with the conditioned taste aversion paradigm. Psychopharmacology 1997; 129(2): 112-20.

[123] St. Andre J, Reilly S. Effects of central and basolateral amygdala lesions on conditioned taste aversion and latent inhibition. Behavioral Neuroscience 2007; 121(1): 90-9.

[124] Bouton ME. Context, time, and memory retrieval in the interference paradigms of Pavlovian learning. Psychological Bulletin 1993; 114(1): 80-99.

[125] Bouton ME, García-Gutiérrez A. Intertrial interval as a contextual stimulus. Behavioural Processes 2006; 71(2-3): 307-17.

[126] Bouton ME, Westbrook RF, Corcoran KA, Maren S. Contextual and temporal modulations of extinction: behavioral and biological mechanisms. Biological Psychiatry 2006; 60(4): 352-60.

[127] Ward-Robinson J, Honey RC. A novel contextual dimension for use with an operant chamber: From simple to hierarchical forms of learning. Journal of Experimental Psychology: Animal Behavior Processes 2000; 26(3): 358-63.

[128] Escobar M, Arcediano F, Miller RR. Latent inhibition and contextual associations. Journal of Experimental Psychology: Animal Behavior Processes 2002; 28(2): 123-36.

[129] Quintero E, Díaz E, Vargas JP, Schmajuk N, López JC, De la Casa LG. Effects of context novelty vs. familiarity on latent inhibition with a conditioned taste aversion procedure. Behavioural Processes 2011; 86(2): 242-9.

[130] Revillo DA, Arias C, Spear NE. The unconditioned stimulus pre-exposure effect in preweanling rats in taste aversion learning: Role of the training context and injection cues. Developmental Psychobiology. In press 2012.

[131] Kwok DW, Boakes RA. Blocking of acquisition of a taste aversion by a context experienced prior to the taste. Behavioural Processes 2012; 89(1): 27-9.

[132] Rosas JM, Bouton ME. Renewal of a conditioned taste aversion upon return to the conditioning context after extinction in another one. Learning and Motivation 1997; 28(2): 216-29.

[133] Pearce JM, Bouton ME. Theories of associative learning in animals. Annual Review of Psychology 2001; 52: 111-39.

[134] Manrique T, Molero A, Ballesteros MA, Morón I, Gallo M, Fenton A. Time of day-dependent latent inhibition taste aversion learning in rats. Neurobiology of Learning & Memory 2004; 82(2): 77–80.

[135] Morón I, Manrique T, Molero A, Ballesteros MA, Gallo M, Fenton A. The contextual modulation of conditioned taste aversions by the physical environment and time of day is similar. Learning & Memory 2002; 9(5): 218–23.

[136] Holland PC, Bouton ME. Hippocampus and context in classical conditioning. Current Opinion in Neurobiology 1999; 9(2): 195-202.

[137] Chen CC, Shen JW, Chung NC, Min MY, Cheng SJ, Liu IY. Retrieval of context-associated memory is dependent on the Ca(v)3.2 T-type calcium channel. PLoS One 2012; 7(1): e29384.

[138] Corcoran KA, Maren S. Hippocampal inactivation disrupts contextual retrieval of fear memory alter extinction. Journal of Neuroscience 2001; 21(5): 1720-6.

[139] de Oliveira Alvares L, Einarsson EO, Santana F, Crestani AP, Haubrich J, Cassini LF, et al. Periodically reactivated context memory retains its precision and dependence on the hippocampus. Hippocampus 2011; 22(5): 1092-5.

[140] Cangioli I, Baldi E, Mannaioni PF, Bucherelli C, Blandina P, Passani MB. Activation of histaminergic H3 receptors in the rat basolateral amygdala improves expression of fear memory and enhances acetylcholine release. European Journal of Neuroscience 2002; 16(3): 521-8.

[141] Hobin JA, Goosens KA, Maren S. Context-dependent neural activity in the lateral amygdala represents fear memories after extinction. The Journal of Neuroscience 2003; 23(23): 8410-6.

[142] Lee HJ, Choi JS, Brown TH, Kim JJ. Amygdalar NMDA receptors are critical for the expression of multiple conditioned fear responses. Journal of Neuroscience 2001; 21(11): 4116-24.

[143] Hetzel A, Meredith GE, Rademacher DJ, Rosenkranz JA. Effect of amphetamine place conditioning on excitatory synaptic events in the basolateral amygdala ex vivo. Neuroscience 2012; 206: 7-16.

[144] Holland PC, Petrovich GD, Gallagher M. The effects of amygdala lesions on conditioned stimulus-potentiated eating in rats. Physiology and Behavior 2002; 76(1): 117-29.

[145] Katz DB, Rogers RF, Steinmetz JE. Novel factors contributing to the expression of latent inhibition. Behavioral Neuroscience 2002; 116(5): 824-36.

[146] Maren S, Holt W. The hippocampus and contextual memory retrieval in Pavlovian conditioning. Behavioural Brain Research 2000; 110(1-2): 97-108.

[147] Molero A, Morón I, Ballesteros MA, Manrique T, Fenton A, Gallo M. Hippocampus, temporal context and taste memories. Chemical Senses 2005; 30(1): 160-1.

[148] Stehberg J, Moraga-Amaro R, Simon F. The role of the insular cortex in taste function. Neurobiology of Learning & Memory 2011; 96(2): 130-5.

[149] Guzmán-Ramos K, Bermúdez-Rattoni F. Post-learning molecular reactivation underlies taste memory consolidation. Frontiers in Systems Neuroscience 2011; 5(79): 1-9.

[150] Roozendaal B, McGaugh JL. Memory modulation. Behavioral Neuroscience 2011; 125(6): 797-824.
[151] McGaugh JL. The amygdala modulates the consolidation of memories of emotionally arousing experiences. Annual Review of Neuroscience 2004; 27: 1-28.
[152] Chavez CM, McGaugh JL, Weinberger NM. The basolateral amygdala modulates specific sensory memory representations in the cerebral cortex. Neurobiology of Learning & Memory 2009; 91(4): 382-92.
[153] Radwanska K, Nikolaev E, Kaczmarek L. Central noradrenergic lesion induced by DSP-4 impairs the acquisition of avoidance reactions and prevents molecular changes in the amygdala. Neurobiology of Learning & Memory 2010; 94(3): 303-11.

Chapter 12

Amygdala, Childhood Adversity and Psychiatric Disorders

Xiaodan Yan

Additional information is available at the end of the chapter

1. Introduction

Above 10% of children in the U.S. are subjected to some form of maltreatment (Table 1) [1]. Childhood adversity can take the form of abuse, neglect, or loss, with examples including but not limited to: sexual abuse, physical abuse, emotional/psychological abuse, neglect, parental death, and bullying. Childhood adversity has been shown to have lifelong impact on the victim's physical and mental well-being (Table 2).

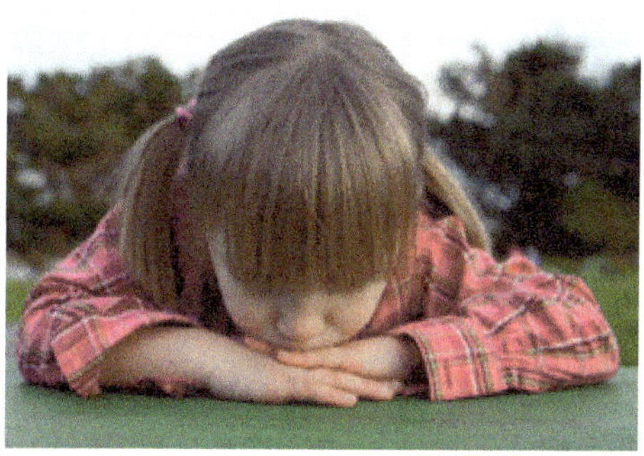

Figure 1. Childhood adversity is prevalent and has pervasive and long term impact on mental and physical health.

In many scientific studies invovling animal or human subjects, childhood trauma has been associated with low resting cortisol levels, altered stress response, increased inflammatory markers, and cognitive impairment [2]. In particular, childhood maltreatment has been linked to a variety of changes in stress-responsive neurobiological systems including brain structure and function [3]. Studies have shown that childhood maltreatment represents a strong risk factor for the development of depression and anxiety disorders in later life [3 - 5].

A presumed mechanism for such association is the persistent sensitization of central nervous system (CNS) circuits, in particular the amygdala, as a consequence of early life stress, which leads to the higher vulnerability to these psychiatric disorders [6].

Childhood abuse	Total N=17,337
Emotional abuse (Did a parent or other adult in the household ...) 1. Often or very often swear at you, insult you, or put you down? 2. Sometimes, often, or very often act in a way that made you fear that you might be physically hurt?	10.6%
Physical abuse (Did a parent or other adult in the household ...) 1. Often or very often push, grab, slap or throw something at you? 2. Often or very often hit you so hard that you had marks or were injured?	28.3%

Table 1. Adverse childhood experience (ACE) score definition and prevalence statistics [1].

2. Childhood adversity and psychiatric vulnerability: Epidemiology studies

It has been shown for a long time that early life adversity significantly increases psychiatric vulnerability in adulthood [7]; such an effect has been replicated in many large sample studies [8,9]. High risk psychiatric conditions include depression [10], anxiety [11], substance abuse [12], as well as psychosis related disorders such as schizophrenia [13,14]. A very large sample (N = 9377) 45-year prospective epidemiologic study has confirmed that such an impact is persistent throughout a person's lifecourse [15]. It has been identified that amygdala hyperactivity and morphological abnoramlity, together with structural and functional abnormality of other brain regions such as the anterior cingulate and prefrontal cortex, could have significant contribution to such heightened risk [16].

		Mental Health Disturbances			
ACE	N	Panic reactions	Depressed affect	Anxiety	Hallucination
0	(6255)	8.3%	18.4%	7.8%	1.3%
1	(4514)	10.9%	25.2%	9.1%	1.5
2	(2758)	13.6%	34.1%	12.4%	2.3%

Table 2. Relationship of the ACE scores (see Table 1 for definition of ACE) to the prevalence of mental health disturbances [1].

What further complicates the picture is the pattern of family risk for psychiatric disorders [17], which goes into a vicious circle, i.e., parents with psychiatric disorders tend to maltreat their children, which increases the psychiatric risk of their children, and such a vicious circle goes on for generations and generations. There are certainly genetic factors in addition to the family enviromental factor in this vicious cycle. Research in recent years are paying more attention on the epi-genetic mechanisms modified by identifiable patterns of childhood maltreatment [18]. Epigenetic mechanisms are mechanisms that regulate gene expression without altering the DNA sequence but rather through changing the biochemical environment of nucleotides. DNA methylation, histone modification, and chromatin remodeling are common epi-genetic mechnisms. However, it should be noted that although epigenetic mechanisms do not involve changing the DNA sequence, they are still inheritable. It is said that every sperm and every egg has a different epigenetic environment, and such differences are maintained during cell divisions for the remainder of the cell's life and may also last for multiple generations. Studies have shown that prenatal maternal stress, postnatal maternal care, and infant neglect/abuse can lead to epigenetic variation, which may have long-term effects on stress responsivity, neuronal plasticity, and behavior [18]. The remainder of this chapter will not elucidate the exact epigenetic mechanisms invovled in the lifelong impact of childhood adversity, since that is an area of research that is still being explored in heavy mist. Instead, we are going to focus our discussion on the neurobiological phenotypes, in particular, the impact of childhood adversity on the structure and functionality of the amygdala, which in turn serves as a significnat risk factor for developing psychiatric disorders in adulthood.

3. Amygdala abnormality due to early life adversity

The amygdala is critically involved in activation of the hypothalamic-pituitary-adrenal (HPA) axis in the face of emotional challenges and threat [19]. The HPA axis is a complex set of interactions in the neuroendocrine system, which controls stress related reactions as well as many other physiological regulations. The amygdala contains a large amount of neurons that produce corticotropin releasing hormone (CRH), as well as endogenous CRH receptors. Stress can increase CRH levels and upregulate CRH receptors in the amygdala so as to initiate fear responses (with behavioral characteristics including *fight, flee or freeze*). Such an effect has been observed in both adult [20] and developing rodents [21]. The critical role of the amygdala in this process has been confirmed by studies on cases with amygdala lesions, in which elevated glucocorticoid levels were absent during stressful situations [22,23]. Furthermore, external infusion of CRH to the amygdala significantly increases typical anxious behaviors [24]; the same effect can also be caused by electrophysiological stimulation of the amygdala [25], and of course, psychobiological stress such as seizure and chronic psychological stress [26,27].

Although stress-induced amygdala abnormality can happen any time in life, developmental studies have found that the amygdala is particularly sensitive to stress in early life such as during infancy and early childhood. Experiencing childhood adversity produces long lasting structural and functional changes in the amygdala during the dynamic processes of endogenous CRH production and regulation. As a behavioral result, the victim's threshold of emotional reaction is lowered, resulting in heightened excitability of the neural system for emotional response, which puts the individual at risk of general anxiety and anxiety-related psychiatric disorders [28]. Such an effect has been observed in many experiments as summarized in Table 3. The rest of this section will discuss these experimental evidences from behavioral neuroscience research with animal models as well as neuroimaging research with humans. At the end of this section, the complex interaction between the amygdala and other brain regions in the context of stress-related neural responses will also be discussed.

Article	N	Subjects	Adversity	Findings
Tottenham *et al.* (2010) [29]	62	Human children	Adverse caregiving	Larger amygdala volume in previously institutionalized group.
Mehta et al. (2009) [30]	25	Human children	Adverse caregiving	Larger amygdala volume in previously institutionalized group.
Bremner et al. (1997) [31]	34	Human adult	Chronic child abuse	Smaller hippocampus and unchanged amygdala volume in PTSD patients
Cohen et al. (2006) [32]	250	Human adult	Various early-life stressors	Differences in hippocampal volume were marginally significant and amygdala were nonsignificant between groups
Driessen et al. (2000) [33]	42	Human adults	Childhood trauma/ BPD	Patients had 16% smaller hippocampal and 8% smaller amygdala volume
Schmahl et al. (2003) [34]	33	Human adult	Childhood trauma/ BPD	Patients had smaller amygdala (~22%) and hippocampal (~14%) volumes
Plotsky et al. (2005) [35]	20	rat	Maternal separation	Elevated CRH mRNA in amygdala
Tsoory et al. (2008) [36]	104	rat	Various	Increased neural cell adhesion molecule in basolateral amygdala
Ono et al. (2008) [37]	148	mice	Early weaning	Precocious development of amygdala at 5 weeks of age
Kikusui et al. (2009)[38]	129	mice	Early weaning	Accelerated amygdala development
Salzberg et al. (2007) [39]	29	rats	Maternal Separation	Amygdala sensitization following maternal separation
Becker et al. (2007) [40]	20	rat	Separation	Higher CRF neuron levels in basolateral with lower levels in central amygdala
Vazquez et al. (2006) [41]	300	rat	Maternal separation	Higher basal CRH gene expression in amygdala than hippocampus.
Moriceau et al. (2004) [42]	108	rat	Predator odor	Exogenously administered cortisol increased amygdala activation
Hatalski et al. (1998) [21]	20	rat	Cold	Increased CRF-mRNA in the central nucleus of the amygdala
Sabatini et al. (2007) [43]	12	rat	Maternal separation	Early separation (more than later), decreased amygdala gene expression

Table 3. Summary of studies about the impact of early life adversity on amygdala. Abbreviation: CRF: corticotropin releasing factor, CRH: Corticotropin-releasing hormone, BPD, borderline personality disorder.

3.1. Evidence from behavioral neuroscience studies

In labaoratory rodents, similar to the case in humans, rodent pups (e.g., baby rats) that experience early life stress also exhibit altered adult behavioral and behavioral responses to stress. There are many ways to introduce early life stress in animal experiments, the most common ones include frequent handling, early weaning, and maternal separation. Chateracteristics of maternal behavior are also commonly used as variables for evaluating early life stress. These characteristics are usually quantified in terms of the frequencies of licking, grooming, arch-back nursing, etc. of the dams (e.g., mom rats) (Figure 2).

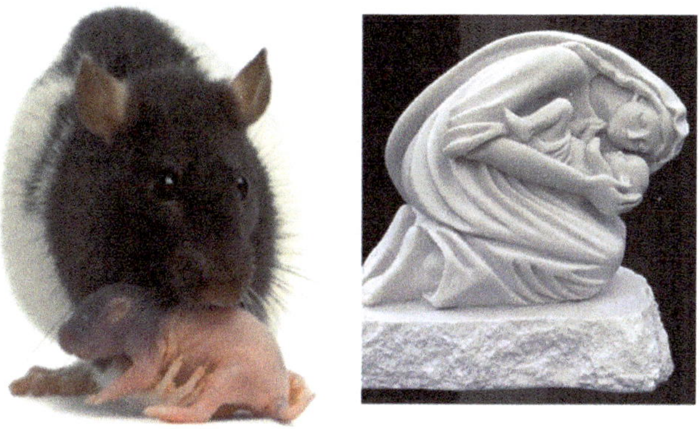

Figure 2. Maternal care patterns have important impact on the mental health of offsprings. In animal models with rats or mice, licking and grooming frequencies of the dam to the pups are common behavioral characteristics of maternal care [44]. This figure depicts rat maternal behavior, in comparison with that of human as represented in an artful sculpture.

By manipulating the caregiving conditions of infant rodents with the above methods, behavioral neuroscience experiments found that early life maltreatment could accelerate amygdala development [38,45,46] in terms of accelerated growth of dendrites, early myelination [37], increases in the amount of CRH-containing neurons [40] (Table 3), and functional sensitization [39]. In the central nucleus of the amygdala, decreased levels of benzodiazepine receptor binding, which plays an important role in inhibition of neuron activity, were observed among rats that received worse maternal care during infancy (Figure 4), and these rats also demonstrated higher anxiety levels behaviorally. The earlier such effects occur, the more devastating they are behaviorally [26], which could include socio-emotional deficits [43]. Experiments have elucidated that the most vulnerable time is the early postnatal period [47]. Compared to exposure to stress in adulthood, it might take 200 times less CRH in the early postnatal period to produce similar behavioral effects [48].

Functionally, accelerated amygdala maturation by early life adversity [49] promotes „aversive learning" (one of the major functions the amygdala is involved in [50]), which can be essential for survival in harsh conditions if seen from an ecological perspective. More importantly, a few studies have shown that amygdala abnormality as a result of adversity may be irreversible, i.e., amygdala cellular growth in response to stress failed to recover even in reversed environment [51,52]. It is possible that during evolution an "over-cautious" mechanism has been adapted to ensure the organism to be prepared for future adversity in an environment that is known to be threatening.

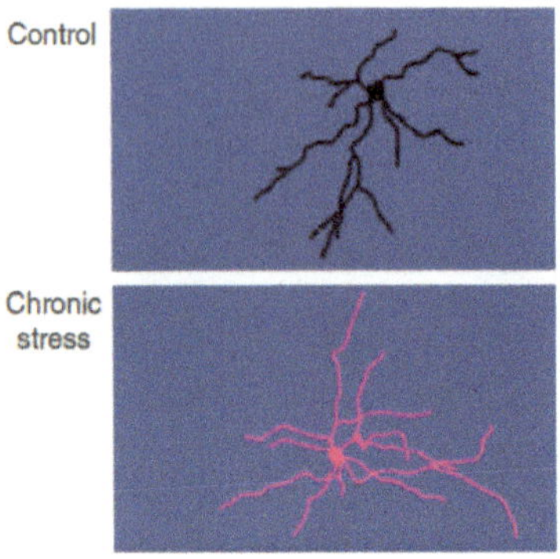

Figure 3. Accelerated amygdala neural growth as a consequence of early life adversity. As illustrated, chronic stress causes increased growth of dendrites (lower pannel compared to the upper panel) in the basolateral amygdala [46].

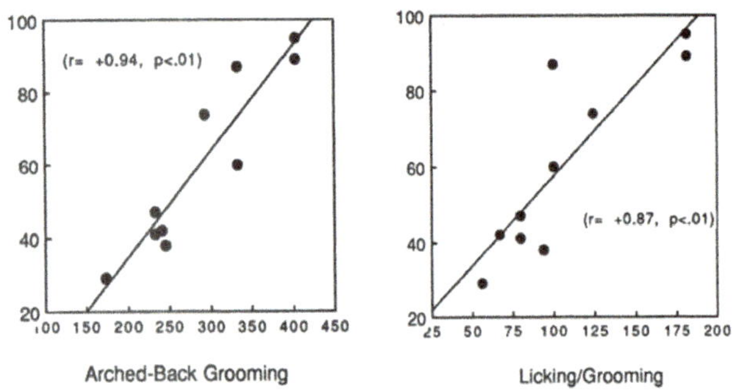

Figure 4. Significant correlations between maternal care characteristics (x-axis) and the level of benzodiazepine receptor binding (y-axis) in the central nucleus of the amygdala [53]. Lower frequencies of maternal care behaviors are associated with lower level of benzodiazepine receptor binding in the central nucleus of the amygdala, indicating less inhibition on neuron activity in the amygdala.

3.2. Amygdala abnormality in human: Neuroimaging studies

Neuroimaging techniques have made it possible to study amygdala morphometric and functional changes *in vivo* in human subjects. Many neuroimaging studies have shown that amygdala is structurally and functionally altered by psychosocial stress. It is usually difficult to study causality from human subjects, yet studies from animal models reviewed above have confirmed that amygdala abnormality follows stress exposure, rather than the other way round (i.e., inborn amygdala abnormality serving as a risk factor for adversity exposure) [54]. Such a conclusion from animal literature is partially applicable to humans.

As a consequence of early life adversity, accelerated amygdala maturation in the form of increased amount of neurons and dendrites can be demonstrated as increased amygdala gross volumes, which is a measure often used in human neuroimaging literature (Table 3). Neuroimaging studies have been conducted on children adopted from orphanages. These studies found increased amygdala volumes [30,48], and children adopted later tend to have larger amygdala (Figure 5). The fact that these children were adopted by families of very high socio-economic status further supported the view that amygdala abnormality as a result of early life adversity may be irreversible.

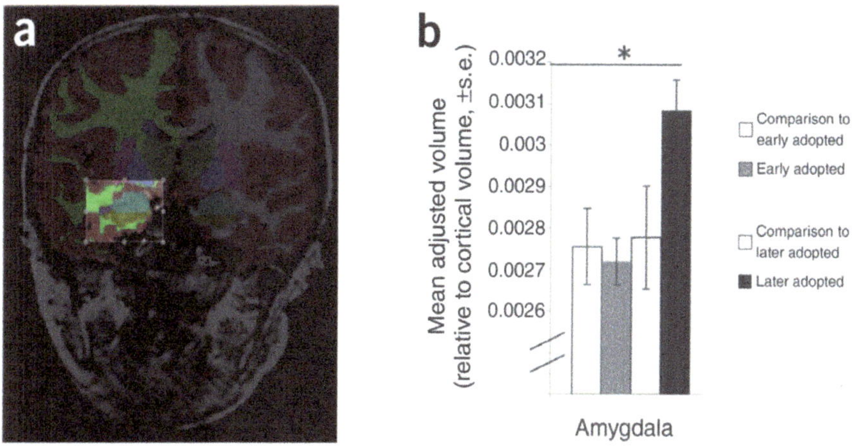

Figure 5. (a) Illustration of amygdala volumetric study with anatomical MRI. In the study presented in (b), it was found that later-adopted post-institutionalized children had larger amygdala volume compared with early adopted and typically developing controls [46].

Some neuroimaging studies might be occluding the picture with results seemingly contradictory with those from animal research. For example, many studies on trauma-exposed adults have demonstrated smaller and hyperactive amygdala [33,34]. Decreased amygdala volumes were also observed in subjects with childhood adversity comorbid with current borderline personality disorder (BPD) (Table 3, [33,34]). It should be noted that the above studies, which used adult subjects, might have been confounded by the effect of aging-related neural atrophy. Given that stress induces acceleration of amygdala development, it is possible a continuation of this effect into late adulthood would be demonstrated as "accelerated aging". This hypothesis is reasonable, given that amygdala hyperactivity has been consistently observed in almost all studies. Besides hyper-responsivity to threatening stimuli has been reported in previous literature [55 - 59], a recent study found amygdala hyperactivity even at *resting state* among individuals with unsuccessful stress coping (Figure 10). Such prolonged hyperactivity is likely to result in cellular atrophy and/or death, as has been seen in terms of reduced brain volumes in MRI studies [60]. Results from some neuroimaging studies also seem to support this hypothesis, in which depression patients showed enlarged amygdala volume at the initial depressive episode [61,62], but decreased amygdala volume after living with depression for extended periods of time [63,64].

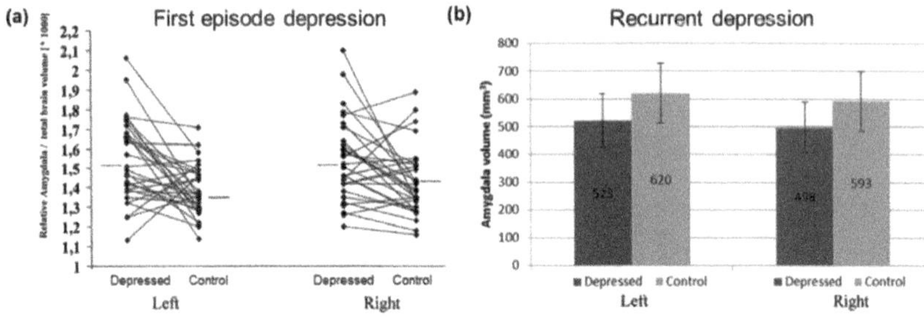

Figure 6. Enlarged versus reduced amygdala volumes in early-state (a) [61] or late stage (b) [63] depression. Note: p values are 0.002 (left amygdala) and 0.024 (right amygdala) in (a) with 30 subjects in each group, and 0.001 (left amygdala) and 0.002 (right amygdala) in (b) with 20 subjects in each group.

Thus it is important to identify the time sensitivity of stress impact on amygdala, which seems to have a dichotomy in early life and late life. It is very difficult to identify specific critical time points in humans, because there are rarely isolated stressors in human life and researchers have limited options to manipulate these stressors compared to what we can do with animals. Nonetheless, identifying the turning time points can be helpful for designing timely intervention programs as demonstrated in section 7. Unlike the case in animal literature [63,64], we might be able to reverse the toxic impact on amygdala through appropriate behavioral intervention programs.

4. Amygdala in the neural network

It is important to keep in mind that amygdala should not be considered in isolation since it is interconnected with other brain regions in a complicated neural network. The amygdala has a large number of connections with a wide range of other brain regions (Figure 7). It sends excitatory signals to the HPA axis through periventricular neurons as well as to other limbic structures (such as the anterior cingulate) and the brain stem. It also receives inhibitory signals from the ventral striatum and frontal cortex (Figure 7).

Due to the complicated network formed by the interactions between the above-mentioned structures, aversive influence from early life stress rarely affects the amygdala alone. Many other structures are also impacted, with the most common ones including the hippocampus, the anterior cingulate cortex, the frontal cortex (especially the ventral medial prefrontal cortex, the orbital frontal cortex as well as inferior frontal gyrus), as well as the right anterior insula. For example, numerous studies have demonstrated reduced volumes of the hippocampus [2,30,33,34,38,48,62,65,66] and anterior cingulate cortex [65,67] as a result of early life stress. Generally speaking, as a consequence of early life adversity, brain regions typically involved in emotional response including the amygdala, anterior cingulate cortex, ventral medial prefrontal cortex, inferior frontal cortex, orbital frontal cortex, as well as the right anterior insula (Figure 8), tend to be *hyperactive*. In the meantime, brain regions typically involved in emotion inhibition and emotion regulation tend to be *hypoactive*, including the dorsal medial prefrontal cortex, the dorsal lateral prefrontal cortex, the posterior cingulate cortex, and the precuneus (Figure 8), which results in reduced inhibition on the amygdala, eventually leading to behavioral patterns demonstrating anxiety. In neuroimaging psychiatric literature, both kinds of brain regions are frequently reported to be associated with anxiety-related psychiatric conditions. Thus, it takes both a *hyperactive* amygdala and a *hypoactive* emotion regulation system to give rise to anxiety-related behaviors.

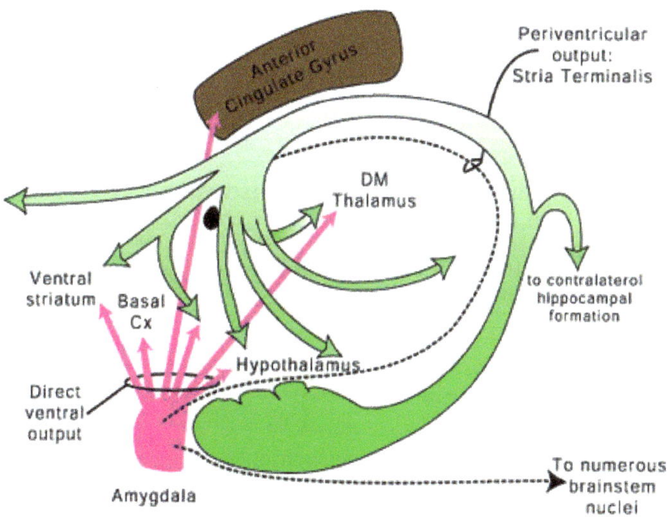

Figure 7. Projections to and from amygdala nuclei to other regions of the brain. Abbreviations: Cx: cortex, DM: dorsal medial.

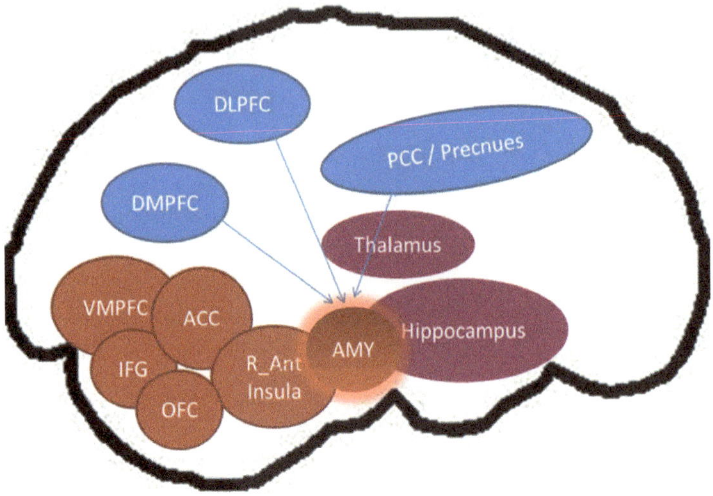

Figure 8. Association of amygdala with brain regions that are actively involved in emotional processing (red) and brain regions that are typically involved in emotion inhibition and regulation (blue), as well as other regions involved in emotional responses (purple). Abnormal morphometry and activity of these brain regions are frequently reported in stress-related psychiatric conditions. Abbreviations: ACC: anterior cingulate cortex, VMPFC: ventral medial prefrontal cortex, IFG: inferior frontal cortex, OFC: orbital frontal cortex, R_Ant_Insula: right anterior insula, DMPFC: dorsal medial prefrontal cortex, DLPFC: dorsal lateral prefrontal cortex, PCC: posterior cingulate cortex.

5. Amygdala abnormality and psychiatric disorders

Amygdala abnormality has been reported in many psychiatric disorders both in pediatric and adult patient population. Most of these disorders are associated with anxiety, such as general anxiety disorder (GAD), panic disorder, posttraumatic stress disorder (PTSD), bipolar disorder and depression. In particular, amygdala abnormality seems to be specifically responsible for the anxiety symptoms, although in the context of comorbid psychiatric disorders, such specificity could be confounded by other comorbid symptoms.

5.1. Amygdala abnormality in pediatric psychiatric disorders

Children with anxiety disorders showed an exaggerated amygdala response to fearful faces compared to healthy children, whereas depressed children showed a blunted amygdala response to these faces [68]. In addition, the magnitude of the amygdala's signal change between fearful and neutral faces was positively correlated with the severity of everyday anxiety symptoms [68]. Figure 9 demonstrates a recent study about the association between childhood maltreatment and amygdala responsiveness to negative facial expressions [69], in which the amount of childhood trauma was positively correlated with the degree of amygdala activity. Such an effect is frequently reported in literature.

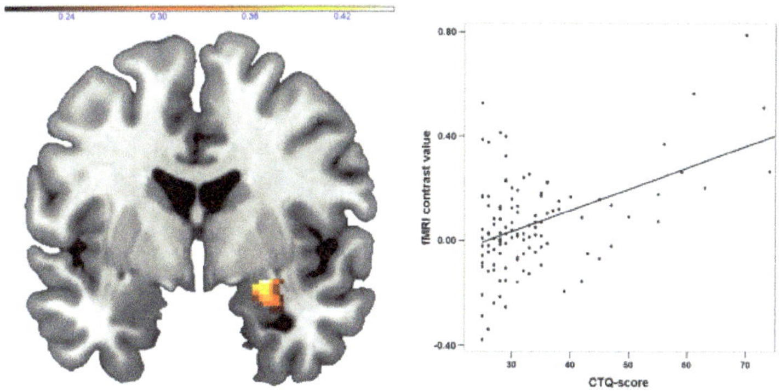

Figure 9. Childhood maltreatment (Childhood Trauma Questionnaire [CTQ] scores) is positively correlated with right amygdala responsiveness to negative facial expressions among 114 adult subjects [69]. The *y* axis stands for the among of fMRI signal change in response to negative facial expressions compared to the control condition.

Amygdala morphmetric changes in pediatric psychiatry literature is more complicated than its functional changes. Children with general anxiety disorder are reported to have enlarged right amygdala volumes [70] (Figure 10). But when anxiety symptoms comorbid with other symptoms, the story gets more complicated. For example, depressed children are reported to have significant reductions of amygdala volumes compared with healthy subjects [71]. Another study found that pediatric depression patients had significantly larger amygdala/hippocampal volume ratios than controls [72]; these increased ratios being associated with increased severity of anxiety but not increased severity of depression or duration of illness [72], suggest that amygdala abnorality was specific to the anxiety symptoms. Patients with a history of childhood trauma and current BPD also have smaller amygdala volumes (Table 3) [33,34]. Such complexity might arise from the timing issue of stress impact on amygdala as discussed in section 3.2, but it may also arise from complicated geneitc and epigenetic variations underlying these comorbid psychiatric disorders.

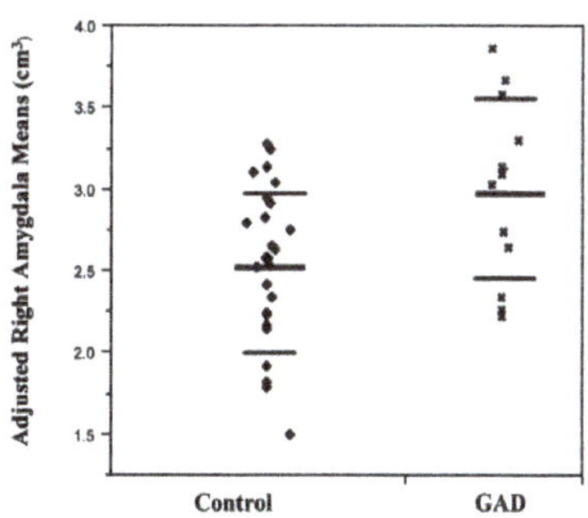

Figure 10. Children with general anxiety disorder (GAD) have an enlarged right amygdala volume compared to healthy developing controls [70]. The *y* axis is the right amygdala volume adjusted for intracranial volume. The horizontal lines stand for group means and standard deviations.

5.2. Amygdala abnormality in adult psychiatric disorders

Amygdala abnoramlity is also frequently reported from studies on adults with stress related psychiatric disorders [73], such as depression, anxiety, BPD, PTSD, etc. Amygdala volume is generally reduced in adult patients, an effect observed with PTSD [74], depression [63] and BPD [33,34]. It is also reported that schizophrenia patients had a left-greater-than-right amygdala asymmetry [75]. Exaggerated amygdala responsivity to threat-related stimuli is also a prevalent effect associated with various kinds of stress-related disorders, such as depression [68,76,77], PTSD [78,79], anxiety [68],etc. A recent study on PTSD using the novel resting state fMRI approach reported that amygdala was hyperactive even in *resting state*, i.e., a state without any prescribed cogntive tasks nor any external stimuli (Figure 11), and it also had reduced functional connectivity with middle frontal cortex, suggesting that amygdala can be constantly hyperactive even without external stimuli, and this is coming along with reduced inhibition from the frontal cortex.

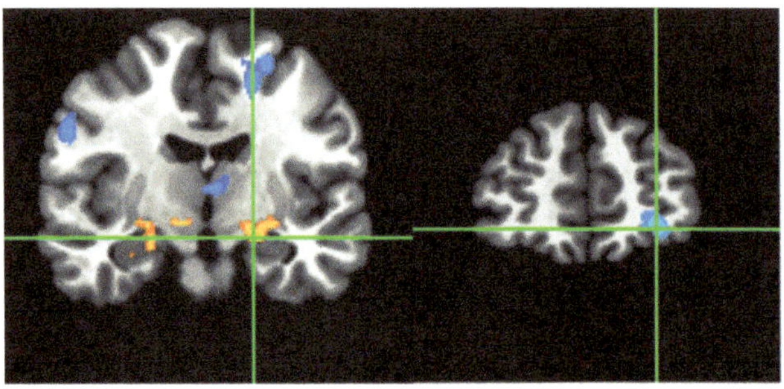

Figure 11. Resting state fMRI revealed higher amygdala spontaneous activity (left) with weaker functional connectivity with middle frontal cortex (right) in PTSD patients.

5.3. Amygdala abnormality as a risk factor for adult psychiatric disorders

In the context of lifelong human develoment, pediatric and adult psychiatric conditions are not isolated from each other. Epidemiology studies have shown that early onset depression and anxiety are highly predicative of adult psychiatric disorders [80]. An important scientific question is to test the following causal link: ealry life adversity → amygdala abnormality (and other neural abnormality) → increased risk for developing psychiatric disorders. Responding to this question is a very difficult scientific challenge. To begin with, it is very hard to identify a causal relationship with emprical experiments involving human subjects, because it is difficult to conduct longitudinal studies across the human lifespan. A common appraoch is to use the cross-sectional research paradigm instead of the longitudinal approach. In order to differentiate the influence of genetic and environmental factors on psychiatric conditions, a common approach is to use twin-studies, in which researchers study monozygotic and/or dizygotic twins, particularly those reared seperatly since brith [81 - 84]. PTSD is a particularly good disease model to address this question, because it has a clear onset and an obviously identifiable external stressor (which may still have complicated interation with other factors in real life). A recent twin study on PTSD identified vulnerability indicators such as smaller hippocampal volumes, low intellectual ability etc, and indicated that higher resting anterior cingulate metabolism could be the consequence rather than a pre-existing risk factor of PTSD [85], although another recent twin study suggest that hyper-responsitivity at dorsal anterior cingulate cortex could be a familial risk factor [86]. However, given the short history of prevelant application of neuroimaging approaches in studies of psychiatric disorders, there has not yet been a neuroimaging study directly establishing the above hypothesized causal link between early life adversity, amygdala abnoramlity and heighted vulnerability to psychiatric disorders in adulthood.

6. The neglected impact of stress from natural environment

Previous studies on childhood adversity have been focused on social stress particularly related to parental relations. However, other factors, such as malnutrition, poverty, crowded housing, urban noise, even industrial pollution and harsh natural environment, can also constitute stress factors during childhood and have equal, if not more, toxic impact on neural substrates including the amygdala, which may in turn have a lifelong influence on mental and physical health. These factors can also induce parental abuse by imposing stress thus elevating the irritability and irrationality of parents. Nonetheless, these factors have been neglected in the literature. In our laboratory, we conducted a series of multi-modal MRI studies on the long term impact of chronic hypoxia on young adults who were born and raised at high altitudes (2500-4000 meters above sea level) regions [87-93]. Our data did not show any effect of hypoxia on the amygdala; however, other regions typically involved in emotion processing such as the insula and hippocampus, were shown to have reduced gray matter volumes and elevated spontaneous activity among the subjects raised at high altitudes compared to control subjects [89]. There is one study that reported smaller amygdala and hippocampal volumes among adult individuals (aged 44-48 years) that suffered from financial hardship during childhood compared to those who did not [94]. These studies suggest a possible impact of factors that constitute childhood adversity on the structure and function of amygdala-related neural circuitry that are not directly linked to parental relationships.

7. What can we do? Neural plasticity and interventions

We hope there are ways to alleviate, if not to reverse, the toxic impact of early life adversity on the amygdala, and eventually, on behavioral patterns. More and more recent studies suggest that neural plasticity can be induced by social, cognitve and behavioral intervention [46]. For example, a study showed that Cognitive Behavioral Therapy (CBT, a common behavioral intervention approach particularly effective for depression) administered to depressive patients, was able to reduce amygdala activity and enhance prefrontal activity [95] (Figure 12). Another study suggested that Mindfulness Based Stress Reduction (MBSR) training (commonly known as "meditation") induced changes in perceived stress level as well as in amygdala gray matter density, while larger decreases in perceived stress were associated with larger decreases in amygdala gray matter density [96] (Figure 13).

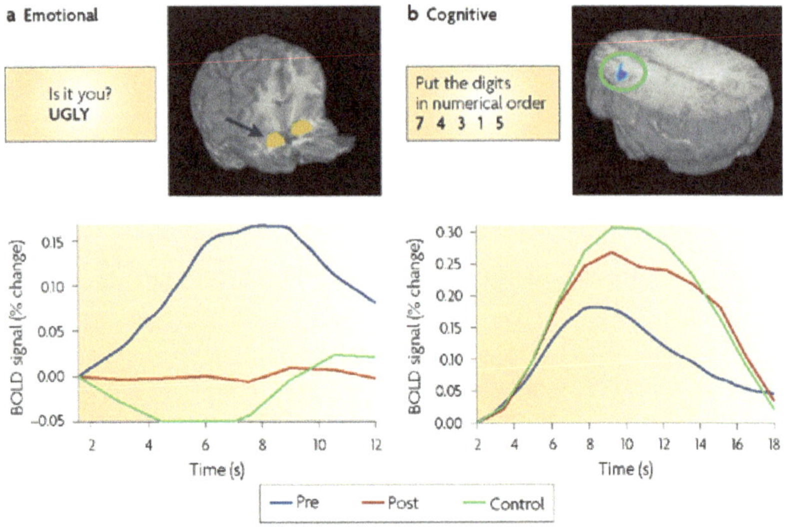

Figure 12. Cognitive behavioral therapy on depressed patients induced reduced amygdala activity in an emotional task and enhanced prefrontal activity in a cognitive task [95]. Panel (a) represents amygdala response in an emotional task (rating the personal relevance of negative words), panel (b) represents prefrontal cortex response in a cognitive task (arranging digits in numerical order). These experiments were conducted on 9 depressed participants before (*pre*) and after (*post*) they had CBT and 24 control participants. As shown in the response profiles, after depressed patients completed CBT (*post* vs. *pre*) they had reduced amgydala response and increased prefrontal response, with the response profile closer to that of the *control* group.

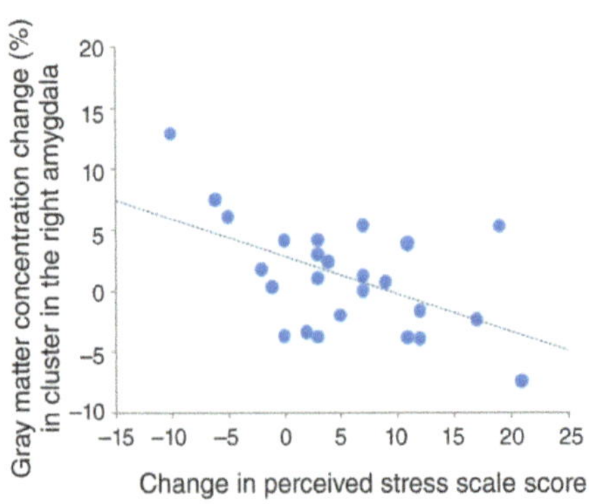

Figure 13. Mindfulness Based Stress Reduction (MBSR) training induced changes in perceived stress level as well as in amygdala gray matter density. Larger decreases in perceived stress were associated with larger decreases in amygdala gray matter density [96].

Other studies indicated that physical exercise was able to modulate aging related neural atrophy [97]. A significant effect was observed at the medial temporal lobe (Figure 14), but there was also a remarkable trend in the amygdala, the volume of which had a significant negative correlation with age in the low-exercise group (r=-0.62, p<0.001) but no significant correlation in the high exercise group (r=-0.21). It is possible that exercise might also help alleviate stress-induced amygdala atrophy, which is a good topic for future study.

In summary, childhood adversity can cause structural and functional changes of the amygdala, which increase the risk of developing psychiatric disorders in adulthood. Nonetheless, some behavioral intervention strategies (Figure 15) might help to promote neural plasticity, thus alleviating the neural toxicity and, thereby, reducing the risk to develop these disorders lately.

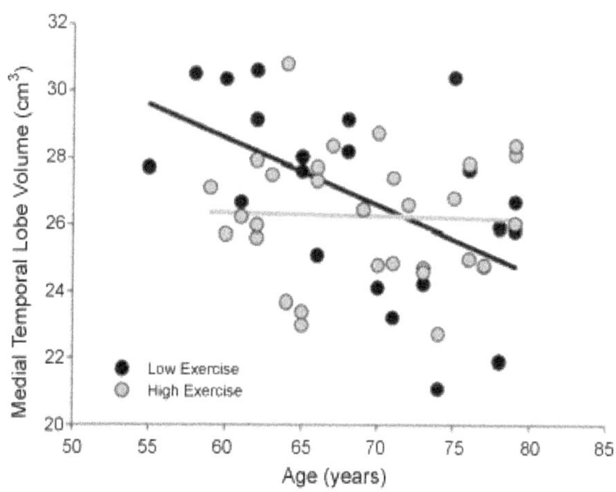

Figure 14. Exercise modulates aging related neural atrophy [97]. There was a significant negative correlation between the medial temporal lobe volume in the low exercise group ($r = -0.65$, $p < 0.001$), which demonstrates aging related atrophy, but such effect was absent in the high exercise group ($r = -0.24$). Such effect was also observed in the amygdala.

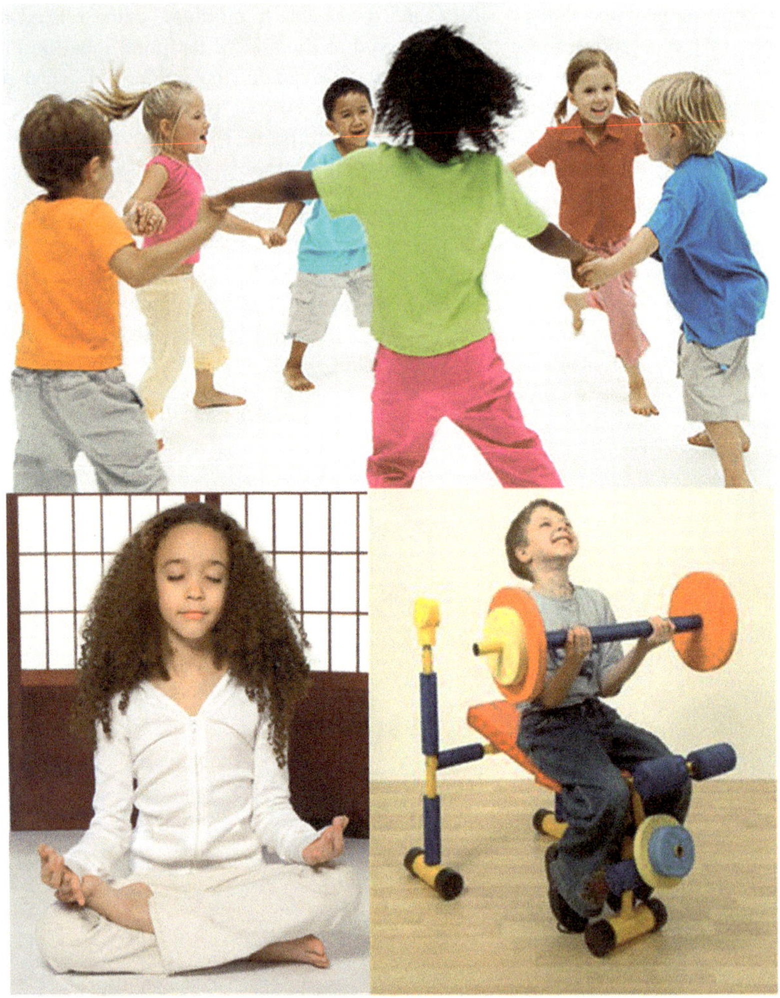

Figure 15. Behavioral intervention can induce neural platicity to protect the toxicity of early life adveristy on neural substracts such as the amygdala, thus reducing the risk of developing psychiatric disorders in later life. There are many easily implementable behavioral interventions, such as prosocial activity [98], meditation [99] or exercise [100], which have been suggested to be helpful in neuroscience literature [95 - 97].

Author details

Xiaodan Yan
Cognitive Science Department, Rensselaer Polytechnic Institute, USA

8. References

[1] Anda RF, Felitti VJ, Bremner JD, Walker JD, Whitfield C, et al. (2006) The enduring effects of abuse and related adverse experiences in childhood. A convergence of evidence from neurobiology and epidemiology. Eur Arch Psychiatry Clin Neurosci 256: 174-186.

[2] Heim C, Newport DJ, Mletzko T, Miller AH, Nemeroff CB (2008) The link between childhood trauma and depression: insights from HPA axis studies in humans. Psychoneuroendocrinology 33: 693-710.

[3] Kaufman J, Charney D (2001) Effects of early stress on brain structure and function: Implications for understanding the relationship between child maltreatment and depression. Development and Psychopathology 13: 451-471.

[4] Heim C, Nemeroff CB (2001) The role of childhood trauma in the neurobiology of mood and anxiety disorders: preclinical and clinical studies. Biol Psychiatry 49: 1023-1039.

[5] Anda RF, Felitti VJ, Bremner JD, Walker JD, Whitfield C, et al. (2006) The enduring effects of abuse and related adverse experiences in childhood. European archives of psychiatry and clinical neuroscience 256: 174-186.

[6] Heim C, Nemeroff CB (2001) The role of childhood trauma in the neurobiology of mood and anxiety disorders: preclinical and clinical studies. Biological Psychiatry 49: 1023-1039.

[7] Brown GW, Harris TO (1993) Aetiology of anxiety and depressive disorders in an inner-city population. 1. Early adversity. Psychol Med 23: 143-154.

[8] van der Vegt EJ, van der Ende J, Ferdinand RF, Verhulst FC, Tiemeier H (2009) Early childhood adversities and trajectories of psychiatric problems in adoptees: evidence for long lasting effects. J Abnorm Child Psychol 37: 239-249.

[9] Schilling EA, Aseltine RH, Jr., Gore S (2007) Adverse childhood experiences and mental health in young adults: a longitudinal survey. BMC Public Health 7: 30.

[10] Gourion D, Arseneault L, Vitaro F, Brezo J, Turecki G, et al. (2008) Early environment and major depression in young adults: a longitudinal study. Psychiatry Res 161: 170-176.

[11] Jolin EM, Weller EB, Weller RA (2008) Anxiety symptoms and syndromes in bipolar children and adolescents. Curr Psychiatry Rep 10: 123-129.

[12] Harrington M, Robinson J, Bolton SL, Sareen J, Bolton J (2011) A longitudinal study of risk factors for incident drug use in adults: findings from a representative sample of the US population. Can J Psychiatry 56: 686-695.

[13] Howes OD, McDonald C, Cannon M, Arseneault L, Boydell J, et al. (2004) Pathways to schizophrenia: the impact of environmental factors. Int J Neuropsychopharmacol 7 Suppl 1: S7-S13.

[14] Varese F, Smeets F, Drukker M, Lieverse R, Lataster T, et al. (2012) Childhood Adversities Increase the Risk of Psychosis: A Meta-analysis of Patient-Control, Prospective- and Cross-sectional Cohort Studies. Schizophrenia Bulletin.

[15] Clark C, Caldwell T, Power C, Stansfeld SA (2010) Does the influence of childhood adversity on psychopathology persist across the lifecourse? A 45-year prospective epidemiologic study. Ann Epidemiol 20: 385-394.

[16] McCrory E Fau - De Brito SA, De Brito Sa Fau - Viding E, Viding E (2012) The link between child abuse and psychopathology: A review of neurobiological and genetic research. J R Soc Med 105: 151-156.
[17] Carballedo A, Lisiecka D, Fagan A, Saleh K, Ferguson Y, et al. (2012) Early life adversity is associated with brain changes in subjects at family risk for depression. World J Biol Psychiatry.
[18] Gudsnuk KM, Champagne FA (2011) Epigenetic effects of early developmental experiences. Clin Perinatol 38: 703-717.
[19] Dedovic K, Duchesne A, Andrews J, Engert V, Pruessner JC (2009) The brain and the stress axis: the neural correlates of cortisol regulation in response to stress. Neuroimage 47: 864-871.
[20] Makino S, Gold PW, Schulkin J (1994) Effects of corticosterone on CRH mRNA and content in the bed nucleus of the stria terminalis; comparison with the effects in the central nucleus of the amygdala and the paraventricular nucleus of the hypothalamus. Brain Res 657: 141-149.
[21] Hatalski CG, Guirguis C, Baram TZ (1998) Corticotropin releasing factor mRNA expression in the hypothalamic paraventricular nucleus and the central nucleus of the amygdala is modulated by repeated acute stress in the immature rat. J Neuroendocrinol 10: 663-669.
[22] Feldman S, Conforti N, Itzik A, Weidenfeld J (1994) Differential effect of amygdaloid lesions on CRF-41, ACTH and corticosterone responses following neural stimuli. Brain Res 658: 21-26.
[23] Herman JP, Cullinan WE (1997) Neurocircuitry of stress: central control of the hypothalamo-pituitary-adrenocortical axis. Trends Neurosci 20: 78-84.
[24] Rosen JB, Schulkin J (1998) From normal fear to pathological anxiety. Psychol Rev 105: 325-350.
[25] Mason JW (1959) Plasma 17-hydroxycorticosteroid levels during electrical stimulation of the amygdaloid complex in conscious monkeys. Am J Physiol 196: 44-48.
[26] Baram TZ, Hatalski CG (1998) Neuropeptide-mediated excitability: a key triggering mechanism for seizure generation in the developing brain. Trends Neurosci 21: 471-476.
[27] Bonaz B, Rivest S (1998) Effect of a chronic stress on CRF neuronal activity and expression of its type 1 receptor in the rat brain. Am J Physiol 275: R1438-1449.
[28] Adamec R, Shallow T (2000) Rodent anxiety and kindling of the central amygdala and nucleus basalis. Physiol Behav 70: 177-187.
[29] Tottenham N, Hare TA, Quinn BT, McCarry TW, Nurse M, et al. (2010) Prolonged institutional rearing is associated with atypically large amygdala volume and difficulties in emotion regulation. Dev Sci 13: 46-61.
[30] Mehta MA, Golembo NI, Nosarti C, Colvert E, Mota A, et al. (2009) Amygdala, hippocampal and corpus callosum size following severe early institutional deprivation: the English and Romanian Adoptees study pilot. J Child Psychol Psychiatry 50: 943-951.
[31] Bremner JD, Randall P, Vermetten E, Staib L, Bronen RA, et al. (1997) Magnetic resonance imaging-based measurement of hippocampal volume in posttraumatic stress disorder related to childhood physical and sexual abuse--a preliminary report. Biol Psychiatry 41: 23-32.

[32] Cohen RA, Grieve S, Hoth KF, Paul RH, Sweet L, et al. (2006) Early life stress and morphometry of the adult anterior cingulate cortex and caudate nuclei. Biol Psychiatry 59: 975-982.
[33] Driessen M, Herrmann J, Stahl K, Zwaan M, Meier S, et al. (2000) Magnetic resonance imaging volumes of the hippocampus and the amygdala in women with borderline personality disorder and early traumatization. Arch Gen Psychiatry 57: 1115-1122.
[34] Schmahl CG, Vermetten E, Elzinga BM, Douglas Bremner J (2003) Magnetic resonance imaging of hippocampal and amygdala volume in women with childhood abuse and borderline personality disorder. Psychiatry Res 122: 193-198.
[35] Plotsky PM, Thrivikraman KV, Nemeroff CB, Caldji C, Sharma S, et al. (2005) Long-term consequences of neonatal rearing on central corticotropin-releasing factor systems in adult male rat offspring. Neuropsychopharmacology 30: 2192-2204.
[36] Tsoory M, Guterman A, Richter-Levin G (2008) Exposure to stressors during juvenility disrupts development-related alterations in the PSA-NCAM to NCAM expression ratio: potential relevance for mood and anxiety disorders. Neuropsychopharmacology 33: 378-393.
[37] Ono M, Kikusui T, Sasaki N, Ichikawa M, Mori Y, et al. (2008) Early weaning induces anxiety and precocious myelination in the anterior part of the basolateral amygdala of male Balb/c mice. Neuroscience 156: 1103-1110.
[38] Kikusui T, Mori Y (2009) Behavioural and neurochemical consequences of early weaning in rodents. J Neuroendocrinol 21: 427-431.
[39] Salzberg M, Kumar G, Supit L, Jones NC, Morris MJ, et al. (2007) Early postnatal stress confers enduring vulnerability to limbic epileptogenesis. Epilepsia 48: 2079-2085.
[40] Becker K, Abraham A, Kindler J, Helmeke C, Braun K (2007) Exposure to neonatal separation stress alters exploratory behavior and corticotropin releasing factor expression in neurons in the amygdala and hippocampus. Dev Neurobiol 67: 617-629.
[41] Vazquez DM, Bailey C, Dent GW, Okimoto DK, Steffek A, et al. (2006) Brain corticotropin-releasing hormone (CRH) circuits in the developing rat: effect of maternal deprivation. Brain Res 1121: 83-94.
[42] Moriceau S, Roth TL, Okotoghaide T, Sullivan RM (2004) Corticosterone controls the developmental emergence of fear and amygdala function to predator odors in infant rat pups. Int J Dev Neurosci 22: 415-422.
[43] Sabatini MJ, Ebert P, Lewis DA, Levitt P, Cameron JL, et al. (2007) Amygdala gene expression correlates of social behavior in monkeys experiencing maternal separation. J Neurosci 27: 3295-3304.
[44] Mosko SS (2012) Epigenetics: Revolutionary New Spin on Nature Versus Nuture.
[45] Sullivan RM, Holman PJ (2010) Transitions in sensitive period attachment learning in infancy: the role of corticosterone. Neurosci Biobehav Rev 34: 835-844.
[46] Davidson RJ, McEwen BS (2012) Social influences on neuroplasticity: stress and interventions to promote well-being. Nat Neurosci 15: 689-695.
[47] Payne C, Machado CJ, Bliwise NG, Bachevalier J (2010) Maturation of the hippocampal formation and amygdala in Macaca mulatta: a volumetric magnetic resonance imaging study. Hippocampus 20: 922-935.
[48] Tottenham N, Sheridan MA (2009) A review of adversity, the amygdala and the hippocampus: a consideration of developmental timing. Front Hum Neurosci 3: 68.

[49] Pechtel P, Pizzagalli DA (2011) Effects of early life stress on cognitive and affective function: an integrated review of human literature. Psychopharmacology 214: 55-70.
[50] Maren S (1999) Long-term potentiation in the amygdala: a mechanism for emotional learning and memory. Trends in neurosciences 22: 561-567.
[51] Vyas A, Pillai AG, Chattarji S (2004) Recovery after chronic stress fails to reverse amygdaloid neuronal hypertrophy and enhanced anxiety-like behavior. Neuroscience 128: 667-673.
[52] Yang J, Hou C, Ma N, Liu J, Zhang Y, et al. (2007) Enriched environment treatment restores impaired hippocampal synaptic plasticity and cognitive deficits induced by prenatal chronic stress. Neurobiol Learn Mem 87: 257-263.
[53] Caldji C, Tannenbaum B, Sharma S, Francis D, Plotsky PM, et al. (1998) Maternal care during infancy regulates the development of neural systems mediating the expression of fearfulness in the rat. Proceedings of the National Academy of Sciences 95: 5335-5340.
[54] Roozendaal B, McEwen BS, Chattarji S (2009) Stress, memory and the amygdala. Nat Rev Neurosci 10: 423-433.
[55] Rauch SL, Whalen PJ, Shin LM, McInerney SC, Macklin ML, et al. (2000) Exaggerated amygdala response to masked facial stimuli in posttraumatic stress disorder: a functional MRI study. Biol Psychiatry 47: 769-776.
[56] Shin LM, Orr SP, Carson MA, Rauch SL, Macklin ML, et al. (2004) Regional cerebral blood flow in the amygdala and medial prefrontal cortex during traumatic imagery in male and female Vietnam veterans with PTSD. Arch Gen Psychiatry 61: 168-176.
[57] Armony JL, Corbo V, Clement MH, Brunet A (2005) Amygdala response in patients with acute PTSD to masked and unmasked emotional facial expressions. Am J Psychiatry 162: 1961-1963.
[58] Liberzon I, Taylor SF, Amdur R, Jung TD, Chamberlain KR, et al. (1999) Brain activation in PTSD in response to trauma-related stimuli. Biol Psychiatry 45: 817-826.
[59] Shin LM, Rauch SL, Pitman RK (2006) Amygdala, medial prefrontal cortex, and hippocampal function in PTSD. Ann N Y Acad Sci 1071: 67-79.
[60] Pantel J, Schroder J, Essig M, Schad LR, Popp D, et al. (1998) [Volumetric brain findings in late depression. A study with quantified magnetic resonance tomography]. Nervenarzt 69: 968-974.
[61] Frodl T, Meisenzahl E, Zetzsche T, Bottlender R, Born C, et al. (2002) Enlargement of the amygdala in patients with a first episode of major depression. Biol Psychiatry 51: 708-714.
[62] Lange C, Irle E (2004) Enlarged amygdala volume and reduced hippocampal volume in young women with major depression. Psychol Med 34: 1059-1064.
[63] Sheline YI, Gado MH, Price JL (1998) Amygdala core nuclei volumes are decreased in recurrent major depression. Neuroreport 9: 2023-2028.
[64] Lee HY, Tae WS, Yoon HK, Lee BT, Paik JW, et al. (2011) Demonstration of decreased gray matter concentration in the midbrain encompassing the dorsal raphe nucleus and the limbic subcortical regions in major depressive disorder: an optimized voxel-based morphometry study. J Affect Disord 133: 128-136.
[65] Dannlowski U, Stuhrmann A, Beutelmann V, Zwanzger P, Lenzen T, et al. (2012) Limbic scars: long-term consequences of childhood maltreatment revealed by functional and structural magnetic resonance imaging. Biol Psychiatry 71: 286-293.

[66] Hart H, Rubia K (2012) Neuroimaging of child abuse: a critical review. Front Hum Neurosci 6: 52.
[67] Treadway MT, Grant MM, Ding Z, Hollon SD, Gore JC, et al. (2009) Early adverse events, HPA activity and rostral anterior cingulate volume in MDD. PLoS One 4: e4887.
[68] Thomas KM, Drevets WC, Dahl RE, Ryan ND, Birmaher B, et al. (2001) Amygdala Response to Fearful Faces in Anxious and Depressed Children. Arch Gen Psychiatry 58: 1057-1063.
[69] Dannlowski U, Stuhrmann A, Beutelmann V, Zwanzger P, Lenzen T, et al. Limbic Scars: Long-Term Consequences of Childhood Maltreatment Revealed by Functional and Structural Magnetic Resonance Imaging. Biological Psychiatry.
[70] De Bellis MD, Casey BJ, Dahl RE, Birmaher B, Williamson DE, et al. (2000) A pilot study of amygdala volumes in pediatric generalized anxiety disorder. Biological Psychiatry 48: 51-57.
[71] Rosso IM, Cintron CM, Steingard RJ, Renshaw PF, Young AD, et al. (2005) Amygdala and hippocampus volumes in pediatric major depression. Biological Psychiatry 57: 21-26.
[72] MacMillan S, Szeszko PR, Moore GJ, Madden R, Lorch E, et al. (2003) Increased Amygdala: Hippocampal Volume Ratios Associated with Severity of Anxiety in Pediatric Major Depression. Journal of Child and Adolescent Psychopharmacology 13: 65-73.
[73] Lupien SJ, McEwen BS, Gunnar MR, Heim C (2009) Effects of stress throughout the lifespan on the brain, behaviour and cognition. Nature Reviews Neuroscience 10: 434-445.
[74] Weniger G, Lange C, Sachsse U, Irle E (2008) Amygdala and hippocampal volumes and cognition in adult survivors of childhood abuse with dissociative disorders. Acta Psychiatrica Scandinavica 118: 281-290.
[75] Levitt JG, Blanton RE, Caplan R, Asarnow R, Guthrie D, et al. (2001) Medial temporal lobe in childhood-onset schizophrenia. Psychiatry Research: Neuroimaging 108: 17-27.
[76] Siegle GJ, Thompson W, Carter CS, Steinhauer SR, Thase ME (2007) Increased amygdala and decreased dorsolateral prefrontal BOLD responses in unipolar depression: related and independent features. Biological Psychiatry 61: 198-209.
[77] Yvette I S (2003) Neuroimaging studies of mood disorder effects on the brain. Biological Psychiatry 54: 338-352.
[78] Rauch SL, Whalen PJ, Shin LM, Mclnerney SC, Macklin ML, et al. (2000) Exaggerated amygdala response to masked facial stimuli in posttraumatic stress disorder: a functional MRI study. Biological Psychiatry 47: 769-776.
[79] Shin LM, McNally RJ, Kosslyn SM, Thompson WL, Rauch SL, et al. (1999) Regional cerebral blood flow during script-driven imagery in childhood sexual abuse-related PTSD: a PET investigation. American Journal of Psychiatry 156: 575-584.
[80] Shanahan L, Copeland WE, Costello EJ, Angold A (2011) Child-, adolescent- and young adult-onset depressions: differential risk factors in development? Psychol Med 41: 2265-2274.
[81] Taylor S (2011) Etiology of obsessions and compulsions: a meta-analysis and narrative review of twin studies. Clin Psychol Rev 31: 1361-1372.

[82] Bierut LJ (2011) Genetic vulnerability and susceptibility to substance dependence. Neuron 69: 618-627.
[83] Naukkarinen J, Rissanen A, Kaprio J, Pietilainen KH (2011) Causes and consequences of obesity: the contribution of recent twin studies. Int J Obes (Lond).
[84] Sartor CE, Grant JD, Lynskey MT, McCutcheon VV, Waldron M, et al. (2012) Common heritable contributions to low-risk trauma, high-risk trauma, posttraumatic stress disorder, and major depression. Arch Gen Psychiatry 69: 293-299.
[85] Kremen WS, Koenen KC, Afari N, Lyons MJ (2012) Twin studies of posttraumatic stress disorder: differentiating vulnerability factors from sequelae. Neuropharmacology 62: 647-653.
[86] Shin LM, Bush G, Milad MR, Lasko NB, Brohawn KH, et al. (2011) Exaggerated activation of dorsal anterior cingulate cortex during cognitive interference: a monozygotic twin study of posttraumatic stress disorder. Am J Psychiatry 168: 979-985.
[87] Zhang J, Yan X, Shi J, Gong Q, Weng X, et al. (2010) Structural modifications of the brain in acclimatization to high-altitude. PLoS One 5: e11449.
[88] Zhang J, Liu H, Yan X, Weng X (2011) Minimal effects on human memory following long-term living at moderate altitude. High Alt Med Biol 12: 37-43.
[89] Yan X, Zhang J, Shi J, Gong Q, Weng X (2010) Cerebral and functional adaptation with chronic hypoxia exposure: a multi-modal MRI study. Brain Res 1348: 21-29.
[90] Yan X, Zhang J, Gong Q, Weng X (2011) Prolonged high-altitude residence impacts verbal working memory: an fMRI study. Exp Brain Res 208: 437-445.
[91] Yan X, Zhang J, Gong Q, Weng X (2011) Appetite at high altitude: an fMRI study on the impact of prolonged high-altitude residence on gustatory neural processing. Exp Brain Res 209: 495-499.
[92] Yan X, Zhang J, Gong Q, Weng X (2011) Adaptive influence of long term high altitude residence on spatial working memory: an fMRI study. Brain Cogn 77: 53-59.
[93] Yan X, Zhang J, Gong Q, Weng X (2011) Cerebrovascular reactivity among native-raised high altitude residents: an fMRI study. BMC Neurosci 12: 94.
[94] Butterworth P, Cherbuin N, Sachdev P, Anstey KJ (2011) The association between financial hardship and amygdala and hippocampal volumes: results from the PATH through life project. Soc Cogn Affect Neurosci.
[95] DeRubeis RJ, Siegle GJ, Hollon SD (2008) Cognitive therapy versus medication for depression: treatment outcomes and neural mechanisms. Nat Rev Neurosci 9: 788-796.
[96] Holzel BK, Carmody J, Evans KC, Hoge EA, Dusek JA, et al. (2010) Stress reduction correlates with structural changes in the amygdala. Social Cognitive and Affective Neuroscience 5: 11-17.
[97] Bugg JM, Head D (2011) Exercise moderates age-related atrophy of the medial temporal lobe. Neurobiology of Aging 32: 506-514.
[98] Teacher (2011) Students Should Be Taught To Be Prosocial.
[99] RAPPIN (2012) Benefits of Meditation for Kids.
[100] Support (2011) Children and Exercise.

Chapter 13

Traumatic Experiences Disrupt Amygdala – Prefrontal Connectivity

Dong Hoon Oh

Additional information is available at the end of the chapter

1. Introduction

Psychological "trauma" refers to a sudden intense surge of anxiety secondary to some external event that exceeds the subject's ability to cope with and to defend against. However, the term "trauma" is actually difficult to define due to its subjective nature. The American Psychiatric Association defines it as "an event or events that involves actual or threatened death or serious injury, or a threat to the physical integrity of self or others." Examples of such events include military combat, violent personal attack, natural or human-made disasters, and torture. For children, sexually traumatic events may include age-inappropriate sexual experiences without violence or injury (American Psychiatric Association. and American Psychiatric Association. Task Force on DSM-IV, 1994).

Unfortunately, traumatic events happen to people all over the world. Estimates of the prevalence of traumatic experiences are likely to vary with the method of assessment (Breslau, 2002, Breslau et al., 1998, Copeland et al., 2007, Finkelhor et al., 2005, Frans et al., 2005, Helzer et al., 1987). In particular, recent epidemiological studies have demonstrated high rates (70%-80%) of lifetime traumatic experiences, suggesting that previous epidemiological surveys may have underestimated the prevalence of traumatic events (de Vries and Olff, 2009, Mills et al., 2011). Although all subjects exposed to traumatic events do not come to exhibit mental disorders, childhood trauma increases the risk of mental disorders during adulthood (Gilbert et al., 2009). Therefore, it is clinically important to understand the biological and psychological changes induced by trauma.

Traumatic experiences induce a wide range of physical and psychological symptoms that affect all aspects of life for survivors. These symptoms can involve clinically significant distress and impairment in social, occupational, and other areas of functioning. Traumatic experiences also lead to significant structural and functional changes in brain regions implicated in emotional and cognitive processing. These brain areas include the medial prefrontal cortex (mPFC), which contains the anterior cingulate cortex (ACC) (Ansell et al., 2012), the hippocampus, and the amygdala (Bremner, 2006, Kolassa et al., 2007, Shin et al., 2006).

Recent advances in neuroimaging have revealed anatomical and functional connectivity between the amygdala and the prefrontal cortex, which is dedicated to emotion regulation. There is accumulating evidence that the amygdala and the prefrontal cortex play critical roles in conditioning and the extinction of memories of traumatic fear. The prefrontal cortex regulates stress-induced fear and anxiety-like behaviors via inhibitory effects on amygdala output and processing (Akirav and Maroun, 2007, Bishop, 2007).

In this chapter, we will describe the structural (volumetric) and functional changes in the amygdala and prefrontal cortex resulting from traumatic stresses. We will argue that there is a structural and functional disconnection between the amygdala and the prefrontal cortex in patients with trauma-related psychiatric disorders but not in controls. We will then present evidence that traumatic experiences can disrupt the normal connectivity between the amygdala and the prefrontal cortex, which suggests that effective interactions between these two brain areas are needed for healthy outcomes of traumatic experiences.

2. Trauma-related structural and functional changes in the amygdala

Anatomically, the amygdala is an almond-shaped mass located above and in front of the temporal horn of the lateral ventricle and anterior to the tail of the caudate nucleus. It is a complex structure containing more than a dozen nuclei that are richly interconnected (Pessoa, 2010). The amygdala also has extensive connections with cortical and subcortical regions (Sah et al., 2003). Functionally, it is an essential component of the circuit involved in implicit emotional learning and memory, emotional modulation of memory, emotional influences on attention and perception, emotion and social behavior, and emotion inhibition and regulation (Phelps and LeDoux, 2005). In particular, the amygdala mediates the acquisition and expression of conditioned fear and the enhancement of emotional memory (Koenigs and Grafman, 2009).

2.1. Traumatic experiences induce changes in amygdala volume

A number of studies have provided evidence of effects of trauma on amygdala volume. Interestingly, the effects of traumatic stress on amygdala volume differ between children and adults. Childhood trauma is associated with increases in amygdala volume, whereas traumatic stress in adulthood is associated with reductions in amygdala volume. Two studies have detected larger amygdala volumes in children and adolescents who have experienced early institutional deprivation and subsequent adoption (Mehta et al., 2009, Tottenham et al., 2010). Mehta et al. (2009) reported larger amygdala volumes in 14 adoptee adolescents who had experienced severe early institutional deprivation in Romania than in a group of non-institutionalized controls (n=11). The conditions of care in the Romanian institutions that these children had experienced varied from poor to appalling. Tottenham et al. (2010) demonstrated that children who had been adopted out of an orphanage at older ages (>15 months old) had larger amygdala volumes than early-adopted children (<15 months old) and non-adopted controls. Similarly, a recent study demonstrated that children exposed to maternal depression (n=17) since birth had significantly larger amygdala volumes than controls (n=21), whereas the two groups did not differ with respect to hippocampal volume (Lupien et al., 2011).

In contrast, the total volume of the amygdala in adult breast cancer survivors (n=35) with a history of cancer-related intrusive recollections was significantly smaller than in control breast cancer survivors who had no such history (n=41) (Matsuoka et al., 2003). A study using a voxel-based morphometry (VBM) method detected smaller amygdala volumes in healthy adults (n=17) who were within a mile and a half of the World Trade Center on September 11, 2001, than in the comparison group (n=19)(Ganzel et al., 2008). Mollica et al. (2009) reported that South Vietnamese ex-political detainees exposed to torture and traumatic head injury had a higher rate of depression than those without traumatic head injury. Trauma/torture events were associated with bilateral loss of amygdala volume (Mollica et al., 2009).

The results of most recent meta-analyses indicate that trauma-related psychiatric disorders such as post-traumatic stress disorder (PTSD), major depressive disorder (MDD) and borderline personality disorder (BPD), are associated with reductions in amygdala volume in the adult. Sacher et al. (2012) analyzed 10 selected studies of adult patients with MDD and found a significant decrease in left amygdala volume in the MDD group. Woon and Hedges (2009) analyzed published data from nine studies comparing amygdala volumes in adult subjects with PTSD, and found no significant effect on amygdala volumes. However, another meta-analysis found significantly smaller left amygdala volumes in adults with PTSD than in either healthy or trauma-exposed controls (Karl et al., 2006). In addition, Nunes et al. (2009) in a meta-analysis of six studies demonstrated significantly reduced volumes of both right and left hippocampi and amygdalae in patients with BPD. One meta-analysis reported that amygdala volume in children with maltreatment-related PTSD did not differ from that in healthy controls (Woon and Hedges, 2008). Thus human data on amygdala volumes in patients with trauma-related psychiatric disorders have thus far yielded conflicting or varied results. Therefore, disease states (or courses), symptom severity and histories of antidepressant medication should be taken into consideration when interpreting the results of volumetric studies on the amygdala in patients with trauma-related psychiatric disorders.

2.2. Traumatic experiences induce changes in amygdala function

In human neuroimaging studies, amygdalar hyper-responsiveness to emotionally negative stimuli has been shown to be associated with trait anxiety (Etkin et al., 2004, Sehlmeyer et al., 2011), PTSD (Shin et al., 2005, Rauch et al., 2000, Francati et al., 2007) and MDD (Sheline et al., 2001, Siegle et al., 2007, Suslow et al., 2010).

A recent functional magnetic resonance imaging (fMRI) study of a large sample of healthy adults (n=148) showed that childhood maltreatment (Childhood Trauma Questionnaire scores) was positively associated with right amygdala responsiveness to negative facial expressions (Dannlowski et al., 2012). In addition, adverse early rearing environments in the postnatal period were followed by heightened amygdala activity during childhood. Tottenham et al. (2011) observed the brain activity of two groups of children while performing an Emotional Face Go/No-Go task. The scanned fMRI obtained in the previously institutionalized group of children showed enhanced activity in the amygdala in comparison to the control (Tottenham et al., 2011). Similarly, the results of another fMRI study comparing unipolar depressed patients with and without a history of significant early life trauma (n=20) and healthy subjects (n=16) provided a robust positive correlation between physical abuse and right amygdalar responses (Grant et al., 2011). Since childhood trauma is a predisposing factor for PTSD and adult depression, the results of these studies suggest that heightened amygdalar response is a mediator between childhood trauma and the development of trauma-related psychiatric disorders such as PTSD and MDD.

3. Trauma-related structural and functional changes in the prefrontal cortex

The prefrontal cortex consists of three major anatomical regions: the dorsolateral prefrontal cortex (dlPFC), the orbitofrontal cortex (OFC), and the medial prefrontal cortex (mPFC). The dorsolateral prefrontal cortex is a multimodal association area that participates in higher cognitive functions (e.g., executive functions), whereas the OFC and the mPFC are considered to make up the limbic (or paralimbic) area that participates in emotional and motivational functions (Ichihara-Takeda and Funahashi, 2007). In particular, the ventromedial prefrontal cortex (vmPFC) mediates the extinction of conditioned fear and the volitional regulation of negative emotion (Koenigs and Grafman, 2009).

3.1. Traumatic experiences induce structural changes in the prefrontal cortex

There are mixed results from studies comparing the volumes of the prefrontal cortex in children with maltreatment-related PTSD and those in non-maltreated children (McCrory et al., 2011). However, reduced prefrontal volume in adults with traumatic experiences has been a consistent finding. For examples, a previous VBM study that compared the gray matter volume of cancer survivors with PTSD with the gray matter volume of those without PTSD and of healthy subjects demonstrated that the gray matter volume of the right OFC was significantly smaller in cancer survivors with PTSD (n=9) than in those without PTSD (n=67) or healthy subjects (n=70) (Hakamata et al., 2007). Chronic exposure to harsh corporal punishment was associated with a marked reduction in gray matter volume in the right mPFC in young adults (18-25 years). There were also possible associations between harsh corporal punishment and reduced gray matter volume in the left dlPFC and the right ACC (Tomoda et al., 2009). Another recent VBM study examined whether healthy control subjects and unmedicated patients with depression and/or anxiety disorders who reported childhood emotional maltreatment before age 16 (n=84) displayed structural brain changes compared with control subjects and patients who reported no childhood abuse (n=97). This study showed that self-reported childhood emotional maltreatment is associated with a profound reduction of mPFC volume, even in the absence of physical or sexual abuse during childhood (van Harmelen et al., 2010). A longitudinal multiwave neuroimaging study in a cohort of direct survivors of a South Korean subway disaster (2003) was conducted as a five-year follow-up case-control study. This study demonstrated that disaster survivors early in the course of PTSD had greater cortical thickness in the dlPFC regions than controls. This greater dlPFC thickness early after the trauma, which was associated with earlier improvement and subsequent recovery from PTSD, gradually reverted to the level of controls (Lyoo et al., 2011).

Based on the results of most recent meta-analyses, prefrontal cortical volume reduction is frequently involved in both MDD and PTSD. A meta-analysis study of 41 studies found significant volume reductions in the prefrontal cortex (especially the OFC) and ACC of patients with MDD (Ansell et al. 2012). In particular, the subgenual ACC and OFC were significantly smaller in antidepressant-free patients compared with medicated patients (Bora et al., 2012). A previous meta-analysis also found significantly smaller ACC in adults with PTSD than in trauma-exposed controls (Karl et al., 2006).

Changes in gray matter volume are associated not only with trauma-related psychiatric disorders but also with recent adverse life events and perceived stress; these associations suggest that some trauma-related changes in gray matter volume may act as vulnerability markers that precede the presence of trauma-related psychiatric disorders (Ansell et al., 2012). However, the exact mechanism that causes prefrontal volume reduction in patients with trauma-related psychiatric disorders and after traumatic events remains unknown. Acute or chronic traumatic stress may induce gray matter volume reduction by several possible mechanisms including glucocorticoid-induced neuronal cell damage, glutamate-mediated neuronal cell death (apoptosis) and decreased neurogenesis (Zhu et al., 2006, Oh et al., 2012).

3.2. Traumatic experiences induce functional changes in the prefrontal cortex

It is known that trauma-related psychiatric disorders are associated with functional abnormalities in the prefrontal cortex. The prefrontal cortex is involved in various affective and cognitive functions supporting the processing of traumatic memories. Traumatic experiences induce structural and functional abnormalities in the prefrontal area, and these are implicated in deficient traumatic memory processing and the subsequent development of trauma-related symptoms (McFarlane et al., 2002).

A recent study compared twelve adopted adolescents who suffered from deprivation of early caregivers (early-life stress group, 9 females) with 21 healthy control adolescents (10 females) who lived with their biological parents. The subjects were tested using a cognitive control task and analyzed using fMRI. The early-life stress group took longer to switch from a prepotent response to an alternative response than the control group. Observation of neural activity revealed greater activation of several regions involved in cognitive control including the dlPFC and the striatum in the early-life stress group than in controls (Mueller et al., 2010). A previous study investigating the functional neuroanatomical correlates of response inhibition in thirty right-handed medication-naive youths (10-16 years, n=16) with post-traumatic symptoms (PTSS) and in a gender-matched control group of healthy youths (n=14) found that the PTSS subjects performed similarly to the control subjects in the Go/No-Go task. However, during the Go-No/Go task, the PTSS group had greater medial frontal activation than the controls (Carrion et al., 2008).

A recent fMRI study in adults examined the relationship between recent negative life stress and regional brain activity in adult subjects with MDD (n=15) and in individually matched healthy controls (n=15). No significant effects of stress on brain activation in response to negative words were found in the controls. However, in the MDD group, negative correlations were found in the right ventrolateral prefrontal cortex (vlPFC), the subgenual cingulate area and the nucleus accumbens. Positive correlations were also found bilaterally in the orbitofrontal areas (Hsu et al. 2010). A previous fMRI study investigated the neural activation patterns during recall of autobiographical traumatic episodes in BPD patients compared with recall of negative (aversive) but nontraumatic episodes. Contrasting between trauma and nontrauma conditions revealed activation of the OFC and Broca's area in all the subjects, as well as activation of the occipital-mesial and temporal-anterior areas (Driessen et al., 2004).

In summary: structural neuroimaging studies have identified volumetric changes in the amygdala and the prefrontal cortex in some subjects exposed to traumatic events. Functional neuroimaging has also revealed activation abnormalities in the same areas in traumatized subjects. These findings have prompted neuroimaging studies aimed at discovering the relationship and interactions between the amygdala and the prefrontal cortex.

4. Trauma and amygdala-prefrontal connectivity

Using the diffusion tensor imaging (DTI) method, it is possible to delineate non-invasively the structural connections between the amygdala and the prefrontal cortex in humans. The amygdala is extensively interconnected with the prefrontal cortex, especially with the OFC (Croxson et al., 2005). Numerous studies have shown that trauma-related psychiatric disorders are associated with abnormal interactions between the amygdala and the prefrontal area (Etkin and Wager, 2007). The prefrontal cortex is thought to be involved in top-down regulation of the amygdala, while the amygdala in turn modulates prefrontal cortical activity. Clarifying the exact neurobiological mechanism of the amygdala-prefrontal dynamic interaction is essential for understanding the pathophysiology of trauma-related psychiatric disorders and for treatment of these disorders.

4.1. Traumatic experiences disrupt amygdala–prefrontal connectivity

The amygdala and the prefrontal cortex are not only structurally but also functionally interconnected. Traumatic experiences induce structural and functional changes in the amygdala and prefrontal cortex, respectively. Changes in amygdala-prefrontal interactions may induce deficits in emotional processing. For examples, a recent DTI study showed that individual differences in trait anxiety scores were negatively correlated with the mean fractional anisotropy (FA) value of the entirety of the identified amygdala–vmPFC pathway. This result suggests that the strength of the anatomical amygdala–prefrontal pathway predicts lower levels of normal trait anxiety (Kim and Whalen, 2009). A previous study analyzed structural and functional MRI data collected from a sample of 20 healthy subjects. It found that greater vmPFC gray matter thickness was associated with greater reductions in activation of the left amygdala during an affect-labeling task. This supports the idea that the vmPFC has a general role in suppression of amygdala activity (Foland-Ross et al., 2010).

Changes in amygdala-prefrontal interactions are involved in the pathophysiology of trauma-related psychiatric disorders. In a positron emission tomography (PET) study examining glucose metabolism, there were significant positive correlations between right OFC and ventral amygdala in healthy control subjects (n=24). BPD patients (n=26) had weak correlations between amygdala and the anterior PFC. This study demonstrated a tight coupling of metabolic activity between right OFC and ventral amygdala in healthy control subjects that was not present in BPD patients (New et al., 2007). Patients with MDD were characterized by decreased interaction between the amygdala and the prefrontal areas (dorsal ACC and dlPFC) during emotional processing compared with healthy subjects. Amygdala–prefrontal connectivity is significantly correlated with the severity of depression. These results suggest that patients with reduced amygdala–dlPFC interaction have a longer and more severe course of disease (Dannlowski et al., 2009). A recent fMRI study showed that both medication-free MDD patients (n=29) and never-depressed subjects with cognitive vulnerability to depression (n=26) displayed similar responses to emotional stimuli, with significantly lower activity in the dlPFC and significantly greater activity in the amygdala than healthy control subjects (n=31) (Zhong et al., 2011).

Numerous neuroimaging studies of PTSD have also revealed a pattern of hyperactivation in regions involved in the generation of emotion (the amygdala and the insula) and corresponding hypoactivation in regions involved in the regulation of emotion (the mPFC and the ACC). Actually, relative to non-traumatized controls, subjects with PTSD showed a marked reduction in activity in the mPFC and a small but significant enhancement in left amygdala activity in response to overtly presented fearful face stimuli. This suggests that traumatic life events disrupt the normal pattern of mPFC and amygdala regulation (Williams et al., 2006). In addition, two other studies reported that the severity of PTSD symptoms was negatively correlated with mPFC activity (Shin et al., 2005, Hopper et al., 2007). Moreover, a recent study investigated the relationship between default mode network connectivity and the severity of PTSD symptoms in subjects who had experienced an acute traumatic event 6–12 weeks before. The results of this study suggest that the resting-state connectivity of the posterior cingulate cortex/precuneus with the perigenual ACC and right amygdala is associated with current PTSD symptoms and that the correlation with the right amygdala predicts future PTSD symptoms (Lanius et al., 2010). Another study measuring resting-state amygdala connectivity in male veterans with PTSD (n=15) and in combat controls (n=14) showed greater positive connectivity between the amygdala and the insula in patients with PTSD than in controls, reduced positive connectivity between the amygdala and the hippocampus, and a reduced anticorrelation between the amygdala and the dorsal and rostral ACC (Sripada et al., 2012).

However, the mechanism underlying the alteration in connectivity between amygdala and prefrontal cortex in trauma-related psychiatric disorders remains unclear. Several lines of evidence have indicated that cortisol could be implicated (Henckens et al., 2010, Kern et al., 2008, Urry et al., 2006, Veer et al., 2012). The strength of the resting-state functional connectivity between the amygdala and the mPFC may be related to individual differences in endogenous cortisol levels under relatively stress-free circumstances (Veer et al., 2012). There is an adaptive mechanism of time-dependent modulation of the amygdala by corticosteroids: rapid nongenomic effects of corticosteroids suppress overall amygdala activity in a nonspecific manner, whereas slow genomic actions of corticosteroids normalize responses to negative input by specifically altering prefrontal control (Henckens et al., 2010). It has been suggested that serotonin (5-hydroxytryptamine) also plays a role in regulating functional interactions between the amygdala and the prefrontal cortex (Davidson et al., 2000, Siever, 2008). A recent neuroimaging study using two complementary methods (psycho-physiological-interaction in a general linear model and dynamic causal modeling) demonstrated that acute tryptophan depletion significantly altered the functional connectivity between the amygdala and the right ventral ACC and the vlPFC when processing angry vs. neutral faces (Passamonti et al., 2012).

4.2. Recovery and the amygdala–prefrontal connectivity

Interestingly, recent findings raise the possibility that more efficient crosstalk between the amygdala and the prefrontal cortex predicts beneficial behavioral outcomes in terms of emotion regulation and anxiety (Kim et al., 2011). It has been found that activity in specific areas of the frontal cortex (dorsolateral, dorsal medial, anterior cingulate, orbital) varies together with amygdala activity and that this functional connectivity is dependent on the reappraisal task. Moreover, the strength of coupling between the amygdala and the OFC/dorsal medial prefrontal cortex predicts the extent of attenuation of negative affect following reappraisal (Banks et al., 2007). In addition, a recent fMRI study investigating the effect of psychotherapy on coping demonstrated that a marked increased in mPFC activity accompanied decreased amygdala activity during traumatic memory retrieval in partial PTSD policemen (n=12) after psychotherapy and these findings were associated with symptom attenuation (Peres et al., 2011).

5. Conclusion

Advances in neuroimaging technology have opened up new ways of understanding human brain function. Numerous studies indicate that the amygdala and the prefrontal cortex are important neuroanatomical structures involved in the response to traumatic stress and its effects on learning and memory. In particular, the amygdala and the prefrontal cortex are structurally and functionally interconnected. Traumatic experiences can be associated with lasting changes in these brain areas. These changes may result in an imbalance between the amygdala and the prefrontal cortex that is typically characterized by hyperactivity of the amygdala and hypoactivity of the prefrontal cortex. Investigations of the connection between the amygdala and prefrontal cortex have provided a deeper understanding of the role of the amygdala–prefrontal circuitry in trauma-related psychiatric disorders. Restoring the imbalance between hyperactivity of the amygdala and hypoactivity of the prefrontal cortex – in the form of robust structural and functional connectivity between the amygdala and the prefrontal cortex – predicts beneficial outcomes in the treatment of trauma-related psychiatric disorders.

Author details

Dong Hoon Oh
Department of Psychiatry, College of Medicine and Institute of Mental Health, Hanyang University, Seoul, Republic of Korea

6. References

[1] Akirav, I. & Maroun, M. 2007. The role of the medial prefrontal cortex-amygdala circuit in stress effects on the extinction of fear. *Neural Plast*, 2007, 30873.
[2] American Psychiatric Association. & American Psychiatric Association. Task Force On DSM-IV. 1994. *Diagnostic and statistical manual of mental disorders : DSM-IV*, Washington, DC, American Psychiatric Association.
[3] Ansell, E. B., Rando, K., Tuit, K., Guarnaccia, J. & Sinha, R. 2012. Cumulative Adversity and Smaller Gray Matter Volume in Medial Prefrontal, Anterior Cingulate, and Insula Regions. *Biol Psychiatry*, 72, 57-64.
[4] Banks, S. J., Eddy, K. T., Angstadt, M., Nathan, P. J. & Phan, K. L. 2007. Amygdala-frontal connectivity during emotion regulation. *Soc Cogn Affect Neurosci*, 2, 303-12.
[5] Bishop, S. J. 2007. Neurocognitive mechanisms of anxiety: an integrative account. *Trends Cogn Sci*, 11, 307-16.
[6] Bora, E., Harrison, B. J., Davey, C. G., Yucel, M. & Pantelis, C. 2012. Meta-analysis of volumetric abnormalities in cortico-striatal-pallidal-thalamic circuits in major depressive disorder. *Psychol Med*, 42, 671-81.
[7] Bremner, J. D. 2006. Traumatic stress: effects on the brain. *Dialogues Clin Neurosci*, 8, 445-61.
[8] Breslau, N. 2002. Epidemiologic studies of trauma, posttraumatic stress disorder, and other psychiatric disorders. *Can J Psychiatry*, 47, 923-9.
[9] Breslau, N., Kessler, R. C., Chilcoat, H. D., Schultz, L. R., Davis, G. C. & Andreski, P. 1998. Trauma and posttraumatic stress disorder in the community: the 1996 Detroit Area Survey of Trauma. *Arch Gen Psychiatry*, 55, 626-32.
[10] Carrion, V. G., Garrett, A., Menon, V., Weems, C. F. & Reiss, A. L. 2008. Posttraumatic stress symptoms and brain function during a response-inhibition task: an fMRI study in youth. *Depress Anxiety*, 25, 514-26.

[11] Copeland, W. E., Keeler, G., Angold, A. & Costello, E. J. 2007. Traumatic events and posttraumatic stress in childhood. *Arch Gen Psychiatry*, 64, 577-84.
[12] Croxson, P. L., Johansen-Berg, H., Behrens, T. E., Robson, M. D., Pinsk, M. A., Gross, C. G., Richter, W., Richter, M. C., Kastner, S. & Rushworth, M. F. 2005. Quantitative investigation of connections of the prefrontal cortex in the human and macaque using probabilistic diffusion tractography. *J Neurosci*, 25, 8854-66.
[13] Dannlowski, U., Ohrmann, P., Konrad, C., Domschke, K., Bauer, J., Kugel, H., Hohoff, C., Schoning, S., Kersting, A., Baune, B. T., Mortensen, L. S., Arolt, V., Zwitserlood, P., Deckert, J., Heindel, W. & Suslow, T. 2009. Reduced amygdala-prefrontal coupling in major depression: association with MAOA genotype and illness severity. *Int J Neuropsychopharmacol*, 12, 11-22.
[14] Dannlowski, U., Stuhrmann, A., Beutelmann, V., Zwanzger, P., Lenzen, T., Grotegerd, D., Domschke, K., Hohoff, C., Ohrmann, P., Bauer, J., Lindner, C., Postert, C., Konrad, C., Arolt, V., Heindel, W., Suslow, T. & Kugel, H. 2012. Limbic scars: long-term consequences of childhood maltreatment revealed by functional and structural magnetic resonance imaging. *Biol Psychiatry*, 71, 286-93.
[15] Davidson, R. J., Putnam, K. M. & Larson, C. L. 2000. Dysfunction in the neural circuitry of emotion regulation--a possible prelude to violence. *Science*, 289, 591-4.
[16] De Vries, G. J. & Olff, M. 2009. The lifetime prevalence of traumatic events and posttraumatic stress disorder in the Netherlands. *J Trauma Stress*, 22, 259-67.
[17] Driessen, M., Beblo, T., Mertens, M., Piefke, M., Rullkoetter, N., Silva-Saavedra, A., Reddemann, L., Rau, H., Markowitsch, H. J., Wulff, H., Lange, W. & Woermann, F. G. 2004. Posttraumatic stress disorder and fMRI activation patterns of traumatic memory in patients with borderline personality disorder. *Biol Psychiatry*, 55, 603-11.
[18] Etkin, A., Klemenhagen, K. C., Dudman, J. T., Rogan, M. T., Hen, R., Kandel, E. R. & Hirsch, J. 2004. Individual differences in trait anxiety predict the response of the basolateral amygdala to unconsciously processed fearful faces. *Neuron*, 44, 1043-55.
[19] Etkin, A. & Wager, T. D. 2007. Functional neuroimaging of anxiety: a meta-analysis of emotional processing in PTSD, social anxiety disorder, and specific phobia. *Am J Psychiatry*, 164, 1476-88.
[20] Finkelhor, D., Ormrod, R., Turner, H. & Hamby, S. L. 2005. The victimization of children and youth: a comprehensive, national survey. *Child Maltreat*, 10, 5-25.
[21] Foland-Ross, L. C., Altshuler, L. L., Bookheimer, S. Y., Lieberman, M. D., Townsend, J., Penfold, C., Moody, T., Ahlf, K., Shen, J. K., Madsen, S. K., Rasser, P. E., Toga, A. W. & Thompson, P. M. 2010. Amygdala reactivity in healthy adults is correlated with prefrontal cortical thickness. *J Neurosci*, 30, 16673-8.
[22] Francati, V., Vermetten, E. & Bremner, J. D. 2007. Functional neuroimaging studies in posttraumatic stress disorder: review of current methods and findings. *Depress Anxiety*, 24, 202-18.
[23] Frans, O., Rimmo, P. A., Aberg, L. & Fredrikson, M. 2005. Trauma exposure and post-traumatic stress disorder in the general population. *Acta Psychiatr Scand*, 111, 291-9.

[24] Ganzel, B. L., Kim, P., Glover, G. H. & Temple, E. 2008. Resilience after 9/11: multimodal neuroimaging evidence for stress-related change in the healthy adult brain. *Neuroimage,* 40, 788-95.

[25] Gilbert, R., Widom, C. S., Browne, K., Fergusson, D., Webb, E. & Janson, S. 2009. Burden and consequences of child maltreatment in high-income countries. *Lancet,* 373, 68-81.

[26] Grant, M. M., Cannistraci, C., Hollon, S. D., Gore, J. & Shelton, R. 2011. Childhood trauma history differentiates amygdala response to sad faces within MDD. *J Psychiatr Res,* 45, 886-95.

[27] Hakamata, Y., Matsuoka, Y., Inagaki, M., Nagamine, M., Hara, E., Imoto, S., Murakami, K., Kim, Y. & Uchitomi, Y. 2007. Structure of orbitofrontal cortex and its longitudinal course in cancer-related post-traumatic stress disorder. *Neurosci Res,* 59, 383-9.

[28] Helzer, J. E., Robins, L. N. & Mcevoy, L. 1987. Post-traumatic stress disorder in the general population. Findings of the epidemiologic catchment area survey. *N Engl J Med,* 317, 1630-4.

[29] Henckens, M. J., Van Wingen, G. A., Joels, M. & Fernandez, G. 2010. Time-dependent effects of corticosteroids on human amygdala processing. *J Neurosci,* 30, 12725-32.

[30] Hopper, J. W., Frewen, P. A., Van Der Kolk, B. A. & Lanius, R. A. 2007. Neural correlates of reexperiencing, avoidance, and dissociation in PTSD: symptom dimensions and emotion dysregulation in responses to script-driven trauma imagery. J Trauma Stress, 20, 713-25.

[31] Hsu, D. T., Langenecker, S. A., Kennedy, S. E., Zubieta, J. K. & Heitzeg, M. M. 2010. fMRI BOLD responses to negative stimuli in the prefrontal cortex are dependent on levels of recent negative life stress in major depressive disorder. Psychiatry Res, 183, 202-8.

[32] Ichihara-Takeda, S. & Funahashi, S. 2007. Activity of primate orbitofrontal and dorsolateral prefrontal neurons: task-related activity during an oculomotor delayed-response task. *Exp Brain Res,* 181, 409-25.

[33] Karl, A., Schaefer, M., Malta, L. S., Dorfel, D., Rohleder, N. & Werner, A. 2006. A meta-analysis of structural brain abnormalities in PTSD. *Neurosci Biobehav Rev,* 30, 1004-31.

[34] Kern, S., Oakes, T. R., Stone, C. K., Mcauliff, E. M., Kirschbaum, C. & Davidson, R. J. 2008. Glucose metabolic changes in the prefrontal cortex are associated with HPA axis response to a psychosocial stressor. *Psychoneuroendocrinology,* 33, 517-29.

[35] Kim, M. J., Gee, D. G., Loucks, R. A., Davis, F. C. & Whalen, P. J. 2011. Anxiety dissociates dorsal and ventral medial prefrontal cortex functional connectivity with the amygdala at rest. *Cereb Cortex,* 21, 1667-73.

[36] Kim, M. J. & Whalen, P. J. 2009. The structural integrity of an amygdala-prefrontal pathway predicts trait anxiety. *J Neurosci,* 29, 11614-8.

[37] Koenigs, M. & Grafman, J. 2009. Posttraumatic stress disorder: the role of medial prefrontal cortex and amygdala. *Neuroscientist,* 15, 540-8.

[38] Kolassa, I. T., Wienbruch, C., Neuner, F., Schauer, M., Ruf, M., Odenwald, M. & Elbert, T. 2007. Altered oscillatory brain dynamics after repeated traumatic stress. *BMC Psychiatry,* 7, 56.

[39] Lanius, R. A., Bluhm, R. L., Coupland, N. J., Hegadoren, K. M., Rowe, B., Theberge, J., Neufeld, R. W., Williamson, P. C. & Brimson, M. 2010. Default mode network connectivity as a predictor of post-traumatic stress disorder symptom severity in acutely traumatized subjects. *Acta Psychiatr Scand,* 121, 33-40.

[40] Lupien, S. J., Parent, S., Evans, A. C., Tremblay, R. E., Zelazo, P. D., Corbo, V., Pruessner, J. C. & Seguin, J. R. 2011. Larger amygdala but no change in hippocampal volume in 10-year-old children exposed to maternal depressive symptomatology since birth. *Proc Natl Acad Sci U S A,* 108, 14324-9.

[41] Lyoo, I. K., Kim, J. E., Yoon, S. J., Hwang, J., Bae, S. & Kim, D. J. 2011. The neurobiological role of the dorsolateral prefrontal cortex in recovery from trauma. Longitudinal brain imaging study among survivors of the South Korean subway disaster. *Arch Gen Psychiatry,* 68, 701-13.

[42] Matsuoka, Y., Yamawaki, S., Inagaki, M., Akechi, T. & Uchitomi, Y. 2003. A volumetric study of amygdala in cancer survivors with intrusive recollections. *Biol Psychiatry,* 54, 736-43.

[43] Mccrory, E., De Brito, S. A. & Viding, E. 2011. The impact of childhood maltreatment: a review of neurobiological and genetic factors. *Front Psychiatry,* 2, 48.

[44] Mcfarlane, A. C., Yehuda, R. & Clark, C. R. 2002. Biologic models of traumatic memories and post-traumatic stress disorder. The role of neural networks. *Psychiatr Clin North Am,* 25, 253-70, v.

[45] Mehta, M. A., Golembo, N. I., Nosarti, C., Colvert, E., Mota, A., Williams, S. C., Rutter, M. & Sonuga-Barke, E. J. 2009. Amygdala, hippocampal and corpus callosum size following severe early institutional deprivation: the English and Romanian Adoptees study pilot. *J Child Psychol Psychiatry,* 50, 943-51.

[46] Mills, K. L., Mcfarlane, A. C., Slade, T., Creamer, M., Silove, D., Teesson, M. & Bryant, R. 2011. Assessing the prevalence of trauma exposure in epidemiological surveys. *Aust N Z J Psychiatry,* 45, 407-15.

[47] Mollica, R. F., Lyoo, I. K., Chernoff, M. C., Bui, H. X., Lavelle, J., Yoon, S. J., Kim, J. E. & Renshaw, P. F. 2009. Brain structural abnormalities and mental health sequelae in South Vietnamese ex-political detainees who survived traumatic head injury and torture. *Arch Gen Psychiatry,* 66, 1221-32.

[48] Mueller, S. C., Maheu, F. S., Dozier, M., Peloso, E., Mandell, D., Leibenluft, E., Pine, D. S. & Ernst, M. 2010. Early-life stress is associated with impairment in cognitive control in adolescence: an fMRI study. *Neuropsychologia,* 48, 3037-44.

[49] New, A. S., Hazlett, E. A., Buchsbaum, M. S., Goodman, M., Mitelman, S. A., Newmark, R., Trisdorfer, R., Haznedar, M. M., Koenigsberg, H. W., Flory, J. & Siever, L. J. 2007. Amygdala-prefrontal disconnection in borderline personality disorder. *Neuropsychopharmacology,* 32, 1629-40.

[50] Nunes, P. M., Wenzel, A., Borges, K. T., Porto, C. R., Caminha, R. M. & De Oliveira, I. R. 2009. Volumes of the hippocampus and amygdala in patients with borderline personality disorder: a meta-analysis. *J Pers Disord,* 23, 333-45.

[51] Oh, D. H., Son, H., Hwang, S. & Kim, S. H. 2012. Neuropathological abnormalities of astrocytes, GABAergic neurons, and pyramidal neurons in the dorsolateral prefrontal cortices of patients with major depressive disorder. *Eur Neuropsychopharmacol,* 22, 330-8.

[52] Passamonti, L., Crockett, M. J., Apergis-Schoute, A. M., Clark, L., Rowe, J. B., Calder, A. J. & ROBBINS, T. W. 2012. Effects of acute tryptophan depletion on prefrontal-amygdala connectivity while viewing facial signals of aggression. *Biol Psychiatry,* 71, 36-43.

[53] Peres JF, Foerster B, Santana LG, Fereira MD, Nasello AG, Savoia M, Moreira-Almeida A, Lederman H. 2011. Police officers under attack: resilience implications of an fMRI study. *J Psychiatr Res,.* 45, 727-34.

[54] Pessoa, L. 2010. Emotion and cognition and the amygdala: from "what is it?" to "what's to be done?". *Neuropsychologia,* 48, 3416-29.

[55] Phelps, E. A. & Ledoux, J. E. 2005. Contributions of the amygdala to emotion processing: from animal models to human behavior. *Neuron,* 48, 175-87.

[56] Rauch, S. L., Whalen, P. J., Shin, L. M., Mcinerney, S. C., Macklin, M. L., Lasko, N. B., Orr, S. P. & Pitman, R. K. 2000. Exaggerated amygdala response to masked facial stimuli in posttraumatic stress disorder: a functional MRI study. *Biol Psychiatry,* 47, 769-76.

[57] Sacher, J., Neumann, J., Funfstuck, T., Soliman, A., Villringer, A. & Schroeter, M. L. 2012. Mapping the depressed brain: A meta-analysis of structural and functional alterations in major depressive disorder. *J Affect Disord.* 140, 142-8

[58] Sah, P., Faber, E. S., Lopez De Armentia, M. & Power, J. 2003. The amygdaloid complex: anatomy and physiology. *Physiol Rev,* 83, 803-34.

[59] Sehlmeyer, C., Dannlowski, U., Schoning, S., Kugel, H., Pyka, M., Pfleiderer, B., Zwitserlood, P., Schiffbauer, H., Heindel, W., Arolt, V. & Konrad, C. 2011. Neural correlates of trait anxiety in fear extinction. *Psychol Med,* 41, 789-98.

[60] Sheline, Y. I., Barch, D. M., Donnelly, J. M., Ollinger, J. M., Snyder, A. Z. & Mintun, M. A. 2001. Increased amygdala response to masked emotional faces in depressed subjects resolves with antidepressant treatment: an fMRI study. *Biol Psychiatry,* 50, 651-8.

[61] Shin, L. M., Rauch, S. L. & Pitman, R. K. 2006. Amygdala, medial prefrontal cortex, and hippocampal function in PTSD. *Ann N Y Acad Sci,* 1071, 67-79.

[62] Shin, L. M., Wright, C. I., Cannistraro, P. A., Wedig, M. M., Mcmullin, K., Martis, B., Macklin, M. L., Lasko, N. B., Cavanagh, S. R., Krangel, T. S., Orr, S. P., Pitman, R. K., Whalen, P. J. & Rauch, S. L. 2005. A functional magnetic resonance imaging study of amygdala and medial prefrontal cortex responses to overtly presented fearful faces in posttraumatic stress disorder. *Arch Gen Psychiatry,* 62, 273-81.

[63] Siegle, G. J., Thompson, W., Carter, C. S., Steinhauer, S. R. & Thase, M. E. 2007. Increased amygdala and decreased dorsolateral prefrontal BOLD responses in unipolar depression: related and independent features. *Biol Psychiatry,* 61, 198-209.

[64] Siever, L. J. 2008. Neurobiology of aggression and violence. *Am J Psychiatry,* 165, 429-42.

[65] Sripada, R. K., King, A. P., Garfinkel, S. N., Wang, X., Sripada, C. S., Welsh, R. C. & Liberzon, I. 2012. Altered resting-state amygdala functional connectivity in men with posttraumatic stress disorder. *J Psychiatry Neurosci,* 37, 241-9.

[66] Suslow, T., Konrad, C., Kugel, H., Rumstadt, D., Zwitserlood, P., Schoning, S., Ohrmann, P., Bauer, J., Pyka, M., Kersting, A., Arolt, V., Heindel, W. & Dannlowski, U. 2010. Automatic mood-congruent amygdala responses to masked facial expressions in major depression. *Biol Psychiatry,* 67, 155-60.

[67] Tomoda, A., Suzuki, H., Rabi, K., Sheu, Y. S., Polcari, A. & Teicher, M. H. 2009. Reduced prefrontal cortical gray matter volume in young adults exposed to harsh corporal punishment. *Neuroimage,* 47 Suppl 2, T66-71.

[68] Tottenham, N., Hare, T. A., Quinn, B. T., Mccarry, T. W., Nurse, M., Gilhooly, T., Millner, A., Galvan, A., Davidson, M. C., Eigsti, I. M., Thomas, K. M., Freed, P. J., Booma, E. S., Gunnar, M. R., Altemus, M., Aronson, J. & Casey, B. J. 2010. Prolonged institutional rearing is associated with atypically large amygdala volume and difficulties in emotion regulation. *Dev Sci,* 13, 46-61.

[69] Tottenham, N., Hare, T. A., Millner, A., Gilhooly, T., Zevin, J. D. & Casey, B. J. 2011. Elevated amygdala response to faces following early deprivation. Dev Sci, 14, 190-204.

[70] Urry, H. L., Van Reekum, C. M., Johnstone, T., Kalin, N. H., Thurow, M. E., Schaefer, H. S., Jackson, C. A., Frye, C. J., Greischar, L. L., Alexander, A. L. & Davidson, R. J. 2006. Amygdala and ventromedial prefrontal cortex are inversely coupled during regulation of negative affect and predict the diurnal pattern of cortisol secretion among older adults. *J Neurosci,* 26, 4415-25.

[71] Van Harmelen, A. L., Van Tol, M. J., Van Der Wee, N. J., Veltman, D. J., Aleman, A., Spinhoven, P., Van Buchem, M. A., Zitman, F. G., Penninx, B. W. & Elzinga, B. M. 2010. Reduced medial prefrontal cortex volume in adults reporting childhood emotional maltreatment. *Biol Psychiatry,* 68, 832-8.

[72] Veer, I. M., Oei, N. Y., Spinhoven, P., Van Buchem, M. A., Elzinga, B. M. & Rombouts, S. A. 2012. Endogenous cortisol is associated with functional connectivity between the amygdala and medial prefrontal cortex. *Psychoneuroendocrinology,* 37, 1039-47.

[73] Williams, L. M., Kemp, A. H., Felmingham, K., Barton, M., Olivieri, G., Peduto, A., Gordon, E. & Bryant, R. A. 2006. Trauma modulates amygdala and medial prefrontal responses to consciously attended fear. *Neuroimage,* 29, 347-57.

[74] Woon, F. L. & Hedges, D. W. 2008. Hippocampal and amygdala volumes in children and adults with childhood maltreatment-related posttraumatic stress disorder: a meta-analysis. *Hippocampus,* 18, 729-36.

[75] Woon, F. L. & Hedges, D. W. 2009. Amygdala volume in adults with posttraumatic stress disorder: a meta-analysis. *J Neuropsychiatry Clin Neurosci,* 21, 5-12.

[76] Zhong, M., Wang, X., Xiao, J., Yi, J., Zhu, X., Liao, J., Wang, W. & Yao, S. 2011. Amygdala hyperactivation and prefrontal hypoactivation in subjects with cognitive vulnerability to depression. *Biol Psychol,* 88, 233-42.

[77] Zhu, M. Y., Wang, W. P. & Bissette, G. 2006. Neuroprotective effects of agmatine against cell damage caused by glucocorticoids in cultured rat hippocampal neurons. *Neuroscience,* 141, 2019-27.

Chapter 14

Amygdala in Alzheimer's Disease

Shira Knafo

Additional information is available at the end of the chapter

1. Introduction

Alzheimer's disease (AD) is a progressive neurodegenerative disease that causes debilitating dementia. For yet unknown reason, AD often leads also to emotional instability. Neuropathologically, AD brains are characterized by the presence of extracellular fibrillar amyloid beta peptide (Aβ) in amyloid plaques, intraneuronal neurofibrillary tangles consisting of aggregated hyperphosphorylated tau, and elevated brain levels of soluble Aβ oligomers. Plaques and neurofibrillary tangles are observed mostly in the cerebral cortex, but subcortical regions such as nucleus basalis, thalamus, locus coeruleus and raphe nuclei are also affected (Price et al., 1991). The amygdala is another important subcortical region that is severely and consistently affected by pathology in AD. This chapter will discuss the neuropathological features of the amygdala affected by AD and the resulting psychological, emotional and cognitive disturbances in AD patients and in model mice of this disease.

2. Emotional disturbances in AD patients

The amygdala is part of the limbic system that plays a major role in the processing and memorizing of emotional reactions (Schafe et al., 2005). The involvement of the amygdala in emotion has been evidenced in monkeys by the overwhelming loss of normal social and affective behavior resulting from bilateral damage to this structure (Izquierdo et al., 2005; Izquierdo and Murray, 2007). The amygdala is affected early in AD and results by neuropsychiatric symptoms leading to functional deficits that greatly contribute to the disability associated with this disease. Due to the early damage to the amygdala, neuropsychiatric symptoms are very common in mild stages of AD. Eventually, approximately 80% of the patients with AD present neuropsychiatric symptoms, such as hallucinations, delusions, paranoia, anxiety, agitation, and affective disturbances during the course of their illness (Mega et al., 1996; Lyketsos et al., 2002). Other symptoms such as dysphoria, irritability, disinhibition and apathy are also common (Kaufer et al., 1998). In addition to these symptoms, AD patients frequently show personality changes that affect their activities of daily living and the interaction with their caregivers. Personality changes may appear in any phase of dementia but often precede other early clinical manifestations of the disease, such as cognitive impairment and mood changes. These changes may therefore help in the clinical diagnosis of AD at early stages (Robins Wahlin and Byrne, 2011). Interestingly, personality changes and some of the neuropsychiatric symptoms (agitation, dysphoria and apathy) are better correlated with the severity of cognitive, functional and behavioral signs than with the patient's age, gender, education or disease duration (Mega et al., 1996; Talassi et al., 2007). Thus, personality changes and neuropsychiatric symptoms may reflect the impact of progressive brain damage in AD (Robins Wahlin and Byrne, 2011).

3. Emotional memory in AD

Emotional memory is a form of episodic memory defined as memory of arousing emotional events. These memories are sometimes referred to as "flashbulb" memories (Hamann et al., 2000). Results from studies in animals and humans have strongly implicated the amygdala in this memory type (LaBar, 2003; Brierley et al., 2004; Richter-Levin, 2004). While it is recognized that normal people better remember events associated with an emotional component, there is a controversy regarding the strength of emotional memory in AD patients (Satler et al., 2007; Schultz et al., 2009; Huijbers et al., 2011; Nashiro and Mather, 2011; Sundstrom, 2011). Since the amygdala is one of the structures damaged in early stages of the AD pathology, it has been hypothesized that emotional memory should be impaired in AD patients. Indeed, data have shown that unlike healthy individuals, AD patients do not show memory enhancement for emotional events (enhanced memory for emotional compared to neutral stimuli) in spite of normal emotional reactions (Hamann et al., 2000). Notably, the degree of emotional memory impairment has positively been correlated with the extent of the amygdaloid atrophy (Mori et al., 1999a, b; Fleming et al., 2003).

4. Pathology of the amygdala in AD patients

While normal aging primarily affects the prefrontal cortex but relatively spares limbic regions, AD mainly affects limbic regions. The amygdala of AD patients shows a considerable shrinkage, distortion and loss of neurons, and widespread gliosis (Vereecken et al.; Herzog and Kemper, 1980; Cuenod et al., 1993). The amygdaloid atrophy in AD is the result of neuronal death (especially in the magnocellular basolateral amygdalar nuclei group) and loss of dendrites and axons. The accumulation of intraneuronal neurofibrillary tangles, Lewy bodies and extracellular Amyloid β peptide (Aβ) deposits in plaques also contribute significantly to the atrophy. Detailed pathological examination of the amygdala of AD patients reveals that many neurofibrillary tangles and Aβ plaques are located in the accessory basal and cortical nuclei and in the cortical transition area, whereas the mediobasal nucleus is less affected (Kromer Vogt et al., 1990). The medial, lateral, laterobasal and central nuclei are relatively free of neurofibrillary tangles and Aβ plaques (Kromer Vogt et al., 1990). Interestingly, it has been observed that the morphological deformation of the amygdala in AD patients is associated with intrinsic damage to its subnuclei and their reciprocal connectivity with other brain areas. Specifically, it has been reported that amygdaloid nuclei receiving input from and giving rise to hippocampal projections are consistently affected by neuropathological alterations in AD. In contrast, amygdaloid nuclei which receive strong cholinergic input from nucleus basalis of Meynert (e.g. laterobasal nucleus) are less affected (Kromer Vogt et al., 1990). To conclude, histological analysis of the amygdala of AD patients allows a thorough examination of this region thus rendering possible to detect nucleus-specific pathologies. Nevertheless, the major limitation of post-mortem analysis is that it is typically performed on brains taken from patients at late stages of the disease. Thus, information is lacking regarding neuropathological alterations in early stages of AD.

5. Imaging of the amygdala *in vivo*

Whereas histological procedures are used to investigate the anatomical complexity of the amygdala in brains from AD patients, a standard magnetic resonance imaging (MRI) technique can only detect few internal details and similar resolution cannot be obtained. The discovery that neuronal loss is a cause of amygdaloid atrophy provided the basis for later studies correlating amygdaloid volumetry, as measured with MRI, with the cognitive status of individual AD patients. Indeed, MRI-based volumetry is now regularly used as a research tool to explore the relationship between amygdaloid volume and the onset and progression of AD (de Leon et al., 1996; Mori et al., 1999a; Vasconcelos et al., 2011). While in the past the use of MRI was limited to clinical studies, the recent rise in MRI accessibility allowed its utilization for non-clinical studies aimed at investigating the involvement of the amygdala in emotion, memory processes and personality (Mori et al., 1999a). The main disadvantage of MRI-based amygdaloid volumetry consists in the difficulty to precisely and reliably delineate the contours of the amygdala *in vivo*. This difficulty arises from the similarity in MRI signal intensities between the amygdala and other temporal lobe structures surrounding it (hippocampus proper, subiculum, entorhinal cortex, claustrum and tail of the caudate)(Convit et al., 1999). Nevertheless, new imaging techniques such as ultrahigh field structural MRI enable clear *in vivo* detection and even segmentation of the amygdala (Solano-Castiella et al., 2011), and might be used to investigate the anatomical features of different amygdaloid nuclei in AD patients.

Numerous studies measuring the amygdaloid volume (normalized to intracranial volume) in AD patients at different clinical stages and in healthy age-matched controls showed a correlation of this factor with the neuropsychological performance of each patient. These studies have consistently demonstrated a decrease in amygdaloid volume in AD patients when compared to healthy controls (Horinek et al., 2007; Beacher et al., 2009; Cherubini et al., 2010; Lehmann et al., 2010; Vasconcelos Lde et al., 2011). Importantly, atrophy of the amygdala was found even in preclinical stages of the disease (Fox et al., 1996; Heun et al., 1997; Golebiowski et al., 1999). In fact, in the very early stages of AD, amygdaloid volume reductions were at least as large as hippocampal volume reductions although at this stage some overlap does exist between patients and healthy controls. Still, the volume of the amygdala has been suggested to be an independent variable in predicting conversion from mild cognitive impairment to AD (Liu et al., 2010).

Functional MRI. Increasing number of neuroimaging studies using functional MRI (fMRI) are used to examine the neuronal activity of the amygdala by detecting changes in local blood perfusion, blood volume or blood oxygenation. Injecting contrast agents are often used in this technique. In some studies, voxel-based morphometry (VBM) on MRI was combined with Positron Emission Tomography (PET) to compare activity in specific brain areas in AD patients and healthy controls (Kawachi et al., 2006). Functional MRI studies showed that the amygdala is excessively responsive to human faces (both novel emotional and familiar neutral expressions) in mild AD patients relative to elderly controls (Wright et al., 2007). On the other hand, AD patients presented deficits in the recognition of some facial expressions of emotion (happy, sad, fearful, and neutral expressions)(Kohler et al., 2005). These alterations in the normal activity of the amygdala probably contribute to the significant social and behavioral defects observed in AD patients.

Positron Emission Tomography (PET). PET is almost exclusively used to image the brain, and may be used to detect functional abnormalities early in the course of AD, way before anatomical changes occur. For example, PET was used to examine acetylcholine esterase activity *in vivo* in the amygdala and cerebral cortex (Shinotoh et al., 2003). To note, levels of acetylcholine are significantly decreased in AD due to degeneration of the cholinergic magnocellular neurons of the nucleus basalis of Meynert (nbM) that send cholinergic projection mainly to the amygdala (Mesulam, 2004). In fact, the degree of the cholinergic loss is positively correlated with the severity of dementia in AD (Perry et al., 1981), probably due to the importance of nbM in emotional memory consolidation. PET measurements of C-11-labeled N-methyl-4-piperidyl-acetate (MP4A, a specific substrate of AChE) have shown that AChE activity is significantly reduced in patients with AD in both the amygdala and cerebral cortex (Shinotoh et al., 2003). Importantly, these deficits are present in mild to moderate AD, supporting the notion that cortical and amygdaloid functional changes of the cholinergic system occur early in AD (Herholz et al., 2004). These functional alterations are therefore suggested to serve as a physiologic and noninvasive marker for certain neuropsychiatric manifestations of mild AD. In addition, these finding suggest that the amygdala should receive an important attention in studies of the mild or even prodromal stages of AD (Basso et al., 2006) even though considerable evidences continue to support the focus on the hippocampus in MRI studies of AD.

6. The use of AD mice model to study the Aβ-dependent changes in the amygdala

In modern AD research, transgenic mice bearing infrequent mutations leading to familial forms of AD are being used to characterize in details the physiological, morphological and behavioral consequences of AD neuropathology in order to understand the anatomical and synaptic basis of dementia (Selkoe, 1996). These mutations include mutations in amyloid precursor protein (APP), the precursor of the Aβ peptide, or in presenilin (PS) 1 or 2, the catalytic subunit of the gamma secretase complex, which cleaves APP to form Aβ. Transgenic AD mice model represents an important tool to examine the consequences of *in vivo* Aβ accumulation and were proved to mimic many of the pathological features of AD (Spires and Hyman, 2005; Spires-Jones and Knafo, 2012). APP and APP/PS1 mice present abundant extracellular Aβ plaques, synaptic dysfunction and loss, astrocytosis, activation of microglia and cognitive deficits (Games et al., 1995). The fact that Aβ plaques occupy a minor fraction (less than 5%) of the neuropil (see Fig. 1) in cognitively impaired transgenic mice (Knafo et al., 2009; Merino-Serrais et al., 2011) and the lack of correlation between the plaque load and the degree of cognitive impairment in AD patients (Terry et al., 1991; Terry, 2000), support the notion that fibrillar Aβ in plaques does not contribute significantly to dementia in AD patients. Instead, soluble Aβ assemblies (i.e. oligomeric or protofibrillary Aβ species that linger in aqueous solution after high-speed centrifugation) seem to be the main factors responsible for the structural, synaptic and cognitive deficits in these mice and probably also in initiating disease in AD patients (Selkoe, 2002).

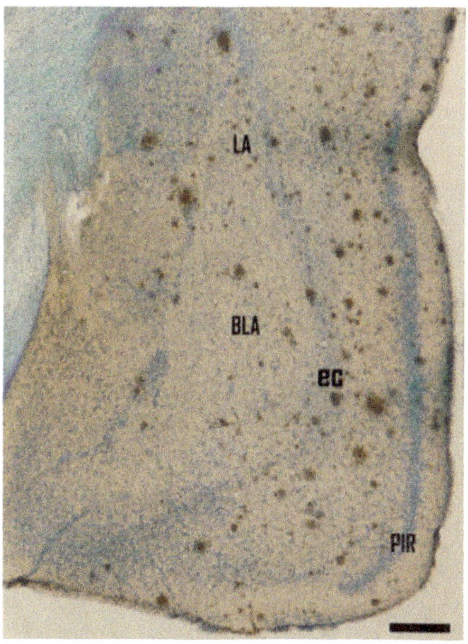

A section stained with the anti-Aβ antibody and Nissl.
BLA = basolateral nucleus of the amygdala; EC = external capsule; LA = lateral nucleus of the amygdala; PIR = piriform cortex. Scale bar, 350 μm (Knafo et al., 2009)

Figure 1. Coronal sections through the amygdala and adjacent regions showing the pattern of distribution of amyloid plaques.

In a recent study, transgenic mice expressing a chimeric mouse/human amyloid precursor protein (Mo/HuAPP695swe) and a mutant human presenilin 1 (PS1-dE9) (APP/PS1, Borchelt et al., 1997) were used to study the morphological basis for amygdala-dependent cognitive impairment (Knafo et al., 2009). In this study, the authors first showed a clear impairment of auditory fear conditioning in APP/PS1 mice, a learning task that depends on the lateral nucleus of the amygdala (LA) (Knafo et al., 2009). Importantly, this cognitive deficit did not result from changes in anxiety or sensitivity to shock. Then, the authors used intracellular injection of Alexa594 into projection neurons in the LA, combined with thioflavin-S plaque staining (Fig. 2) and three-dimensional reconstructions of the dendritic trees and spines. The results of this study show that in APP/PS1 mice the morphology of projection neurons in the amygdala is modified, as reflected by changes in dendritic complexity, and that there is a

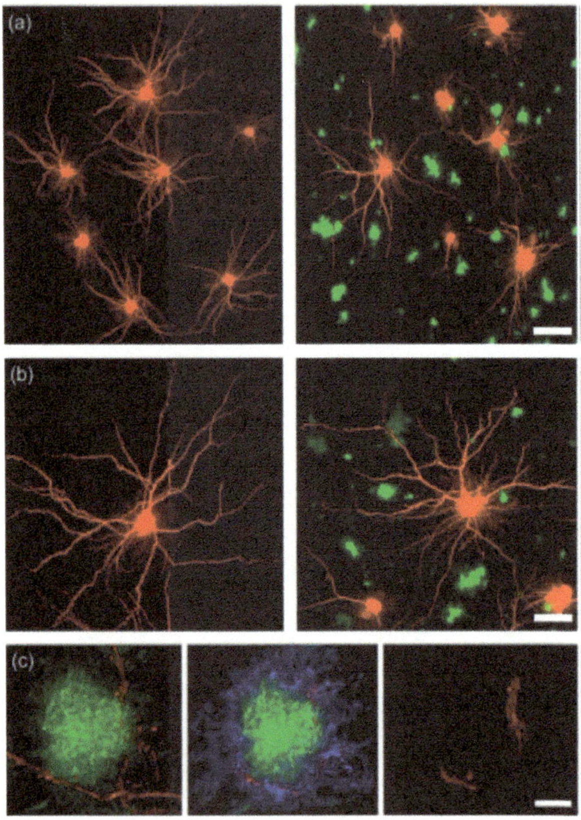

(a) Panoramic confocal (10x) views of the lateral amygdala showing Alexa594-injected neurons and thioflavin-s-positive plaques in a Tg- mouse (left) and an APP/PS1 mouse (right).
(b) Representative images of projection neurons from a Tg- mouse (left) and an APP/PS1 mouse (right).
(c) The method used to distinguish dendrites and spines within and outside plaques. Left: a plaque suspected of containing a dendrite due to the rotation of its three-dimensional image. Center: the plaque surface is marked with the aid of the IsoSurface tool of Imaris software. Right: the voxels outside the surface are set to zero, leaving only the dendritic segment within the plaque (Knafo et al., 2009).

Figure 2. Intracellular injections

significant decrease in number of large spines on these neurons (Knafo et al., 2009). The authors emphasized the finding that the morphological alteration in dendrites and spines occur mainly in plaque-free areas that occupy most of the neuropil. Thus, as spines are main postsynaptic elements of excitatory synapses in the brain (Gray, 1959) and are fundamental in memory, learning and cognition (Lamprecht and LeDoux, 2004) the authors suggested that these changes, rather than changes detected within plaques contribute to the cognitive impairment seen in APP/PS1 mice.

To summarize, amygdala is significantly and consistently affected by Aβ both in patients with AD and in mouse models of this disease. Therefore, this region is a central participant in the pathology of AD (Unger et al., 1991) and its damage may be the structural substrate to the frequent emotional, psychological, and memory disturbances seen in this devastating disorder.

Author details

Shira Knafo
Severo Ochoa Center for Molecular Biology, Spanish National Research Council (CSIC)/Autonomous University of Madrid, Madrid, Spain

7. References

Basso M, Yang J, Warren L, MacAvoy MG, Varma P, Bronen RA, van Dyck CH (2006) Volumetry of amygdala and hippocampus and memory performance in Alzheimer's disease. Psychiatry Research: Neuroimaging 146:251-261.

Beacher F, Daly E, Simmons A, Prasher V, Morris R, Robinson C, Lovestone S, Murphy K, Murphy DG (2009) Alzheimer's disease and Down's syndrome: an in vivo MRI study. Psychological medicine 39:675-684.

Borchelt DR, Ratovitski T, van Lare J, Lee MK, Gonzales V, Jenkins NA, Copeland NG, Price DL, Sisodia SS (1997) Accelerated amyloid deposition in the brains of transgenic mice coexpressing mutant presenilin 1 and amyloid precursor proteins. Neuron 19:939-945.

Brierley B, Medford N, Shaw P, David AS (2004) Emotional memory and perception in temporal lobectomy patients with amygdala damage. Journal of neurology, neurosurgery, and psychiatry 75:593-599.

Cherubini A, Peran P, Spoletini I, Di Paola M, Di Iulio F, Hagberg GE, Sancesario G, Gianni W, Bossu P, Caltagirone C, Sabatini U, Spalletta G (2010) Combined volumetry and DTI in subcortical structures of mild cognitive impairment and Alzheimer's disease patients. J Alzheimers Dis 19:1273-1282.

Convit A, McHugh P, Wolf OT, de Leon MJ, Bobinski M, De Santi S, Roche A, Tsui W (1999) MRI volume of the amygdala: a reliable method allowing separation from the hippocampal formation. Psychiatry Res 90:113-123.

Cuenod C-A, Denys A, Michot J-L, Jehenson P, Forette F, Kaplan D, Syrota A, Boller F (1993) Amygdala Atrophy in Alzheimer's Disease: An In Vivo Magnetic Resonance Imaging Study. In, pp 941-945.

de Leon MJ, Convit A, George AE, Golomb J, de Santi S, Tarshish C, Rusinek H, Bobinski M, Ince C, Miller D, Wisniewski H (1996) In vivo structural studies of the hippocampus in normal aging and in incipient Alzheimer's disease. Annals of the New York Academy of Sciences 777:1-13.

Fleming K, Kim SH, Doo M, Maguire G, Potkin SG (2003) Memory for emotional stimuli in patients with Alzheimer's disease. Am J Alzheimers Dis Other Demen 18:340-342.

Fox NC, Warrington EK, Freeborough PA, Hartikainen P, Kennedy AM, Stevens JM, Rossor MN (1996) Presymptomatic hippocampal atrophy in Alzheimer's disease. A longitudinal MRI study. Brain 119 (Pt 6):2001-2007.

Games D et al. (1995) Alzheimer-type neuropathology in transgenic mice overexpressing V717F [beta]-amyloid precursor protein. Nature 373:523-527.

Golebiowski M, Barcikowska M, Pfeffer A (1999) Magnetic resonance imaging-based hippocampal volumetry in patients with dementia of the Alzheimer type. Dement Geriatr Cogn Disord 10:284-288.

Gray EG (1959) Electron microscopy of synaptic contacts on dendrite spines of the cerebral cortex. Nature 183:1592-1593.

Hamann SB, Monarch ES, Goldstein FC (2000) Memory enhancement for emotional stimuli is impaired in early Alzheimer's disease. Neuropsychology 14:82-92.

Herholz K, Weisenbach S, Z√ºndorf G, Lenz O, Schröder H, Bauer B, Kalbe E, Heiss WD (2004) In vivo study of acetylcholine esterase in basal forebrain, amygdala, and cortex in mild to moderate Alzheimer disease. Neuroimage 21:136-143.

Herzog AG, Kemper TL (1980) Amygdaloid Changes in Aging and Dementia. In, pp 625-629.

Heun R, Mazanek M, Atzor KR, Tintera J, Gawehn J, Burkart M, Gansicke M, Falkai P, Stoeter P (1997) Amygdala-hippocampal atrophy and memory performance in dementia of Alzheimer type. Dement Geriatr Cogn Disord 8:329-336.

Horinek D, Varjassyova A, Hort J (2007) Magnetic resonance analysis of amygdalar volume in Alzheimer's disease. Current opinion in psychiatry 20:273-277.

Huijbers MJ, Bergmann HC, Olde Rikkert MG, Kessels RP (2011) Memory for emotional pictures in patients with Alzheimer's dementia: comparing picture-location binding and subsequent recognition. Journal of aging research 2011:409364.

Izquierdo A, Murray EA (2007) Selective Bilateral Amygdala Lesions in Rhesus Monkeys Fail to Disrupt Object Reversal Learning. The Journal of Neuroscience 27:1054-1062.

Izquierdo A, Suda RK, Murray EA (2005) Comparison of the Effects of Bilateral Orbital Prefrontal Cortex Lesions and Amygdala Lesions on Emotional Responses in Rhesus Monkeys. The Journal of Neuroscience 25:8534-8542.

Kaufer DI, Cummings JL, Christine D, Bray T, Castellon S, Masterman D, MacMillan A, Ketchel P, DeKosky ST (1998) Assessing the impact of neuropsychiatric symptoms in Alzheimer's disease: the Neuropsychiatric Inventory Caregiver Distress Scale. Journal of the American Geriatrics Society 46:210-215.

Kawachi T, Ishii K, Sakamoto S, Sasaki M, Mori T, Yamashita F, Matsuda H, Mori E (2006) Comparison of the diagnostic performance of FDG-PET and VBM-MRI in very mild Alzheimer's disease. European journal of nuclear medicine and molecular imaging 33:801-809.

Knafo S, Venero C, Merino-Serrais P, Fernaud-Espinosa I, Gonzalez-Soriano J, Ferrer I, Santpere G, DeFelipe J (2009) Morphological alterations to neurons of the amygdala and impaired fear conditioning in a transgenic mouse model of Alzheimer's disease. The Journal of pathology 219:41-51.

Kohler CG, Anselmo-Gallagher G, Bilker W, Karlawish J, Gur RE, Clark CM (2005) Emotion-Discrimination Deficits in Mild Alzheimer Disease. American Journal of Geriatric Psych 13:926-933.

Kromer Vogt LJ, Hyman BT, Van Hoesen GW, Damasio AR (1990) Pathological alterations in the amygdala in Alzheimer's disease. Neuroscience 37:377-385.

LaBar KS (2003) Emotional memory functions of the human amygdala. Current neurology and neuroscience reports 3:363-364.

Lamprecht R, LeDoux J (2004) Structural plasticity and memory. Nature reviews 5:45-54.

Lehmann M, Douiri A, Kim LG, Modat M, Chan D, Ourselin S, Barnes J, Fox NC (2010) Atrophy patterns in Alzheimer's disease and semantic dementia: a comparison of FreeSurfer and manual volumetric measurements. Neuroimage 49:2264-2274.

Liu Y, Paajanen T, Zhang Y, Westman E, Wahlund LO, Simmons A, Tunnard C, Sobow T, Mecocci P, Tsolaki M, Vellas B, Muehlboeck S, Evans A, Spenger C, Lovestone S, Soininen H (2010) Analysis of regional MRI volumes and thicknesses as predictors of conversion from mild cognitive impairment to Alzheimer's disease. Neurobiology of aging 31:1375-1385.

Lyketsos CG, Lopez O, Jones B, Fitzpatrick AL, Breitner J, DeKosky S (2002) Prevalence of neuropsychiatric symptoms in dementia and mild cognitive impairment: results from the cardiovascular health study. Jama 288:1475-1483.

Mega MS, Cummings JL, Fiorello T, Gornbein J (1996) The spectrum of behavioral changes in Alzheimer's disease. Neurology 46:130-135.

Merino-Serrais P, Knafo S, Alonso-Nanclares L, Fernaud-Espinosa I, DeFelipe J (2011) Layer-specific alterations to CA1 dendritic spines in a mouse model of Alzheimer's disease. Hippocampus 21:1037-1044.

Mesulam M (2004) The Cholinergic Lesion of Alzheimer's Disease: Pivotal Factor or Side Show? Learning & Memory 11:43-49.

Mori E, Ikeda M, Hirono N, Kitagaki H, Imamura T, Shimomura T (1999a) Amygdalar volume and emotional memory in Alzheimer's disease. Am J Psychiatry 156:216-222.

Mori E, Ikeda M, Hirono N, Kitagaki H, Imamura T, Shimomura T (1999b) Amygdalar volume and emotional memory in Alzheimer's disease. The American journal of psychiatry 156:216-222.

Nashiro K, Mather M (2011) Effects of emotional arousal on memory binding in normal aging and Alzheimer's disease. The American journal of psychology 124:301-312.

Perry EK, Blessed G, Tomlinson BE, Perry RH, Crow TJ, Cross AJ, Dockray GJ, Dimaline R, Arregui A (1981) Neurochemical activities in human temporal lobe related to aging and Alzheimer-type changes. Neurobiology of aging 2:251-256.

Price JL, Davis PB, Morris JC, White DL (1991) The distribution of tangles, plaques and related immunohistochemical markers in healthy aging and Alzheimer's disease. Neurobiology of aging 12:295-312.

Richter-Levin G (2004) The amygdala, the hippocampus, and emotional modulation of memory. The Neuroscientist : a review journal bringing neurobiology, neurology and psychiatry 10:31-39.

Robins Wahlin TB, Byrne GJ (2011) Personality changes in Alzheimer's disease: a systematic review. Int J Geriatr Psychiatry 26:1019-1029.

Satler C, Garrido LM, Sarmiento EP, Leme S, Conde C, Tomaz C (2007) Emotional arousal enhances declarative memory in patients with Alzheimer's disease. Acta neurologica Scandinavica 116:355-360.

Schafe GE, Doyere V, LeDoux JE (2005) Tracking the fear engram: the lateral amygdala is an essential locus of fear memory storage. J Neurosci 25:10010-10014.

Schultz RR, de Castro CC, Bertolucci PH (2009) Memory with emotional content, brain amygdala and Alzheimer's disease. Acta neurologica Scandinavica 120:101-110.

Selkoe DJ (1996) Amyloid beta-protein and the genetics of Alzheimer's disease. The Journal of biological chemistry 271:18295-18298.

Selkoe DJ (2002) Alzheimer's disease is a synaptic failure. Science (New York, NY 298:789-791.

Shinotoh H, Fukushi K, Nagatsuka S, Tanaka N, Aotsuka A, Ota T, Namba H, Tanada S, Irie T (2003) The Amygdala and Alzheimer's Disease. Annals of the New York Academy of Sciences 985:411-419.

Solano-Castiella E, Schäfer A, Reimer E, Türke E, Pröger T, Lohmann G, Trampel R, Turner R (2011) Parcellation of human amygdala in vivo using ultra high field structural MRI. Neuroimage 58:741-748.

Spires TL, Hyman BT (2005) Transgenic models of Alzheimer's disease: Learning from animals. NeuroRx 2:423-437.

Spires-Jones T, Knafo S (2012) Spines, Plasticity, and Cognition in Alzheimer's Model Mice. Neural Plasticity 2012.

Sundstrom M (2011) Modeling recall memory for emotional objects in Alzheimer's disease. Neuropsychology, development, and cognition Section B, Aging, neuropsychology and cognition 18:396-413.

Talassi E, Cipriani G, Bianchetti A, Trabucchi M (2007) Personality changes in Alzheimer's disease. Aging Ment Health 11:526-531.

Terry RD (2000) Cell Death or Synaptic Loss in Alzheimer Disease. Journal of Neuropathology & Experimental Neurology 59:1118-1119.

Terry RD, Masliah E, Salmon DP, Butters N, DeTeresa R, Hill R, Hansen LA, Katzman R (1991) Physical basis of cognitive alterations in alzheimer's disease: Synapse loss is the major correlate of cognitive impairment. Annals of neurology 30:572-580.

Unger JW, Lapham LW, McNeill TH, Eskin TA, Hamill RW (1991) The amygdala in Alzheimer's disease: neuropathology and Alz 50 immunoreactivity. Neurobiology of aging 12:389-399.

Vasconcelos Lde G, Jackowski AP, Oliveira MO, Flor YM, Bueno OF, Brucki SM (2011) Voxel-based morphometry findings in Alzheimer's disease: neuropsychiatric symptoms and disability correlations - preliminary results. Clinics (Sao Paulo) 66:1045-1050.

Vasconcelos LdG, Jackowski AP, Oliveira MOd, Flor YMR, Bueno OFA, Brucki SMD (2011) Voxel-based morphometry findings in Alzheimer's disease: neuropsychiatric symptoms and disability correlations - preliminary results. Clinics 66:1045-1050.

Vereecken THLG, Vogels OJM, Nieuwenhuys R Neuron loss and shrinkage in the amygdala in Alzheimer's disease. Neurobiology of aging 15:45-54.

Wright CI, Dickerson BC, Feczko E, Negeira A, Williams D (2007) A Functional Magnetic Resonance Imaging Study of Amygdala Responses to Human Faces in Aging and Mild Alzheimer's Disease. Biological Psychiatry 62:1388-1395.

Chapter 15

The Irritable Bowel Syndrome: How Stress Can Affect the Amygdala Activity and the Brain-Gut Axis

Bruno Bonaz, Sonia Pellissier, Valérie Sinniger, Didier Clarençon,André Peinnequin and Frédéric Canini

Additional information is available at the end of the chapter

1. Introduction

Irritable bowel syndrome (IBS) is a functional digestive disorder characterized by abdominal pain, bloating and altered bowel habits without any organic cause (Drossman 1999b; Mulak and Bonaz 2004). Patients with IBS exhibit enhanced perception of visceral sensation to colonic distension which is associated with hypervigilance at the origin of visceral hypersensitivity (VHS) (Ritchie 1973; Bradette, et al. 1994; Elsenbruch, et al. 2010). VHS is a clinical marker of IBS considered to play a major role in its pathophysiology. The exact cause of VHS is unknown but a number of mechanisms are evoked as represented by neuroplastic changes in primary afferent terminals (peripheral sensitization) due to peripheral inflammation or infection of the gut (i.e. post-infectious IBS) but also in the spinal cord (central sensitization) and in the brain (supraspinal pain modulation) or in descending pathways that modulate spinal nociceptive transmission (Bonaz 2003; Mulak and Bonaz 2004). In addition, stress is able to increase visceral sensitivity either at the central and/or peripheral level (Mulak and Bonaz 2004; Larauche, et al. 2011).

There is a bidirectional communication between the central nervous system (CNS) and the gastrointestinal (GI) tract, i.e. the brain-gut axis, such as signals from the brain can modify the motor, sensory, secretory, and immune functions of the GI tract and, conversely, visceral messages from the GI tract can influence brain functions in a top-down and bottom-up relation. Numerous data argue for a dysfunction of this brain-gut axis in the pathophysiology of IBS (Mulak and Bonaz 2004; Bonaz and Sabate 2009; Tillisch, et al. 2011).

Stress, through the corticotrophin-releasing factor (CRF) system (CRF, urocortins and their receptors CRF1,2), is a key factor involved in the pathophysiology of IBS. Indeed, stress is able to modify visceral sensitivity as well as GI motility, permeability, intestinal microbiota, and immunity of the GI tract, all mechanisms that are involved in the pathophysiology of IBS. In addition, stress is able to modulate the hypothalamic pituitary adrenal (HPA) axis and the autonomic nervous system (ANS) which is the link between the gut and the CNS and an imbalance of the ANS is observed in IBS patients (Pellissier, et al. 2010a; Mazurak, et al. 2012). The main brain areas involved in stress are the prefrontal cortex, the limbic system (e.g. the hippocampus and the amygdala) and the hypothalamus. Relations between the prefrontal cortex and the limbic system are important in the management of stress response.

The amygdala is a key structure involved in the stress effect on the GI tract. Indeed, the amygdala is involved in brain-gut and gut-brain interactions. *i)* The amygdala receives informations from the gut through the parabrachial (PB) nucleus, a sensitive nucleus, and the dorsal vagal complex. The latter, composed of the nucleus tractus solitaries (NTS), is the main entrance of the vagus nerve (vagal afferents) and sends projections to the amygdala. The amygdala is therefore a relay of somatic and visceral nociceptive and non-nociceptive afferents through ascending inputs from the spinal cord and the NTS to the insula which is the main cortical area involved in sensitive information processing. *ii)* The amygdala controls the ANS which is a key element in the neuro-endocrine and autonomic responses to stress of the organism to maintain homeostasis. On the one hand, the amygdala projects to the dorsal motor nucleus of the vagus nerve (DMNV) at the origin of the parasympathetic branch of the vagus nerve (vagal efferents); this makes the amygdala able to modulate the functioning of the parasympathetic system through the vagus nerve. On the other hand, the amygdala projects to the intermediolateral column cells of the spinal cord, at the origin of the sympathetic nerves, and locus coeruleus (LC) in the pons. It makes the amygdala able to modulate the sympathetic nervous system, the other branch of the ANS, and thus to modulate the sympatho-vagal balance, a marker of brain-gut interactions (Mazurak, et al. 2012). *iii)* The amygdala controls the HPA axis activation either directly or indirectly via the hippocampus (i.e. inhibition), known to inhibit the HPA axis, and thus to decrease stress response. *iv)* The amygdala is also involved in childhood psycho-traumatic experiences which are key elements in the pathophysiology of IBS. Indeed, early life stress, as represented by sexual abuse in infancy or adolescence, is present in 30 to 50% of IBS patients (Chitkara, et al. 2008; Bradford, et al. 2012). The amygdala is particularly vulnerable to stressors in early life. The amygdala contains all the elements of the CRFergic system (e.g. CRF, Ucns, CRF1,2) and early life stress induces persistent changes of the CRFergic system in the amygdala leading to an increased stress sensitivity in adulthood. This has been well modelled in the maternally separated (MS) rat model where morphological modifications of the amygdala (e.g. enlarged amygdala volumes and increases in CRF-containing neurons) are induced. *v)* The amygdala (central nucleus; CeA) and the bed nucleus of the stria terminalis (BNST) are highly interconnected with limbic regions (Bienkowski and Rinaman 2012). These two regions are frequently referred as a "central extended amygdala", which shares similar connectivity with other brain regions (e.g. hypothalamus and brainstem) that coordinate behavioural and physiological responses to interoceptive and exteroceptive stressors. It makes the amygdala able to link pain and emotional processings. Furthermore, the amygdala is sensitive to stress-induced increase in glucocorticoids since the existence of elevated glucocorticoid level in the amygdala is associated with anxiety-like behavior and visceral hypersensitivity (Myers and Greenwood-Van Meerveld 2007b; 2010). The amygdala is therefore at the cross-road of anxiety, stress, and visceral sensitivity. The role of the amygdala in IBS is therefore crucial since IBS patients reported higher score of state and trait anxiety than healthy volunteers or in inflammatory bowel disease (IBD) patients in remission with IBS symptoms (Drossman 1999b; Pellissier, et al. 2010a). *vi)* The prefrontal cortex (PFC), and particularly its medial part (mPFC), is able to modulate the functioning of the amygdala. Indeed, the mPFC involvement in fear extinction process (Sotres-Bayon, et al. 2004; Quirk, et al. 2006a) has been shown to be indirectly mediated by its inhibitory action on the amygdala output (Vidal-Gonzalez, et al. 2006). *vii)* Brain imaging techniques (fMRI, PET) have contributed to a better understanding of the pathophysiology of IBS. During rectal distention, an activation of most of the brain structures referenced above, and in particular the amygdala, have been observed in healthy volunteers (Baciu, et al. 1999) while an abnormal brain processing (i.e. abnormal loci of cerebral activation) of pain was observed in IBS patients (Bonaz, et al. 2002; Agostini, et al. 2011). In addition, brain structural changes of the HPA axis and limbic structures have been recently reported in IBS patients (Blankstein, et al. 2010; Seminowicz, et al. 2010).

At the present time, the only medical treatment of IBS is directed at GI motor/sensory or CNS processing. Unfortunately, this treatment is poorly effective and often associated with high placebo effects, thus revealing the importance of the overlap between pain and placebo neurobiological pathways. The therapeutic approach is essentially focused on the symptoms as represented by anti-spasmodics for pain, laxatives or bulking agents, 5-HT4 agonists and guanylate cyclase-C agonist for intestinal transit regulation and anti-depressives/anxiolytics drugs. Placebo has a $\approx$ 40% efficacy in IBS patients (Patel, et al. 2005) and pronounced placebo analgesia is coupled with prominent changes of brain activity in visceral pain matrix, as represented by the amygdala (Lu, et al. 2010). Non-pharmacological therapies are of special interest. Cognitive behavioral therapy is associated with reduced limbic activity (e.g. reduced neural activity in the amygdala), GI symptoms, and anxiety (Lackner, et al. 2006). Hypnosis has shown efficacy in IBS (Whorwell, et al. 1984) and is known to modify the activity of the amygdala (Drossman 1999b). All methods focused on stress reduction such as mindfulness-based stress reduction should reduce pain perception (Drossman 1999a). Repetitive transcranial magnetic stimulation of the PFC that decreases the activity of the amygdala (Baeken, et al. 2010) would also be of interest in IBS patients. In this context, vagal nerve stimulation, used for the treatment of refractory epilepsy and depression, should be of interest in the treatment of IBS by modulating the amygdala. Indeed, an inhibitory action of vagal nerve stimulation on amygdala-mPFC neurotransmission, probably due to the deactivation of the amygdala, has been described under VNS (Kraus, et al. 2007). Consequently, new methods aimed at modifying the activity of the amygdala represent a therapeutic challenge in the management of IBS patients.

2. Irritable bowel syndrome

2.1. Definition-background

The irritable bowel syndrome (IBS) is the most common disorder encountered by gastroenterologists. IBS is defined as "a functional bowel disorder in which abdominal pain is associated with defecation or a change in bowel habit with features of disordered defecation and distension"(Drossman 1999b). Classically the syndrome is considered as functional since biological as well as morphological (e.g. colonoscopy) investigations are not able to evidence any detectable organic lesions or anatomical abnormalities (colonic polyps or diverticulosis…) relative to symptomatology of the affected patients. The syndrome has been defined according to Rome III criteria (Longstreth, et al. 2006). There is a female predominance in a ratio of 2:1 (Drossman, et al. 1993). IBS affects up to 10–15% of the population with an estimated 1.7 billion dollars in annual direct cost (Talley, et al. 1991). Generally patients suffer from the absence of a real diagnostic and from the consideration that they have a psychosomatic disease. Pain is perceived by patients as the most distressing symptom and constitutes their major reason for consulting a physician (Sandler, et al. 1984). Extra-intestinal manifestations are also frequently described by the patients (e.g. headache, low back pain, chronic fatigue, interstitial cystitis…) (Whitehead, et al. 2002).

2.2. Pathophysiology

The pathophysiology of IBS is multifactorial. Altered bowel motility, sensory disorders, psychosocial factors are evoked (Drossman, et al. 1999c; Gaynes and Drossman 1999; Bonaz and Sabate 2009). Local features have also been considered as important. The role of food is often evoked by patients and a number of them are intolerant to lactose, fructose, gluten, polyols (Dapoigny, et al. 2004; Morcos, et al. 2009) with an enhancement of their symptoms following an eviction of such foods from diet. There is also good evidence for a role of the GI microbiota in its pathogenesis (Parkes, et al. 2008). Neuroimmune interactions are also involved, based on the development of IBS after infectious gastroenteritis (i.e. post-infectious IBS) (Gwee 2001) or in patients with IBD in clinical remission (i.e. post-inflammatory IBS) (Long and Drossman 2010). A low grade inflammation has been observed in IBS patients with a predominance of mastocytes in close contact with neural fibers explaining why IBS is assimilated to an IBD by some authors (Ford and Talley 2011).

Sensory disorders, and especially VHS, have also been evoked in the pathophysiology of IBS. VHS, represented by the increased sensation of pain when the pelvic colon is distended with an inflated rectal balloon, is a clinical marker of IBS which is observed in most of IBS patients. The exact location of the abnormal processing of visceral pain is unknown, and can have a peripheral origin, i.e. in the digestive tract by altered peripheral functioning of visceral afferents (i.e. bottom-up model), a spinal origin, e.g. spinal hyperalgesia by a defect of the gate control, or a defect of descending inhibitory controls or an altered central processing of afferent information from the gut, i.e. top-down model or a combination of all these hypotheses. IBS patients have an alteration in the spinal modulation of nociceptive process by the inhibitory descending pain modulation systems (Wilder-Smith, et al. 2004) in which the amygdala could be involved.

Psychosocial factors are often found in IBS patients. Among 20 to 50% of IBS patients have psychiatric disorders, such as major depression, anxiety, and somatoform disorders (Garakani, et al. 2003). Low dose of tricyclic antidepressants have shown efficacy in ameliorating the symptoms in patients (Rahimi, et al. 2009). IBS is also frequently associated with fibromyalgia in 30% to 70% of the cases. This syndrome is characterized by somatic hyperalgesia, the physiopathology of which is close to IBS (Mathieu 2009). IBS and fibromyalgia are classified by some authors as central sensitization syndromes (Woolf 2011). A majority of IBS patients associate stressful life events with initiation or exacerbation of their symptoms (Whitehead, et al. 1992) and stress is able to act at all levels of the physiopathology of IBS (see below). Globally, a concept has emerged that IBS is the result of a dysfunction of the brain-gut interplay, as conceptualized in the brain-gut axis. The ANS is, with the HPA axis, the link between the CNS and the gut and an autonomic dysfunction is observed in IBS patients which could be of top-down or bottom-up origin, as observed for VHS.

3. The brain-gut axis

3.1. Definition

The brain talks to the gut and conversely through a bidirectional communication under normal conditions and especially during perturbations of homeostasis. The CNS and the gut communicate through the ANS and the circumventricular organs and the gut contains a "little brain" as represented by the enteric nervous system which is a target of the ANS.

3.2. The enteric nervous system

The enteric nervous system can control functions of the intestine even when it is completely separated from the CNS (Bayliss and Starling 1899). The enteric nervous system contains three categories of neurons, identified as sensory, associative, and motor neurons (both excitatory and inhibitory) which are the final common pathways for the control of signals to the musculature, submucosa, mucosa, and vasculature, both blood and lymphatic. The enteric nervous system contains as many neurons as in the spinal cord (400–600 million) and confers an autonomy to the digestive tract such as the enteric nervous system can function independently of the CNS for the programming of motility and secretion (Furness 2012). Some neuropeptides and receptors are present in both the enteric nervous system and the CNS. The function of the GI tract is modulated by both the enteric nervous system and the ANS.

3.3. The autonomic nervous system (The afferent system)

The ANS is composed of the sympathetic (i.e. the splanchnic nerves) and parasympathetic nervous system (i.e. the vagus nerves and the sacral parasympathetic nucleus represented by the pelvic nerves) which are mixed systems.

The vagus nerve contains essentially 80-90% of afferent fibers vehiculating informations from the abdominal organs to the brain (Altschuler, et al. 1989) with the exception of the pelvic viscera for which informations are vehiculated to S2-S4 levels of the spinal cord by the pelvic nerves with central projections similar to other spinal visceral afferents. The vagus nerve carries mainly mechanoreceptor and chemosensory informations from the gut. If classically vagal afferents do not encode painful stimuli, they are able to modulate nociceptive processing in the spinal cord and the brain (Randich and Gebhart 1992).

The sympathetic nerves contain 50% afferent fibers. Visceral afferents that enter via spinal nerves (i.e; splanchnic and pelvic nerves), at thoracic 5 - lumbar 2 segments of the spinal cord, carry information concerning temperature as well as nociceptive visceral inputs related to mechanical, chemical, or thermal stimulation through C and Aδ fibers, which will reach conscious perception.

The afferent informations of the ANS reach the CNS at the spinal cord level, for the splanchnic nerves, the nucleus tractus solitarius (NTS) level in the dorsal medulla for the vagus nerve, and the sacral parasympathetic (S2-S4) level for the pelvic nerves. At the level of the spinal cord, sympathetic afferents are integrated at the level of laminae I, II outer, V, VII (indirectly) and X. Then the information is sent to the upper level through the spino-thalamic and spino-reticular tracts, the dorsal column with projection to the thalamus (ventral posterolateral nucleus, intralaminar nucleus) and the cerebral cortex (insular, anterior-cingulate, dorsolateral PFC…). Neurons from laminae I, IV, and V responding to visceral stimuli also receive nociceptive cutaneous inputs (Foreman 1999).

At the level of the NTS, vagal afferents are integrated in subnuclei according to visceral somatotopy (e.g. medial, commissural, gelatinosus) (Altschuler, et al. 1993) and then projections to the PB nucleus, in the pons, according to a viscerotopic organization, which in turn projects to numerous structures in the brainstem, hypothalamus, basal forebrain, thalamus, and cerebral cortex (Fulwiler and Saper 1984). In the cerebral cortex, the insular cortex acts as a visceral (e.g. GI) cortex through a NTS-PB-thalamo-cortical pathway according to a viscerotopic map. The insular cortex is connected with the limbic system (bed nucleus of the stria terminalis and CeA) and with the lateral frontal cortical system (Saper 1982). The NTS also sends projections to the ventrolateral medulla, the hypothalamus, and the amygdala/bed nucleus of the stria terminalis contributing to visceral perception. The NTS receives convergent afferents from both the spinal cord (i.e. laminae I, V, VII, and X) and the vagus nerve; some of these afferents probably being at the origin of autonomic reflex responses. This convergence is also observed at the level of the PB and ventrolateral medulla (Saper 2002) thus arguing for a relationship of pain with visceral sensations.

At the forebrain level, the spinal visceral sensory system constitutes a postero-lateral continuation of the cranial nerve to the visceral sensory thalamus and cortex (Saper 2000). There is also a spino-PB pathway since about 80% of lamina I spinothalamic axons send collaterals to the PB (Hylden, et al. 1989) and a spino–parabrachio–amygdaloid pain pathway which implicates the transmission of nociceptive information to the amygdala. Spinal nociceptive neurons in laminae I, IV, V, VII, and X directly innervate the hypothalamus and medial prefrontal cortex (Cliffer, et al. 1991; Burstein 1996). The messages coming from the gut are integrated in the central autonomic network (see below), which, in turn, adapts the response of the digestive tract through the efferent ANS through reflex loops which are essentially unconscious or become conscious in pathological conditions such as VHS observed in IBS. There is also descending pathways that control somatic as well as visceral pain by modulating visceral informations at the spinal cord level. These pathways are both inhibitory, thus producing analgesia as represented by projections from the periaqueductal gray to the rostroventral medulla, and LC descending fibers to the spinal cord as well as facilitatory producing hyperalgesia (rostroventral medulla and OFF and ON cells) (Tsuruoka, et al. 2010).

3.4. The circumventricular organs

The circumventricular organs are highly vascularized structures with fenestrated capillaries located around the 3rd and 4th ventricles. They are characterized by the lack of a blood–brain barrier and represent points of communication between the blood, the brain, and the cerebrospinal fluid (Benarroch 2011). They are represented by the subfornical organ, median eminence, pineal gland, area postrema, organum vasculosum of the lamina terminalis. The circumventricular organs are sensitive to the vascular content (e.g. circulating interleukins, electrolytes). They activate dendritic cells releasing prostaglandins acting on PGE2 receptor of neurons located closely to these circumventricular organs. These neurons send projections to the hypothalamus, activating the HPA axis, and to the central autonomic network represented by the DMNV and the sympathetic pre-ganglionar neurons of the intermediolateralis column. The circumventricular organs are consequently involved in the central integration of a peripheral message to maintain homeosthasis. For example, they are involved in sodium and water balance, cardiovascular regulation, metabolic and energetic balance, immune function, regulation of body temperature, vomiting, reproduction. During an immune challenge represented by systemic inflammation, cytokines released in the circulation talk to the brain through two routes i.e. neural (vagal afferents) and humoral (circumventricular organs) to activate the HPA axis.

3.5. The central autonomic nervous system

The central autonomic nervous system integrates and modulates afferent informations from the gut and sends reversible inputs to the gut. In the CNS, visceral informations are integrated in the central autonomic nervous system via brain regions involved in the autonomic, endocrine, motor, and behavioral responses (Saper 2002). The brain network can be roughly divided into executive structures, mainly hypothalamic, coordinating structures, mainly included in the limbic system, and high level control structures, mainly the frontal cortex.

The hypothalamus e.g. paraventricular nucleus (PVN), lateral hypothalamus, arcuate nucleus and adjacent retrochiasmatic area innervate the parasympathetic and sympathetic preganglionic neurons. The principal neuromediators are oxytocin and vasopressin

(Hallbeck, et al. 2001). Through the release of CRF, the neuromediator of stress, the PVN is involved in the HPA axis response to stress. The limbic system is represented by the amygdala and its nuclei, the bed nucleus of the stria terminalis, considered as the extended amygdala, the septum and the hippocampus. The limbic system modulates the endocrine system and the ANS, two major components of the brain-gut axis. Classically, the amygdala is involved in the integration of emotions and the emotional conditioning which is represented by the association of a conditioned stimulus (i.e. a sound) with an unconditioned stimulus (the reinforcement) (Henke, et al. 1991; Benarroch 2006; LeDoux 2007). The amygdala receives afferents from the NTS, PB nucleus, frontal cortex, and LC and sends projection to the ANS, the frontal cortex and the hippocampus. The amygdala inhibits the DMNV, stimulates the sympathetic nervous system and the stress response through the HPA axis. The amygdala is a CRF-containing nucleus.

The prefrontal, insular, and anterior cingulate cortices are involved in the integration of visceral informations, attention, emotions and in the regulation of humor. The anterior cingulate cortex is divided in a cognitive dorsal part and an affective ventral part i.e. the perigenual part which has been frequently activated in brain imaging by numerous emotional stimuli. Most of these structures (ANS, HPA axis, limbic system, endogenous pathways that modulate pain and discomfort…) are part of the emotional motor system that mediates the effect of emotional states on the GI function, modulates gut functions and communicates emotional changes via the ANS to the gut. The threshold for visceral perception is dependent on the individual's emotional and cognitive state (Mayer 2000; Mayer 2011).

Visceral as well as stressful informations activate the LC, a nucleus belonging to central noradrenergic system localized in the pons. The LC is the largest group of noradrenergic neurones. It is involved in emotional arousal, autonomic, and behavioural responses to stress and attention-related processes through its dense projections to most areas of the cerebral cortex and alertness-modulating nuclei (e.g. majority of the cerebral cortex, cholinergic neurones of the basal forebrain, cortically-projecting neurones of the thalamus, serotoninergic neurones of the dorsal raphe and cholinergic neurones of the pedunculopontine and laterodorsal tegmental nucleus). The LC also exerts an indirect action on autonomic activity via projections to the PVN and to the cerebral cortex and amygdala, structures which are known to influence the activity of premotor sympathetic neurones in the PVN. LC activation leads to anxiety through an activation of the amygdala (Tasan, et al. 2010).

4. Stress and the gut

4.1. Background

Stress is defined as the response of the organism to a solicitation of the challenging environment. The body engages a "fight or flight" response when exposed to an acute challenge with a sympathetic activation leading to an increase of heart rate and respiration, increased arousal, alertness, and inhibition of acutely non adaptive vegetative functions (feeding, digestion, growth and reproduction). The time course of the reaction corresponds to the general syndrome of adaptation defined by Hans Selye in 1950 (Selye 1950). The reaction of stress is physiological but may become pathological following an unbalance between the capacities of adaptation and the requirement of the environment, thus leading to functional, metabolic, and even lesional disorders.

4.2. The CRFergic system

CRF is a 41-amino acid peptide derived from a 191-amino acid preprohormone. CRF is secreted by the paraventricular nucleus (PVN) of the hypothalamus in response to stress (Vale et al. in 1981) as well as its related peptides the urocortines (Ucn) i.e. Ucn 1, Ucn 2 (also known as stresscopin-related peptide), and Ucn 3 (also known as stresscopin). CRF and the Ucns exert their biological actions on target cells through activation of two 7–transmembrane-domain G protein–coupled receptors, known as CRF receptor type 1 (CRF1) and CRF receptor type 2 (CRF2) which are encoded by 2 distinct genes [for review (Gravanis and Margioris 2005)]. CRF and Ucn 1 have equal affinity for the CRF1 receptor, although Ucn 1 is 40 times more potent than CRF in binding CRF2. In contrast, Ucns 2 and 3 bind selectively to CRF2. The population of CRF synthetizing neurons is predominantly expressed in the parvocellular part of the PVN of the hypothalamus and projects via the external zone of the median eminence to the anterior pituitary. In addition to its role as a hypothalamic hypophysiotropic hormone, CRF acts as a neurotransmitter in several brain areas. CRF has predominantly excitatory actions on neurons in the hippocampus, cortex, LC, and hypothalamic nuclei (Siggins, et al. 1985). CRF1 mediates anxiety-like behaviors whereas CRF2 mediates anxiolytic effects in the defensive withdrawal test (Heinrichs, et al. 1997). Competitive CRF receptor antagonists have been developed to determine the functions of CRF receptors under basal and stress conditions (Bonaz and Tache 1994b). The CRF system plays a critical role in coordinating the autonomic, endocrine, and behavioural responses to stress (Dunn and Berridge 1990).

The effect of stress on the GI tract is now well characterized. Stress induces modifications of motility, secretion, visceral sensitivity, local inflammatory responses (Delvaux 1999; Mawdsley and Rampton 2006; Tache and Bonaz 2007) through a central and/or peripheral action through CRF1,2 related receptors. Alterations of this complex system in humans are linked to a variety of anxiety-related psychiatric disorders and stress-sensitive pain syndromes, including IBS. Dysfunction in the HPA axis regulation attributable to overactivation of CRF/CRF1 signaling in response to chronic stress has been implicated in the pathophysiology of IBS symptoms (Chang, et al. 2009).

4.3. Stress effect on GI functions

4.3.1. Motility and secretion

Stress is known to decrease gastric emptying, lengthen small bowel motility and increase colonic motility (Tache and Bonaz 2007). The effects of stress on gut function are mediated by the ANS represented by the sympathetic, vagal and pelvic parasympathetic innervation of the enteric nervous system (Grundy 2006). At the central level, stress inhibits the parasympathetic nervous system and activates the sympathetic nervous system through the effect of PVN projections on the DMNV and intermediolateral column cells of the spinal cord.

CRF signaling is a key component in the alterations of gut motor function in response to stress in both the brain and the gut. The CRF/CRF1 signalling pathway is involved in stress-induced anxiety/depression (Holsboer and Ising 2008) and alterations of colonic motor and visceral pain while both central and peripheral CRF2 receptor activation may exert a counteracting influence (Tache, et al. 2005; Million, et al. 2006). At the level of the GI tract, stress delays gastric emptying through CRF2 while increasing colonic motility and secretion through CRF1 (Tache and Bonaz 2007). In the small bowel, CRF-like peptides stimulate the contractile activity of the duodenum through CRF1 receptor while inhibiting phasic contractions of the ileum through CRF2 receptor (Porcher, et al. 2005).

Stress also induces an activation of the sacral parasympathetic nucleus through the projections of the Barrington nucleus through CRF activation thus stimulating recto-colonic motility (Tache and Bonaz 2007). Numerous data have established the involvement of peripheral CRF signalling in the modulation of secretory function under stress conditions via activation of both CRF1 and CRF2 receptors, activation of cholinergic enteric neurons, mast cells and possibly serotonergic pathways (Larauche, et al. 2009).

4.3.2. Intestinal permeability

An increase of intestinal permeability is observed in the colon of IBS patients, associated with visceral or somatic hypersensitivity (Zhou and Verne 2011). Stress is able to disrupt the intestinal epithelial barrier thus increasing the penetration of luminal antigens into the lamina propria, leading to nociceptors sensitization and favoring the development of visceral hypersensitivity (Ait-Belgnaoui, et al. 2005). This increase of intestinal permeability is due to an activation of peripheral CRF signaling involving both CRF2 and CRF1 (Buckinx, et al. 2011) as well as mast cell activation (Santos, et al. 2001).

4.4. Stress effect on intestinal inflammation

Stress is able to increase intestinal inflammation by increasing intestinal permeability (see above) thus activating mast cells and visceral afferents in a local loop. Stress favours intestinal inflammation by stimulating the sympathetic nervous system and inhibiting the vagus nerve thus decreasing the cholinergic anti-inflammatory pathway. Stress, through its immune-suppressive function also favours inflammation (Ghia, et al. 2006; Mawdsley, et al. 2006; Bonaz 2010).

4.5. Stress effect on the microbiota

Bacteria in the gut (400–1,000 different bacterial species) have an important role in the immune response, including inflammation (Lee and Mazmanian 2010). Stress is able to modify the intestinal microbiota (Bailey, et al. 2010). Alteration of the microbiota favors translocation of bacteria from the intestinal lumen to the interior of the body where they can stimulate the immune system (Clarke, et al. 2010). This can in turn have significant impact on the host and affect behavior, visceral sensitivity and inflammatory susceptibility (Collins and Bercik 2009).

4.6. Stress effect on visceral sensitivity

Stress is known to increase visceral sensitivity [(Larauche, et al. 2012) for review]. Either acting at the central and/or peripheral (e.g. digestive) level, stress is able to increase visceral perception and emotional response to visceral events by a disturbance of the brain-gut axis at its different levels, central, gut and the ANS. Genetic model of depression or anxiety, such as the high-anxiety Wistar-Kyoto (WKY) rats or Flinders Sensitive Line rats have shown increased sensitivity to colorectal distension (Overstreet and Djuric 2001). In the same way genetic models deleting CRF1 exhibit a decrease in colonic sensitivity to colonic distension (Trimble, et al. 2007) while models overexpressing CRF1 exhibit enhanced response to colonic distension (Million, et al. 2007). These data argue for the filiation stress-anxiety-inflammation and visceral hypersensitivity.

Again, the CRF signalling, at both the central and peripheral level, is a key element involved in stress-induced visceral hypersensitivity. Recent data argue for an equally important contribution of the peripheral CRF/CRF1 signalling pathway locally expressed in the gut to the GI stress response (Larauche, et al. 2009). At the peripheral level, mast cells degranulation observed in the colon following stress and peripheral administration of CRF (Wallon, et al. 2008) induces visceral hypersensitivity via the release of mediators (histamine, tryptase, prostaglandin E2, nerve growth factor) that can stimulate or sensitize sensory afferents (van den Wijngaard, et al. 2009; 2010). Intravenous administration of CRF increases GI motility and visceral pain sensitivity in IBS patients compared with healthy controls, whereas administration of a non-selective CRF receptor antagonist improved these responses (Million, et al. 2005; Tache, et al. 2005; Tsukamoto, et al. 2006).

4.7. Gut pathologies are engineered by stress

The GI tract is a sensitive target to stress. Numerous data argue for a role of stress in the pathophysiology of IBS. Patients with IBS report more stressful life events than medical comparison groups or healthy subjects (Drossman, et al. 1996; 2000; Drossman 2011). Stress is strongly associated with symptom onset and symptom severity in IBS patients. Illness experience, health care-seeking behavior, and treatment outcome are adversely affected by stressful life events, chronic social stress, anxiety disorders, maladaptive coping style. A history of emotional, sexual, or physical abuse is often found in IBS patients [(Chitkara, et al. 2008) for review]. For example, there is a significantly higher prevalence (i.e. 44%) of sexual or physical abuse in patients with functional GI disorders than in controls with organic GI disorders (Drossman, et al. 1990). Psychiatric comorbidity, especially major depression, anxiety, and somatoform disorders, occur in 20 to 50% of IBS patients (Garakani, et al. 2003) and more likely precede the onset of the GI symptoms, thus suggesting a role for psychiatric disorders in functional GI disorder development (Sykes, et al. 2003).

Functional brain imaging studies have shown that there is a major influence of cognitive-affective processes on GI sensations and its CNS correlates in health and functional digestive disorders as IBS (Mayer, et al. 2006; Van Oudenhove, et al. 2007). Cognitive-affective processes including arousal, attention and negative emotions strongly influence visceral pain perception through modulation of its neural correlates (Mayer 2011). Feeling emotions requires the participation of brain regions, such as the somatosensory cortices and the upper brainstem nuclei that are involved in the mapping and/or regulation of internal organism states (Damasio, et al. 2000). This has led to the biopsychosocial concept of IBS (Drossman 1996b). These data are in agreement with the role of hypervigilance in the visceral hypersensitivity observed in IBS patients (Naliboff, et al. 2008). Spence et al. (Spence and Moss-Morris 2007) have characterized predictors of post-infectious IBS such as perceived stress, anxiety, somatisation and negative illness beliefs at the time of infection in favor of a cognitive-behavioural model of IBS. The importance of psychosocial factors and somatisation compared to gastric sensorimotor function is most pronounced in hypersensitive patients with functional dyspepsia, another functional GI disorder (Van Oudenhove, et al. 2008).

5. Gut and emotional memories

Early life trauma (neglect, abuse, loss of caregiver or life threatening situation) increases susceptibility to develop later affective disorders such as depression, anxiety, and is a key factor in the development of IBS (Bradford, et al. 2012). Traumatic events, such as war, environmental disasters, physical abuse or a bad accident in adulthood can induce post-traumatic stress disorder (PTSD) with increased prevalence of GI symptoms, such as IBS (Cohen, et al. 2006).

The role of stress sensitization is also reproduced in preclinical studies. Adults rats previously subjected to neonatal maternal separation (MS) exhibit visceral hypersensitivity to colorectal distension in basal conditions (Ren, et al. 2007). This visceral hypersensitivity is exacerbated in acute stress (e.g. water avoidance stress: WAS; Avoidance to water for 1 h by standing on a small platform; Bonaz & Taché 1994b) conditions (Coutinho, et al. 2002). Chronic exposure to repeated WAS is used to study visceral hypersensitivity and is very close to clinical conditions. However, habituation of the CRFergic system is observed in chronic conditions (Bonaz and Rivest 1998) and may induce analgesia. It seems that these conflicting data are influenced by the basal state conditions of the animals before applying the repeated stressor (surgery and single housing) (Larauche, et al. 2010).

6. The amygdala in IBS pathophysiology

The amygadala is a key element in the pathogeny of IBS.

6.1. Anatomical and functional basis

6.1.1. Amygdala structures

The amygdala is divided into a primitive group of nuclei associated with the olfactory system (central, medial and cortical nuclei, and nucleus of the lateral olfactory tract), and a phylogenetically new group of nuclei (lateral and basal) (Knapska, et al. 2007). The lateral (LA), basolateral (BLA), and central nuclei (CeA) are important for sensory processing (Neugebauer 2006; LeDoux 2007). The amygdala is part of the central autonomic nervous system that is involved in the brain-gut axis. The amygdala is a key element in emotional/affective behavior (LeDoux 2007), including the emotional responses to pain such as anxiety and fear of pain (Gauriau and Bernard 2002; Neugebauer, et al. 2004; Neugebauer 2006) as well as in the reciprocal relationship between pain and affective state (Meagher, et al. 2001; Rhudy and Meagher 2003). Affective content is attached to sensory information through associative processing in the LA–BLA circuitry and is then transmitted to the CeA which is the output nucleus for major amygdala functions (Maren 2005; Phelps and LeDoux 2005). The CeA serves to attach emotional significance to afferent nociceptive transmission and coordinates appropriate autonomic, affective and motor behavioral responses through its outputs to the hypothalamus, cortex and brainstem (Neugebauer, et al. 2004).

6.1.2. Amygdala inputs

The CeA receives numerous sensory informations from descending cortical, thalamic (perigeniculate, paraventricular) and brainstem inputs (Whalen and Kapp 1991), as well as from the olfactory system, medial PFC, insula, brainstem viscerosensory and nociceptive centers (NTS, PB), and from all parts of the amygdala. The amygdala increases the excitability of CNS sites regulating behavioral, neuroendocrine, and autonomic responses to stress (LeDoux, et al. 1988) and thus is able to modify GI functions. The amygdala is involved in the affective processing of sensory information and in the generation of anxiety and fear (Davis 1997), elements which are involved in the pathogeny of IBS.

6.1.3. CRF as a key mediator in amygdala

The amygdala, and particularly the CeA, is a major site of extrahypothalamic CRF, in cell bodies and terminals as well as CRF1 and, to a lesser extent, CRF2 receptors. The amygdala is a key element of the extrahypothalamic circuits through which CRF contributes to anxiety-like behavior and affective disorders (Aguilera, et al. 1987; Sajdyk, et al. 1999; Reul and Holsboer 2002; Fu and Neugebauer 2008). Excepting the hypothalamus, the amygdala is the major site of urocortin III (the endogenous ligands for CRF2 receptors) expression (Li, et al. 2002). In particular, activation of CRF neurons in the CeA that project to the LC increase its firing thus resulting in a noradrenaline release in the structures it is projecting to (Bouret, et al. 2003). LC activation leads to anxiety through the activation of the amygdala and, conversely, anxiety producing stimuli (stressful and fear-inducing stimuli) that increase the activity of the amygdala lead to LC activation (Samuels and Szabadi 2008).

6.1.4. Amygdala output to gut

The CEA is involved in the modulation of the ANS because of its brainstem projections to the DMNV, NTS, PB and the periaqueductal gray (Rizvi, et al. 1991), known to modulate the spinal cord processing of noxious information through descending inhibitory controls (Le Bars, et al. 1992). The CEA innervates hypothalamic nuclei, modulating the HPA axis (Rodrigues, et al. 2009). The CeA also projects to the medial peri-LC dendritic region, resulting in increased norepinephrine release and other monoamine systems in the brainstem and forebrain (Gray 1993; Fudge and Emiliano 2003; Pare 2003) which are involved in arousal and hypervigilance.

6.1.5. Modulators of amygdala

The LC has an inhibitory effect on the BLA and the activation of this pathway leads to a disinhibition of the CeA, since the BLA has a predominantly inhibitory influence over the CeA (Rosenkranz, et al. 2006). The LC is involved in the stress response through CRF1 receptors as well as CRF afferent fibers from the Barrington nucleus which is ventro-laterally located to the LC. The Barrington nucleus projects to the sacral parasympathetic nucleus to increase the motility of the distal recto-colon (Valentino, et al. 1993). Colorectal distension increases the firing of the LC through CRF1 through a LC-Barrington nucleus pathway (Rouzade-Dominguez, et al. 2001). In addition, the LC is involved in the brain noradrenergic modulation of the GI tract motility (Bonaz, et al. 1992a; 1992b; 1995). Consequently, the Barrington-LC-amygdalo complex is ideally positioned to bidirectionally coordinate brain-gut interactions.

6.2. Amygdala and the pathophysiology of IBS

6.2.1. Amygdala and visceral hyperalgesia

The use of C-Fos expression as a marker of neuronal activation has shown that somato-visceral (Bonaz and Fournet 2000; Sinniger, et al. 2004; 2005), and visceral (Wang, et al. 2009) pain as well as stress- or abdominal surgery-induced GI disturbances (Bonaz and Tache 1994a; 1994b; 1997; Bonaz and Rivest 1998) and colitis (Porcher, et al. 2004) induced the activation of the amygdala. In addition, the amygdala is one of the central areas from where digestive sensations are elicited in epileptic patients (Mulak, et al. 2008) during intracerebral electrical stimulations. In a model of visceral pain induction such as inflating a balloon into the rectum, an activation of the amygdala is observed in healthy volunteers (Baciu, et al. 1999) while aberrant functional responses (e.g. deactivation of the amygdala) to noxious rectal stimulation was observed in areas of the brain involved in emotional sensory processing, particularly the amygdala, insula, and prefrontal cortex in IBS patients (Bonaz, et al. 2002; Elsenbruch, et al. 2010; Tillisch, et al. 2011) thus arguing for an abnormal brain processing of visceral pain following rectal distension.

Activation of corticosteroid receptor (both glucocorticoid and mineralocorticoid receptors) in the CeA is involved in the induction of anxiety and visceral hypersensitivity (Myers and Greenwood-Van Meerveld 2007b). High levels of glucocorticoids result in CRF mRNA level increases in the amygdala (Makino, et al. 1994). The group of Greenwood-Van Meerveld) have shown that implants of corticosterone micropellets in the CeA increase anxiety-like behavior as well as visceral hypersensitivity to colonic distension and increased responsiveness of viscera-sensitive lumbosacral spinal neurons that mediate visceromotor reflexes to colo-rectal distension (Greenwood-Van Meerveld, et al. 2001; Myers, et al. 2005; Greenwood-van Meerveld, et al. 2006; Myers and Greenwood-Van Meerveld 2007a). Indeed, exposure of the amygdala to corticosterone-releasing micropellets caused an increase in action potential frequency in the dorsal horn neurons in the L6-S1 spinal segments suggesting that a descending neuronal pathway, originating in the amygdala, could be triggered by continuous activation by corticosterone. The neurons responding with excitation to colorectal distension were short-lasting and long-lasting excitatory neurons based on the duration of the reponse (Venkova et al. 2009). Mineralocorticoid receptors but not glucocorticoid receptors in the amygdala trigger descending pathways facilitating viscero-nociceptive processing in the spinal cord (Venkova, et al. 2009). In addition, a WAS known to activate the amygdala (Bonaz and Tache 1994b), performed during 7 consecutive days induced VHS that was abolished by glucocorticoid receptor and mineralocorticoid receptor antagonists in the amygdala. These results argue for a role of amygdaloid glucocorticoid receptor and mineralocorticoid receptor in IBS.

The CRF signaling is also involved in pain processing. WKY is a rat strain for studying anxiety and IBS. WKY express a greater amount of CRF and CRF1 mRNA in the CeA and the PVN (Bravo, et al. 2011). In this model, it has been shown that colonic hypersensitivity to luminal distension is reversed by peripheral administration of a CRF1 antagonist (O'Malley, et al. 2011). Infusion of CRF1 antagonist into the CeA attenuates the hypersensitivity to colonic distension in the WKY rats, thus confirming the role of CRF1 receptor in the amygdala in VHS mechanism (Johnson, et al. 2012). The basal expression of CRF in the LC is increased in WKY rats and a selective CRF1 receptor antagonist abolished the activation of LC neurons by colorectal distension and intracisternal CRF in rats (Kosoyan, et al. 2005). These data strengthen the role of the CeA and LC in VHS through CRF1 which is in agreement with the interactions between both nuclei involved in emotional-arousal circuit. Indeed, CRF neurons in the CeA project directly to the LC and increase the firing rate of LC neurons thus increasing noradrenaline release in the vast terminal fields of this ascending noradrenergic system. In humans, oral administration of a selective CRF1 antagonist (GW876008) is followed by a significant BOLD signal reductions within the amygdala during pain expectation in IBS patients (Hubbard, et al. 2011). CRF1 receptors in the amygdala contribute to pain-related sensitization, whereas the normally inhibitory function of CRF2 receptors is suppressed in the arthritis pain model. Thus, due to the opposing effect of CRF1 and CRF2 receptors, CRF can induce a dual effect in the amygdala. The differential effects of CRF1 and CRF2 receptor antagonists on pain-related processing in the amygdala have reciprocal opposing influences on anxiety-like behaviors. CRF1 and CRF2 receptors in the amygdala mediate opposing effects on nociceptive processing (Ji and Neugebauer 2007).

Numerous data argue for a role of CRF1 and CRF2 to mediate pro- and anti-nociceptive effects of CRF respectively. It has been shown that low concentrations of CRF facilitate nociceptive processing in the CeA neurons through CRF1 while higher concentrations of CRF have inhibitory effects through CRF2 receptors. This is in agreement with the concept that CRF2 receptors serve to dampen or reverse CRF1-initiated responses (Tache and Bonaz 2007). These results clarify the controversial role of CRF in pain modulation and show that the CRFergic system in the amygdala may be a key link between pain and affective states and disorders.

6.3. Amygdala and stress conditioning

6.3.1. The synchronic stress engineering

Systemic cortisol is a classical marker of the HPA axis activation. The amygdala and hippocampus have numerous receptors for cortisol and are consequently highly susceptible to the products of the HPA axis. Glucocorticoid occupation of hippocampal receptors has a suppressive effect on the HPA axis (van Haarst, et al. 1997) whereas glucocorticoid occupation of amygdala receptors have a facilitating effect on the HPA axis, often increasing CRF expression within the amygdala (Makino, et al. 1994). CRF receptors are greatly expressed in the amygdala and hippocampus early in development (Baram and Hatalski 1998), thus explaining why young animals are especially vulnerable to threat. In agreement, early-life stress induces a decrease of hippocampal volume and functional alterations when measured in adulthood (Nemeroff, et al. 2006). Structural changes have also been observed in IBS patients using brain imaging (Blankstein, et al. 2010; Seminowicz, et al. 2010). Also, circulating glucocorticoids can have contrasting effects in the amygdala and hippocampus, and these two structures can play contrasting roles in the activity of the HPA axis. In the context of an overactivity of the HPA axis due to an enhanced stress responsiveness, greater basal levels of systemic cortisol have been reported in IBS patients (Chang, et al. 2009). Circulating cortisol regulates the HPA axis and is also able to act within the amygdala by binding to selective glucocorticoid and mineralocorticoid receptors, highly expressed in the amygdala (Sapolsky, et al. 1983) to facilitate behavioral and psychological stress responses including GI motility.

6.3.2. Amygdala and stress memorisation

Functional imaging studies indicate that the mPFC is engaged in fear extinction process in relation with the amygdala (Phelps, et al. 2004). The amygdala is an important region involved in the acquisition of fear conditioning, a learning that corresponds to the association between a conditioned stimulus andan unconditioned stimulus. The infralimbic region of the mPFC participates in the mechanism of fear extinction (Rosenkranz, et al. 2003; Quirk and Vidal-Gonzalez 2006b) and also in the recall of fear extinction with an active inhibition of the previous fear condition responses. This is mediated by a down regulation of amygdala outputs with mPFC neurons exciting (glutamate) inhibitory neurons (GABA) within the BLA or in the intercalated region inhibiting in turn amygdala outputs from the

CeA (Vidal-Gonzalez, et al. 2006). The activity of intentional regulation of treat related-cues by the PFC is decreased in anxious patients and the conditioned fear extinction is also less active, in PTSD-anxious patients and this is associated with symptoms provocations (Bradette, et al. 1994). The amygdala is also activated by uncertainty and the capacity of the PFC to regulate attention, (re) interpretation of the situation will modulate the level of the response of amygdala to uncertainty. In IBS, uncertainty plays an important role in the perception of pain. Therefore it seems important to study the fronto-amygdalar relations in IBS patients. The inhibitory control of the mPFC on CeA would maintain an homeostatic state with an equilibrated sympatho-vagal balance and low glucocorticoids circulating levels. In the case of a deficit in PFC activity with a lack of inhibitory regulatory communications with the amygdala, a chronic imbalance of the ANS with an increase sympathetic activity should appear as we have observed in IBS patients exhibiting a low heart rate variability and a high score of anxiety (Pellissier, et al. 2010a). Moreover, there is a strong relation between the activity of the ANS and the immune system as recently shown by the cholinergic anti-inflammatory pathway (Huston and Tracey 2011). Hence, when the parasympathetic system is hypoactive as a consequence of anxiety for instance, it could facilitate inflammation which could be deleterious for health and well-being (Bonaz 2003). The hypoactivity of the PFC and the enhancement of amygdala (re)-activity are strongly influenced by stress as demonstrated by a number of studies. It has recently been shown an increase in the dendritic arborization, and synaptic connectivity in the LA/B neurons under chronic stress conditions (Vyas, et al. 2002; Vyas, et al. 2006). LA/B neurons from stressed animals display increased firing rates and greater responsiveness (Kavushansky and Richter-Levin 2006) since the mediators of stress i.e. norepinephrine, and glucocorticoids decrease GABA inhibition (Rodriguez Manzanares, et al. 2005), thereby allowing for increased excitability in LA/B. In the meantime, an atrophy and spine loss of neurons in the mPFC following stress and glucocorticoid exposition is observed (Czeh, et al. 2008) allowing an over-activation of amygdala under chronic stress exposition.

6.3.3. Amygdala and early stress

Environmental events during early postnatal life can influence the formation of neural circuits that provide limbic and cortical control over autonomic emotional motor output since a differential timing of hypothalamic and limbic forebrain synaptic inputs to autonomic neurons has been observed during the first 1–2 weeks postnatal (Rinaman, et al. 2011). This provides a potential structural correlate for early experience-dependent effects on later responsiveness to emotionally evocative stimuli and an enhanced risk for the development of psychopathologies such as mood and aggressive disorders. MS is classically used as a model of brain-gut axis dysfunction (O'Mahony, et al. 2011) and early life trauma are often observed in IBS patients (Bradford, et al. 2012). The amygdala is functionally active early in life and demonstrates continued refinement, through increased cortical connections, throughout childhood and adolescence. The amygdala is particularly vulnerable to stressors early in life. Reduced hippocampal volumes (Woon, et al. 2010) and increased amygdala volumes (Tottenham, et al. 2010) have been associated with early life stress.

6.3.4. The maternal separation model (MS)

Numerous studies have shown that the HPA axis of MS rodents shows hyperactivity in the PVN and amygdala (Plotsky and Meaney 1993; Coutinho, et al. 2002; Plotsky, et al. 2005; Schwetz, et al. 2005). Offspring of mothers that exhibit more licking and grooming of pups show reduced plasma ACTH and corticosterone responses to acute stress and decreased levels of hypothalamic CRF mRNA in correlation with the frequency of maternal licking and grooming during the first 10 days of life (Plotsky, et al. 2005). Thus, it is likely that a major part of the alterations associated with early life stress are related to CRF hyperproduction that account for amygdala hyperactivity. Maternal care during the first week of life is associated with increased GABAergic inhibition of amygdala activity (Diorio and Meaney 2007). These data reflect the importance of early environmental factors in regulating the development of the hypothalamic CRF system in relation with amygdala activity and the vulnerability to stress. Moreover, there is a sex-specific difference in the effects of early life stress on HPA axis activity consistent with the higher prevalence of major depression with hypercortisolism in women than in men. Moreover, women who experienced early life stress are more likely to develop depression as well as IBS (Bradford, et al. 2012). Sex-hormones influence amygdala development in human populations (Rose, et al. 2004). An alteration in the central CRF system has been evidenced in two different rat models of comorbid depression and functional GI disorders (e.g. IBS) represented by neonatal MS and the WKY rat, a genetically stress-sensitive rat strain, that display increased visceral hypersensitivity and alterations in the HPA axis. These rat strains express a greater amount of CRF and CRF1 mRNA in the amygdala (CeA) as well as in the PVN (Bravo, et al. 2011). They also present a positive correlation between increased central CRF and CRF1 receptor expression, with elevated anxiety-like behavior and colonic hypersensitivity (Gunter, et al. 2000; Shepard and Myers 2008). An increase of CRF1 mRNA was observed in the PVN and amygdala while CRF2 mRNA, classically counteracting CRF1 in the CNS, was lower in the amygdala of MS rats. Such modifications, by affecting the HPA axis regulation, may contribute to behavioral changes associated with stress-related disorders, and alter the affective component of visceral pain modulation, which is enhanced in IBS patients (Bravo, et al. 2011).

6.4. The alteration of amygdala control in IBS

The amygdala has interconnections with the anterior cingulate cortex, the PFC, the hippocampus, the hypothalamus (e.g. PVN), the bed nucleus of the stria terminalis, the lateral septum, the thalamus, the periacqueductal gray, the PB, the LC, the raphe nuclei, and the dorsal vagal complex (area postrema, nucleus tractus solitarius and DMNV) (Knapska, et al. 2007). All these regions have been shown to be activated in experimental models of stress, inflammation, and pain as represented by c-fos expression and/or CRF receptor mRNA induction (Bonaz and Tache 1994a; Bonaz and Rivest 1998; Bonaz, et al. 2000; Porcher, et al. 2004; Sinniger, et al. 2004; 2005) or electrical stimulations (Mulak, et al. 2008).

In addition, brain imaging techniques (fMRI, PET), have contributed to the better understanding of IBS. An activation of most of the brain structures referenced above, and particularly the amygdala, has been observed in healthy volunteers following rectal pain while an abnormal brain processing of pain was observed in IBS and IBD patients (Baciu, et al. 1999; Bonaz, et al. 2002; Agostini, et al. 2011). In addition, brain structural changes of the HPA axis and limbic structures have been recently reported in IBS patients (Blankstein, et al. 2010; Seminowicz, et al. 2010). Because psycho- or pharmacotherapy tends to result in normalization of activity of key structures such as the PFC including anterior cingulate cortex, hippocampus, or amygdala, either through a top-down or bottom-up effect (Quide, et al. 2012), the determination of psycho-physiological vulnerability in IBS patients should be a flag to consider the psychological needs in the follow-up of such patients in the prevention of relapses of such diseases (Pellissier, et al. 2010b).

7. Therapeutic implications-treatment targeting amygdala activity reduction in IBS

The effect of stress on amygdala functioning has therapeutic implications both with non-pharmacological and pharmacological treatment to reduce stress perception. Psychological mind-body interventions including psychotherapy, cognitive behavioral therapy, hypnotherapy, relaxation exercises or mindfulness mediation have been shown to improve symptoms of IBS patients (Kearney and Brown-Chang 2008; Ford 2009; Whorwell 2009). Repetitive transcranial magnetic stimulation of the PFC, based on the central role of the mPFC in cognitive theory of mind, can cause changes in acute pain perception and has been used in a model of central sensitization syndrome such as fibromyalgia (Mhalla, et al. 2011; Short, et al. 2011) but no data have been currently published in IBS patients. Modulation of the ANS by restoring the sympatho-vagal balance (DeBenedittis, et al. 1994; Nishith, et al. 2003; Gemignani, et al. 2006) as well as modifying coping strategies vigilance state and globally the restoration of a functional brain-gut axis, are at the origin of the efficacy of these treatments. Brain imaging techniques have shown modulation of brain activation, as for example in the amygdala, by such treatments (Goldin and Gross 2010; Lawrence, et al. 2011). Conventional treatment as represented by anti-depressives, anxiolytics, drug targeting the central sensitization syndrome [$\alpha 2\delta$ ligand (pregabalin, gabapentin); tachykinin receptor antagonists] either directly and/or indirectly are supposed to target the hyperfunctioning of the amygdala (Ghaith, et al. 2010; Gale and Houghton 2011; Trinkley and Nahata 2011; Larauche, et al. 2012). In the context of the microbiota-brain-gut axis, probiotics, prebiotics, antibiotics such as rifaximin, an antibacterial agent that is virtually unabsorbed after oral administration and is devoid of systemic side effects, are of interest (Bercik, et al. 2011; Fukudo, et al. 2011; Fukudo and Kanazawa 2011). If targeting CRF signaling with CRF1 receptor antagonists, based on pre-clinical and/or clinical data (brain imaging) has been used successfully in humans to treat depression and anxiety (Kunzel, et al. 2003) their efficacy is still matter of debate in the treatment of IBS patients (Sweetser, et al. 2009).

8. Conclusion

A growing body of evidence argues for an important role of stress, through the HPA axis, limbic system activity (e.g. the amygdala), and the ANS, i.e. the sympathetic and the parasympathetic (e.g. the vagus nerve) nervous system, in the initiation and perpetuation of IBS. Stress, pain, and immune activation are common risk factors involved in the pathogenesis of IBS which are able to act through this neuro-endocrine-immune axis. The amygdala, through its connections with the PFC, LC, hippocampus, HPA axis, and ANS is a key structure involved in the pathogeny of IBS. Animal models of activation of the CRFergic system in the amygdala, as represented by maternal separation stress or WKY rats, developed VHS as observed in most of IBS patients. Thereofore, a therapeutic targeting of the amygdala either through pharmacological or non-pharmacological approach should be of interest for the treatment of IBS.

Author details

Bruno Bonaz*
Clinique Universitaire d'Hépato-Gastroentérologie, CHU de Grenoble, BP217, France
Stress et Interactions Neuro-Digestives, Grenoble Institut des Neurosciences (GIN), Centre de Recherche INSERM U836-UJF-CEA-CHU, CHU de Grenoble, BP217, France

Sonia Pellissier
Stress et Interactions Neuro-Digestives, Grenoble Institut des Neurosciences (GIN), Centre de Recherche INSERM U836-UJF-CEA-CHU, CHU de Grenoble, BP217, France
Département de Psychologie, Université de Savoie, France

Valérie Sinniger
Stress et Interactions Neuro-Digestives, Grenoble Institut des Neurosciences (GIN), Centre de Recherche INSERM U836-UJF-CEA-CHU, CHU de Grenoble, BP217, France

Didier Clarençon, André Peinnequin and Frédéric Canini
Stress et Interactions Neuro-Digestives, Grenoble Institut des Neurosciences (GIN), Centre de Recherche INSERM U836-UJF-CEA-CHU, CHU de Grenoble, BP217, France
Institut de Recherche Biomédicale des Armées – CRSSA-Antenne La Tronche, BP 87, France

9. References

Agostini, A., N. Filippini, D. Cevolani, R. Agati, C. Leoni, R. Tambasco, C. Calabrese, F. Rizzello, P. Gionchetti, M. Ercolani, M. Leonardi and M. Campieri (2011). "Brain functional changes in patients with ulcerative colitis: a functional magnetic resonance imaging study on emotional processing." Inflammatory bowel diseases 17(8): 1769-1777.

* Corresponding Author

Aguilera, G., M.A. Millan, R.L. Hauger and K.J. Catt (1987). "Corticotropin-releasing factor receptors: distribution and regulation in brain, pituitary, and peripheral tissues." Annals of the New York Academy of Sciences 512: 48-66.

Ait-Belgnaoui, A., S. Bradesi, J. Fioramonti, V. Theodorou and L. Bueno (2005). "Acute stress-induced hypersensitivity to colonic distension depends upon increase in paracellular permeability: role of myosin light chain kinase." Pain 113(1-2): 141-147.

Altschuler, S.M., X.M. Bao, D. Bieger, D.A. Hopkins and R.R. Miselis (1989). "Viscerotopic representation of the upper alimentary tract in the rat: sensory ganglia and nuclei of the solitary and spinal trigeminal tracts." The Journal of comparative neurology 283(2): 248-268.

Altschuler, S.M., J. Escardo, R.B. Lynn and R.R. Miselis (1993). "The central organization of the vagus nerve innervating the colon of the rat." Gastroenterology 104(2): 502-509.

Baciu, M.V., B.L. Bonaz, E. Papillon, R.A. Bost, J.-F. Le Bas, J. Fournet and C.M. Segebarth (1999). "Central processing of rectal pain: A functional MR imaging study." AJNR Am J Neuroradiol. 20(10):1920-1924.

Baeken, C., R. De Raedt, P. Van Schuerbeek, M.A. Vanderhasselt, J. De Mey, A. Bossuyt and R. Luypaert (2010). "Right prefrontal HF-rTMS attenuates right amygdala processing of negatively valenced emotional stimuli in healthy females." Behav Brain Res 214(2): 450-455.

Bailey, M.T., S.E. Dowd, N.M. Parry, J.D. Galley, D.B. Schauer and M. Lyte (2010). "Stressor exposure disrupts commensal microbial populations in the intestines and leads to increased colonization by Citrobacter rodentium." Infection and immunity 78(4): 1509-1519.

Baram, T.Z. and C.G. Hatalski (1998). "Neuropeptide-mediated excitability: a key triggering mechanism for seizure generation in the developing brain." Trends in neurosciences 21(11): 471-476.

Bayliss, W.M. and E.H. Starling (1899). "The movements and innervation of the small intestine." The Journal of physiology 24(2): 99-143.

Benarroch, E.E. (2006). "Pain-autonomic interactions." Neurological Science 27: S130-S133.

Benarroch, E.E. (2011). "Circumventricular organs: receptive and homeostatic functions and clinical implications." Neurology 77(12): 1198-1204.

Bercik, P., A.J. Park, D.A. Sinclair, A. Khoshdel, J. Lu, X. Huang, Y. Deng, P.A. Blennerhasset, M. Fahnestock, D. Moine, B. Berger, J.D. Huizinga, W. Kunze, P.G. McLean, G.E. Bergonzelli, S.M. Collins and E.F. Verdu (2011). "The anxiolytic effect of Bifidobacterium longum NCC3001 involves vagal pathways for gut-brain communication." Neurogastroenterology Motility 23: 1132-e1544.

Bienkowski, M.S. and L. Rinaman (2012). "Common and distinct neural inputs to the medial central nucleus of the amygdala and anterior ventrolateral bed nucleus of stria terminalis in rats." Brain structure & function.

Blankstein, U., J. Chen, N.E. Diamant and K.D. Davis (2010). "Altered brain structure in irritable bowel syndrome: potential contributions of pre-existing and disease-driven factors." Gastroenterology 138(5): 1783-1789.

Bonaz, B., L. Martin, E. Beurriand, J. Hostein and C. Feuerstein (1992a). "Involvement of hypothalamic noradrenergic systems in the modulation of intestinal motility in rats." Brain Res 583(1-2): 332-335.

Bonaz, B., L. Martin, E. Beurriand, M. Manier, J. Hostein and C. Feuerstein (1992b). "Locus ceruleus modulates migrating myoelectric complex in rats." Am J Physiol 262(6 Pt 1): G1121-1126.

Bonaz, B. and Y. Tache (1994a). "Induction of Fos immunoreactivity in the rat brain after cold-restraint induced gastric lesions and fecal excretion." Brain Res 652(1): 56-64.

Bonaz, B. and Y. Tache (1994b). "Water-avoidance stress-induced c-fos expression in the rat brain and stimulation of fecal output: role of corticotropin-releasing factor." Brain Res 641(1): 21-28.

Bonaz, B., L. Martin, E. Beurriand, J. Hostein and C. Feuerstein (1995). "Brain noradrenergic systems modulate the ceco-colonic myoelectric activity in rats." Neurogastroenterology and motility : the official journal of the European Gastrointestinal Motility Society 7(2): 101-110.

Bonaz, B. and Y. Tache (1997). "Corticotropin-releasing factor and systemic capsaicin-sensitive afferents are involved in abdominal surgery-induced Fos expression in the paraventricular nucleus of the hypothalamus." Brain Res 748(1-2): 12-20.

Bonaz, B. and S. Rivest (1998). "Effect of a chronic stress on CRF neuronal activity and expression of its type 1 receptor in the rat brain." Am J Physiol 275(5 Pt 2): R1438-1449.

Bonaz, B. and J. Fournet (2000). "[Acid-sensitive esophagus: a model of abnormal visceroception]." Gastroenterologie clinique et biologique 24(10): 903-905.

Bonaz, B., P.J. Riviere, V. Sinniger, X. Pascaud, J.L. Junien, J. Fournet and C. Feuerstein (2000). "Fedotozine, a kappa-opioid agonist, prevents spinal and supra-spinal Fos expression induced by a noxious visceral stimulus in the rat." Neurogastroenterology and motility : the official journal of the European Gastrointestinal Motility Society 12(2): 135-147.

Bonaz, B., M. Baciu, E. Papillon, R. Bost, N. Gueddah, J.F. Le Bas, J. Fournet and C. Segebarth (2002). "Central processing of rectal pain in patients with irritable bowel syndrome: an fMRI study." Am J Gastroenterol 97(3): 654-661.

Bonaz, B. (2003). "Visceral sensitivity perturbation integration in the brain-gut axis in functional digestive disorders." Journal of physiology and pharmacology : an official journal of the Polish Physiological Society 54 Suppl 4: 27-42.

Bonaz, B. and J.M. Sabate (2009). "[Brain-gut axis dysfunction]." Gastroenterologie clinique et biologique 33 Suppl 1: S48-58.

Bonaz, B. (2010). "[Brain-gut interactions]." La Revue de medecine interne / fondee ... par la Societe nationale francaise de medecine interne 31(8): 581-585.

Bouret, S., A. Duvel, S. Onat and S.J. Sara (2003). "Phasic activation of locus ceruleus neurons by the central nucleus of the amygdala." The Journal of neuroscience : the official journal of the Society for Neuroscience 23(8): 3491-3497.

Bradette, M., M. Delvaux, G. Staumont, J. Fioramonti, L. Bueno and J. Frexinos (1994). "Evaluation of colonic sensory thresholds in IBS patients using a barostat. Definition of optimal conditions and comparison with healthy subjects." Dig Dis Sci 39(3): 449-457.

Bradford, K., W. Shih, E.J. Videlock, A.P. Presson, B.D. Naliboff, E.A. Mayer and L. Chang (2012). "Association between early adverse life events and irritable bowel syndrome." Clinical gastroenterology and hepatology : the official clinical practice journal of the American Gastroenterological Association 10(4): 385-390 e383.

Bravo, J.A., T.G. Dinan and J.F. Cryan (2011). "Alterations in the central CRF system of two different rat models of comorbid depression and functional gastrointestinal disorders." Int J Neuropsychopharmacol 14(5): 666-683.

Buckinx, R., D. Adriaensen, L.V. Nassauw and J.P. Timmermans (2011). "Corticotrophin-releasing factor, related peptides, and receptors in the normal and inflamed gastrointestinal tract." Frontiers in neuroscience 5: 54.

Burstein, R. (1996). "Somatosensory and visceral input to the hypothalamus and limbic system." Progress in brain research 107: 257-267.

Chang, L., S. Sundaresh, J. Elliott, P.A. Anton, P. Baldi, A. Licudine, M. Mayer, T. Vuong, M. Hirano, B.D. Naliboff, V.Z. Ameen and E.A. Mayer (2009). "Dysregulation of the hypothalamic-pituitary-adrenal (HPA) axis in irritable bowel syndrome." Neurogastroenterology and motility : the official journal of the European Gastrointestinal Motility Society 21(2): 149-159.

Chitkara, D.K., M.A.L. van Tilburg, N. Blois-Martin and W.E. Whitehead (2008). "Early life risk factors that contribute to irritable bowel syndrome in adults: a systematic review." The American Journal of Gastroenterology 103: 765-774.

Clarke, T.B., K.M. Davis, E.S. Lysenko, A.Y. Zhou, Y. Yu and J.N. Weiser (2010). "Recognition of peptidoglycan from the microbiota by Nod1 enhances systemic innate immunity." Nature medicine 16(2): 228-231.

Cliffer, K.D., R. Burstein and G.J. Giesler, Jr. (1991). "Distributions of spinothalamic, spinohypothalamic, and spinotelencephalic fibers revealed by anterograde transport of PHA-L in rats." The Journal of neuroscience : the official journal of the Society for Neuroscience 11(3): 852-868.

Cohen, H., A. Jotkowitz, D. Buskila, S. Pelles-Avraham, Z. Kaplan, L. Neumann and A.D. Sperber (2006). "Post-traumatic stress disorder and other co-morbidities in a sample population of patients with irritable bowel syndrome." European journal of internal medicine 17(8): 567-571.

Collins, S.M. (2001). "Stress and the gastrointestinal tract. IV. Modulation of intestinal inflammation by stress: basic mechanisms and clinical relevance." The American Journal of Physiology 280: G315-G318.

Collins, S.M. and P. Bercik (2009). "The relationship between intestinal microbiota and the central nervous system in normal gastrointestinal function and disease." Gastroenterology 136(6): 2003-2014.

Coutinho, S.V., P.M. Plotsky, M. Sablad, J.C. Miller, H. Zhou, A.I. Bayati, J.A. McRoberts and E.A. Mayer (2002). "Neonatal maternal separation alters stress-induced responses to viscerosomatic nociceptive stimuli in rat." American journal of physiology. Gastrointestinal and liver physiology 282(2): G307-316.

Czeh, B., C. Perez-Cruz, E. Fuchs and G. Flugge (2008). "Chronic stress-induced cellular changes in the medial prefrontal cortex and their potential clinical implications: does hemisphere location matter?" Behav Brain Res 190(1): 1-13.

Damasio, A.R., T.J. Grabowski, A. Bechara, H. Damasio, L.L. Ponto, J. Parvizi and R.D. Hichwa (2000). "Subcortical and cortical brain activity during the feeling of self-generated emotions." Nat Neurosci 3(10): 1049-1056.

Dapoigny, M., J. Bellanger, B. Bonaz, S. Bruley des Varannes, L. Bueno, B. Coffin, P. Ducrotte, B. Flourie, M. Lemann, A. Lepicard and O. Reigneau (2004). "Irritable bowel syndrome in France: a common, debilitating and costly disorder." Eur J Gastroenterol Hepatol 16(10): 995-1001.

Davis, M. (1997). "Neurobiology of fear responses: the role of the amygdala." The Journal of neuropsychiatry and clinical neurosciences 9(3): 382-402.

DeBenedittis, G., M. Cigada, A. Bianchi, M.G. Signorini and S. Cerutti (1994). "Autonomic changes during hypnosis: a heart rate variability power spectrum analysis as a marker of sympatho-vagal balance." The International journal of clinical and experimental hypnosis 42(2): 140-152.

Delvaux, M.M. (1999). "Stress and visceral perception." Canadian journal of gastroenterology = Journal canadien de gastroenterologie 13 Suppl A: 32A-36A.

Diorio, J. and M.J. Meaney (2007). "Maternal programming of defensive responses through sustained effects on gene expression." Journal of psychiatry & neuroscience : JPN 32(4): 275-284.

Drossman, D.A., J. Leserman, G. Nachman, Z.M. Li, H. Gluck, T.C. Toomey and C.M. Mitchell (1990). "Sexual and physical abuse in women with functional or organic gastrointestinal disorders." Annals of internal medicine 113(11): 828-833.

Drossman, D.A., Z. Li, E. Andruzzi, R.D. Temple, N.J. Talley, W.G. Thompson, W.E. Whitehead, J. Janssens, P. Funch-Jensen, E. Corazziari and et al. (1993). "U.S. householder survey of functional gastrointestinal disorders. Prevalence, sociodemography, and health impact." Dig Dis Sci 38(9): 1569-1580.

Drossman, D.A., Z. Li, J. Leserman, T.C. Toomey and Y.J. Hu (1996a). "Health status by gastrointestinal diagnosis and abuse history." Gastroenterology 110(4): 999-1007.

Drossman, D.A. (1996b). "Gastrointestinal illness and the biopsychosocial model." Journal of clinical gastroenterology 22(4): 252-254.

Drossman, D.A. (1999a). "Do psychosocial factors define symptom severity and patient status in irritable bowel syndrome?" The American journal of medicine 107(5A): 41S-50S.

Drossman, D.A. (1999b). "The Rome criteria process: diagnosis and legitimization of irritable bowel syndrome." Am J Gastroenterol 94(10): 2803-2807.

Drossman, D.A., F.H. Creed, K.W. Olden, J. Svedlund, B.B. Toner and W.E. Whitehead (1999c). "Psychosocial aspects of the functional gastrointestinal disorders." Gut 45 Suppl 2: II25-30.

Drossman, D.A., W.E. Whitehead, B.B. Toner, N. Diamant, Y.J. Hu, S.I. Bangdiwala and H. Jia (2000). "What determines severity among patients with painful functional bowel disorders?" Am J Gastroenterol 95(4): 974-980.

Drossman, D.A. (2011). "Abuse, trauma, and GI illness: is there a link ?" The American Journal of Gastroenterology 106: 14–25.

Dunn, A.J. and C.W. Berridge (1990). "Physiological and behavioral responses to corticotropin-releasing factor administration: is CRF a mediator of anxiety or stress responses?" Brain research. Brain research reviews 15(2): 71-100.

Elsenbruch, S., C. Rosenberger, P. Enck, M. Forsting, M. Schedlowski and E.R. Gizewski (2010). "Affective disturbances modulate the neural processing of visceral pain stimuli in irritable bowel syndrome: an fMRI study." Gut 59(489e495): 10.1136/gut.2008.175000.

Ford, A.C. (2009). "Management of irritable bowel syndrome." Minerva gastroenterologica e dietologica 55(3): 273-287.

Ford, A.C. and N.J. Talley (2011). "Mucosal inflammation as a potential etiological factor in irritable bowel syndrome: a systematic review." Journal of gastroenterology 46(4): 421-431.

Foreman, R.D. (1999). "Mechanisms of cardiac pain." Annu Rev Physiol 61: 143-167.

Fu, Y. and V. Neugebauer (2008). "Differential mechanisms of CRF1 and CRF2 receptor functions in the amygdala in pain-related synaptic facilitation and behavior." The Journal of neuroscience : the official journal of the Society for Neuroscience 28(15): 3861-3876.

Fudge, J.L. and A.B. Emiliano (2003). "The extended amygdala and the dopamine system: another piece of the dopamine puzzle." The Journal of neuropsychiatry and clinical neurosciences 15(3): 306-316.

Fukudo, S., M. Hongo, H. Kaneko and R. Ueno (2011). "Efficacy and safety of oral lubiprostone in constipated patients with or without irritable bowel syndrome: a randomized, placebo-controlled and dose-finding study." Neurogastroenterology and motility : the official journal of the European Gastrointestinal Motility Society 23(6): 544-e205.

Fukudo, S. and M. Kanazawa (2011). "Gene, environment, and brain-gut interactions in irritable bowel syndrome." J Gastroenterol Hepatol 26 Suppl 3: 110-115.

Fulwiler, C.E. and C.B. Saper (1984). "Subnuclear organization of the efferent connections of the parabrachial nucleus in the rat." Brain Res 319(3): 229-259.

Furness, J.B. (2012). "The enteric nervous system and neurogastroenterology." Nature reviews. Gastroenterology & hepatology.

Gale, J.D. and L.A. Houghton (2011). "Alpha 2 Delta (alpha(2)delta) Ligands, Gabapentin and Pregabalin: What is the Evidence for Potential Use of These Ligands in Irritable Bowel Syndrome." Frontiers in pharmacology 2: 28.

Garakani, A., T. Win, S. Virk, S. Gupta, D. Kaplan and P.S. Masand (2003). "Comorbidity of irritable bowel syndrome in psychiatric patients: a review." American journal of therapeutics 10(1): 61-67.

Gauriau, C. and J.F. Bernard (2002). "Pain pathways and parabrachial circuits in the rat." Experimental physiology 87(2): 251-258.

Gaynes, B.N. and D.A. Drossman (1999). "The role of psychosocial factors in irritable bowel syndrome." Bailliere's best practice & research. Clinical gastroenterology 13(3): 437-452.

Gemignani, A., L. Sebastiani, A. Simoni, E.L. Santarcangelo and B. Ghelarducci (2006). "Hypnotic trait and specific phobia: EEG and autonomic output during phobic stimulation." Brain Res Bull 69(2): 197-203.

Ghaith, O., M. El-Halabi, J.G. Hashash and A.I. Sharara (2010). "Investigational agents for the irritable bowel syndrome." Expert opinion on investigational drugs 19(10): 1161-1178.

Ghia, J.-E., P. Blennerhassett, H. Kumar-Ondiveeran, E.F. Verdu and S.M. Collins (2006). "The vagus nerve: a tonic inhibitory influence associated with inflammatory bowel disease in a murine model." Gastroenterology 131: 1122-1130.

Goldin, P.R. and J.J. Gross (2010). "Effects of mindfulness-based stress reduction (MBSR) on emotion regulation in social anxiety disorder." Emotion 10(1): 83-91.

Gravanis, A. and A.N. Margioris (2005). "The corticotropin-releasing factor (CRF) family of neuropeptides in inflammation: potential therapeutic applications." Current medicinal chemistry 12(13): 1503-1512.

Gray, T.S. (1993). "Amygdaloid CRF pathways. Role in autonomic, neuroendocrine, and behavioral responses to stress." Annals of the New York Academy of Sciences 697: 53-60.

Greenwood-Van Meerveld, B., M. Gibson, W. Gunter, J. Shepard, R. Foreman and D. Myers (2001). "Stereotaxic delivery of corticosterone to the amygdala modulates colonic sensitivity in rats." Brain Res 893(1-2): 135-142.

Greenwood-van Meerveld, B., A.C. Johnson, J. Schulkin and D.A. Myers (2006). "Long-term expression of corticotropin-releasing factor (CRF) in the paraventricular nucleus of the hypothalamus in response to an acute colonic inflammation." Brain Research 1071: 91-96.

Grundy, D. (2006). "Signalling the state of the digestive tract." Autonomic Neuroscience: Basic and Clinical 125: 76-80.

Gunter, W.D., J.D. Shepard, R.D. Foreman, D.A. Myers and B. Greenwood-Van Meerveld (2000). "Evidence for visceral hypersensitivity in high-anxiety rats." Physiol Behav 69(3): 379-382.

Gwee, K.A. (2001). "Postinfectious Irritable Bowel Syndrome." Current treatment options in gastroenterology 4(4): 287-291.

Hallbeck, M., D. Larhammar and A. Blomqvist (2001). "Neuropeptide expression in rat paraventricular hypothalamic neurons that project to the spinal cord." The Journal of comparative neurology 433(2): 222-238.

Heinrichs, S.C., J. Lapsansky, T.W. Lovenberg, E.B. De Souza and D.T. Chalmers (1997). "Corticotropin-releasing factor CRF1, but not CRF2, receptors mediate anxiogenic-like behavior." Regulatory peptides 71(1): 15-21.

Henke, P.G., A. Ray and R.M. Sullivan (1991). "The amygdala. Emotions and gut functions." Digestive Diseases and Sciences 36(11): 1633-1643.

Holsboer, F. and M. Ising (2008). "Central CRH system in depression and anxiety--evidence from clinical studies with CRH1 receptor antagonists." Eur J Pharmacol 583(2-3): 350-357.

Hubbard, C.S., J.S. Labus, J. Bueller, J. Stains, B. Suyenobu, G.E. Dukes, D.L. Kelleher, K. Tillisch, B.D. Naliboff and E.A. Mayer (2011). "Corticotropin-releasing factor receptor 1 antagonist alters regional activation and effective connectivity in an emotional-arousal circuit during expectation of abdominal pain." The Journal of neuroscience : the official journal of the Society for Neuroscience 31(35): 12491-12500.

Huston, J.M. and K.J. Tracey (2011). "The pulse of inflammation: heart rate variability, the cholinergic anti-inflammatory pathway and implications for therapy." Journal of internal medicine 269(1): 45-53.

Hylden, J.L., F. Anton and R.L. Nahin (1989). "Spinal lamina I projection neurons in the rat: collateral innervation of parabrachial area and thalamus." Neuroscience 28(1): 27-37.

Ji, G. and V. Neugebauer (2007). "Differential effects of CRF1 and CRF2 receptor antagonists on pain-related sensitization of neurons in the central nucleus of the amygdala." Journal of neurophysiology 97(6): 3893-3904.

Johnson, A.C., L. Tran, J. Schulkin and B.G. Meerveld (2012). "Importance of stress receptor-mediated mechanisms in the amygdala on visceral pain perception in an intrinsically anxious rat." Neurogastroenterology and motility : the official journal of the European Gastrointestinal Motility Society.

Kavushansky, A. and G. Richter-Levin (2006). "Effects of stress and corticosterone on activity and plasticity in the amygdala." Journal of neuroscience research 84(7): 1580-1587.

Kearney, D.J. and J. Brown-Chang (2008). "Complementary and alternative medicine for IBS in adults: mind-body interventions." Nature clinical practice. Gastroenterology & hepatology 5(11): 624-636.

Knapska, E., K. Radwanska, T. Werka and L. Kaczmarek (2007). "Functional internal complexity of amygdala: focus on gene activity mapping after behavioral training and drugs of abuse." Physiological reviews 87(4): 1113-1173.

Kosoyan, H.P., D.E. Grigoriadis and Y. Tache (2005). "The CRF(1) receptor antagonist, NBI-35965, abolished the activation of locus coeruleus neurons induced by colorectal distension and intracisternal CRF in rats." Brain Res 1056(1): 85-96.

Kraus, T., K. Hosl, O. Kiess, A. Schanze, J. Kornhuber and C. Forster (2007). "BOLD fMRI deactivation of limbic and temporal brain structures and mood enhancing effect by transcutaneous vagus nerve stimulation." J Neural Transm 114(11): 1485-1493.

Kunzel, H.E., A.W. Zobel, T. Nickel, N. Ackl, M. Uhr, A. Sonntag, M. Ising and F. Holsboer (2003). "Treatment of depression with the CRH-1-receptor antagonist R121919: endocrine changes and side effects." Journal of psychiatric research 37(6): 525-533.

Lackner, J.M., M. Lou Coad, H.R. Mertz, D.S. Wack, L.A. Katz, S.S. Krasner, R. Firth, T.C. Mahl and A.H. Lockwood (2006). "Cognitive therapy for irritable bowel syndrome is associated with reduced limbic activity, GI symptoms, and anxiety." Behav Res Ther 44(5): 621-638.

Larauche, M., C. Kiank and Y. Tache (2009). "Corticotropin releasing factor signaling in colon and ileum: regulation by stress and pathophysiological implications." Journal of physiology and pharmacology : an official journal of the Polish Physiological Society 60 Suppl 7: 33-46.

Larauche, M., G. Gourcerol, M. Million, D.W. Adelson and Y. Tache (2010). "Repeated psychological stress-induced alterations of visceral sensitivity and colonic motor functions in mice: influence of surgery and postoperative single housing on visceromotor responses." Stress 13(4): 343-354.

Larauche, M., A. Mulak and Y. Tache (2011). "Stress-related alterations of visceral sensation: animal models for irritable bowel syndrome study." Journal of neurogastroenterology and motility 17(3): 213-234.

Larauche, M., A. Mulak and Y. Tache (2012). "Stress and visceral pain: from animal models to clinical therapies." Experimental neurology 233(1): 49-67.

Lawrence, J.M., F. Hoeft, K.E. Sheau and S.C. Mackey (2011). "Strategy-dependent dissociation of the neural correlates involved in pain modulation." Anesthesiology 115(4): 844-851.

Le Bars, D., L. Villanueva, D. Bouhassira and J.C. Willer (1992). "Diffuse noxious inhibitory controls (DNIC) in animals and in man." Patologicheskaia fiziologiia i eksperimental'naia terapiia(4): 55-65.

LeDoux, J.E., J. Iwata, P. Cicchetti and D.J. Reis (1988). "Different projections of the central amygdaloid nucleus mediate autonomic and behavioral correlates of conditioned fear." The Journal of neuroscience : the official journal of the Society for Neuroscience 8(7): 2517-2529.

LeDoux, J. (2007). "The amygdala." Current Biology 17(20): R868-R874.

Lee, Y.K. and S.K. Mazmanian (2010). "Has the microbiota played a critical role in the evolution of the adaptive immune system?" Science 330(6012): 1768-1773.

Li, C., J. Vaughan, P.E. Sawchenko and W.W. Vale (2002). "Urocortin III-immunoreactive projections in rat brain: partial overlap with sites of type 2 corticotrophin-releasing factor receptor expression." The Journal of neuroscience : the official journal of the Society for Neuroscience 22(3): 991-1001.

Long, M.D. and D.A. Drossman (2010). "Inflammatory bowel disease, irritable bowel syndrome, or what?: A challenge to the functional-organic dichotomy." Am J Gastroenterol 105(8): 1796-1798.

Longstreth, G.F., W.G. Thompson, W.D. Chey, L.A. Houghton, F. Mearin and R.C. Spiller (2006). "Functional bowel disorders." Gastroenterology 130(5): 1480-1491.

Lu, H.C., J.C. Hsieh, C.L. Lu, D.M. Niddam, Y.T. Wu, T.C. Yeh, C.M. Cheng, F.Y. Chang and S.D. Lee (2010). "Neuronal correlates in the modulation of placebo analgesia in experimentally-induced esophageal pain: a 3T-fMRI study." Pain 148(1): 75-83.

Makino, S., P.W. Gold and J. Schulkin (1994). "Corticosterone effects on corticotropin-releasing hormone mRNA in the central nucleus of the amygdala and the parvocellular region of the paraventricular nucleus of the hypothalamus." Brain Res 640(1-2): 105-112.

Maren, S. (2005). "Synaptic mechanisms of associative memory in the amygdala." Neuron 47(6): 783-786.

Mathieu, N. (2009). "[Somatic comorbidities in irritable bowel syndrome: fibromyalgia, chronic fatigue syndrome, and interstitial cystitis]." Gastroenterologie clinique et biologique 33 Suppl 1: S17-25.

Mawdsley, J.E., M.G. Macey, R.M. Feakins, L. Langmead and D.S. Rampton (2006). "The effect of acute psychologic stress on systemic and rectal mucosal measures of inflammation in ulcerative colitis." Gastroenterology 131: 410–419.

Mawdsley, J.E. and D.S. Rampton (2006). "The role of psychological stress in inflammatory bowel disease." Neuroimmunomodulation 13(5-6): 327-336.

Mayer, E.A. (2000). "The neurobiology of stress and gastrointestinal disease." Gut 47: 861-869.

Mayer, E.A., B.D. Naliboff and A.D.B. Craig (2006). "Neuroimaging of the brain-gut axis: from basic understanding to treatment of functional GI disorders." Gastroenterology 131: 1925-1942.

Mayer, E.A. (2011). "Gut feelings: the emerging biology of gut–brain communication." Nature Neuroscience 12: 453-466.

Mazurak, N., N. Seredyuk, H. Sauer, M. Teufel and P. Enck (2012). "Heart rate variability in the irritable bowel syndrome: a review of the literature." Neurogastroenterology and motility : the official journal of the European Gastrointestinal Motility Society 24(3): 206-216.

Meagher, M.W., R.C. Arnau and J.L. Rhudy (2001). "Pain and emotion: effects of affective picture modulation." Psychosom Med 63(1): 79-90.

Mhalla, A., S. Baudic, D. Ciampi de Andrade, M. Gautron, S. Perrot, M.J. Teixeira, N. Attal and D. Bouhassira (2011). "Long-term maintenance of the analgesic effects of transcranial magnetic stimulation in fibromyalgia." Pain 152(7): 1478-1485.

Million, M., C. Maillot, D.A. Adelson, T. Nozu, A. Gauthier, J. Rivier, G.P. Chrousos, A. Bayati, H. Mattsson and Y. Tache (2005). "Peripheral injection of sauvagine prevents repeated colorectal distension-induced visceral pain in female rats." Peptides 26(7): 1188-1195.

Million, M., L. Wang, Y. Wang, D.W. Adelson, P.Q. Yuan, C. Maillot, S.V. Coutinho, J.A. McRoberts, A. Bayati, H. Mattsson, V. Wu, J.Y. Wei, J. Rivier, W. Vale, E.A. Mayer and Y. Tache (2006). "CRF2 receptor activation prevents colorectal distension induced visceral pain and spinal ERK1/2 phosphorylation in rats." Gut 55(2): 172-181.

Million, M., L. Wang, M.P. Stenzel-Poore, S.C. Coste, P.Q. Yuan, C. Lamy, J. Rivier, T. Buffington and Y. Tache (2007). "Enhanced pelvic responses to stressors in female CRF-overexpressing mice." American journal of physiology. Regulatory, integrative and comparative physiology 292(4): R1429-1438.

Morcos, A., T. Dinan and E.M. Quigley (2009). "Irritable bowel syndrome: role of food in pathogenesis and management." Journal of digestive diseases 10(4): 237-246.

Mulak, A. and B. Bonaz (2004). "Irritable bowel syndrome: a model of the brain-gut interactions." Medical science monitor : international medical journal of experimental and clinical research 10(4): RA55-62.

Mulak, A., P. Kahane, D. Hoffmann, L. Minotti and B. Bonaz (2008). "Brain mapping of digestive sensations elicited by cortical electrical stimulations." Neurogastroenterology and motility : the official journal of the European Gastrointestinal Motility Society 20(6): 588-596.

Myers, D.A., M. Gibson, J. Schulkin and B. Greenwood Van-Meerveld (2005). "Corticosterone implants to the amygdala and type 1 CRH receptor regulation: effects on behavior and colonic sensitivity." Behav Brain Res 161(1): 39-44.

Myers, B. and B. Greenwood-Van Meerveld (2007a). "Corticosteroid receptor-mediated mechanisms in the amygdala regulate anxiety and colonic sensitivity." American journal of physiology. Gastrointestinal and liver physiology 292(6): G1622-1629.

Myers, B. and B. Greenwood-Van Meerveld (2007b). "Corticosteroid receptor-mediated mechanisms in the amygdala regulate anxiety and colonic sensitivity." The American Journal of Physiology 292: G1622-G1629.

Myers, B. and B. Greenwood-Van Meerveld (2010). "Elevated corticosterone in the amygdala leads to persistant increases in anxiety-like behavior and pain sensitivity." Behavioural Brain Research.

Naliboff, B.D., A.M. Waters, J. Labus, L. Kilpatrick, M.G. Craske, L. Chang, H. Negoro, H. Ibrahimovic, E.A. Mayer and E. Ornitz (2008). "Increased acoustic startle responses in IBS patients during abdominal and nonabdominal threat." Psychosomatic Medicine 70: 920-927.

Nemeroff, C.B., J.D. Bremner, E.B. Foa, H.S. Mayberg, C.S. North and M.B. Stein (2006). "Posttraumatic stress disorder: a state-of-the-science review." Journal of psychiatric research 40(1): 1-21.

Neugebauer, V., W. Li, G.C. Bird and J.S. Han (2004). "The amygdala and persistent pain." The Neuroscientist : a review journal bringing neurobiology, neurology and psychiatry 10(3): 221-234.

Neugebauer, V. (2006). "Chapter 11 Subcortical processing of nociceptive information: basal ganglia and amygdala." Handbook of clinical neurology / edited by P.J. Vinken and G.W. Bruyn 81: 141-158.

Nishith, P., S.P. Duntley, P.P. Domitrovich, M.L. Uhles, B.J. Cook and P.K. Stein (2003). "Effect of cognitive behavioral therapy on heart rate variability during REM sleep in female rape victims with PTSD." Journal of traumatic stress 16(3): 247-250.

O'Mahony, S.M., N.P. Hyland, T.G. Dinan and J.F. Cryan (2011). "Maternal separation as a model of brain-gut axis dysfunction." Psychopharmacology 214(1): 71-88.

O'Malley, D., T.G. Dinan and J.F. Cryan (2011). "Neonatal maternal separation in the rat impacts on the stress responsivity of central corticotropin-releasing factor receptors in adulthood." Psychopharmacology 214(1): 221-229.

Overstreet, D.H. and V. Djuric (2001). "A genetic rat model of cholinergic hypersensitivity: implications for chemical intolerance, chronic fatigue, and asthma." Annals of the New York Academy of Sciences 933: 92-102.

Pare, D. (2003). "Role of the basolateral amygdala in memory consolidation." Progress in neurobiology 70(5): 409-420.

Parkes, G.C., J. Brostoff, K. Whelan and J.D. Sanderson (2008). "Gastrointestinal microbiota in irritable bowel syndrome: their role in its pathogenesis and treatment." Am J Gastroenterol 103(6): 1557-1567.

Patel, S.M., W.B. Stason, A. Legedza, S.M. Ock, T.J. Kaptchuk, L. Conboy, K. Canenguez, J.K. Park, E. Kelly, E. Jacobson, C.E. Kerr and A.J. Lembo (2005). "The placebo effect in irritable bowel syndrome trials: a meta-analysis." Neurogastroenterology and motility : the official journal of the European Gastrointestinal Motility Society 17(3): 332-340.

Pellissier, S., C. Dantzer, F. Canini, N. Mathieu and B. Bonaz (2010a). "Psychological adjustment and autonomic disturbances in inflammatory bowel diseases and irritable bowel syndrome." Psychoneuroendocrinology 35(5): 653-662.

Pellissier, S., C. Dantzer, F. Canini, N. Mathieu and B. Bonaz (2010b). "Toward a definition of a global psycho-physiological criterion of vulnerability to relapse in inflammatory bowel diseases." The American Journal of Gastroenterology 105: 1446-1447.

Phelps, E.A., M.R. Delgado, K.I. Nearing and J.E. LeDoux (2004). "Extinction learning in humans: role of the amygdala and vmPFC." Neuron 43(6): 897-905.

Phelps, E.A. and J.E. LeDoux (2005). "Contributions of the amygdala to emotion processing: from animal models to human behavior." Neuron 48(2): 175-187.

Plotsky, P.M. and M.J. Meaney (1993). "Early, postnatal experience alters hypothalamic corticotropin-releasing factor (CRF) mRNA, median eminence CRF content and stress-induced release in adult rats." Brain research. Molecular brain research 18(3): 195-200.

Plotsky, P.M., K.V. Thrivikraman, C.B. Nemeroff, C. Caldji, S. Sharma and M.J. Meaney (2005). "Long-term consequences of neonatal rearing on central corticotropin-releasing factor systems in adult male rat offspring." Neuropsychopharmacology : official publication of the American College of Neuropsychopharmacology 30(12): 2192-2204.

Porcher, C., V. Sinniger, A. Juhem, P. Mouchet and B. Bonaz (2004). "Neuronal activity and CRF receptor gene transcription in the brains of rats with colitis." American journal of physiology. Gastrointestinal and liver physiology 287(4): G803-814.

Porcher, C., A. Juhem, A. Peinnequin, V. Sinniger and B. Bonaz (2005). "Expression and effects of metabotropic CRF1 and CRF2 receptors in rat small intestine." American journal of physiology. Gastrointestinal and liver physiology 288(5): G1091-1103.

Quide, Y., A.B. Witteveen, W. El-Hage, D.J. Veltman and M. Olff (2012). "Differences between effects of psychological versus pharmacological treatments on functional and morphological brain alterations in anxiety disorders and major depressive disorder: a systematic review." Neurosci Biobehav Rev 36(1): 626-644.

Quirk, G.J., R. Garcia and F. Gonzalez-Lima (2006a). "Prefrontal mechanisms in extinction of conditioned fear." Biol Psychiatry 60(4): 337-343.

Quirk, G.J. and I. Vidal-Gonzalez (2006b). "Keeping the memories flowing." Nat Neurosci 9(10): 1199-1200.

Rahimi, R., S. Nikfar, A. Rezaie and M. Abdollahi (2009). "Efficacy of tricyclic antidepressants in irritable bowel syndrome: a meta-analysis." World journal of gastroenterology : WJG 15(13): 1548-1553.

Randich, A. and G.F. Gebhart (1992). "Vagal afferent modulation of nociception." Brain research. Brain research reviews 17(2): 77-99.

Ren, T.-H., J. Wu, D. Yew, E. Ziea, L. Lao, W.-k. Leung, B. Berman, P.-j. Hu and J.J.Y. Sung (2007). "Effects of neonatal maternal separation on neurochemical and sensory response to colonic distension in a rat model of irritable bowel syndrome." The American Journal of Physiology 292: G849-G856.

Reul, J.M. and F. Holsboer (2002). "On the role of corticotropin-releasing hormone receptors in anxiety and depression." Dialogues in clinical neuroscience 4(1): 31-46.

Rhudy, J.L. and M.W. Meagher (2003). "Negative affect: effects on an evaluative measure of human pain." Pain 104(3): 617-626.

Rinaman, L., L. Banihashemi and T.J. Koehnle (2011). "Early life experience shapes the functional organization of stress-responsive visceral circuits." Physiology & Behavior 104: 632-640.

Ritchie, J. (1973). "Pain from distension of the pelvic colon by inflating a balloon in the irritable colon syndrome." Gut 14(2): 125-132.

Rizvi, T.A., M. Ennis, M.M. Behbehani and M.T. Shipley (1991). "Connections between the central nucleus of the amygdala and the midbrain periaqueductal gray: topography and reciprocity." The Journal of comparative neurology 303(1): 121-131.

Rodrigues, S.M., J.E. LeDoux and R.M. Sapolsky (2009). "The influence of stress hormones on fear circuitry." Annual review of neuroscience 32: 289-313.

Rodriguez Manzanares, P.A., N.A. Isoardi, H.F. Carrer and V.A. Molina (2005). "Previous stress facilitates fear memory, attenuates GABAergic inhibition, and increases synaptic plasticity in the rat basolateral amygdala." The Journal of neuroscience : the official journal of the Society for Neuroscience 25(38): 8725-8734.

Rose, A.B., D.P. Merke, L.S. Clasen, M.A. Rosenthal, G.L. Wallace, A.C. Vaituzis, J.D. Fields and J.N. Giedd (2004). "Effects of hormones and sex chromosomes on stress-influenced regions of the developing pediatric brain." Annals of the New York Academy of Sciences 1032: 231-233.

Rosenkranz, J.A., H. Moore and A.A. Grace (2003). "The prefrontal cortex regulates lateral amygdala neuronal plasticity and responses to previously conditioned stimuli." The Journal of neuroscience : the official journal of the Society for Neuroscience 23(35): 11054-11064.

Rosenkranz, J.A., D.M. Buffalari and A.A. Grace (2006). "Opposing influence of basolateral amygdala and footshock stimulation on neurons of the central amygdala." Biol Psychiatry 59(9): 801-811.

Rouzade-Dominguez, M.L., A.L. Curtis and R.J. Valentino (2001). "Role of Barrington's nucleus in the activation of rat locus coeruleus neurons by colonic distension." Brain Res 917(2): 206-218.

Sajdyk, T.J., D.A. Schober, D.R. Gehlert and A. Shekhar (1999). "Role of corticotropin-releasing factor and urocortin within the basolateral amygdala of rats in anxiety and panic responses." Behav Brain Res 100(1-2): 207-215.

Samuels, E.R. and E. Szabadi (2008). "Functional neuroanatomy of the noradrenergic locus coeruleus: its roles in the regulation of arousal and autonomic function part I: principles of functional organisation." Current neuropharmacology 6(3): 235-253.

Sandler, R.S., D.A. Drossman, H.P. Nathan and D.C. McKee (1984). "Symptom complaints and health care seeking behavior in subjects with bowel dysfunction." Gastroenterology 87(2): 314-318.

Santos, J., P.C. Yang, J.D. Soderholm, M. Benjamin and M.H. Perdue (2001). "Role of mast cells in chronic stress induced colonic epithelial barrier dysfunction in the rat." Gut 48(5): 630-636.

Saper, C.B. (1982). "Convergence of autonomic and limbic connections in the insular cortex of the rat." The Journal of comparative neurology 210(2): 163-173.

Saper, C.B. (2000). "Hypothalamic connections with the cerebral cortex." Progress in brain research 126: 39-48.

Saper, C.B. (2002). "The central autonomic nervous system: conscious visceral perception and autonomic pattern generation." Annual review of neuroscience 25: 433-469.

Sapolsky, R.M., B.S. McEwen and T.C. Rainbow (1983). "Quantitative autoradiography of [3H]corticosterone receptors in rat brain." Brain Res 271(2): 331-334.

Schwetz, I., J.A. McRoberts, S.V. Coutinho, S. Bradesi, G. Gale, M. Fanselow, M. Million, G. Ohning, Y. Tache, P.M. Plotsky and E.A. Mayer (2005). "Corticotropin-releasing factor receptor 1 mediates acute and delayed stress-induced visceral hyperalgesia in maternally separated Long-Evans rats." American journal of physiology. Gastrointestinal and liver physiology 289(4): G704-712.

Selye, H. (1950). "Stress and the general adaptation syndrome." British medical journal 1(4667): 1383-1392.

Seminowicz, D.A., J.S. Labus, J.A. Bueller, K. Tillisch, B.D. Naliboff, M.C. Bushnell and E.A. Mayer (2010). "Regional gray matter density changes in brains of patients with irritable bowel syndrome." Gastroenterology 139(1): 48-57 e42.

Shepard, J.D. and D.A. Myers (2008). "Strain differences in anxiety-like behavior: association with corticotropin-releasing factor." Behav Brain Res 186(2): 239-245.

Short, E.B., J.J. Borckardt, B.S. Anderson, H. Frohman, W. Beam, S.T. Reeves and M.S. George (2011). "Ten sessions of adjunctive left prefrontal rTMS significantly reduces fibromyalgia pain: a randomized, controlled pilot study." Pain 152(11): 2477-2484.

Siggins, G.R., D. Gruol, J. Aldenhoff and Q. Pittman (1985). "Electrophysiological actions of corticotropin-releasing factor in the central nervous system." Federation proceedings 44(1 Pt 2): 237-242.

Sinniger, V., C. Porcher, P. Mouchet, A. Juhem and B. Bonaz (2004). "c-fos and CRF receptor gene transcription in the brain of acetic acid-induced somato-visceral pain in rats." Pain 110(3): 738-750.

Sinniger, V., P. Mouchet and B. Bonaz (2005). "Effect of nor-trimebutine on neuronal activation induced by a noxious stimulus or an acute colonic inflammation in the rat." Life sciences 77(23): 2927-2941.

Sotres-Bayon, F., D.E. Bush and J.E. LeDoux (2004). "Emotional perseveration: an update on prefrontal-amygdala interactions in fear extinction." Learn Mem 11(5): 525-535.

Spence, M.J. and R. Moss-Morris (2007). "The cognitive behavioural model of irritable bowel syndrome: a prospective investigation of patients with gastroenteritis." Gut 56(8): 1066-1071.

Sweetser, S., M. Camilleri, S.J. Linker Nord, D.D. Burton, L. Castenada, R. Croop, G. Tong, R. Dockens and A.R. Zinsmeister (2009). "Do corticotropin releasing factor-1 receptors influence colonic transit and bowel function in women with irritable bowel syndrome?"

American journal of physiology. Gastrointestinal and liver physiology 296(6): G1299-1306.

Sykes, M.A., E.B. Blanchard, J. Lackner, L. Keefer and S. Krasner (2003). "Psychopathology in irritable bowel syndrome: support for a psychophysiological model." Journal of behavioral medicine 26(4): 361-372.

Tache, Y., M. Million, A.G. Nelson, C. Lamy and L. Wang (2005). "Role of corticotropin-releasing factor pathways in stress-related alterations of colonic motor function and viscerosensibility in female rodents." Gend Med 2(3): 146-154.

Tache, Y. and B. Bonaz (2007). "Corticotropin-releasing factor receptors and stress-related alterations of gut motor function." The Journal of clinical investigation 117(1): 33-40.

Talley, N.J., A.R. Zinsmeister, C. Van Dyke and L.J. Melton, 3rd (1991). "Epidemiology of colonic symptoms and the irritable bowel syndrome." Gastroenterology 101(4): 927-934.

Tasan, R.O., N.K. Nguyen, S. Weger, S.B. Sartori, N. Singewald, R. Heilbronn, H. Herzog and G. Sperk (2010). "The central and basolateral amygdala are critical sites of neuropeptide Y/Y2 receptor-mediated regulation of anxiety and depression." The Journal of neuroscience : the official journal of the Society for Neuroscience 30(18): 6282-6290.

Tillisch, K., E.A. Mayer and J.S. Labus (2011). "Quantitative meta-analysis identifies brain regions activated during rectal distension in irritable bowel syndrome." Gastroenterology 140: 91-100.

Tottenham, N., T.A. Hare, B.T. Quinn, T.W. McCarry, M. Nurse, T. Gilhooly, A. Millner, A. Galvan, M.C. Davidson, I.M. Eigsti, K.M. Thomas, P.J. Freed, E.S. Booma, M.R. Gunnar, M. Altemus, J. Aronson and B.J. Casey (2010). "Prolonged institutional rearing is associated with atypically large amygdala volume and difficulties in emotion regulation." Developmental science 13(1): 46-61.

Trimble, N., A.C. Johnson, A. Foster and B. Greenwood-van Meerveld (2007). "Corticotropin-releasing factor receptor 1-deficient mice show decreased anxiety and colonic sensitivity." Neurogastroenterology and motility : the official journal of the European Gastrointestinal Motility Society 19(9): 754-760.

Trinkley, K.E. and M.C. Nahata (2011). "Treatment of irritable bowel syndrome." Journal of clinical pharmacy and therapeutics 36(3): 275-282.

Tsukamoto, K., Y. Nakade, C. Mantyh, K. Ludwig, T.N. Pappas and T. Takahashi (2006). "Peripherally administered CRF stimulates colonic motility via central CRF receptors and vagal pathways in conscious rats." The American Journal of Physiology 290: R1537-R1541.

Tsuruoka, M., D. Wang, J. Tamaki and T. Inoue (2010). "Descending influence from the nucleus locus coeruleus/subcoeruleus on visceral nociceptive transmission in the rat spinal cord." Neuroscience 165(4): 1019-1024.

Vale, W., J. Spiess, C. Rivier, and J. Rivier (1981). Characterization of a 41-residue ovine hypothalamic peptide that stimulates secretion of corticotropin and beta-endorphin. Science 213(4514): 1394-1397.

Valentino, R.J., S.L. Foote and M.E. Page (1993). "The locus coeruleus as a site for integrating corticotropin-releasing factor and noradrenergic mediation of stress responses." Annals of the New York Academy of Sciences 697: 173-188.

van den Wijngaard, R.M., T.K. Klooker, O. Welting, O.I. Stanisor, M.M. Wouters, D. van der Coelen, D.C. Bulmer, P.J. Peeters, J. Aerssens, R. de Hoogt, K. Lee, W.J. de Jonge and G.E. Boeckxstaens (2009). "Essential role for TRPV1 in stress-induced (mast cell-dependent) colonic hypersensitivity in maternally separated rats." Neurogastroenterology and motility : the official journal of the European Gastrointestinal Motility Society 21(10): 1107-e1194.

van den Wijngaard, R.M., T.K. Klooker, W.J. de Jonge and G.E. Boeckxstaens (2010). "Peripheral relays in stress-induced activation of visceral afferents in the gut." Autonomic neuroscience : basic & clinical 153(1-2): 99-105.

van Haarst, A.D., M.S. Oitzl and E.R. de Kloet (1997). "Facilitation of feedback inhibition through blockade of glucocorticoid receptors in the hippocampus." Neurochemical research 22(11): 1323-1328.

Van Oudenhove, L., S.J. Coen and Q. Aziz (2007). "Functional brain imaging of gastrointestinal sensation in health and disease." World journal of gastroenterology : WJG 13(25): 3438-3445.

Van Oudenhove, L., J. Vandenberghe, B. Geeraerts, R. Vos, P. Persoons, B. Fischler, K. Demyttenaere and J. Tack (2008). "Determinants of symptoms in functional dyspepsia: gastric sensorimotor function, psychosocial factors or somatisation?" Gut 57(12): 1666-1673.

Venkova, K., R.D. Foreman and B. Greenwood-Van Meerveld (2009). "Mineralocorticoid and glucocorticoid receptors in the amygdala regulate distinct responses to colorectal distension." Neuropharmacology 56(2): 514-521.

Vidal-Gonzalez, I., B. Vidal-Gonzalez, S.L. Rauch and G.J. Quirk (2006). "Microstimulation reveals opposing influences of prelimbic and infralimbic cortex on the expression of conditioned fear." Learn Mem 13(6): 728-733.

Vyas, A., R. Mitra, B.S. Shankaranarayana Rao and S. Chattarji (2002). "Chronic stress induces contrasting patterns of dendritic remodeling in hippocampal and amygdaloid neurons." The Journal of neuroscience: the official journal of the Society for Neuroscience 22(15): 6810-6818.

Vyas, A., S. Jadhav and S. Chattarji (2006). "Prolonged behavioral stress enhances synaptic connectivity in the basolateral amygdala." Neuroscience 143(2): 387-393.

Wallon, C., P.C. Yang, A.V. Keita, A.C. Ericson, D.M. McKay, P.M. Sherman, M.H. Perdue and J.D. Soderholm (2008). "Corticotropin-releasing hormone (CRH) regulates macromolecular permeability via mast cells in normal human colonic biopsies in vitro." Gut 57(1): 50-58.

Wang, L., V. Martinez, M. Larauche and Y. Tache (2009). "Proximal colon distension induces Fos expression in oxytocin-, vasopressin-, CRF- and catecholamines-containing neurons in rat brain." Brain Res 1247: 79-91.

Whalen, P.J. and B.S. Kapp (1991). "Contributions of the amygdaloid central nucleus to the modulation of the nictitating membrane reflex in the rabbit." Behavioral neuroscience 105(1): 141-153.

Whitehead, W.E., M.D. Crowell and J.C. Robinson (1992). "Effects of stressful life events on bowel symptoms: subjects with irritable bowel syndrome compared with subjects without bowel dysfunction." Gut 33: 825-830.

Whitehead, W.E., O. Palsson and K.R. Jones (2002). "Systematic review of the comorbidity of irritable bowel syndrome with other disorders: what are the causes and implications?" Gastroenterology 122(4): 1140-1156.

Whorwell, P.J., A. Prior and E.B. Faragher (1984). "Controlled trial of hypnotherapy in the treatment of severe refractory irritable-bowel syndrome." Lancet 2(8414): 1232-1234.

Whorwell, P.J. (2009). "Behavioral therapy for IBS." Nature clinical practice. Gastroenterology & hepatology 6(3): 148-149.

Wilder-Smith, C.H., D. Schindler, K. Lovblad, S.M. Redmond and A. Nirkko (2004). "Brain functional magnetic resonance imaging of rectal pain and activation of endogenous inhibitory mechanisms in irritable bowel syndrome patient subgroups and healthy controls." Gut 53: 1595–1601.

Woolf, C.J. (2011). "Central sensitization: implications for the diagnosis and treatment of pain." Pain 152(3 Suppl): S2-15.

Woon, F.L., S. Sood and D.W. Hedges (2010). "Hippocampal volume deficits associated with exposure to psychological trauma and posttraumatic stress disorder in adults: a meta-analysis." Progress in neuro-psychopharmacology & biological psychiatry 34(7): 1181-1188.

Zhou, Q. and G.N. Verne (2011). "New insights into visceral hypersensitivity - clinical implications in IBS." Nature Reviews Gastroenterology & Hepatology 8: 349-355.

Chapter 16

The Ventral Striatopallidum and Extended Amygdala in Huntington Disease

Elisabeth Petrasch-Parwez, Hans-Werner Habbes,
Marlen Löbbecke-Schumacher, Carsten Saft and Jennifer Niescery

Additional information is available at the end of the chapter

1. Introduction

In the mammalian basal forebrain, two overlapping systems provide a complex morphological substrate for the investigation of emotion-associated functions (de Olmos et al., 2004; Heimer & Van Hoesen, 2006) and are, therefore, crucial for elucidating the pathophysiology of neuropsychiatric diseases. The ventral striatopallidum (VSP) consists of the nucleus accumbens, the olfactory tubercle, the ventral parts of the caudate nucleus and the putamen (caudatoputamen in rodents) and the ventral pallidum, which integrates emotional, cognitive and sensory information and is implicated in linking motivation to behaviour (Heimer et al., 2008; Waraczynski, 2006). The extended amygdala (EA) is a cell continuum emerging from the central or medial amygdaloid nuclei via the sublenticular region up to the bed nuclei of the stria terminalis. The medial EA has a strong influence on emotional, social and sexual behaviour and stress responses. The central EA is associated with fear-related behaviour, hormonal responses and the modulation of affective reactions to stress, and is also involved in alcohol dependence behaviour. The dysfunction of both systems is associated with various neurodegenerative and/or psychiatric diseases, including Parkinson's disease, Alzheimer's disease, schizophrenia, autism and Huntington's disease (HD). HD is a hereditary neurodegenerative disorder with early and marked striatal atrophy (Vonsattel et al., 1985) and the accumulation of huntingtin (htt) aggregates in selected brain areas (Difiglia et al., 1997; Gutekunst et al., 1999). The underlying pathogenesis is still a matter of debate. Clinically, HD is characterized by a triad of motor, cognitive and psychiatric impairments. The morphological correlates of psychiatric-associated symptoms are poorly defined in HD, but there is increasing evidence that the ventral striatum (Enzi et al., 2012; Majid et al., 2011) and the amygdala (Klöppel et al., 2010) are involved in the psychiatric affection of the disease. In this chapter, we introduce the structural components of the VSP and the EA and present the main characteristics of the disorder, with a focus on emotional affection. We include our previous results in a rat transgenic for Huntington's disease (tgHD), which is unique in its limbic impact (Niescery et al., 2009; Petrasch-Parwez et al., 2007), and add recent results in the respective areas of the human HD brain (Petrasch-Parwez et al., 2012).

2. The Ventral Striatopallidal System

The ventral striatum is a term which was initially introduced in the rat on the basis of cytoarchitectural, chemoarchitectonic and projection studies which, clearly provide evidence, that the topographically organized corticostriatal input contains an overlapping ventral and dorsal division (Heimer & Wilson, 1975). The dorsal (motor) striatum receives input from the isocortex, while the ventral (limbic) striatum is mainly related to allocortical and nonisocortical areas including the piriform, enthorhinal and anterior cingulate cortices, the insula as well as large parts of the orbitomedial prefrontal cortex and the hippocampus (Heimer & Van Hoesen, 2006). The ventral striatum comprises the nucleus accumbens as its major component, the olfactory tubercle, cell bridges connecting both parts and the ventrally located areas of the caudatoputamen in rodents and the putamen and caudate nucleus in primates respectively (Mai et al., 2008; Paxinos & Watson, 2007). The rodent nucleus accumbens with a centrally located core and a shell surrounding the core on its medial and ventrolateral aspects forms the main part of the ventral striatum and is continuus with the overlying caudatoputamen. The core is similar to the caudatoputamen and more associated with motor function such as movement initiation, whereas the shell is a crucial GABAergic output area to the ventral pallidum, which itself projects to the mediodorsal thalamus (Heimer et al., 1987) and is therefore associated with the prefrontal cortex. Functionally, the nucleus accumbens is related to somatic motor function, motivation and the control of vigor (Heimer et al., 2008). The continuity between the nucleus accumbens and the dorsolaterally located caudatoputamen is observed in Nissl sections (Fig. 1A) and clearly identified by various markers including tyrosin hydroxylease (TH; Fig. 1B), which is enormously enriched in these areas due to the strong dopaminergic input from the midbrain. Strong TH-immunoreactivity is also observed in the olfactory tubercle and the connecting cell bridges confirming the continuity of the VSP to the brain surface. The olfactory tubercle as a ventral extension of the VSP indicates the close association with olfactory-related areas, which has led to the term olfactostriatum initially introduced by Herrick (1926) and still used in the corresponding areas of nonmammalian vertebrates. The morphology of the rodent olfactory tubercle (Fig. 1) is intermediate between cortical, striatal and pallidal structures and obviously constitutes a relay station between olfaction and the VSP. It is trilaminated as the other olfactory cortices with an overall olfactory input, however, in nonprimates the dense cell layer exhibits a corrugated appearance with dwarf cell caps towards the molecular layer and the polymorph layer is penetrated by ventral pallidal extensions. Finally the area comprises the islands of Calleja, aggregations of small granule cells, which are characteristic for the ventral striatum of all mammals including humans. The ventral pallidum is located ventrally to the anterior commissure. It receives in addition to the ventral striatal input dopaminergic input from the ventral tegmental area, a pathway, which is functionally involved in addiction (Pierce & Kumaresan, 2006). The close relation of the ventral striatum and ventral pallidum within the limbic loop of the basal ganglia led to the term VSP. The VSP may function as a crossroad between emotional content (amygdala), motivational behavior (dopaminergic input from the ventral tegmental area), locomotor behaviour (output to caudal mesencephalon), cognition and executive functions (via mediodorsal thalamic nuclei to the prefrontal cortex) and olfaction (olfactory bulb input).

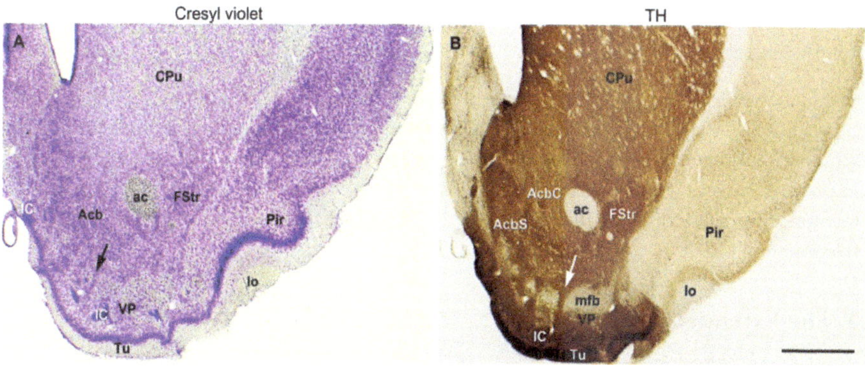

Figure 1. Cresyl violet stained (A) and Tyrosin hydroxylase (TH)-immunolabelled (B) frontal rat brain vibratome sections showing the main components of the ventral striatopallidum. The nucleus accumbens (Acb) and the fundus striati (FStr) are detected in the cresyl violet section (A) by dense accumulation of neurons in contrast to the overlying caudatoputamen (CPu). Note the continuum of the Acb and FStr with the olfactory tubercle (Tu) and the sharp medial and lateral border of the Acb and Tu in the TH-labelled section (B). The piriform cortex (Pir) lacks significant TH-immunoreactivity. The Acb can be distinguished into a shell (AcbS) and a core (AcbC) area. Cell bridges (arrow) traverse the medial forebrain bundle (mfb) and connect the Acb with the Tu. Islands of Calleja (IC) are dispersed in the Tu and associated with ventral pallidal extensions (VP). Anterior commissure (ac); lateral olfactory tract (lo); Bar in B for A and B = 1000μm..

In the primate brain the nucleus accumbens is located where the putamen and the caudate nucleus meet rostrally ventral to the anterior part of the internal capsule. It is impossible to define the boundaries between these three structures and therefore the nucleus accumbens and adjacent ventral parts of the caudate nucleus and putamen form together the main components of primate ventral striatum. Whereas the morphological, neurochemical and electrophysiological division into a shell and core region is widely accepted in rodents, in primates the core-shell dichotomy is more difficult to define. Attempts have been made for a differentiation of the area by comparing various primates including the human brain using Calbindin immunohistochemistry (Meredith et al., 1996). In humans, the shell begins rostrally as a narrow Calbindin-poor irregular outlined stripe, which expands at more caudal levels medially towards the ventricle and laterally towards the adjacent putamen to occupy the major part of the nucleus accumbens. However, the Calbindin immunoreactivity is unevenly distributed in both zones, therefore it can only be assumed that the core is generally Calbindin-rich and the shell Calbindin-poor. Furthermore, interspecious differences complicate the primate core-shell-dichotomy and may have led to a more topographically differentiation into a medial, central and lateral part as used by Mai et al., (2008).

The clear identification of the striatal, pallidal and olfactory structural components within the olfactory tubercle in primates and especially in the human brain is difficult. The olfactory tubercle is localized in the anterior perforated space caudally to the olfactory trigone, bordered laterally by the piriform cortex and medially by the diagonal band. It is continuous with the overlying nucleus accumbens more rostrally and with the ventral parts of the putamen and pallidum more caudally. Calleja islands are frequent, the major Calleja island between the nucleus accumbens and septal nuclei is the largest island among all mammalian brains.

The nucleus accumbens has attracted much interest in the field of psychiatry in recent years especially as the dysfunction of this area has been related with various disorders, including schizophrenia and obsessive-compulsive disorder. The nucleus accumbens is also an important target of antipsychotic drugs, which may respond differentially in the sub-territories, a matter which is frequently discussed in the neuronal circuit of addiction (Heimer et al., 2008).

3. The Extended Amygdala

Based on biochemical, morphological and ontogenetic criteria, the term EA was introduced for a system closely associated with the VSP in the overlapping limbic basal forebrain circuits. The first description of the EA dates back to Johnston (1923), who detected that the amygdala extends from caudolateral to rostromedial in the basal forebrain. Starting from the central and medial amygdaloid nucleus, the EA extends via the sublenticular region up to the bed nuclei of the stria terminalis and returns back to the central and medial amygdaloid nuclei. In consideration of morphological and functional aspects, the EA can be divided into a central and a medial part. The two divisions show a strongly pronounced symmetry between the medial and the central amygdaloid nuclei and the central and medial stria terminals respectively (Aldheid & Heimer, 1988; de Olmos et al., 2004; Heimer et al., 1997; 2008). The EA receives major afferents from the laterobasal amygdaloid complex and the cingulate cortex. Projections lead to autonomic and somatomotor centers in the hypothalamus and brain stem (central division) and to endocrine-associated areas in the medial hypothalamus (medial division).

The components of the medial division of the EA include the medial amygdaloid nucleus, the medial and intraamygdaloid bed nucleus of the stria terminalis, the medial sublenticular EA and the medial division of the supracapsular bed nucleus of the stria terminalis. The medial amygdaloid nucleus is located medially to the nucleus of the lateral olfactory tract and expands caudally to the temporal horn of the lateral ventricle. Laterally it extends to the basolateral amygdala. Based on the cytoarchitectual criteria, the medial amygdaloid nucleus can be subdivided into a principal body, a smaller anteroventral part and a posterodorsal part at the caudal end. Functionally, it may be involved in odor discrimination and in mediating sexual behavior (delBarco-Trillo et al., 2009; Holder et al., 2010). The medial bed nucleus of the stria terminalis can be divided into an anterior, a ventral and a posterior part. The medial nucleus may influence social approach between individuals, as well as social aversion (Goodson & Wang, 2006) via Vasotoxin-positive neurons. The intraamygdaloid bed nucleus of the stria terminalis contains only a few cells bordering the dorsal part of the medial nucleus laterally. It is interspersed by fibers projecting to the stria terminalis. The medial sublenticular EA is a homogeneous complex of medium-sized neurons that borders the globus pallidus dorsally. Due to its prominent projections to dopaminergic neurons in the substantia nigra pars compacta, the medial sublenticular EA has been suggested to influence the dopamine metabolism (Fudge & Emiliano, 2003). The neurons of the medial division of the supracapsular bed nucleus of the stria terminalis form a cell continuum that follows the stria terminalis and penetrates the dorsal part of the internal capsule. This subnucleus receives afferents from the medial (endocrine-associated) hypothalamus (Shammah-Lagnado et al., 2000).

Comparable to the medial division of the EA, the central EA contains the central amygdaloid nucleus, the lateral bed nucleus of the stria terminalis, the central sublenticular EA, the central division of the supracapsular bed nucleus of the stria terminalis and the interstitial nucleus of the posterior limb of the anterior commissure (IPAC). The IPAC is a general term for neurons being located above and below the posterior part of the anterior commissure ventral to the striatum in rodents (Paxinos & Watson, 2007) and primates (Fudge & Tucker, 2009). The IPAC, which may also be subdivided into a lateral and medial part, is considered as part of the VSP and also of the EA (Shammah-Lagnado et al., 2001), as this area receives afferents from various autonomic and limbic areas as the insular cortex, the amygdala, lateral hypothalamus and the bed nucleus of the stria terminalis suggesting the close limbic association.

The central amygdala is a continuum of cells in the dorsocentral part of the amygdala. It is located between the striatum (amygdalostriatal transition area) dorsolaterally and the interstitial nucleus of the ansa lenticularis at its dorsomedial side. The central nucleus can further be subdivided into a medial, lateral and lateral capsular central nucleus. Functionally, the central nucleus is involved in mediating the behavioral and physiological responses associated with fear and anxiety, it modulates hormonal responses to stress and plays an important role in learning Pavlovian conditioning (Kalin et al., 2004; Liubashina et al., 2000). It has recently been proposed, that while the central nucleus of the amygdala is involved in acute fear responses, the bed nucleus of the stria terminalis is more related to anxiety responses (Pitts et al., 2009). The lateral bed nucleus of the stria terminalis is a heterogeneous cell continuum expanding from the internal capsule on the medial side to the nucleus accumbens rostrally, it borders the caudate nucleus dorsally and reaches the IPAC at its caudal end. Based on morphological, structural and immunohistochemical data, the lateral division of the bed nucleus of the stria terminalis can be separated into a dorsal, posterior, ventral, intermediate and juxtacapsular part. It seems to be important for the expression of anxiety and fear through the integration of autonomic and behavioral responses as well as by modulation of affective responses to stress (Bartfai et al., 1992; Davis & Shi, 1999). The central sublenticular EA expands from the lateral bed nucleus of the stria terminalis in a dorsomedial and ventrolateral direction until it borders the central nucleus. With regard to their neurochemistry, the medial and central sublenticular subdivisions are very similar to each other, which suggests that the majority of cells interact with the medial central nucleus (Fallon et al., 1992). The central division of the supracapsular bed nucleus of the stria terminalis borders the lateral bed nucleus of the stria terminalis rostrally and the central amygdaloid nucleus caudally.

The EA is functionally associated with emotion, motivation and social behavior because of its morphological and neurochemical composition as well as its projections and pathways. Therefore, it is not surprising that the EA is involved in diverse psychiatric and neurodegenerative diseases such as depression, anxiety and chronic stress, schizophrenia and HD. In recent years scientists discussed the role of the amygdala in terms of addiction, loss of control in limiting drug intake as well as dysphoria and anxiety after drug abuse. Therefore, they often focused on the central amygdaloid nucleus, as it has a key function in reinforcing actions of drug abuse. In the rat, lesions of this nucleus block oral self-administration of alcohol and the cocaine self-administration can be blocked by microinjections of dopamine D1 receptor antagonists into the area (Caine et al., 1995; McGregor & Roberts, 1993). Additionally, closely related functional effects could be detected for the central EA in terms of withdrawl and negative affects after drug abuse. Especially an acute withdrawl may lead to an increased release of norepinephrine (brain stress system) in the bed nucleus of the stria terminalis and an inactivation of Neuropeptid Y (antistress system), which may cause a negative emotional state (Kobb, 2008). Accessorily, changes in the gene expression of alcohol-preferring rats within the EA have been detected (McBride et al., 2010).

In summary, the EA comprises a complex system of multiple subdivisions with a close crucial pharmacological relationship, which makes this area a valuble target for investigating pathophysiological pathways and pharmacological approaches.

4. Huntington Disease

HD is a hereditary neurodegenerative disorder caused by a cytosine-adenine-guanine (CAG) repeat expansion in exon 1 of the *huntingtin* gene (*HTT*), (Huntington's Disease Collaborative Research Group, 1993). Patients with 36 to 39 CAG repeats have an increasing risk to develop HD, repeats of 40 and more will always lead to the disorder within a normal lifespan (Bates, 2003). The mean age of onset is around 35-50 years with marked individual variations; the duration is around 15-20 years with no differences between the sexes (Hayden, 1981). The most characteristic brain pathology is the atrophy of the caudate nucleus and putamen, which is accompanied by a secondary enlargement of the lateral ventricles (Roos et al., 1985; Vonsattel et al., 1985). The striatal atrophy is due to the progressive loss of medium-sized GABAergic striatal neurons (Heinsen et al., 1994), which comprise approximately 90% of all neurons in the striatum. Cortical, subcortical and brainstem areas with grey and white matter changes are also affected (de la Monte et al., 1988; Dumas et al., 2012; Heinsen et al., 1996; Heinsen et al., 1999; Rosas et al., 2003; Rüb et al., 2009; Schmitz et al. 1999; Tabrizi et al., 2011). Up to now, there is no cure for HD.

Histopathological hallmark is the accumulation of htt aggregates in affected brains (Difiglia et al., 1997; Gutekunst et al., 1999; Maat-Schiemann, 2007) which can be identified by immunohistochemistry with the so-called EM48, a widely used antibody which specifically detects N-terminal htt aggregates in brains of HD individuals and HD animal models (Gutekunst et al., 1999; Hodgson et al., 1999; Li et al., 1999; 2001; Nguyen et al., 2006; von Hörsten et al., 2003). The role of htt aggregates and neurodegeneration is still controversial. They may be toxic by a direct influence on cellular processing (Bates, 2003) or, conversely, could also be neuroprotective by sequestering toxic fragments into an insoluble form in order to prevent them from interacting with key cellular proteins (Arrasate et al., 2004).

Clinically, HD is characterized by cognitive impairments, motor dysfunctions and psychiatric changes, the latter often preceding the onset of the other symptoms. The early detection of psychiatric affection is essential in HD, as these changes are mainly accessable to symptomatic treatment. Psychiatric symptoms have been reported to affect 35-75% of HD individuals (van Duijn et al., 2007). They are more variable than motor and cognitive impairments and do not follow a progressive course, except apathy (with loss of initiation and motivation), which is discussed to be the most frequent personality change in HD (Caine et al., 1978; Craufurd & Snowden, 2003; Paulsen et al., 2001; Thomson et al., 2002). Depression is also a common feature; irritability, aggression and outbursts are frequent (Burns et al., 1990) and often observed in presymptomatic HD patients (Klöppel et al., 2010). Anxiety and reduced ability to recognize negative face expressions as disgust, fear and anger have also been reported in several studies (Hayes et al., 2009; Johnson et al., 2007; Sprengelmeyer at al., 2006). Heining et al. (2003) found an increase in the activity of the ventral striatum in response to disgusting odors in HD patients. Interestingly, HD patients exhibit lower fear and higher anger ratings in response to fear stimuli than control individuals, reflecting dysfunctions within the frontostriatal circuit and the amygdala (Eddy et al., 2011).

Neuropathological analyses of limbic associated regions in human HD brains (such as the nucleus accumbens and the amygdala) are relatively sparse, areas as the olfactory tubercle, the bed nucleus of the stria terminalis and the IPAC are rarely mentioned. Striatal degeneration occurs gradually, starting dorsomedially and extending ventrolaterally. The caudate nucleus is initially more affected than the putamen, the nucleus accumbens appears relatively preserved (Vonsattel et al., 1985; Kassubek et al., 2005). However, when compared with control brains, the nucleus accumbens shows significant volume shrinkage already at preHD stages as detected by magnetic resonance imaging (MRI) and voxel based morphometry (van den Bogaard et al., 2011a; 2011b; Majid et al., 2011). These methods can be applied in large cohorts of HD-affected patients in presymptomatic and early stages as well as follow-up studies and are therefore valuable tools for detecting changes of and in specific brain areas.

In HD individuals the amygdaloid complex is also affected. Cross section analysis of the amygdala has shown a reduced area (Mann et al., 1993) and amygdaloid volume atrophy was detected by MRI studies, which may occur at a very early stage of the disease (Van den

Bogaard et al., 2011; Rosas et al., 2003). It should be noted that the reduction of D2/D3 receptor binding and a microglia activation has been observed in the bed nucleus of the stria terminalis, the ventral striatum and the amygdala of premanifest and symptomatic HD gene carriers (Politis et al., 2011). In contrast, Enkephalin, Neuropeptid Y and Neurotensin immunohistochemistry in the central nucleus of the amygdala showed no obvious changes (Zech et al., 1986). In addition, a reduction in the activity of Cholinacetyltransferase in the olfactory tubercle has been reported in some HD cases (Simpson et al., 1984).

In summary, the human HD individuals show a broad spectrum of psychiatric symptoms which may occur at all stages of the disease, often prior to movement and cognitive disturbances. Structural alterations in the nucleus accumbens and amygdala have also been described, suggesting that their dysfunction may explain some of the psychiatric symptoms. To date, the distribution of htt aggregates has not been investigated in the VSP and EA.

5. The Transgenic Huntington Rat - a `Limbic Huntington Model´

As HD occurs only in humans, the creation of genetically engineered HD animal models represents an important step for elucidation of genetic and behavioral aspects as well as testing new therapeutic strategies. Since the mutation that causes HD was identified in 1993, numerous rodent models for HD have been generated all of which reproducing more or less HD-like behavioral and/or neuropathological features of the disease.

The first transgenic mouse model, the R6/2 mouse, expresses an exon 1 of the human HD gene containing around 141 to 157 CAG repeats (Mangiarini et al., 1996). From the third week after birth, R6/2 mice develop an early phenotype with severe behavioral and motor dysfunctions. Tremors, lack of coordination and enormous loss of weight is accompanied by a severe general atrophy of the brain leading finally to death within 12 - 15 weeks of age (Crook & Housman, 2011; Heng et al., 2008). The R6/2 mice show an early and overall distribution of htt aggregates in many brain areas including the hippocampus, the cerebellum and the spinal cord as detected by the EM48 antibody (Li et al., 1999; 2001). A focus on the limbic associated areas did not reveal any special abnormalities. According to the rapid and reproducible phenotype, the R6/2 mice have been extensively studied and gave important results on the pathogenesis, however, R6/2 mice mimic the juvenile form of HD, which only affects approximately 10% of all HD individuals with onset before age 20 and repeats typically exceeding 50 CAGs (Rasmussen et al., 2000).

Another well studied and widely used transgenic HD animal model is the yeast artificial chromosome mouse model YAC128 (Hodgson et al., 1999; Slow et al., 2003). The YAC128 transgenic mouse expresses the full-length human *HTT* gene with 128 CAG repeats under the control of the endogenous *HTT* promoter. This animal model also exhibits motor abnormalities and cognitive dysfunction. In YAC128 mice, the HD-like phenotype progresses slowly, and is fully developped over the course of 12-18 months. Mild cognitive impairments and motor deficits begin with hyperactivity at two month of age followed by hypokinesis from the fourth month onwards. Behavioral abnormalities can also be detected at the age of two months followed by a depressive-like behavior at the early stage of three months of age. Between nine to twelve months of age, animals show an atrophy of the striatum, the globus pallidus and the cortex, which extends to a global atrophy at the age of two years. Htt aggregates are localized in various brain areas including the striatum, the cortex and the hippocampus with a prominent nuclear localization (Hodgson et al., 1999; Van Raamsdonk et al., 2005).

The first tgHD rat model harbors a human cDNA fragment with 51 CAG repeats in a truncated htt spanning exon 1 to exon 15 under the control of the native rat htt promotor (von Hörsten et al., 2003). TgHD rats show adult-onset neurological HD-like phenotype with an early reduced anxiety, followed by later onset of cognitive impairments and slowly progressive motor dysfunction (von Hörsten et al., 2003; Cao et al., 2006) closely resembling the adult-onset neurological phenotype of human HD. Among all Huntington animal models generated until now (and including the two extensively studied R6/2 and YAC128 mice), the tgHD rat is unique as it shows most prominent accumulation of htt aggregates in structures of the VSP and the EA (Niescery et al., 2009; Petrasch-Parwez et al., 2007). Moreover, it presents very early and ongoing emotional changes, which partly may be associated with dysfunctions of the VSP and EA (Bode et al., 2008; Faure et al., 2011; Nguyen et al., 2006). The distribution of htt accumulates in the medioventral striatum including the olfactory tubercle (Fig. 2A-C), which receives topographically organized input from the ventral tegmental area in the midbrain. In detail, at advanced age htt aggregates are abundantly expressed in the nucleus accumbens (more expressed in the shell than in the core), in the ventral parts of the caudatoputamen, in the cell bridges and in the olfactory tubercle, more expressed in the medial part. The prominent distribution of htt in the medial olfactory tubercle and the medial shell may reflect two mesolimbic dopamine reward circuitries to the accumbens-olfactory tubercle complex (Ikemoto, 2007). According to the midbrain input, the htt-rich medial olfactory tubercle is a continuum of the medial shell, whereas the lateral olfactory tubercle with minor aggregates is related to the core and lateral shell of the nucleus accumbens. Furthermore, the special htt distribution in the olfactory tubercle corresponds to the subdivision into a medial striatal-associated and a lateral more olfactory-related part, as has been reported in various studies (Ikemoto et al., 2007; Meyer & Wahle, 1986; Wahle & Meyer, 1986).

The htt composition in the ventral striatum shows highly heterogeneous aggregates varying in size suggesting that htt is localized in all cell compartments, whereas in the projection area (the ventral pallidum) it is homogenously and finely structured and mainly localized in synaptic terminals, suggesting a production in the ventral striatum and a projection to the ventral pallidum (Petrasch-Parwez et al., 2007). The pronounced localization of htt aggregates in the ventral (limbic) striatum, lacking in the dorsal (motor) striatum, suggests a strong neuropathological affection of the ventral striatum in the tgHD rat. This observation correlates with the behavioral phenotype of the tgHD rat, which shows early onset of emotional changes followed later by motor dysfunction and cognitive decline.

Blunting of emotional oro-facial perception, which were recently described in tgHD rats (Faure et al., 2011), may also be related to ventral striatal circuits.

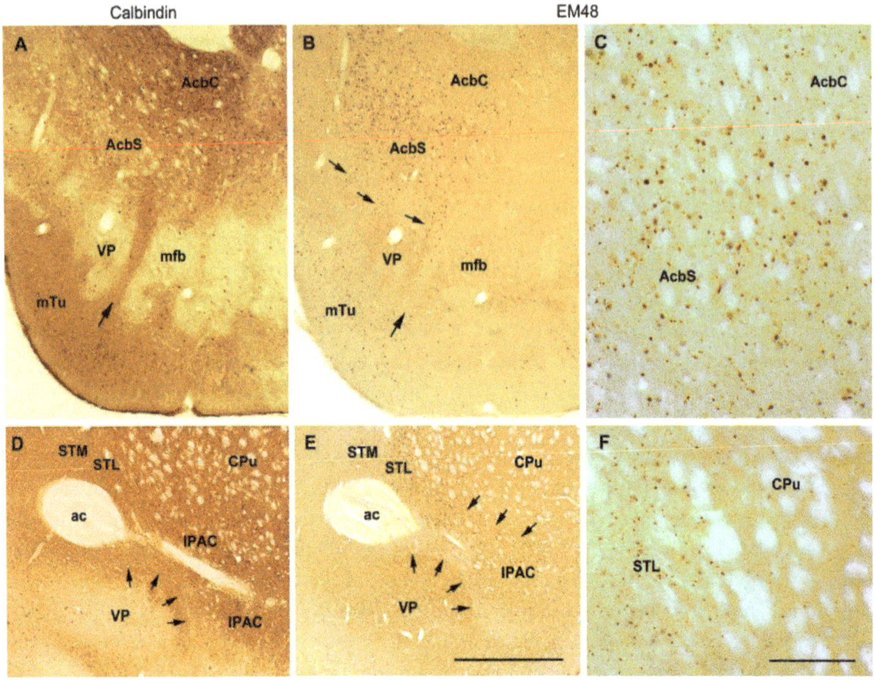

Figure 2. Calbindin (A, D) and EM48 (B, C, E, F) immunostained adjacent vibratome sections showing structures of the ventral striatopallidum (A, B, C) and the extended amygdala (D, E, F) of a tgHD rat, 19 months of age. The Calbindin section shows the nucleus accumbens with the shell (AcbS) and core region (AcbC), the medial olfactory tubercle (mTu) and the connecting cell bridges (arrow) traversing between the medial forebrain bundle (mfb). B. Note the strong huntingtin (htt) immunoreactivity in the AcbS, the cell bridges (arrows) and the mTu. C. Aggregates are less abundant in the AcbC than in the AcbS. D. The medial (STM) and lateral bed nucleus of the stria terminalis (STL) and the interstitial nucleus of the posterior part of the anterior commissure (IPAC) adjacent to the anterior commissure (ac) are distinguished by Calbindin immunohistochemistry and display abundant htt aggregates as detected in the EM-48-stained section (E). F. Higher enlargement shows the dense accumulation of aggregates in the STL as compared with the caudatoputamen (CPu). Ventral pallidum (VP). Bar in E for A, B, D, E=1000μm; bar in F for C and F=100μm.

Htt has also been shown in the EA, more precisely in the bed nuclei of the stria terminalis adjacent to the lateral ventricle (Fig. 2 D, E, F). The distribution follows the posterior part of the anterior commissure and ends in the central amygdaloid nucleus, where aggregates are abundantly expressed (Fig. 3). The dichotomy of the medial and central part of the EA is also reflected by the htt distribution. The aggregates in the central part are larger and more heterogeneously, whereas the aggregates of the medial part are smaller and more homogenously distributed (Niescery et al., 2009; Petrasch-Parwez et al., 2007).

In the tgHD rat, the special affection of the central amygdaloid nucleus is also supported by a recent investigation of Faure et al. (2011), who assessed a significant shrinkage of the central nucleus at 15 months of age. Additionally, the central EA has prominent projections to autonomic and somatomotor centers in the hypothalamus and brainstem (Heimer & Van Hoesen, 2006) and may therefore elucidate the autonomic dysfunction observed in HD patients (Andrich et al., 2002). Within the medial EA, the aggregates are very fine and tiny. The emotional blunting and hypersensitivity to negative situations observed in tgHD rat (Faure et al., 2011) may reflect corresponding emotional blunting and dyscontrol observed in HD patients (Paradiso et al., 2008; Snowden et al., 2008; Spengelmeyer et al., 1996).

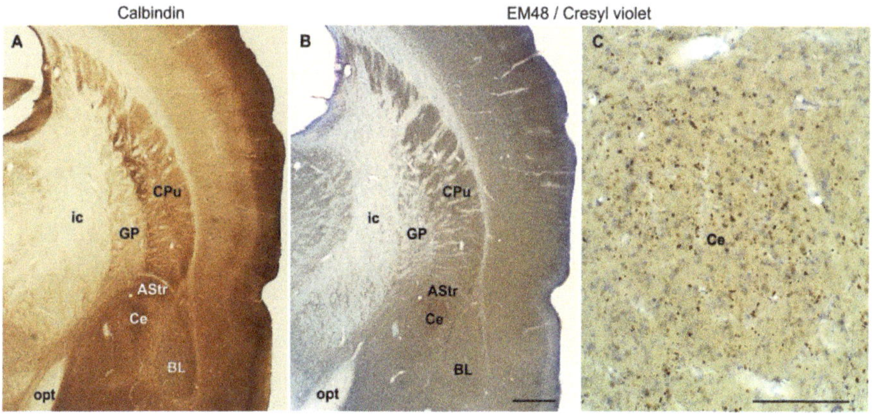

Figure 3. Calbindin (A) and EM48 immunohistochemistry, the latter counterstained with Cresyl violet (B, C) of a tgHD rat brain vibratome section of the central amygdaloid nucleus (Ce). A. The strongly Calbindin-stained Ce ventrally to the amygdalostriatal transition area (AStr) is also detected in the adjacent EM48 section by the dense accumulation of aggregates, clearly identified at higher enlargement in C. Basolateral amygdala nucleus (BL); caudatoputamen (CPu); globus pallidus (GP); internal capsule (ic); optic tract (opt). Bar in B for A and B=1000μm; bar in C=100μm.

In conclusion, the pronounced accumulation of htt in the VSP and EA observed in the tgHD rat is unique among the HD animal models. The tgHD rat is therefore an extremely valuable model to investigate behavioral and neuropathological aspects of emotional dysfunction in HD.

6. The Ventral Striatopallidum and Extended Amygdala in Huntington Brains

Though animal models are valuable tools for investigating the mechanism of a disease and their generation have lead to great progresses during the last decades, the pathogenetic pathway from the HD gene mutation to neurodegeneration and neuronal dysfunction is still unknown. An important criterium for the validity of an animal model is whether and how far the pathological features in the animal models may represent the corresponding pathological features in human HD. In order to determine whether the accumulation of aggregates in the tgHD rat forebrain reflects a pathological feature of human HD, the distribution of htt aggregates were investigated in the VSP and EA of HD brains by EM48 immunohistochemistry. Post-mortem study of human HD brains showed abundantly distributed htt aggregates in the nucleus accumbens and the most ventral parts of the caudate nucleus and putamen (Fig. 4). The aggregates accumulate in patches, but are neither consistent with the distribution of Calbindin-poor nor with Calbindin-rich areas. The localization and heterogenous form and size closely resemble the pattern of aggregates, which were observed in the tgHD rat. In the dorsal caudate nucleus and putamen, where atrophy is mostly expressed, aggregates were sparse. The pronounced distribution of htt aggregates in the ventral striatum is in agreement with a previous report (Kümmerle et al., 2003), though not shown before. Some patch- or stripe-like accumulations of aggregates were also identified in the olfactory tubercle, but not in the ventral pallidum nor in the globus pallidus.

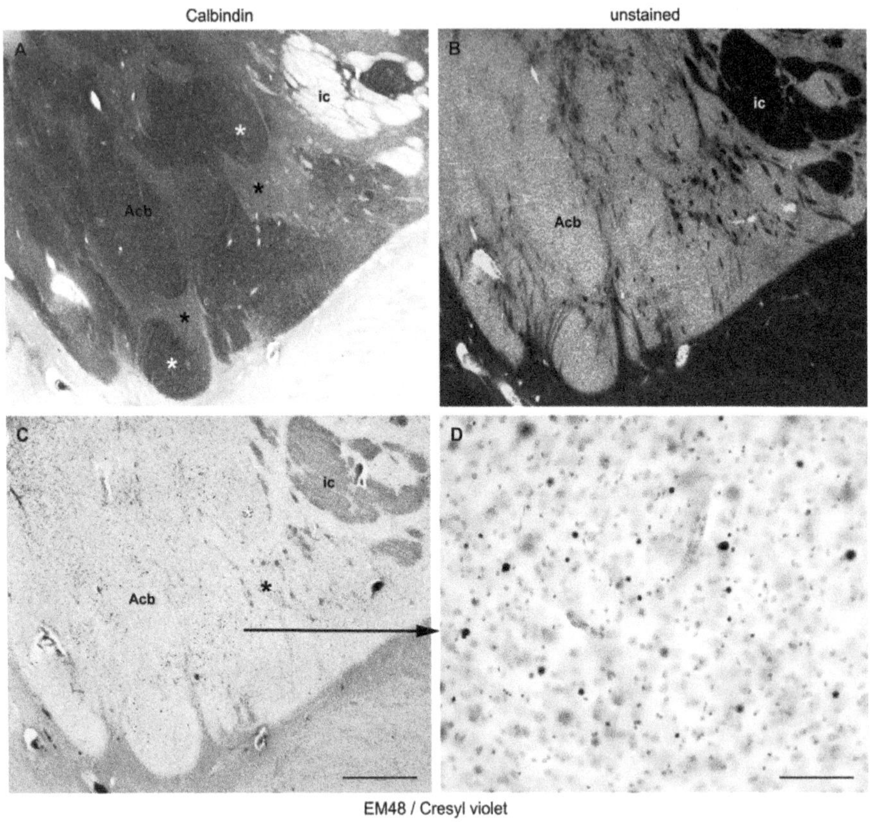

Figure 4. Micrographs of adjacent vibratome sections of the human HD nucleus accumbens (Acb). A. Calbindin-poor (black asterisks) and Calbindin–rich zones (white asterisks) are distinguished. B. The unstained section prior to Calbindin immunohistochemistry shows the fiber distribution. C. The adjacent EM48-immunostained section exhibits the patch-like distribution pattern of huntingtin (htt) aggregates in the Acb, which does not match neither to Calbindin-rich nor Calbindin-poor areas in A. D. Enlargement of a htt-rich area (arrow) shows numerous aggregates varing in size and form. Internal capsule (ic). Bar in C for A-C=1000µm; bar in D=200µm.

The nuclei of the stria terminalis also showed abundantly distributed htt aggregates in HD brains, which were detected in the angle between the anterior commissure and the internal capsule (not shown). More laterally adjacent and ventrally to the posterior part of the anterior commissure, many aggregates were present in the so-called amygdalostriatal transition area, which extends far ventrally adjacent to the amygdaloid complex. Inspecting the amygdaloid complex of HD individuals, aggregates were mainly distributed in the central amygdaloid nucleus, and most prominently in the lateral subdivision (Fig. 5).

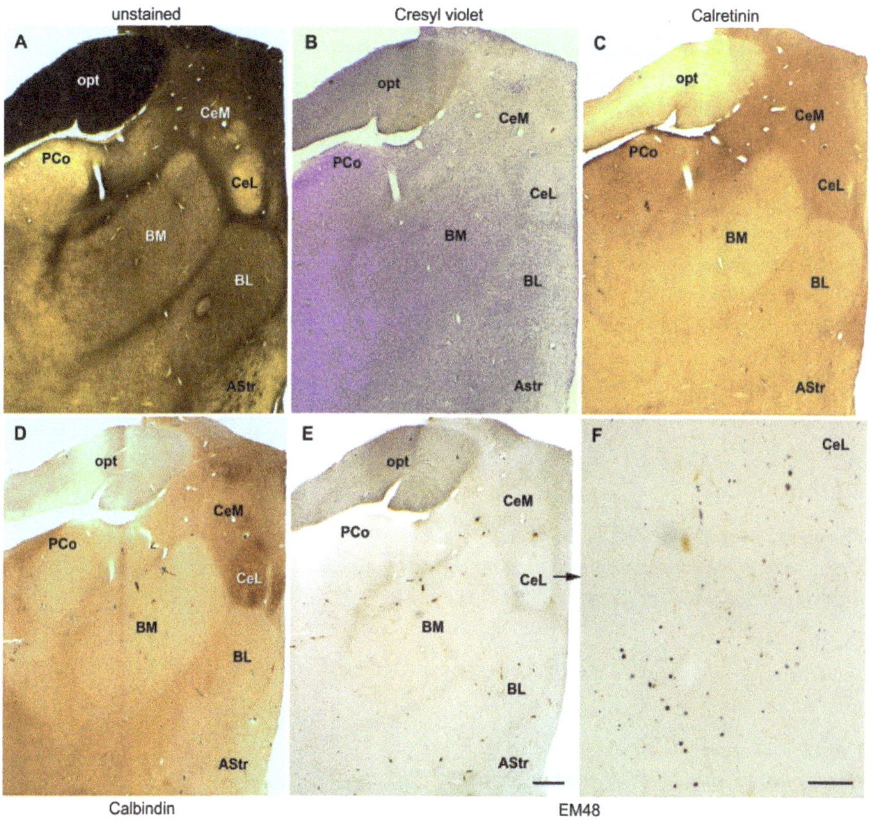

Figure 5. Micrograph of vibratome sections of a human HD amygdala. The overviews show adjacent sections unstained (A), stained for Cresyl violet (B), immunolabelled for Calretinin. (C) Calbindin (D) and EM48 (E) at the level of the medial (CeM) and lateral part of the central amygdaloid nucleus (CeL). F. Higher enlargement of the CeL shows many unevenly distributed htt aggregates. Amygdalostriatal transition area (AStr); basomedial amygdaloid nucleus (BM); basolateral amygdaloid nucleus (BL); posterior cortical amygdaloid nucleus (PCo); optic tract (opt). Bar in E for A-E=500μm; bar in F=100μm.

In summary, the distribution pattern of htt aggregates in the human HD brain is comparable to the pattern reported in the tgHD rat (Fig. 2; 3); Petrasch-Parwez et al., 2007). The pronounced localization within defined limbic forebrain structures give hints for affected circuits, which demand further investigations.

7. Conclusion

The introduction of the two interacting basal forebrain systems VSP and EA four decades ago paved the way for better understanding the complex organization of the mammalian forebrain. Both systems are now accepted as functional-anatomical entities and may act as an interface between motor, limbic and olfactory areas. The discovery had an enormous impact in the field of psychiatry, as both systems are involved in personality and behavioral changes, which are common in neurodegenerative disorders. HD is a neurodegenerative disease characterized by motor dysfunction, cognitive decline and a broad spectrum of psychiatric impairments. The disease is often seen as a motor-related illness, but a majority of patients develop psychiatric symptoms long before motor dysfunction can be detected. To date, the areas associated with motor functions are intensively investigated, but morphological correlates to psychiatric disturbances are poorly understood. Our studies on HD brains have shown a clear and important accumulation of N-terminal htt aggregates in the VSP and EA, which closely resemble the distribution pattern previously published in the tgHD rat. The affection of both limbic forebrain systems may help elucidating the emotional regulation and the psychiatric aspects of HD disorder.

Author details

Elisabeth Petrasch-Parwez, Hans-Werner Habbes and Marlen Löbbecke-Schumacher
Department of Neuroanatomy and Molecular Brain Research,
Ruhr-University Bochum, Germany

Carsten Saft
Department of Neurology, Huntington-Center NRW, St. Josef's Hospital,
Ruhr-University Bochum, Germany

Jennifer Niescery
Department of Anaesthesiology and Intensive Care, St. Josef's Hospital,
Ruhr-University Bochum, Germany

8. References

Alheid, G.F. & Heimer, L. (1988). New perspectives in basal forebrain organization of special relevance for neuropsychiatric disorders: The striatopallidal, amygydaloid and corticopetal components of substantia innominata. *Neuroscience,* 27(1):1-39.

Andrich, J., Schmitz, T., Saft, C., Postert, T., Kraus, P., Epplen, J.T., Przuntek, H. & Angelik, M.W. (2002). Autonomic nervous system function in Huntington's disease. *J. Neurol Neurosurg Psychiatry*, 72(6):726-731.

Arrasate, M., Mitra, S., Schweitzer, E..S., Segal, M.R. & Finkbeiner, S. (2004). Inclusion body formation reduces levels of mutant huntingtin and the risk of neuronal death. *Nature*, 431(7010):805-10.

Bates, G. (2003). Huntingtin aggregation and toxicity in Huntington's disease. *Lancet*, 361(9369):1642-4.

Bartfai,T., Fisone, G. & Langel, U. (1992). Galanin and galanin antagonists: molecular and biochemical perspectives. *Trends Pharmacol Sci*, 13 (8):312-317.

Bode, F., Stephan, M., Suhling, H., Papst, R., Straub, R.H., Raber, K.H., Bonin, M., Nguyen, H.P., Riess, O., Bauer, A., Sjoberg, C., Petersén, A. & von Hörsten, S. (2008). Sex differences in a transgenic rat model of Huntington's disease: decreased 17beta-estradiol levels correlate with reduced numbers of DARPP32+ neurons in males. *Hum Mol Genet*, 17(17):2595-609.

Burns, A., Folstein, S., Brandt, J., Folstein, M. (1990). Clinical assessment of irritability, aggression, and apathy in Huntington and Alzheimer disease. *J. Nerv. Ment. Dis*, 178(1):20-6.

Caine, E.D., Hunt, R.D., Weingartner, H. & Ebert, M.H. (1978). Huntington's dementia. Clinical and neuropsychological features. *Arch Gen Psychiatry*, 135(2):241-3.

Caine, S.B., Heinrichs, S.C., Coffin, V.L. & Koob, G.F. (1995). Effects of the dopamine D-1 antagonist SCH 23390 microinjected into the accumbens, amygdala or striatum on cocaine self-administration in the rat. *Brain Res*, 692(1-2):47–56.

Cao, C., Temel, Y., Blokland, A., Ozen, H., Steinbusch, H.W., Vlamings, R., Nguyen, H.P, von Hörsten, S., Schmitz, C. & Visser-Vandewalle, V. (2006). Progressive deterioration of reaction time performance and choreiform symptoms in a new Huntington's disease transgenic rat model. *Behav Brain Res*, 170(2):257-61.

Craufurd, D. & Snowden, J. (2003). Neuropsychological and neuropsychiatric aspects of Huntington disease. In: *Huntington's Disease*, Bates, G., Harper, P., Jones, L. (eds), pp. 62-94, Oxford Monographs on Genetic 45, Oxford University Press, ISBN 019851060 8, Oxford.

Crook, Z.R. & Housman, D. (2011). Huntington's Disease: can mice lead the way to treatment. *Neuron*, 69(5):423-435.

Davis, M. & Shi, C. (1999). The extended amygdala: are the central nucleus of the amygdala and the bed nucleus of the stria terminalis differentially involved in fear versus anxiety? *Ann N Y Acad Sci*. 29(877):281-91.

De Olmos, J.S., Betramino, C.A. & Alheid, G. (2004). Amygdala and extended amygdala of the rat : a cytoarchitectonical, fibroarchitectonical, and chemoarchitectonical survey. In: *The rat nervous system*, Paxinos, G.F., (ed), pp.509-603, (3rd edition), Elsevier Academic Press. ISBN: 0-12-547638-8, Amsterdam.

De la Monte, S.M., Vonsattel, J.P. & Richardson, E.P. Jr. (1988). Morphometric demonstration of atrophic changes in the cerebral cortex, white matter and neostriatum in Huntington's disease. *J Neuropathol Exp Neurol*, 47(5):516-25.

Del Barco-Trillo, J., Gulewicz, K. & Johnston, R.E. (2009). Medial amygdala involvement in discrimination of same-species and closely-related-species male stimuli in estrous female Mesocricetus hamsters. *Behav Neurosci*. 123(4):758-63.

DiFiglia, M., Sapp, E., Chase, K.O., Davies, S.W., Bates, G.P., Vonsattel, J. P. & Aronin, N. (1997). Aggregation of huntingtin in neuronal intranuclear inclusions and dystrophic neurites in brain. *Science*, 277(5334):1990-3.

Dumas, E.M., van den Bogaard, S.J.A., Ruber, M.E., Reilmann, R.R., Stout, J.C., Craufurd, D., Hicks, S.L., Kennard, C., Tabrizi, S.J., van Buchem, M.A., van der Grond, J. & Roos, R.A. (2012). Early changes in the white matter pathway of the sensorimotor cortex in premanifest Huntington's disease. *Hum Brain Mapping*, 33(1):203-12.

Eddy, C.M., Mitchell, I.J., Beck, S.R., Cavanna, A.E. & Rickards, H.E. (2011). Altered subjective fear responses in Huntington's disease. *Parkinsonism Relat Disord*, 17(5):386-9.

Enzi, B., Edel, M.A., Lissek, S., Peters, S., Hoffmann, R., Nicolas, V., Tegenthoff, M. Juckel, G. & Saft, C. (2012). Altered ventral striatal activation during reward and punishment processing in premanifest Huntington's disease : A functional magnetic resonance study. *Exp Neurol* 235(1):256-64.

Faure, A., Höhn, S., von Hörsten, S., Delatour, B., Raber, K., Le Blanc, P., Desvignes, N., Doyère, V. & El Massioui, N. (2011). Altered emotional and motivational processing in the transgenic rat model for Huntington's disease. *Neurobiol Learn Mem* 95(1):92-101.

Fallon, J.H., Di Salvo, J., Loughlin, S.E., Gimenez-Gallego, G., Seroogy, K.B., Bradshaw, R.A., Morrison, R.S., Ciofi, P. & Thomas, K.A. (1992). Localization of acidic fibroblast growth factor within the mouse brain using biochemical and immunocytochemical techniques. *Growth Factors*, 6(2):139-57.

Fudge, J.L. & Emiliano, A.B. (2003). The extended amygdala and the dopamine system: another piece of the dopamine puzzle. *J Neuropsychiatry Clin Neurosci*, 15(3):306-16.

Fudge, J.L. & Tucker, T. (2009). Amygdala projections to central amygdaloid nucleus subdivisions and transition zones in the primate. *Neuroscience*, 159(2):819-41.

Goodson, J.L. & Wang, Y. (2006). Valence-sensitive neurons exhibit divergent functional profiles in gregarious and asocial species. *Proc Natl Acad Sci U S A*, 103(45):17013-7.

Gutekunst, C.A., Li, S.H., Yi, H., Mulroy, J.S., Kuemmerle, S., Jones, R., Rye, D., Ferrante, R.J., Hersch, S.M. & Li, X.J. (1999). Nuclear and neuropil aggregates in Huntington's disease: relationship to neuropathology. *J Neu*rosci, 19(7):2522-34.

Hayden, M.R. (1981). Huntington's Chorea. In Scriver CS, Beaudet A, Valle D (eds.) : McGraw Hill N Y

Hayes, C.J., Stevenson, R.J. & Cotheart, M. (2009). The processing of emotion in patients with Huntington's disease: variability and differential deficits in disgust. *Cogn Behav Neurol*, 22(4):249-57.

Heimer, L., Harlan, R.E., Alheid, G.F., Garcia, M.M. & de Olmos, J. (1997). Substantia innominata: a notion which impedes clinical-anatomical correlations in neuropsychiatric disorders. *Neuroscience,* 76(4):957-1006.

Heimer, L. & Wilson, R.D. (1975). The subcortical projection of allocortex : Similarities in the neuronal association of the hippocampus, the piriform cortex and the neocortex. In: *Golgi Centennial Symposium Proceedings,* Santini, M. (Ed), pp. 173-193, Raven Press, New York.

Heimer, L., Zaborszky, L., Zahm, D.S. & Alheid, G.F. (1987). The ventral striatopallidothalamic projection : I. The striatopallidal link originating in the striatal parts of the olfactory tubercle. *J Comp Neurol,* 255(4):571-91.

Heimer, L. & van Hoesen, G.W. (2006). The limbic lobe and its output channels : implication for emotional functions and adaptive behavior. *Neurosci Biobehav Rev,* 30(2):126-147.Heimer, L., van Hoesen, G.W., Trimble, M. & Zahm, D.D. (2008). *Anatomy of Neuropsychiatry,* The New Anatomy of the Basal Forebrain and its implications for Neuropsychiatric Illness. Academic Press, Elsevier, ISBN 978-0-12-374239-1, Amsterdam.

Heining, M., Young, A.W., Ioannou, G., Andrew, C.M., Brammer, M.J., Gray, J.A. & Phillips, M.L. (2003). Disgusting smells activate human anterior insula and ventral striatum. *Ann NY Acad Sci,* 1000:380-4.

Heinsen, H., Strik, M., Bauer, M., Luther, K., Ulmar, G., Gangnus, D., Jungkunz, G., Eisenmenger, W. & Götz, M. (1994). Cortical and striatal neuron number in Huntington's disease. *Acta Neuropathol,* 88(4):320-33.

Heinsen, H., Rüb, U., Gangnus, D., Jungkunz, G., Bauer, M., Ulmar, G., Bethke, B., Schüler, M., Böcker, F., Eisenmenger, W., Götz, M., & Strik, M. (1996). Nerve cell loss in the thalamic centromedian parafascicular complex in patients with Huntington's disease. *Acta Neuropathol,* 91(2):161-8.

Heinsen, H., Rüb, U., Bauer, M., Ulmar, G., Bethke, B., Schüler, M., Böcker, F., Eisenmenger, W., Götz, M., Korr, H., Schmitz, C. (1999). *Acta Neuropathol,* 97(6):613-22.

Heng, M.Y, Detleff, P.J. & Albin, R.L. (2008). Rodent genetic models of Huntington disease. *Neurobiol Dis,* 32 (1):1-9.

Herrick, C.J. (1926). Brains of rats and men. Chicago: University of Chicago Press.

Hodgson, J.G., Agopyan, N., Gutekunst, C.A., Leavitt, B.R., LePiane, F., Singaraja, R., Smith, D.J., Bissada, N., McCutcheon, K., Nasir, J., Jamot, L., Li, X.J., Stevens, M.E., Rosemond, E., Roder, J.C., Philips, A.G., Rubin, E.M., Hersch, S.M. & Hayden, M.R. (1999). A YAC mouse model for Huntington's disease with full-length mutant huntingtin, cytoplasmic toxicity, and selective striatal neurodegeneration. *Neuron,* 23(1):181-92.

Holder, M.K., Hadjimarkou, M.M., Zup, S.L., Blutstein, R.S., McCarthy, M.M. & Mong, J.A. (2010). Methamphetamine facilitates female sexual behavior and enhances neuronal activation in the medial amygdala and ventromedial nucleus of the hypothalamus. *Psychoneuroendocrinology,* 35(2):197-208.

Huntington's Disease Collaborative Research group. (1993). A novel gene containing a trinucleotide repeat that is expanded and unstable on Huntington's disease chromosomes. *Cell*, 72(6):971-983.

Ikemoto, S. (2007). Dopaminergic reward circuitry: Two projection systems from the ventral midbrain to the nucleus accumbens-olfactory tubercle complex. *Brain Res Reviews*, 56(1):27-78.

Johnson, S.A., Stout, J.C., Solomon, A.C., Langbehn, D.R., Aylward, E.H., Cruce, C.B., Ross, C.A., Nance, M., Kayson, E., Julian-Baros, E, Hayden, M.R., Kieburtz, K., Guttman, M., Oakes, D., Shoulson, I., Beglinger, L., Duff, K., Penzinger, E., Paulsen, J.S., & Predict HD Investigators of the Huntington Study Group. (2007). Beyond disgust: impaired recognition of negative emotions prior to diagnosis in Huntington's disease. *Brain*, 130 (Pt 7):1732-44.

Johnston, J.B. (1923). Further contributions to the study oft the evolution oft the forebrain. *J Comp Neurol*, 35(5):337-481.

Kalin, N.H., Shelton, S.E. & Davidson, R.J. (2004). The role of the central nucleus of the amygdala in mediating fear and anxiety in the primate. *J Neurosci*, 24(24):5506-15.

Kassubek, J., Juengling, F.D., Kioschies, T., Henkel, K., Karitzky, J., Kramer, B., Ecker, D., Andrich, J., Saft, C., Kraus, P., Aschoff, A.J., Ludolph, A.C. & Landwehrmeyer, G.B. (2004). Topography of brain atrophy in early Huntington's disease: a voxel based morphometric MRI study. *J Neurol Neurosurg Psychiatry*, 75(2):213-20.

Klöppel, S., Stonnington, C.M., Petrovic, P., Mobbs, D., Tuescher, O., Craufurd, D., Tabrizi, S.J. & Frackowiak, R.S.J. (2010). Irritability in pre-clinical Huntington's disease. *Neuropsychologica*, 48(2):549-57.

Koob, G.F. (2008) A role for brain stress systems in addiction. *Neuron*, 59(1):11–34.

Kümmerle, S. (2003). Pathogenetische Bedeutung von intrazellulären Huntingtinaggregaten beim Morbus Huntington. Thesis. Technische University, München.

Li, H., Li, S.H., Zhao-Xue Y, Shelbourne, P., Li, X.J. (2001). Huntingtin aggregate-associated axonal degeneration is an early pathological event in Huntington's disease mice. *J Neurosci*, 21(21):8473-81.

Li, Liubashina, O., Jolkkonen, E. & Pitkänen, A. (2000). Projections from the central nucleus of the amygdala to the gastric related area of the dorsal vagal complex: a Phaseolus vulgaris-leucoagglutinin study in rat. *Neurosci Lett*, 291(2):85-9.

Maat-Schiemann, M., Roos, R., Loosekot, M., Dorsman, J., Welling-Graafland, C., Hegemann-Klein, I., Broeyer, F., Breuning, M. & van Duinen, S. (2007). Neuronal intranuclear and neuropil inclusions for pathological assessment of Huntington's disease. *Brain Pathol*, 17(1):31-7.

Mai, J.K., Paxinos, G. & Voss, T. (2008). *Atlas of the Human Brain* (3rd edition) Elsevier, Academic Press, ISBN978-0-12-373603-1, Amsterdam.

Majid, D.S., Aron, A.R., Thompson, W., Sheldon, S., Hamza, S., Stoffers, D., Holland, D., Goldstein, J., Corey-Bloom, J. & Dale, A.M. (2011). Basal ganglia atrophy in prodromal

Huntington's disease is detectable over one year using automatic segmentation. *Mov Disord*, 26(8):1481-8.

Mangiarini, L., Sathasivam, K., Seller, M., Cozens, B., Harper, A., Hetherington, C., Lawton, M., Trottier, Y., Lehrach, H., Davies, S.W.& Bates, G.P. (1996). Exon 1 of the HD gene with an expanded CAG repeat is sufficient to cause a progressive neurological phenotype in transgenic mice. *Cell* 87(3): 493-506.

Mann, D.M, Oliver, R. & Snowden, J.S. (1993). The topographic distribution of brain atrophy in Huntington's disease and progressive supranuclear palsy. *Acta Neuropathol*, 85(5):553-9.

McBride, W.J., Kimpel, M.W., Schultz, J.A., McClintick, J.N., Edenberg, H.J.& Bell, R.L. (2010). Changes in gene expression in regions of the extended amygdala of alcohol-preferring rats after binge-like alcohol drinking. *Alcohol*, 44(2):171-83.

McGregor, A. & Roberts, D.C. (1993). Dopaminergic antagonism within the nucleus accumbens or the amygdala produces differential effects on intravenous cocaine self-administration under fixed and progressive ratio schedules of reinforcement. *Brain Res*, 624(1-2):245–52.

Meredith, G.E., Pattiselanno, A., Groenwegen, H.J. & Haber, S.N. (1996). Shell and core in monkey and human nucleus accumbens identified with antibodies to calbindin-D28k. *J Comp Neurol*, 365(4):621-39.

Meyer, G & Wahle, P. (1986). The olfactory tubercle of the cat. I. Morphological components. *Exp Brain Res*. 62(3):515-27.

Nguyen, H.P., Kobbe, P., Rahne, H., Wörpel, T., Jäger, B., Stephan, M., Papst, R., Holzmann, C., Riess, O., Korr, H., Kántor, O., Petrasch-Parwez, E., Wetzel, R., Osmand, A. & von Hörsten, S. (2006). Behavioral abnormalities precede neuropathological markers in rats transgenic for Huntington's disease. *Hum Mol Genet*, 15(21):3177-94.

Niescery, J., Nguyen, H.-P., von Hörsten, S., Arning, L., Dermietzel, R. & Petrasch-Parwez, E. (2009). A limbic Huntington rodent model: Huntingtin aggregates accumulate in the ventral striatopallidum and extended amygdala. *Clinical Genetics*, 76 (Suppl. 1):83.

Paradiso, S., Turner, B.M., Paulsen, J.S., Jorge, R., Ponto, L.L., Robinson, R.G. (2008). Neural bases of dysphoria in early Huntington's disease. *Psychiatry Res*, 162(1):73-87.

Paulsen, J.S., Ready, R.E., Hamilton, J.M., Mega, M.S. & Cummings, J.L. (2001). Neuropsychiatric aspects of Huntington's disease. *J Neurol Neurosurg Psychiatr*, 71(3):310-4.

Paxinos, G. & Watson, C. (2007). *The rat brain in stereotaxic coordinates*, 6th edition, Elsevier, Academic Press. ISBN13:978-0-12-547612-6 , Amsterdam.

Petrasch-Parwez, E., Nguyen, H.P., Löbbecke-Schumacher, M., Habbes, H.W., Wieczorek, S., Riess, O., Andres, K.H., Dermietzel, R. & von Hörsten, S. (2007). Cellular and subcellular localization of Huntingtin (corrected) aggregates in the brain of a rat transgenic for Huntington disease. *J Comp Neurol*, 501(5):716-30.

Petrasch-Parwez, E., Epplen J.T., Saft C. (2012). Neuropathology of the ventral striatum and extended amygdala in Huntington disease. *J Neurol Neurosurg Psychiatr,* 83 (Suppl.1):A38-39.

Pierce, R. C. & Kumaresan, V. (2006). The mesolimbic dopamine system: the final common pathway for the reinforcing effect of drugs of abuse? *Neurosci Biobehav Revs,* 30(2):215-38.

Pitts, M.W., Todorovic, C., Blank, T. & Takahashi, L.K. (2009). The central nucleus of the amygdala and Corticotropin-Releasing Factor: insights into contextual fear memory. *J Neurosci,* 29(22):7379-88.

Politis, M., Pavese, N., Tai, Y.F., Kiferle, L., Mason, S.L., Brooks, D.J., Tabrizi, S.J., Barker, R.A. & Piccini, P. (2011). Microglia activation in regions related to cognitive function predicts disease onset in Huntington's disease: A multimodale Imaging study. *Human Brain Mapping,* 32(2):258-70.

Rasmussen, A., Macias, R., Yescas, P., Ochoa, A., Davila, G. & Alonso, E. (2000). Huntington disease in children: genotype-phenotype correlation. *Neuropediatrics,* 31(4):190-4.

Roos, R., Pruyt, J.F., de Vries, J.& Bots, G.T. (1985). Neuronal distribution in the putamen in Huntington's disease. *J Neurol, Neurosurg Psychiatry,* 48(5):422-25.

Rosas, H.D., Koroshetz, W.J., Chen, Y.I., Skeuse, C., Vangel, M., Cudkowicz, M.E., Caplan, K., Marek, K., Seidman, L.J., Makris, N., Jenkins, B.G. & Goldstein, J.M. (2003). Evidence for more widespread cerebral pathology in early HD: an MRI-based morphometric analysis. *Neurology,* 60 (10):1615-20.

Rüb, U., Heinsen, H., Brunt, E.R., Landwehrmeyer, B., Den Dunnen, W.F., Gierga, K. & Deller, T. (2009). The human premotor oculomotor brainstem system – can it help to understand oculomotor symptoms in Huntington's disease? *Neuropathol Appl Neurobiol,* 35(1):4-15.

Schmitz, C., Rüb, U., Korr, H. & Heinsen, H. (1999). Nerve cell loss in the thalamic mediodorsal nucleus in Huntington's disease. II. Optimization of a stereological estimation procedure. *Acta Neuropathol* 97(6):623-8.

Shammah-Lagnado, S.J., Beltramino, C.A., McDonald, A.J., Miselis, R.R.,Yang, M., de Olmos, J., Heimer, L & Alheid, G.F. (2000). Supracapsular bed nucleus of the stria terminalis contains central and medial extended amygdala elements: evidence from anterograde and retrograde tracing experiments in the rats. *J Comp Neurol,* 422(4):533-55.

Shammah-Lagnado, S.J., Alheid, G.F. & Heimer, L. (2001). Striatal and central extended amygdala of the interstitial nucleus of the posterior limb of the anterior commissure: evidence from tract-tracing techniques in the rat. *J Comp Neurol,* 439(1):104-26.

Simpson, J., Yates, C.M., Gordon, A. & St. Clair, D.M. (1984). Olfactory tubercle choline acetyltransferase activity in Alzheimer-type dementia, Down's syndrome and Huntington's chorea. *J Neurol Neurosurg Psychiatry,* 47(10):1138-9.

Slow, E.J., van Raamsdonk, J., Rogers, D., Coleman, S.H., Graham, R.K., Deng, Y., Oh R., Bissada N., Hossain S.M., Yang Y.Z., Li X.J., Simpson E.M., Gutekunst C.A., Leavitt B.R.

& Hayden M.R. (2003) Selective striatal neuronal loss in a YAC128 mouse model of Huntington disease. *Hum Mol Genet*, 12(13):1555-67.
Sprengelmeyer, R., Young, A.W., Calder, A.J., Karnat, A., Lange, H., Hömberg, V., Perrett, D.I. & Rowland, D. (1996). Loss of disgust. Perception of faces and emotions in Huntington's disease. *Brain*, 119 (pt5):1647-65.
Sprengelmeyer, R., Schroeder, U., Young, A.W. & Epplen, J.T. (2006). Disgust in pre-clinal Huntington's disease. A longitudinal study. *Neuropsychologica*, 44(4):518-33.
Snowden, J.S., Austin, N.A., Sembi, S., Thomson, J.C., Craufurd, D. & Neary, D. (2008). Emotion recognition in Huntington's disease and frontotemporal dementia. *Neuropsychologica*, 46(11):2638-49.
Stevens, J.R. (1973). An anatomy of schizophrenia. *Arch Gen Psychiatry*, 29(2):177-89.
Tabrizi, S.J., Scahill , R.I., Durr, A., Roos, R.A., Leavitt, B.R., Jones, R, Landwehrmeyer, G.B., Fox, N.C., Johnson, H., Hicks, S.L., Kennard, C., Craufurd, D., Frost, C., Langbehn, D.R., Reilmann, R., Stout, J.C. & the TRACK-HD investigators. (2011). Biological and clinical changes in premanifest and early stage Huntington's disease in the TRACK-HD study: the 12-month longitudinal analysis. *Lancet Neurol*, 10(1):31-42.
Thomson, J.C., Snowden, J.S., Craufurd, D., Neary D. (2002). Behavior in Huntington's disease: dissociating cognition-based and mood-based changes. (2002). *J Neuropsychiatry Clin Neurosci* 14(1):37-43.
Van den Bogaard, S.J.A., Dumas, E.M., Acharya, T.B., Johnson, H., Langbehn, D.R., Scahill, R.I., Tabrizi, S.J., van Buchem, M.A., van der Grond, R., Roos, R.A., [1] & TRACK-HD Investigator Group. (2011a). Early atrophy of pallidum and accumbens nucleus in Huntington's disease. *J Neurol*, 258(3):412–20.
Van den Bogaard, S.J.A., Dumas, E.M., Ferrarini, L., Milles, J., van Buchem, M.A., van der Grond, J. & Roos, A. (2011b). Shape analysis of subcortical nuclei in Huntington's disease, global versus local atrophy--results from the TRACK-HD study. *J Neurol Sci*, 307(1-2):60-8.
Van Ramsdonk, J.M., Murphy, Z., Slow, E.J., Leavitt, B.R.& Hayden, M.R. (2005). Selective degeneration and nuclear localization of mutant huntingtin in the YAC128 mouse model of Huntington disease. *Hum Mol Genet*, 14(24):3823-35.
Vonsattel, J.P., Myers, R.H., Stevens, T.J., Ferrante, R.J., Bird, E.D. & Richarson, E.P.Jr. (1985). Neuropathological classification of Huntington's disease. *J Neuropathol Exp Neurol*, 44(6):559-77.
Von Hörsten, S., Schmitt, I., Nguyen, H.P., Holzmann, C., Schmidt, T., Walther, T., Bader, M., Papst, R., Kobbe, P., Krotova, J., Stiller, D., Kask, A., Vaarmann, A., Rathke-Hartlieb, S., Schulz, J.B., Grasshoff, U., Bauer, I., Vieira-Saecker, A.M., Paul, M., Jones, L., Lindenberg, K.S., Landwehrmeyer, B., Bauer, A., Li, X.J. & Riess, O. (2003). Transgenic rat model of Huntington's disease. *Hum Mol Genet*, 12(6):617-24.
Wahle, P. & Meyer, G. (1986). The olfactory tubercle of the cat. II. Immunohistochemical compartmentation. *Exp Brain Res*, 62(3) 528-40.

Waraczynski, M.A. (2006). The central extended amygdala network as a proposed circuit underlying reward valuation. *Neurosci Biobehav Rev*, 30(4):472-96.

Zech, M., Roberts, G.W., Bogerts, B., Crow, T.J. & Polak, J.M. (1986). Neuropeptides in the amygdala of controls, schizophrenics and patients suffering from Huntington's chorea: An immunohistochemical study. *Acta Neuropathol*, 71(3-4):259-66.

Permissions

The contributors of this book come from diverse backgrounds, making this book a truly international effort. This book will bring forth new frontiers with its revolutionizing research information and detailed analysis of the nascent developments around the world.

We would like to thank Barbara Ferry, Ph.D., for lending her expertise to make the book truly unique. She has played a crucial role in the development of this book. Without her invaluable contribution this book wouldn't have been possible. She has made vital efforts to compile up to date information on the varied aspects of this subject to make this book a valuable addition to the collection of many professionals and students.

This book was conceptualized with the vision of imparting up-to-date information and advanced data in this field. To ensure the same, a matchless editorial board was set up. Every individual on the board went through rigorous rounds of assessment to prove their worth. After which they invested a large part of their time researching and compiling the most relevant data for our readers. Conferences and sessions were held from time to time between the editorial board and the contributing authors to present the data in the most comprehensible form. The editorial team has worked tirelessly to provide valuable and valid information to help people across the globe.

Every chapter published in this book has been scrutinized by our experts. Their significance has been extensively debated. The topics covered herein carry significant findings which will fuel the growth of the discipline. They may even be implemented as practical applications or may be referred to as a beginning point for another development. Chapters in this book were first published by InTech; hereby published with permission under the Creative Commons Attribution License or equivalent.

The editorial board has been involved in producing this book since its inception. They have spent rigorous hours researching and exploring the diverse topics which have resulted in the successful publishing of this book. They have passed on their knowledge of decades through this book. To expedite this challenging task, the publisher supported the team at every step. A small team of assistant editors was also appointed to further simplify the editing procedure and attain best results for the readers.

Our editorial team has been hand-picked from every corner of the world. Their multi-ethnicity adds dynamic inputs to the discussions which result in innovative outcomes. These outcomes are then further discussed with the researchers and contributors who give their valuable feedback and opinion regarding the same. The feedback is then collaborated with the researches and they are edited in a comprehensive manner to aid the understanding of the subject.

Apart from the editorial board, the designing team has also invested a significant amount of their time in understanding the subject and creating the most relevant covers. They scrutinized every image to scout for the most suitable representation of the subject and create an appropriate cover for the book.

The publishing team has been involved in this book since its early stages. They were actively engaged in every process, be it collecting the data, connecting with the contributors or procuring relevant information. The team has been an ardent support to the editorial, designing and production team. Their endless efforts to recruit the best for this project, has resulted in the accomplishment of this book. They are a veteran in the field of academics and their pool of knowledge is as vast as their experience in printing. Their expertise and guidance has proved useful at every step. Their uncompromising quality standards have made this book an exceptional effort. Their encouragement from time to time has been an inspiration for everyone.

The publisher and the editorial board hope that this book will prove to be a valuable piece of knowledge for researchers, students, practitioners and scholars across the globe.

List of Contributors

Juan Pedro Vargas, Juan Carlos López and Manuel Portavella
Laboratory of Behavioral Neuroscience, Department of Experimental Psychology, University of Seville, Spain

Miguel Ángel Bertoni
East Kent Hospitals University NHS Foundation Trust, University of Kent, UK

Ryong-Moon Shin
National Institute of Radiological Sciences, Japan

Gina L. Forster, Andrew M. Novick, Jamie L. Scholl and Michael J. Watt
Division of Basic Biomedical Sciences, Sanford School of Medicine, University of South Dakota, Vermillion, SD, USA

Sodikdjon A. Kodirov
Pavlov Institute of Physiology, Russian Academy of Sciences, Saint Petersburg, Russia
I. P. Pavlov Department of Physiology, State Research Institute of Experimental Medicine, Russian Academy of Medical Sciences, Saint Petersburg, Russia
Department of Molecular Physiology & Biophysics, University of Iowa, Iowa City, USA

Candice M. Chavez, James L. McGaugh and Norman M. Weinberger
Center for the Neurobiology of Learning and Memory, and Department of Neurobiology and Behavior, University of California, Irvine, CA, USA

Satish S. Nair
Department of Electrical and Computer Engineering, University of Missouri - Columbia, Columbia, MO, USA

Barbara Ferry
Center for Research in Neuroscience, LYON (CRNL), CNRS UMR 5292 - INSERM U 1028, University Claude Bernard, Lyon 1, France

Gina L. Quirarte
Behavioral and Cognitive Neurobiology Department, Institute of Neurobiology, National Autonomous University of México, Campus Querétaro, Qro, México

Rodrigo Moraga-Amaro
Laboratorio de Neurobiología, Facultad de Ciencias Biológicas y Medicina, Universidad Andres Bello, Santiago, Chile

Jimmy Stehberg
Laboratorio de Neurobiología, Facultad de Ciencias Biológicas y Medicina, Universidad Andres Bello, Santiago, Chile
Centro de Investigaciones Biomédicas, Universidad Andrés Bello, Santiago, Chile

Trevor H. Gilbert
Centre for Psychology, Faculty of Humanities & Social Sciences, Athabasca University, Canada

Andrés Molero Chamizo
University of Huelva, Spain

Xiaodan Yan
Cognitive Science Department, Rensselaer Polytechnic Institute, USA

Dong Hoon Oh
Department of Psychiatry, College of Medicine and Institute of Mental Health, Hanyang University, Seoul, Republic of Korea

Shira Knafo
Severo Ochoa Center for Molecular Biology, Spanish National Research Council (CSIC)/ Autonomous University of Madrid, Madrid, Spain

Bruno Bonaz
Clinique Universitaire d'Hépato-Gastroentérologie, CHU de Grenoble, BP217, France
Stress et Interactions Neuro-Digestives, Grenoble Institut des Neurosciences (GIN), Centre de Recherche INSERM U836-UJF-CEA-CHU, CHU de Grenoble, BP217, France

Sonia Pellissier
Stress et Interactions Neuro-Digestives, Grenoble Institut des Neurosciences (GIN), Centre de Recherche INSERM U836-UJF-CEA-CHU, CHU de Grenoble, BP217, France
Département de Psychologie, Université de Savoie, France

Valérie Sinniger
Stress et Interactions Neuro-Digestives, Grenoble Institut des Neurosciences (GIN), Centre de Recherche INSERM U836-UJF-CEA-CHU, CHU de Grenoble, BP217, France

Didier Clarençon, André Peinnequin and Frédéric Canini
Stress et Interactions Neuro-Digestives, Grenoble Institut des Neurosciences (GIN), Centre de Recherche INSERM U836-UJF-CEA-CHU, CHU de Grenoble, BP217, France
Institut de Recherche Biomédicale des Armées – CRSSA-Antenne La Tronche, BP 87, France

Elisabeth Petrasch-Parwez, Hans-Werner Habbes and Marlen Löbbecke-Schumacher
Department of Neuroanatomy and Molecular Brain Research, Ruhr-University Bochum, Germany

Carsten Saft
Department of Neurology, Huntington-Center NRW, St. Josef´s Hospital, Ruhr-University Bochum, Germany

Jennifer Niescery
Department of Anaesthesiology and Intensive Care, St. Josef´s Hospital, Ruhr-University Bochum, Germany